Signs and Symptoms in Emergency Medicine

Signs and Symptoms in Pediatrics:
Urgent and Emergent Care

EDITOR-IN-CHIEF
Karen D. Gruskin, MD

EDITORS
Vincent W. Chiang, MD
Shannon Manzi, PharmD

Signs and Symptoms in Emergency Medicine

Literature–Based Approach to Emergent Conditions

2nd Edition

Editors

SCOTT R. VOTEY, MD

Professor of Medicine/Emergency Medicine
Assistant Dean for Graduate Medical Education
David Geffen School of Medicine at UCLA
UCLA Emergency Medicine Center, Los Angeles, California

MARK A. DAVIS, MD, MS

Director, Institute for International Emergency Medicine
   and Health
Department of Emergency Medicine
Brigham and Women's Hospital
Harvard Medical School;
Boston, Massachusetts

Consulting Editors:

JEROME R. HOFFMAN, MD, MA

Professor of Medicine/Emergency Medicine
David Geffen School of Medicine at UCLA
UCLA Emergency Medicine Center, Los Angeles, California

MICHAEL I. ZUCKER, MD

Professor of Radiological Sciences
Chief, Trauma and Emergency Radiology
David Geffen School of Medicine at UCLA
UCLA Center for the Health Sciences, Los Angeles, California

Series Editor:

MARK A. DAVIS, MD, MS

MOSBY
ELSEVIER

1600 John F. Kennedy Blvd.
Ste 1800
Philadelphia, PA 19103-2899

SIGNS AND SYMPTOMS IN EMERGENCY MEDICINE   ISBN-13: 978-0-323-03645-0
Copyright © 2006, 1999 by Mosby, Inc., an affiliate   ISBN-10: 0-323-03645-7
of Elsevier Inc.

Notice

Great efforts have been made to check the accuracy of the information in this book; however, practitioners should use only those treatments, drugs, and drug dosages with which they have experience and for which they have cross-referenced dosages from other sources. In addition, knowledge and best practice in this field are constantly changing. As new research and experience broaden our knowledge, changes in practice, treatment and drug therapy may become necessary or appropriate. Readers are advised to check the most current information provided (i) on procedures featured or (ii) by the manufacturer of each product to be administered, to verify the recommended dose or formula, the method and duration of administration, and contraindications. It is the responsibility of the practitioner, relying on their own experience and knowledge of the patient, to make diagnoses, to determine dosages and the best treatment for each individual patient, and to take all appropriate safety precautions. To the fullest extent of the law, neither the Publisher nor the Editors assumes any liability for any injury and/or damage to persons or property arising out of or related to any use of the material contained in this book.

The Publisher

Library of Congress Cataloging-in-Publication Data
Signs and symptoms in emergency medicine : literature-based approach to emergent conditions / [edited by] Scott R. Votey, and Mark A. Davis.—2nd ed.
p. ; cm.
Includes bibliographical references and index.
ISBN 0-323-03645-7
1. Emergency medicine—Handbooks, manuals, etc. 2. Symptoms—Handbooks, manuals, etc. I. Votey, Scott R. II. Davis, Mark A.
[DLNM: 1. Emergencies—Handbooks. 2. Diagnosis—Handbooks. 3. Emergency Medicine—Handbooks. WB 39 S5785 2006]
RC86.8.S575 2006
616.02'5—dc22
2005058438

Working together to grow
libraries in developing countries
www.elsevier.com | www.bookaid.org | www.sabre.org
ELSEVIER   BOOK AID International   Sabre Foundation

Acquisitions Editor: James Merritt
Developmental Editor: Carla Holloway, Andrea Deis
Publishing Services Manager: Linda Van Pelt
Project Manager: Melanie Peirson Johnstone
Design Direction: Karen O'Keefe Owens

Printed and bound by CPI Group (UK) Ltd, Croydon, CR0 4YY

To the memory of my mother. A teacher by vocation,
she taught me a love of learning that has shaped my life.
And to my wife Lisa and my son Max who each in their own way
have taught me much about love and life.

Scott R. Votey

With great appreciation to my friend, mentor, and colleague,
Scott; to our wonderful authors and those who work every day
to care for the sick and injured; and with much love to Eric,
Michael, Sigalit, Ruth, and Joe.

Mark A. Davis

Contributors

JACOB COBI ASSAF, MD
Chairman, Judy and Sidney Swartz Center for
    Emergency Medicine
Director, Diagnostic & Preoperative Evaluation Unit
Hadassah University Hospital
Jerusalem, Israel

BEVERLY BAUMAN, MD, FAAP, FACEP
Emergency Medicine
Oregon Health and Science University
Portland, Oregon

DAVID F. M. BROWN, MD
Vice Chair, Department of Emergency Medicine
Massachusetts General Hospital;
Assistant Professor, Division of Emergency Medicine
Harvard Medical School
Boston, Massachusetts

MICHAEL J. BURNS, MD, FACEP, FACMT
Co-Director, Division of Medical Toxicology, Department of
    Emergency Medicine
Beth Israel Deaconess Medical Center;
Assistant Professor of Medicine, Harvard Medical School
Boston, Massachusetts

ELIZABETH A. CHAR, MD, FACEP
Assistant Clinical Professor, Surgery
    (Emergency Medicine)
University of Hawaii, School of Medicine
Honolulu, Hawaii

YI-MEI CHNG, MD, MPH
Attending Physician, Department of Emergency Medicine
Kaiser Permanente
Santa Clara, California

RICHELLE J. COOPER, MD, MSHS
Assistant Clinical Professor, Department of
    Medicine/Emergency Medicine
David Geffen School of Medicine at UCLA
UCLA Emergency Medicine Center
Los Angeles, California

HILARIE HARTEL CRANMER, MD, MPH, FACEP
Faculty of Harvard Humanitarian Initiative
Associate Fellowship Director of the International Emergency
    Medicine and Health Fellowship
Division of International Health and Humanitarian Programs
Brigham & Women's Hospital
Boston, Massachusetts

GERIANNE E. DUDLEY, MD, DTMH
Clinical Faculty
Attending Physician, Department of Emergency Medicine
Olive View-UCLA Medical Center
Sylmar, California

PAMELA L. DYNE, MD
Associate Clinical Professor of Medicine/Emergency Medicine
David Geffen School of Medicine at UCLA
Los Angeles, California;
Residency Program Director, Olive View-UCLA/Emergency
    Medicine Residency;
Co-Director, Olive View-UCLA Combined Emergency
    and Internal Medicine Residency Program;
Attending Physician, Department of Emergency Medicine
Olive View-UCLA Medical Center
Sylmar, California

JONATHAN A. EDLOW, MD
Vice-Chairman, Department of Emergency Medicine
Beth Israel Deaconess Medical Center;
Associate Professor of Medicine, Harvard Medical School
Boston, Massachusetts

JOSEPH S. ENGLANOFF, MD
Assistant Clinical Professor of Medicine/Emergency
    Medicine
David Geffen School of Medicine at UCLA
UCLA Emergency Medicine Center
Westwood, California

STEPHEN K. EPSTEIN, MD, MPP
Department of Emergency Medicine
Beth Israel Deaconess Medical Center;
Instructor in Medicine, Division of Emergency Medicine
Harvard Medical School
Boston, Massachusetts

STEVEN GO, MD
Assistant Dean for Medical Education, Department
    of Emergency Medicine
University of Missouri-Kansas City School of Medicine
Kansas City, Missouri

JOSHUA N. GOLDSTEIN, MD, PHD
Instructor of Medicine, Harvard Medical School;
Department of Emergency Medicine
Brigham & Women's Hospital;
Department of Vascular and Critical Care Neurology
Massachusetts General Hospital
Boston, Massachusetts

THOMAS P. GRAHAM, MD
Associate Professor of Medicine/Emergency Medicine
David Geffen School of Medicine at UCLA
UCLA Emergency Medicine Center
Los Angeles, California

ZACHARY A. GRAY, MD
Attending Physician, Emergency Department
Torrance Memorial Medical Center
Torrance, California;
Associate Attending
UCLA Emergency Medicine Center
Los Angeles, California

MYLES D. GREENBERG, MD, MBA
Attending Physician, Department of Emergency Medicine
Norwalk Hospital
Norwalk, Connecticut;
Partner, CHL Medical Partners
Stamford, Connecticut

RICHARD T. GRIFFEY, MD, MPH
Director of Quality and Patient Safety
Director of Information Systems
Department of Emergency Medicine
Brigham & Women's Hospital
Boston, Massachusetts

DANIEL GROSSMAN, MD, FACEP
Physician Specialist, Emergency Medicine
Saint John's Health Center
Santa Monica, California;
Assistant Clinical Professor of Medicine/Emergency Medicine
David Geffen School of Medicine at UCLA
UCLA Emergency Medicine Center
Los Angeles, California

WILLIAM F. HANING III, MD
Associate Dean for Graduate Affairs
John A. Burns School of Medicine, University of Hawaii
Honolulu, Hawaii

MEL E. HERBERT, MBBS, BMEDSCI, MD, FACEP, FAAEM
Associate Professor of Clinical Emergency Medicine,
    Department of Emergency Medicine
KECK School of Medicine
Los Angeles, California;
Editor, EMRAP: Emergency Medicine Reviews
    and Perspectives
Woodland Hills, California

JONATHAN S. ILGEN, MD
Resident, Department of Emergency Medicine
Massachusetts General Hospital;
Resident, Department of Emergency Medicine
Brigham & Women's Hospital
Boston, Massachusetts

MICHELLE KALINSKI, MD, FACEP
Emergency Physician
Emergency Medicine Director of Trauma, Pediatrics,
    and EMS
Community Hospital of the Monterey Peninsula
Monterey, California

RICK G. KULKARNI, MD
Director of Informatics, Department of Emergency Medicine
Olive View-UCLA Medical Center
Sylmar, California;
Assistant Professor of Medicine/Emergency Medicine
David Geffen School of Medicine at UCLA
Los Angeles, California

MARY LANCTOT-HERBERT, NP
Staff NP, Department of Emergency Medicine
Olive View–UCLA Medical Center
Sylmar, California;
Assistant Professor of Nursing, Acute Care Division
UCLA School of Nursing
Los Angeles, California

ERIC LEGOME, MD
Attending Physician, Emergency Medicine
New York University;
Attending Physician, Emergency Medicine
Bellevue Hospital Center;
Director, NYU/Bellevue Emergency Medicine Residency
New York University;
Assistant Professor of Emergency Medicine
New York University School of Medicine
New York, New York

MICHAEL LEVINE, MD
Resident, Department of Emergency Medicine
Harvard-Affiliated Emergency Medicine Residency
Brigham & Women's/Massachusetts General Hospitals
Boston, Massachusetts

RESA E. LEWISS, MD, RDMS
Director of Emergency Ultrasound
Attending Physician, Emergency Medicine
St. Luke's – Roosevelt Hospital Center;
Columbia University
New York, New York

JULIAN G. LIS, MD, MPH
Quality Assurance Director, Department of
    Emergency Medicine
Scripps Mercy Hospital
San Diego, California

MARK S. LOUDEN, MD, FACEP, FAAEM
Emergency Department
Duke Health Raleigh Hospital
Raleigh, North Carolina

LUIS M. LOVATO, MD
Director of Critical Care, Department of Emergency Medicine
Olive View – UCLA Medical Center
Sylmar, California;
Assistant Clinical Professor of Medicine/Emergency Medicine
David Geffen School of Medicine at UCLA
Los Angeles, California

SCOTT LUNDBERG, MD
Faculty Physician Specialist, Department of Internal Medicine,
    Department of Emergency Medicine
Associate Program Director, UCLA Combined Emergency
    Medicine and Internal Medicine Residency
Olive View – UCLA Medical Center
Sylmar, California;
Assistant Clinical Professor of Medicine, Department
    of Internal Medicine
David Geffen School of Medicine at UCLA
Los Angeles, California

FRANCES MCCABE, MD
Emergency Physician
St. Charles Medical Center
Bend, Oregon

MAUREEN MCCOLLOUGH, MD, FACEP, FAAEM
Associate Professor of Clinical Emergency Medicine and Pediatrics
Keck USC School of Medicine;
Director, Pediatric Emergency Department
Director, Major Trauma and Resuscitation
Los Angeles County USC Medical Center
Los Angeles, California

LYNNE MCCULLOUGH, MD, FACEP
Associate Director, Emergency Medicine Residency
Assistant Clinical Professor of Medicine/Emergency Medicine
David Geffen School of Medicine at UCLA
UCLA Emergency Medicine Center
Los Angeles, California

ALISA MCQUEEN, MD
Fellow in Pediatric Emergency Medicine, Division of
    Emergency Medicine
Children's Hospital Boston;
Clinical Fellow in Pediatrics, Harvard Medical School
Boston, Massachusetts

MICHAEL MENCHINE, MD
Clinical Instructor of Medicine/Emergency Medicine
David Geffen School of Medicine at UCLA
UCLA Emergency Medicine Center
Los Angeles, California

BENJAMIN T. MILLIGAN, MD
Emergency Medicine
New York University/Bellevue Hospital Center
New York, New York

BRIAN ROBERT MIURA, MD, FACEP
Attending Physician, Emergency Department
Torrance Memorial Medical Center
Torrance, California;
Visiting Assistant Professor of Medicine/Emergency Medicine
David Geffen School of Medicine at UCLA
Los Angeles, California

GREGORY J. MORAN, MD
Department of Emergency Medicine, Division of
    Infectious Disease
Olive View – UCLA Medical Center
Sylmar, California;
Clinical Professor of Medicine
David Geffen School of Medicine at UCLA
Los Angeles, California

SAMUEL ONG, MD
Attending Physician, Department of Emergency Medicine
Olive View – UCLA Medical Center
Sylmar, California

NEAL PEEPLES, MD
Emergency Physician
St. Charles Medical Center
Bend, Oregon

CHARLES N. POZNER, MD
Director, STRATUS Center for Medical Stimulation
Director of Prehospital Care, Department of Emergency Medicine
Brigham & Women's Hospital;
Assistant Professor of Medicine/Emergency Medicine,
    Harvard Medical School
Boston, Massachusetts

VIRGINIA M. RIBEIRO, MD, FACEP
Physician, Department of Emergency Medicine
MetroWest Medical Center
Framingham, Massachusetts

VENA RICKETTS, MD, FACEP
Associate Chief, Department of Emergency Medicine
Olive View – UCLA Medical Center;
Professor of Medicine
David Geffen School of Medicine at UCLA
Sylmar, California

SCOTT W. RODI, MD, MPH
Assistant Professor of Medicine, Department of Medicine,
    Section of Emergency Medicine
Dartmouth Hitchcock Medical Center
Lebanon, New Hampshire

CAROLYN J. SACHS, MD, MPH
Associate Professor of Medicine/Emergency Medicine
David Geffen School of Medicine at UCLA
UCLA Emergency Medicine Center
Los Angeles, California

ERIC A. SAVITSKY, MD
Director, UCLA Center for International Emergency Medicine;
Associate Professor of Medicine/Emergency Medicine
David Geffen School of Medicine at UCLA
UCLA Emergency Medicine Center
Los Angeles, California

RICHARD SONNER, MD
Director of Pediatric Emergency Services
Attending Physician in Emergency Medicine
Torrance Memorial Medical Center
Torrance, California;
Visiting Assistant Professor, Department of Medicine/Emergency
    Medicine
David Geffen School of Medicine at UCLA
Los Angeles, California

SUKHJIT S. TAKHAR, MD
Department of Emergency Medicine
Olive View – UCLA Medical Center
Sylmar, California

ATILLA UNER, MD, MPH, FAAEM
Assistant Professor of Medicine/Emergency Medicine
David Geffen School of Medicine at UCLA
UCLA Emergency Medicine Center
Los Angeles, California

CARIN VAN ZYL, MD
Resident Physician
UCLA Medical Center/Olive View Medical Center Emergency
   Medicine Residency
David Geffen School of Medicine at UCLA
Los Angeles, California

MICHAEL WEITZ, MD, FACEP
Associate Director of Emergency Services
Saint John's Health Center
Santa Monica, California;
Assistant Professor of Medicine/Emergency Medicine
David Geffen School of Medicine at UCLA
Attending Physician, Department of Emergency Medicine
Olive View – UCLA Medical Center;
Sylmar, California

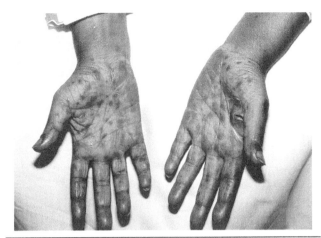

Fig. 30-1 Erythema multiforme. "Target" lesions on the palms. (Courtesy of Anthony J. Mancini, MD, Chicago.)

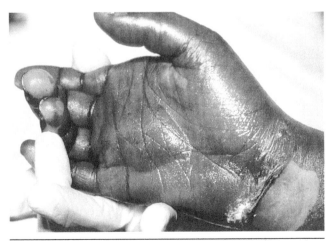

Fig. 30-2 Toxic epidermal necrolysis. Blisters and epidermal sloughing. (Courtesy of Anthony J. Mancini, MD, Chicago.)

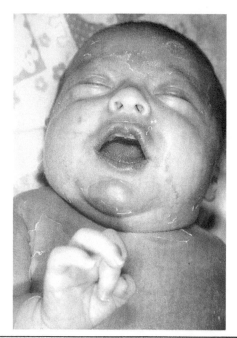

Fig. 30–3 Staphylococcal scalded skin syndrome. Epidermolysis in a 3-week-old infant. (Courtesy of Anthony J. Mancini, MD, Chicago.)

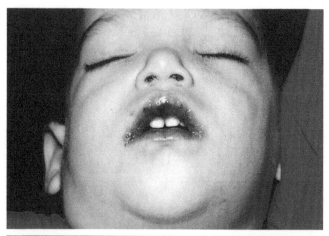

Fig. 30–4 Kawasaki's disease. Dry, fissured lips. (Courtesy of Anthony J. Mancini, MD, Chicago.)

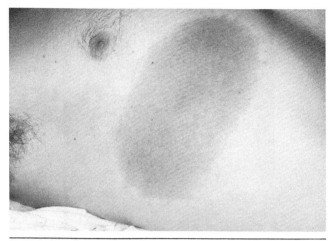

Fig. 30-5 Lyme disease, erythema migrans.

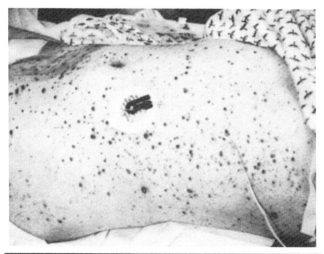

Fig. 30-6 Meningococcemia. Purpura and petechiae. (Courtesy of Javier Gonzalez del Rey, MD.)

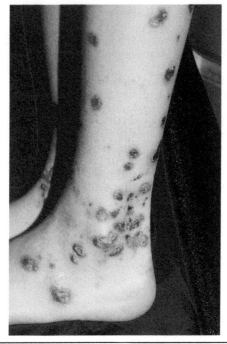

Fig. 30-7 Henoch-Schönlein purpura. Raised, palpable hemorrhagic lesions on a child's leg. (Courtesy of Anthony J. Mancini, MD, Chicago.)

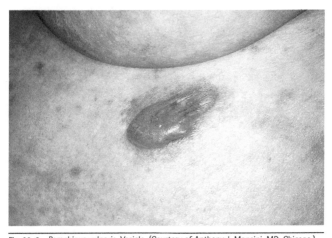

Fig. 30-8 Pemphigus vulgaris. Vesicle. (Courtesy of Anthony J. Mancini, MD, Chicago.)

Preface

We have been pleased by the enthusiastic reception to the first
edition of *Signs and Symptoms in Emergency Medicine*. It has
been gratifying to hear how this text has been used in patient care,
personal review, and teaching. We hope this second edition, with
its updates and new chapters, will be even more useful than the
first, and that the expansion of the series to Pediatrics and other
specialties will be helpful in many clinical environments.

In designing these texts, we realize that patients come to the
emergency department (ED) with symptoms, not diagnoses.
Practitioners of emergency medicine must consider whether
a patient's symptoms represent a serious disease before making
the diagnosis of a more benign condition. Migraine is not
diagnosed without consideration of subarachnoid hemorrhage,
nor is spontaneous abortion diagnosed before evaluation for
ectopic pregnancy. Although we always consider the most
serious conditions before the most common, in most cases all
that is necessary to effectively rule out life-threatening disease
are history, physical examination, and knowledge of the disease
under consideration.

This pocket text provides a symptom-based approach to
ED patient care based on current literature. Created for use in the
ED and written by practicing emergency physicians, its approach
is pertinent anywhere emergency care is provided. It is also a
time-efficient study guide to many presenting complaints and
emergent conditions. This text is not a "cookbook" for patient care.
Nor is it possible in a text of this size to provide a comprehensive
differential diagnosis of disease. This text is designed to stimulate
the practitioner to consider the important conditions that could
be responsible for the presenting problems of ED patients. Most
chapters are based on presenting symptoms, such as Abdominal
Pain or Shortness of Breath. In a few instances chapters are based
on specific patient characteristics, such as having HIV/AIDS or

being a solid organ transplant recipient, which are of sufficient magnitude that they influence all aspects of a patient's care.

For each diagnosis listed within a chapter, associated symptoms, signs, workup, and treatment considerations are addressed.

The authors and editors have tried, where possible, to provide a literature-based assessment of the frequency with which symptoms, signs, and diagnostic tests are positive when the disease is present (i.e., sensitivity). The following system has been used:

+	(< 5%)
++	(6% to 30%)
+++	(31% to 69%)
++++	(70% to 94%)
+++++	(95% to 100%)

If a finding or a test is highly sensitive, it is likely to be positive if the disease is present. However, as sensitivity rises, specificity (the frequency of negative results in those without the disease) usually falls, which increases the likelihood of false positive results. It is also important to remember the importance of pre-test probability of disease on the decision to order and final interpretation of the results of a test. Due to imperfect specificity and sensitivity most medical tests show a high frequency of false positive results in populations of patients with low prevalence of disease; and conversely show a high frequency of false negative results in populations with high prevalence of disease.

Experienced practitioners and decision scientists alike understand that the thoughtful application of literature-based decision-making requires a thorough understanding of the literature applied in conjunction with the recognition of patterns in presentation. We hope that the information framing each discussion of symptoms and diagnoses will help in this regard.

Although diagnosis is the principle focus of this text, it must be remembered that a diagnosis is only useful in so far as it guides therapy, and that the goal of any therapeutic intervention is to improve patient outcome. Recommendations for therapy are provided in general terms, but therapy should be individualized for each patient. Optimal therapeutic decision-making requires consideration of the value of each possible outcome that may occur, given treatment alternatives. For example, it is prudent to admit to the hospital a patient thought to be at moderately low risk for myocardial infarction (MI), when failure to do so could result in the patient's demise if discharged from the ED with an MI in progress. Conversely it may be appropriate not to treat a suspected otitis media in a child, since in this generally low-risk condition the choice of treatment versus non-treatment is unlikely to have a significant impact on the child's welfare. Ideally treatment decisions would include the value (utility) patients place on the treatment alternatives, including their views on risk. In practice, patients' preferences are only occasionally considered in decision making, and then incompletely. Unfortunately, there is no validated framework currently available for routinely measuring patient utilities or integrating them formally into medical decisions.

Given the shortcomings of the medical literature, the variability in patient presentations, and the limitations of diagnostic testing, how should ED patient care decisions be made? A careful problem-oriented history and directed physical examination are essential. Always consider the most serious condition that the presentation could represent, and decide if the information at hand is sufficient to exclude each serious diagnosis. Determine whether the information is adequate to make the necessary therapeutic decisions. If uncertainty remains, choose diagnostic tests judiciously, selecting tests that can provide needed data most efficiently. Interpret test results with an understanding of their shortcomings. Choose among management alternatives based on the expected outcomes and, if practical, the preferences of the patient. Remember that you may be wrong, and weigh the consequences. In the minority of patients for whom a serious diagnosis remains a possibility, thoughtful use of additional diagnostic tests, consultation, or observation is appropriate to "rule in" or "rule out" the entities of concern.

Although as emergency medicine practitioners we will establish a diagnosis in most patients at risk for significant complications, at times we will miss a critical diagnosis in those with emergent conditions. We can protect our patients (and ourselves) by providing discharge instructions that specifically inform them of events that should lead to their return to the ED. We should arrange for patients to be re-examined in an appropriate time frame and prescribe a follow-up physician visit to ensure the adequacy of our intervention and to provide for further evaluation as indicated. Patients should be instructed to seek further medical attention if their symptoms worsen or persist for longer than a specified time interval. It is perhaps most important that we be honest with our patients and ourselves. We can limit risk to patients through a careful, informed evaluation, but risk can never be completely eliminated.

Caring for ED patients is an awesome responsibility and a wonderful opportunity. We hope that this text adds to your ability to effectively diagnose and treat the patients entrusted to your care.

Scott R. Votey, MD
Editor-in-Chief

Mark A. Davis, MD, MS
Series Editor

Acknowledgments

While still a resident Mark Davis identified the need for a signs and symptoms oriented, literature-based emergency medicine text that could be used in the emergency department as care was given. This text, and the growing series of texts of which it is the cornerstone, would not exist without his vision, determination, and hard work. Thank you for the years of effort, your generosity, and above all your friendship.

Scott R. Votey, MD

Occasionally in our pursuits we meet someone whose intellect, insight, and strength of character change us and the world in which we live. On behalf of the legions of students, colleagues, patients, and friends who have benefited from his tireless efforts, we want to thank Jerry Hoffman.

In creating the first edition of *Signs and Symptoms in Emergency Medicine*, many individuals gave of their time and talents. We wish to recognize their important contributions, which serve as the foundation for this second edition and the series of which it is a part.

Jeremy Brown	Chapter 10, Ear Pain
Victor A. Candioty	Chapter 34, Shortness of Breath
Hilarie Cranmer	Chapter 40, Trauma, Burns
Jonathan Edlow	Chapter 30, Rash
P. Gregg Greenough	Associate Editor
	Chapter 35, Sore Throat
John Halamka	Appendix A
Kenneth R. Lawrence	Appendices B and C
Resa Lewiss	Chapter 39, Trauma, Approach to
Laura Macnow	Chapter 18, Headache
Richard Oh	Chapter 37, Toxic Exposure, Approach to

Jolie Hall Pfahler	Chapter 30, Rash
Eric Salk	Chapter 23, Jaundice
Richard M. Schwartzenstein	Consulting Editor
Jorge Vournas	Chapter 44, Weakness and Fatigue
John Wong	Chapter 1, Abdominal Pain

This text is the product of tremendous effort on the part of many friends and colleagues who served as authors and editors. We appreciate their dedication to the project. Special thanks to Jim Merritt, Carla Holloway, and Andrea Deis at Elsevier for their insight and support in keeping this project on track.

Scott R. Votey, MD   **Mark A. Davis, MD, MS**

Contents

Signs and Symptoms in Emergency Medicine

Abdominal Pain
Elizabeth A. Char and William F. Haning III

Abdominal pain is a common complaint of emergency department (ED) patients. Although in most cases the cause of the pain is benign, great care must be taken not to miss emergent conditions requiring treatment. Elderly patients and those with comorbid conditions are especially at high risk for having a serious abdominal condition. Medical and surgical emergencies arising from pathologic conditions outside the abdomen must also be considered.

 ABDOMINAL AORTIC ANEURYSM

An abdominal aortic aneurysm (AAA) is caused by dilation of the aorta secondary to weakening of all layers of the aortic wall. Risk factors include hypertension, male sex, smoking, coronary artery disease, age older than 50, and a first-degree relative with AAA.

SYMPTOMS
- Severe abdominal pain ++++
- Flank or back pain with radiation to the groin or legs
- Syncope

SIGNS
- Pulsatile abdominal mass ++++
- Diffuse abdominal tenderness
- Abdominal bruit ++
- Hypotension (late finding) +++
- Hematuria ++
- Evidence of peripheral embolization +
- Ischemic lower extremities
- High-output cardiac failure (rare)
- Gastrointestinal (GI) bleed (rare)

WORKUP

- A computed tomography (CT) scan should be obtained for the hemodynamically stable patient because it is highly sensitive and specific and also can demonstrate retroperitoneal hemorrhage, rupture, leakage, and other potential diagnoses.
- An ED ultrasound can be used in the hemodynamically unstable patient as arrangements are being made for transfer to the operating room. Ultrasound has good overall sensitivity if the entire aorta is visualized as it can generally evaluate for enlarged aortic diameter, but it is unreliable in visualizing leakage or rupture.

COMMENTS AND TREATMENT CONSIDERATIONS

Femoral pulses usually are normal even after rupture. If the patient is unstable, consult with the surgery department to prepare for immediate transfer to the operating room as these unstable patients generally do not require, or benefit from, delays associated with CT scanning. AAAs are often asymptomatic until they rapidly expand, leak, or rupture. The classic triad of abdominal pain/back pain, pulsatile abdominal mass, and hypotension is present in less than 50% of patients. Suspect AAA in older people presenting with symptoms suggestive of renal colic or diverticulitis.

REFERENCES

Hendrickson M, Naparst TR: Abdominal surgical emergencies in the elderly, *Emerg Med Clin North Am* 21:937, 2003.

Kuhn M, Bonnin RL, Davey MJ, et al: Emergency department ultrasound scanning for abdominal aortic aneurysm: accessible, accurate and advantageous, *Ann Emerg Med* 36:219, 2000.

Lynch RM: Ruptured abdominal aortic aneurysm presenting as groin pain, *Br J Gen Pract* 52:320, 2002.

Marston WA, Ahlquist R, Johnson G Jr, Meyer AA: Misdiagnosis of ruptured abdominal aortic aneurysms, *J Vasc Surg* 16:17, 1992.

Rogers RL, McCormack R: Aortic disasters, *Emerg Med Clin North Am* 22:887, 2004.

Shergill IS, Bosse D: Abdominal aortic aneurysm, *Br J Gen Pract* 52:584, 2002.

Siegel C, Cohan R: CT of abdominal aortic aneurysm, *AJR Am J Roentgenol* 163:17, 1994.

 MESENTERIC ISCHEMIA

Ischemic disease of the intestines (small bowel is most common) can be hyperacute, chronic recurrent, or an acute exacerbation of a chronic condition. The classic symptoms and signs attributed to ischemia are actually those of infarction. Diagnosis after infarction is associated with a high mortality rate. Mesenteric ischemia should be considered for patients at risk, such as elderly patients with vascular disease or atrial fibrillation, valvular disease, or a history of an embolic event, and for those who have severe abdominal pain that cannot be adequately explained.

SYMPTOMS

Symptoms vary depending on which segment of the bowel is involved.

- Superior mesenteric artery embolism (50%): acute onset of severe, poorly localized, unrelenting abdominal pain followed by nausea, vomiting, and diarrhea. Patients usually have a history of cardiovascular disease (myocardial infarct, dysrhythmia, or valvular disease), a previous embolism ++, or evidence of embolism elsewhere ++.
- Superior mesenteric artery thrombosis (15% to 20%): gradual onset of abdominal pain. Patients may have a history of intestinal angina (postprandial abdominal pain relieved by vomiting), weight loss, and diarrhea or a history of vasculitis, prothrombic disorder, or atherosclerosis, diabetes, and hypertension.
- Nonocclusive mesenteric ischemia (20%): Abdominal pain is typically of gradual onset; 25% have no pain and manifest only as distention or bloating. Typically occurs in association with a low-flow state or vasospasm of mesenteric vessels related to excessive sympathetic activity during sepsis, cardiogenic shock, congestive heart failure, hypotension, hemodialysis or hypovolemia, or previous treatment with vasopressors, digoxin, or beta-blockers.
- Mesenteric vein thrombosis (5% to 15%): progressive onset of abdominal pain, nausea, and vomiting and history of venous thrombosis +++, hypercoagulable state, or malignancy.

SIGNS

- Pain is typically out of proportion to physical findings.
- Abdominal examination varies depending on the stage of ischemia. Often, physical findings occur late in the course of the illness and range from mild localized or generalized tenderness to peritoneal signs. Occult fecal blood may precede other signs, but its absence does not rule out the diagnosis.
- Usually afebrile with stable vital signs until becoming hypovolemic or septic
- Vomiting +++
- Diarrhea

WORKUP

- Angiography is considered the "gold standard," but in some centers the diagnosis is increasingly made by CT angiography, especially if three-dimensional reconstructions are used.

CHAPTER 1

- CT with triple contrast may show dilated fluid-filled loops of thick-walled bowel, luminal dilatation, pneumatosis intestinalis (intramural gas), or mesenteric or portal venous gas as the disease progresses. CT is the test of choice for demonstrating mesenteric venous thrombosis.
- Plain abdominal radiographs are rarely helpful but may show thumbprinting (smooth indentations on the colon); dilated, thickened bowel loops; gasless abdomen or ileus; or gas in the bowel wall or portal vein (late signs).
- Laboratory abnormalities, such as metabolic acidosis and leukocytosis, occur late in the ischemic process.

COMMENTS AND TREATMENT CONSIDERATIONS

Early diagnosis is critical and is based primarily on the history and physical examination. Early angiographic or surgical intervention (especially if the patient is exhibiting peritoneal signs) is necessary to prevent serious morbidity or death. Treatment modalities include heparin (timing is controversial), antibiotics (for bacterial translocation), and intravenous (IV) hydration. Intra-arterial thrombolytics have been beneficial in certain subsets of patients.

REFERENCES

Bassiouny HS: Nonocclusive mesenteric ischemia, *Surg Clin North Am* 77:319, 1997.

Bradbury A, McBride B, Ruckley C: Mesenteric ischemia: a multidisciplinary approach, *Br J Surg* 82:1446, 1995.

Hendrickson M, Naparst TR: Abdominal surgical emergencies in the elderly, *Emerg Med Clin North Am* 21:937, 2003.

Lee R, Tung HK, Tung PH, et al: CT in acute mesenteric ischaemia, *Clin Radiol* 58:279, 2003.

Martinez JP, Hogan GJ: Mesenteric Ischemia, *Emerg Med Clin North Am* 22:909, 2004.

Schneider TA, Longo WE, Ure T, Vernava AM III: Mesenteric ischemia: acute arterial syndromes, *Dis Colon Rectum* 37:1163, 1994.

Walker JS, Dire DJ: Vascular abdominal emergencies, *Emerg Med Clin North Am* 14:571, 1996.

 ACUTE MYOCARDIAL INFARCTION

See Chapter 7, Chest Pain.

COMMENTS AND TREATMENT CONSIDERATIONS

Elderly patients, women, and those with diabetes or congestive heart failure may present without the chest pain or tightness typical of acute myocardial infarction (AMI). Many of these patients complain of dyspnea +++, but a significant number have gastrointestinal complaints alone, usually consisting of abdominal pain, epigastric discomfort or "heartburn" ++, or nausea and vomiting. Patients may also have silent or asymptomatic AMIs. The percentage of patients with atypical presentations of acute MI increases with age.

REFERENCES

Brieger D, Eagle KA, Goodman SG, et al: Acute coronary syndromes without chest pain, an underdiagnosed and undertreated high-risk group: insights from the Global Registry of Acute Coronary Events, *Chest* 126:461, 2004.

Lusiani L, Perrone A, Pesavento R, et al: Prevalence, clinical features, and acute course of atypical myocardial infarction, *Angiology* 45:49, 1994.

Patel H, Rosegren A, Ekman I: Symptoms in acute coronary syndromes: does sex make a difference? *Am Heart J* 148:27, 2004.

Pellicia F, Cartoni D, Verde M, et al: Comparison of presenting features, diagnostic tools, hospital outcomes, and quality of care indicators in older (>65 years) to younger, men to women, and diabetics to non-diabetics with acute chest pain triaged in the emergency department, *Am J Cardiol* 94:216, 2004.

 PERFORATED ULCER

Perforated ulcers are commonly caused by nonsteroidal anti-inflammatory drug use or by *Helicobacter pylori* disease, but up to one third of patients lack either risk factor. Smoking has also been identified as a risk factor. Perforation with spillage of gastric or duodenal contents into the abdomen can lead to severe peritonitis.

SYMPTOMS
- Severe abdominal pain of sudden onset ++++; back pain in posterior penetrating ulcer
- Older patients may have only minimal pain +++.
- Nausea
- Vomiting

SIGNS
- Diffuse abdominal pain with diminished bowel sounds
- Acute peritonitis
- Rigid abdomen +++
- Hypovolemia
- Hypotension
- Tachycardia
- Fever

CHAPTER 1

WORKUP

- Abdominal series to look for free air ++++. Plain films can detect as little as 1 to 2 ml of free air, but the patient must be in a left lateral decubitus position for 10 to 20 minutes and then upright for 10 minutes.
- CT scans identify free air in the abdomen and can rule out other diagnoses that may mimic the presentation of a perforated viscus.
- An elevated white blood cell (WBC) count is insensitive +++, as are elevated amylase and alkaline phosphatase levels.

COMMENTS AND TREATMENT CONSIDERATIONS

The duration of perforation is an independent risk factor for death, so patients who have an acute abdominal condition should have perforated ulcer diagnosed expeditiously. Signs and symptoms become more pronounced over time as sepsis and peritonitis develop. Elderly patients may present with nonspecific complaints or minimal signs and symptoms.

Treatment should include antibiotics, a nasogastric tube, and surgical repair.

REFERENCES

Chen CH, Yang CC, Yeh YH: Role of upright chest radiography and ultrasonography in demonstrating air of perforated peptic ulcers, *Hepatogastroenterology* 48:1082, 2001.

Grassi R, Roman S, Pinto A, et al: Gastro-duodenal perforations: conventional plain film, US and CT findings in 166 consecutive patients, *Eur J Radiol* 50:30, 2004.

Hermansson M, Stael von Holstein C, Zilling T: Peptic ulcer perforation before and after introduction of H2 receptor blockers and proton pump inhibitors, *Scand J Gastroenterol* 32:523, 1997.

Lin CK, Lee T: Perforated duodenal ulcer, *Gastrointest Endosc* 60:266, 2004.

Newton M, Mandavia S: Surgical complications of selected gastrointestinal emergencies: pitfalls in management of the acute abdomen, *Emerg Med Clin North Am* 21:873, 2003.

Svanes C: Trends in perforated peptic ulcer: incidence, etiology, treatment and prognosis, *World J Surg* 24:277, 2000.

Yoshizumi T, Ikeda T, Ohta S, et al: Abdominal ultrasonography reveals the perforation site of duodenal ulcers, *Surg Endosc* 15:758, 2001

 VOLVULUS

See also Malrotation and Volvulus in Chapter 43, Vomiting Child. The following discussion pertains to adults.

Location: sigmoid colon, 55% to 60%; cecal, 40%; small bowel, very rare.

SYMPTOMS
- Generally severe, colicky abdominal pain but may be less pronounced, especially in debilitated patients.
- Abdominal distention
- Recurrent episodes +++
- Constipation
- Nausea
- Vomiting

SIGNS
- Diffuse, generally lower, abdominal tenderness
- Tympanic and distended abdomen
- Peritoneal signs, fever, and shock if ischemic

WORKUP
- Abdominal plain films identify the dilated loop of bowel in 80% of sigmoid volvulus and 50% of cecal volvulus (Fig. 1–1).
- CT has high negative predictive value.
- Sigmoidoscopy (diagnosis and reduction in 60% to 90% of sigmoid volvulus)
- Barium enema (BE)

COMMENTS AND TREATMENT CONSIDERATIONS
Surgical consultation is required for adults with volvulus. Detorsion with sigmoidoscopy is usually successful, but recurrence is common and (elective or emergent) resection is often required.

REFERENCES
Dulger M, Canturk NZ, Utkan NZ, et al: Management of sigmoid colon volvulus, *Hepatogastroenterology* 47:1280, 2000.

Echenique EM, Amondarian AJ: Colonic volvulus, *Rev Esp Enferm Dig* 94:201, 2002.

Frizelle F, Wolff B: Colonic volvulus, *Adv Surg* 29:131, 1996.

Montes H, Wolf J: Cecal volvulus in pregnancy, *Am J Gastroenterol* 94:2554, 1999.

Raveenthiran V: Emptiness of the left iliac fossa: a new clinical sign of sigmoid volvulus, *Postgrad Med J* 76:638, 2000.

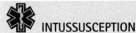 **INTUSSUSCEPTION**

Intussusception—a "telescoping" of intestine usually occurring at the junction of the terminal ileum and ileocecal valve—occurs most commonly in children younger than 2 years. Approximately 5% of

CHAPTER 1

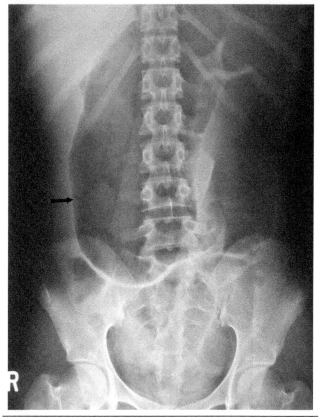

Fig. 1–1 Sigmoid volvulus. Anteroposterior supine view of abdomen reveals markedly distended sigmoid colon *(arrow)*.

cases occur in adults (usually enteroenteric), and in 70% to 90% of these patients a lead point is found for the intussusception (polyp, tumor, adhesions, and edema). Less than 50% of patients have the classic clinical triad of abdominal pain, currant jelly stools, and a palpable abdominal mass. Some studies list nausea and vomiting as the third component of the triad. Lethargy may be a predominant finding in some younger pediatric patients.

SYMPTOMS
- Episodic colicky abdominal pain ++++ in an otherwise healthy child (90% to 95% of cases) or in an adult (5% to 10% of cases)

- Nausea and vomiting ++++
- Bloody stool +++
- Diarrhea ++
- Poor oral feeding by a child and episodes of crying and drawing up the legs

SIGNS
- Palpable abdominal mass +++ classically described as sausage shaped
- Abdominal tenderness +++
- Deydration, pallor, and altered mental status (particularly lethargy) between episodes of pain may be the only signs of intussusception in young children.
- Occult blood in stool ++++
- Currant jelly (bloody, mucoid) stool ++

WORKUP
- Abdominal series lacks sensitivity and may be normal ++ or may show evidence of a bowel obstruction +++, mass effect +++, or the classic target sign or soft tissue density +++ (Fig. 1–2).
- BE has long been the gold standard for diagnosing and sometimes treating and reducing ++++ intussusception.
- In recent years, air or gas enema (GE) has become the preferred study (improved reduction rate, less risk in the event of perforation). BE and GE are commonly not recommended in adults (and are generally contraindicated in patients with peritonitis or shock) because both the high likelihood of a pathologic condition (lead points and malignancy) and the higher risk of perforation with an enema under pressure are indications for operation.
- Routine laboratory tests are not helpful in the diagnosis of intussusception.
- Ultrasound has also been useful in the diagnosis of intussusception, especially in children (sensitivity up to +++++, specificity 88%).
- CT may demonstrate an intraluminal mass or may be helpful in ruling out other causes of acute abdominal conditions, especially in adults.
- Magnetic resonance imaging may be helpful in stable adults to identify the intussusception and the lead point.

COMMENTS AND TREATMENT CONSIDERATIONS
Consider intussusception whenever evaluating a young child with a possible abdominal process, altered mental status, or a septic appearance. The recurrence rate is 6% to 12%.

CHAPTER 1

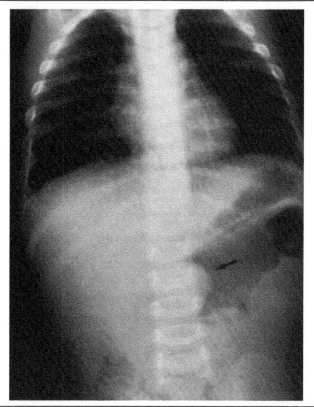

Fig. 1–2 Intussusception. Anteroposterior supine view of abdomen demonstrates soft tissue density (*arrow*) in distended small bowel. (From Rosen P: *Diagnostic radiology in emergency medicine*, St Louis, 1992, Mosby.)

REFERENCES

Byrne AT, Goegehan T, Govender P, et al: The imaging of intussusception, *Clin Radiol* 60:39, 2005.

D'Agostino J: Common abdominal emergencies in children, *Emerg Med Clin North Am* 20:139, 2002.

Daneman A, Alton DJ: Intussusception: issues and controversies related to diagnosis and reduction, *Radiol Clin North Am* 34:743, 1996.

Gayer G, Hertz M, Zissin R: CT findings of intussusception in adults, *Semin Ultrasound CT MR* 24:377, 2003.

McCollough M, Sharieff GQ: Abdominal surgical emergencies in infants and young children, *Emerg Clin North Am* 21:909, 2003.

Prater JM, Olshenki FC: Adult intussusception, *Am Fam Physician* 47:447, 1993.

Roeyen, G, Jansen M, Hubens G: Intussusception in infants: an emergency in diagnosis and treatment, *Eur J Emerg Med* 6:73, 1999.

 OVARIAN TORSION

Ovarian torsion is a twisting of an ovary that compromises ovarian blood supply, leading to ovarian infarction if not rapidly diagnosed and treated. Torsion is more likely to occur in patients with an enlarged ovary or prior pelvic surgery and in patients in the second half of the menstrual cycle. Fifteen percent to 20% of the cases occur during pregnancy.

SYMPTOMS
- Abrupt onset of severe unilateral or nonlocalized lower abdominal or pelvic pain +++
- Nausea ++++
- Vomiting ++++
- Recurrent episodes +++
- Urinary symptoms

SIGNS
- Unilateral lower abdominal or pelvic tenderness, tender adnexal mass +++
- Progression to peritoneal signs (not common)
- Low-grade fever

WORKUP
- Pregnancy test
- Transvaginal ultrasound without delay is the imaging study of choice. Addition of color Doppler may increase specificity.
- Laparoscopy can be used for diagnosis and treatment.

COMMENTS AND TREATMENT CONSIDERATIONS
In infants and small children, the reproductive organs are higher in the abdomen, and torsion may mimic renal colic.

REFERENCES
Dolgin SE: Acute ovarian torsion in children, *Am J Surg* 183:95, 2002.

Houry D, Abbott JT: Ovarian torsion: a fifteen year review, *Ann Emerg Med* 38:156, 2001.

Kokoska ER, Keller MS, Weber TR: Acute ovarian torsion in children, *Am J Surg* 180:462, 2000.

CHAPTER 1

Lambert MJ, Villa M: Gynecologic ultrasound in emergency medicine, *Emerg Med Clin North Am* 22:683, 2004.

Rha SE, Byun JY, Jung SE, et al: CT and MR imaging features of adnexal torsion, *Radiographics* 22:283, 2002.

TESTICULAR TORSION

See Chapter 31, Scrotal Pain.

ECTOPIC PREGNANCY

See Chapter 41, Vaginal Bleeding. Always consider ectopic pregnancy in women of childbearing age who have lower abdominal pain.

BOWEL OBSTRUCTION

In developed countries, approximately 50% to 70% of all small bowel obstructions are caused by adhesions, 5% to 15% by incarcerated or strangulated hernias, and 10% to 15% by neoplasms.

SYMPTOMS
- Abdominal pain ++++++
- Nausea ++++
- Vomiting ++++
- No flatus or stool passage
- Bloating ++++
- Inguinal pain or a bulge or mass in the scrotum if an incarcerated hernia is the cause of the obstruction

SIGNS
- Abdominal distention ++++
- Abdominal tenderness ++++
- Fever ++
- Tender palpable mass if hernia is present
- Peritonitis if hernia is strangulated or perforated

WORKUP
- Abdominal series ++++ but may be negative early
- CT has high sensitivity and specificity in complete small bowel obstruction. It may be useful if the cause of the obstruction is unclear or if there is a question of partial obstruction versus ileus.
- An elevated white blood cell (WBC) count is neither sensitive nor specific for bowel obstruction +++

- Levels of creatine phosphokinase (CPK), lactate dehydrogenase (LDH), alkaline phosphatase, and amylase have not shown any consistent correlation with the diagnosis of small bowel obstruction.

COMMENTS AND TREATMENT CONSIDERATIONS

Treatment of small bowel obstruction includes insertion of a nasogastric tube, intravenous fluids with the patient NPO, surgical consultation (although rarely requires emergent surgical intervention), and hospital admission.

REFERENCES

Anderson VT, Humphrey CT: Contrast radiography in small bowel obstruction: a prospective randomized trial, *Mil Med* 162:749, 1997.

Burkill G, Bell J, Healy J: Small bowel obstruction: the role of computed tomography in its diagnosis and management with reference to other imaging modalities, *Eur Radiol* 11:1405-1422, 2001.

Delabrousse E, Destrumelle N, Brunelle S, et al: CT of small bowel obstruction in adults, *Abdom Imaging* 28:257, 2003.

Frager D: Intestinal obstruction role of CT, *Gastroenterol Clin North Am* 31:777, 2002.

Hendrickson M, Naparst TR: Abdominal surgical emergencies in the elderly, *Emerg Med Clin North Am* 21:937, 2003.

Simpson A, Sandeman D, Nixon SJ, et al: The value of an erect abdominal radiograph in the diagnosis of intestinal obstruction, *Clin Radiol* 36:41, 1985.

CHOLECYSTITIS, CHOLANGITIS, AND COMMON BILE DUCT OBSTRUCTION

Gallbladder disease generally presents as biliary colic, a "benign" condition in which gallstones cause colicky right upper quadrant pain that is easily treated with analgesics. Cholelithiasis is most common in obese women in their fourth decade.

It is important not to miss patients who have cholecystitis (inflammation of the gallbladder), common bile duct obstruction, or cholangitis (inflammation of the biliary duct system), for which hospital admission and specific treatments are required. Approximately 10% of cholecystitis occurs in the absence of documented gallstones.

SYMPTOMS

- Acute onset of colicky severe right upper quadrant or epigastric pain
- Nausea and vomiting +++
- Fever is variably present with cholecystitis and cholangitis.

SIGNS

- Right upper quadrant or epigastric tenderness ++++
- Localized peritonitis
- Murphy's sign (arrest of respiration with palpation of the right upper quadrant)
- Low-grade fever and tachycardia are variably present in cholecystitis.

WORKUP

- Ultrasound is sensitive in identifying stones and can confirm clinical suspicion of cholecystitis ++++. It may demonstrate cholelithiasis, dilated gallbladder, thickened wall, pericholecystic fluid, or sonographic Murphy's sign. It has limited sensitivity for acute ductal dilatation +++ associated with obstruction.
- Radionuclide cholescintigraphy (HIDA scan) has sensitivity similar to or better than that of ultrasound for cholecystitis ++++ but is more specific. It is more sensitive for detecting obstruction. False positive results are seen in severely ill patients.
- Hepatic aminotransferase, alkaline phosphatase, bilirubin, and amylase levels may be elevated.
- CT is limited in detecting gallstones but is useful in visualizing pericholecystic changes, a thickened gallbladder wall, and distention of the gallbladder.

COMMENTS AND TREATMENT CONSIDERATIONS

Radionuclide cholescintigraphy is the most sensitive and specific test to rule out cholecystitis and common bile duct obstruction. Ultrasound is quicker and noninvasive, is generally more readily available, can be done at the bedside, and offers more anatomic detail of the hepatic ducts and pancreas. Radionuclide cholescintigraphy is occasionally required when concern remains for cholecystitis or obstruction and ultrasound studies are negative. Treatment should include IV fluids, antibiotics, and surgical consultation.

REFERENCES

Babb R: Acute acalculous cholecystitis, *J Clin Gastroenterol* 15:238, 1992.

Bennett GL, Balthazar EJ: Ultrasound and CT evaluation of emergent gallbladder pathology, *Radiol Clin North Am* 41:1203, 2003.

Davis L, McCarroll K: Correlative imaging of the liver and hepatobiliary system, *Semin Nucl Med* 3:208, 1994.

Hendrickson M, Naparst TR: Abdominal surgical emergencies in the elderly, *Emerg Med Clin North Am* 21:937, 2003.

Trowbridge RL, Rutkowski NK, Shojania KG: Does this patient have acute cholecystitis? *JAMA* 289:80, 2003.

Zeisman H: Acute cholecystitis, biliary obstruction and biliary leakage, *Semin Nucl Med* 33:279, 2003.

 ACUTE APPENDICITIS

The most important factors in diagnosing appendicitis are the history and physical examination. Because patients come to the ED at various times in the course of the disease and may have atypical symptoms, a period of observation and reexamination may be necessary.

SYMPTOMS
- Abdominal pain that begins periumbilically or diffusely and localizes to the right lower quadrant over the next 12 to 48 hours ++++
- Anorexia ++++
- Nausea and vomiting +++
- Diarrhea ++

SIGNS
- Abdominal tenderness +++++
- Fever +++
- Rebound tenderness +++
- Rovsing sign (peritoneal irritation producing right lower quadrant pain with palpation of the left lower quadrant)
- Psoas sign (pain with active flexion against resistance or passive extension of the right hip) ++
- Obturator sign (pain with passive internal rotation of the flexed right hip) ++
- Voluntary or involuntary guarding
- Cervical motion tenderness ++

WORKUP
- Appendicitis is a clinical diagnosis.
- Although the sensitivity of an elevated WBC count is reasonably high ++++, the specificity (40% to 75%) is inadequate for the test to have much clinical usefulness, and there is poor correlation with the severity of the illness.
- Analysis of C-reactive protein, erythrocyte sedimentation rate (ESR), WBC differential, and abdominal x-rays has unproven value.
- CT scan with contrast ++++; specificity, 92% to 98%. CT use has led to a decreased negative appendicitis rate at surgery from around 15% to 4%.
- Abdominal ultrasound; accuracy varies widely according to experience.
- CT and ultrasound may be helpful in diagnosing other causes of abdominal pain when the diagnosis of acute appendicitis is in doubt.

COMMENTS AND TREATMENT CONSIDERATIONS

Elderly patients and children are more likely to have atypical presentations and are more likely to have appendiceal perforation at the time of presentation to the ED.

REFERENCES

Coleman C, Thompson JE Jr, Bennion RS, et al: White blood cell count is a poor predictor of severity of disease in the diagnosis of appendicitis, *Am Surg* 64:983, 1998.

Hershko DD, Sroka G, Bahouth H, et al: The role of selective computed tomography in the diagnosis and management of suspected acute appendicitis, *Am Surg* 68:1003, 2002.

Izbicki JR, Knoefel WT, Wilker DK, et al: Accurate diagnosis of acute appendicitis: a retrospective analysis of 686 patients, *Eur J Surg* 158:227, 1992.

Kamel IR: Right lower quadrant pain and suspected appendicitis: non-focal appendiceal review of 100 cases, *Radiology* 217:159, 2000.

Kraemer M, Franke C, Ohman C, et al: Acute appendicitis in late adulthood: incidence, presentation, and outcome. Review of a prospective multicenter acute abdominal pain study and a review of the literature, *Arch Surg* 385:470, 2000.

Morris KT, Kavanagh M, Hansen P, et al: The rational use of computed tomography scans in the diagnosis of appendicitis, *Am J Surg* 183:547, 2002.

Reynolds SL: Missed appendicitis in a pediatric emergency department, *Pediatr Emerg Care* 9:1, 1993.

Snyder B, Hayden SR: Accuracy of leukocyte count in the diagnosis of acute appendicitis, *Ann Emerg Med* 32:565, 1999.

 COLONIC DIVERTICULITIS

Diverticulitis is generally a disease of older adults caused by diminished elasticity of the colon. The incidence of diverticula is approximately 50% in those 70 years and older and increases to 80% in those older than 80. Approximately 25% have an episode of acute diverticulitis. Most commonly it affects the sigmoid colon (70%), but cecal diverticulitis is also well documented (30%). A low-fiber diet, lack of activity, and increasing age have all been identified as risk factors.

SYMPTOMS

- Abdominal pain, usually in the left lower quadrant ++++
- Nausea and vomiting
- Constipation
- Diarrhea

SIGNS

- Left lower and less commonly right lower quadrant tenderness ++++
- Guarding or rebound tenderness
- Fever may be present.
- Generalized peritonitis and signs of sepsis (high fever, tachycardia, hypotension) if colonic perforation occurs
- Stools occult blood positive ++

WORKUP

- Diverticulitis is primarily a clinical diagnosis.
- A CT scan with intravenous and oral contrast can demonstrate pericolic inflammation, abscess (both at the site of perforation and at distant sites in the abdomen), and involvement of other organs.
- WBC is of limited value +++.
- Abdominal x-rays may be useful for ruling out free air or bowel obstruction but otherwise provide little diagnostic information and are generally not indicated.

COMMENTS AND TREATMENT CONSIDERATIONS

Treatment involves oral antibiotics and close outpatient follow-up for stable patients and IV antibiotics and admission for those who have severe pain or cannot tolerate oral intake. Emergent surgical consult is necessary for anyone with signs of perforation or peritonitis. Elective resection of the segment of the colon with diverticula may be required when infection has been treated, particularly with recurrent episodes.

REFERENCES

Buckley O, Geoghegan T, O'Riordain DS, et al: Computed tomography in the imaging of colonic diverticulitis, *Clin Radiol* 59:977, 2004.

Farrell RJ, Farrell JJ, Morrin MM: Diverticular disease in the elderly, *Gastroenterol Clin North Am* 30:475, 2001.

Keidar S, Pappo I, Shperber Y, et al: Cecal diverticulitis: a diagnostic challenge, *Dig Surg* 17:508, 2000.

Marinella MA, Mustafa M: Acute diverticulitis in patients 40 years of age and younger, *Am J Emerg Med* 18:140, 2000.

ACUTE PANCREATITIS

Pancreatitis can be acute or chronic. Diagnosis is generally clinical and can be confirmed by ancillary testing. The most common causes of acute pancreatitis are biliary obstruction and toxins (alcohol and medications), which account for 70% to 80% of all cases. Approximately 10% to 20% of cases are idiopathic.

CHAPTER 1

SYMPTOMS
- Epigastric or left upper quadrant pain ++++
- Back pain ++

SIGNS
- Abdominal tenderness ++++
- Vomiting ++++
- Abdominal distention
- Guarding
- Dehydration (as a result of third spacing and occasionally hemorrhage in severe pancreatitis)

WORKUP
- Amylase ++++; specificity, 70% to 95%
- Lipase ++++; specificity, 87% to 99%
- CT scan (contrast enhanced) ++++; specificity, near 100%; CT is generally not required in the ED.
- Ultrasound is useful for viewing the biliary tract but is unable to visualize the pancreas because of overlying bowel gas in 25% to 40%.
- Plain x-ray films (abdominal series) may be useful to check for free air (perforated viscus) if the diagnosis is in doubt.

COMMENTS AND TREATMENT CONSIDERATIONS
Severe pancreatitis is life threatening (5% mortality) and can lead to many complications, including hemorrhage, hypocalcemia, coagulation abnormalities, hypoxia, adult respiratory distress syndrome (ARDS), cardiovascular decompensation, and renal failure. Generally, patients with acute pancreatitis must be admitted for IV hydration, analgesia, and observation. Consider IV antibiotics in severe pancreatitis or septic-appearing patients.

REFERENCES
Bohidar NP, Garg PK, Khanna S, Tandon RK: Incidence, etiology, and impact of fever in patients with acute pancreatitis, *Pancreatology* 3:9, 2003.

Calleja GA, Barkin JS: Acute pancreatitis, *Med Clin North Am* 77: 1037, 1993.

Frank B, Gottleib K: Amylase normal, lipase elevated: is it pancreatitis? A case series and review of the literature, *Am J Gastroenterol* 94:463, 1999.

Gumaste V, Dave P, Sereny G: Serum lipase: a better test to diagnose acute alcoholic pancreatitis, *Am J Med* 92:239, 1992.

Jacobs JE, Birnbaum BA: Computed tomography evaluation of acute pancreatitis, *Semin Roentgenol* 36:92, 2001.

Newton E, Mandavia S: Surgical complications of selected gastrointestinal emergencies: pitfalls in management of the acute abdomen, *Emerg Med Clin North Am* 21:873, 2003.

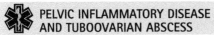

PELVIC INFLAMMATORY DISEASE AND TUBOOVARIAN ABSCESS

Risk factors for pelvic inflammatory disease (PID) and tuboovarian abscess (TOA) include younger age, multiple sex partners, history of PID or sexually transmitted disease (STD), nonuse of contraceptives, recent (within 3 months) insertion of an intrauterine device (IUD), and douching. TOA can be a complication of PID, occurring in up to 30% of the patients hospitalized with PID.

SYMPTOMS
- Lower abdominal or pelvic pain for more than 48 hours that is dull, constant, and poorly localized +++++
- Vaginal discharge ++++
- Abnormal vaginal bleeding ++
- Urinary symptoms ++
- Dyspareunia

SIGNS
- Lower abdominal tenderness ++++
- Adnexal mass or tenderness ++++
- Cervical motion tenderness
- Mucopurulent endocervical discharge
- Fever
- Endocervix that is erythematous, edematous, or friable in association with temperature of >38°C +++

WORKUP
- Pregnancy test
- Cervical cultures for gonorrhea and *Chlamydia*
- Wet mount for clue cells (bacterial vaginosis) and *Trichomonas*
- Pelvic ultrasound to rule out tuboovarian abscess in select cases
- Consider syphilis and human immunodeficiency virus (HIV) testing
- Laparoscopy may occasionally be required when the diagnosis is in doubt or when other conditions (such as appendicitis) remain in the differential diagnosis after clinical and radiologic evaluation.

COMMENTS AND TREATMENT CONSIDERATIONS
There is no good diagnostic test. Because of the potential complications of untreated PID, the empirical use of antibiotics is common after a presumptive diagnosis is made on clinical examination. The patient should be hospitalized for IV antibiotics and

CHAPTER 1

19

observation if she appears ill (peritonitis), if she is pregnant, if the diagnosis is unclear (possible appendicitis or other gastrointestinal pathologic condition), if she is unable to tolerate oral antibiotics, or if there is failure of outpatient therapy. Current U.S. Centers for Disease Control and Prevention outpatient recommendations include ofloxacin or levofloxacin for *Chlamydia* and gonorrhea plus metronidazole for coverage of anaerobes. An alternative is intramuscular (IM) ceftriaxone plus oral doxycycline, with or without metronidazole.

REFERENCES

Beigi RH, Wiesenfeld HC: Pelvic inflammatory disease: new diagnostic criteria and treatment, *Obstet Gynecol Clin North Am* 30:777, 2003.

Gaitan H, Angel E, Diaz R, et al: Accuracy of five different diagnostic techniques in mild-to-moderate pelvic inflammatory disease, *Infect Dis Obstet Gynecol* 10:171, 2002.

Marks C, Tideman RL, Estcourt CS, et al: Diagnosing PID—getting the balance right, *Int J STD AIDS* 11:545, 2000.

Newkirk G: Pelvic inflammatory disease: a contemporary approach, *Am Fam Physician* 53:112, 1996.

Simms I, Warburton F, Westrom L: Diagnosis of pelvic inflammatory disease: time for a rethink, *Sex Transm Infect* 79:491, 2003.

Varras M, Polyzos D, Perouli E, et al: Tubo-ovarian abscesses: spectrum of sonographic findings with surgical and pathological correlations, *Clin Exp Obstet Gynecol* 30:117, 2002.

Zeger W, Holt K: Gynecologic infections, *Emerg Med Clin North Am* 21:631, 2003.

 SPLENIC SEQUESTRATION IN SICKLE CELL PATIENTS

In patients with hemoglobin SS genotype, acute splenic sequestration crisis (ASSC) is a pediatric disease (6 months to 3 years) because the patients usually become functionally asplenic by adulthood from repeated infarctions. Occasionally one can see ASSC in an adult, but it usually involves hemoglobin SC genotype or hemoglobin S–thalassemia genotype. Sequestration crisis can also be brought about by high altitude and low ambient oxygen tension.

SYMPTOMS

- Abdominal pain
- Acute weakness
- Syncope
- Thirst

SIGNS
- Abdominal fullness or tenderness in the left upper quadrant
- Splenomegaly
- Pallor
- Tachycardia
- Hypotension

WORKUP
- Hemoglobin: rapid fall of >2 g/dl despite an elevated reticulocyte count
- Platelets: mild to moderate thrombocytopenia

COMMENTS AND TREATMENT CONSIDERATIONS
Sequestration crisis may lead to hemodynamic instability and hypotension because of a severe decrease in circulating blood volume. Sequestration may resemble sepsis, and patients may receive antibiotics while cultures are pending, but these patients are not infected. Treatment includes blood transfusions and supportive care (IV fluids, oxygen, and pain medication). Hospital admission is required.

REFERENCES
Franklin QJ: Splenic syndrome in sickle cell trait: four case presentations and a review of the literature, *Mil Med* 164:230, 1999.

Pollack C: Emergencies in sickle cell disease, *Emerg Med Clin North Am* 11:365, 1993.

Sheth S, Ruzal-Shapiro C, Piomelli S, et al: CT imaging of splenic sequestration in sickle cell disease, *Pediatr Radiol* 30:830, 2000.

Wang-Gillam A, Lee R, Hsi E, et al: Acute splenic sequestration crisis resembling sepsis in an adult with hemoglobin SC disease, *South Med J* 97:413, 2004.

CHAPTER 1

 DIABETIC KETOACIDOSIS

See Chapter 27, Mental Status Change and Coma.

Abdominal pain can be a symptom of a precipitant of diabetic ketoacidosis (DKA) or a symptom of DKA itself. Abdominal processes should be considered and thoroughly ruled out.

 VIRAL HEPATITIS

See Chapter 23, Jaundice.

BLACK WIDOW (LATRODECTUS) SPIDER ENVENOMATION

Muscle pain and fasciculations can result from excessive stimulation of the motor end plates by the envenomated neurotoxin. Muscle spasms may involve the abdomen (latrodectism) and can lead to the erroneous diagnosis of an acute surgical condition.

SYMPTOMS
- Severe muscle pain and muscle spasms of the involved area, which may progress to the abdomen, back, and other areas
- Pain usually begins within 30 minutes to 2 hours at the site of the bite and is followed by painful regional and abdominal muscle cramping in 3 to 4 hours, peaking at 8 to 12 hours, and enduring as long as several days.
- Associated symptoms include headache, nausea/emesis, and dyspnea.

SIGNS
- Muscle fasciculations
- Abdominal rigidity
- Diaphoresis
- Hypertension
- Bite site characterized by paired punctures (··)

WORKUP
- A history of likely exposure (working in a cool, dark place or on a construction site or in a wood pile)
- The physical examination may uncover the spider bite.
- Hemolysis and rhabdomyolysis (uncommon) may be tracked with serial complete blood counts and myoglobins.

COMMENTS AND TREATMENT CONSIDERATIONS
Treatment consists of benzodiazepines and analgesia. Administration of 10% calcium gluconate (adults, 10 to 20 ml; children, 0.2 to 0.3 ml/kg) for pain is controversial; it may provide transient relief and can be repeated as necessary. Antivenom, if used, should be preceded by a test dose for allergy; as there have been no recorded U.S. deaths from arachnid envenomations since 1968, the risks of antivenom use may outweigh the benefit.

REFERENCES
Frundle TC: Management of spider bites, *Air Med J* 23:24, 2004.
Jelinek GA: Widow spider envenomation (latrodectism): a worldwide problem, *Wilderness Environ Med* 8:226, 1997.

Pearigen PD: Unusual causes of abdominal pain, *Emerg Clin North Am* 14:593, 1996.

Saucier JR: Arachnid envenomation, *Emerg Med Clin North Am* 22:405, 2004.

GENERAL REFERENCES

D'Agostino J: Common abdominal emergencies in children, *Emerg Med Clin North Am* 20:139, 2002.

Hendrickson M, Naparst TR: Abdominal surgical emergencies in the elderly, *Emerg Med Clin North Am* 21:937, 2003.

McCollough M, Sharieff GQ: Abdominal surgical emergencies in infants and young children, *Emerg Clin North Am* 21:909, 2003.

CHAPTER 1

Agitation and Psychosis
Eric Legome and Benjamin T. Milligan

Agitated or violent behavior can be caused by a medical disorder ("organic"), a psychiatric disorder ("functional"), or both. Although the distinction between organic and functional is somewhat artificial, it provides a useful model for evaluating an agitated patient. The differential diagnosis of each includes emergent conditions that may require different treatment strategies. Many medical illnesses have the capability to alter CNS functioning and produce delusions, dementia, delirium, and other disordered thinking. Psychosis is a psychiatric disorder characterized by a gross distortion or disorganization of a person's mental capacity, affective response, and capacity to recognize reality, communicate, and relate to others in a way that meets the demands of everyday life. New "psychiatric" patients may have an unrecognized medical illness that caused or exacerbated their psychiatric symptoms. Furthermore, patients with psychiatric diseases manifesting as psychosis have a higher incidence of medical illness and die of medical diseases at a rate higher than that of the general population.

The goal in the ED is to conduct a brief but thorough examination to exclude the most common and dangerous physical disorders mimicking psychiatric illness and to control dangerous behaviors.

Although by no means definite, certain physical and historical factors favor an organic rather than a functional etiology. Aspects that suggest an organic etiology include autonomic disturbances, including severe hypertension or hypotension, hyperthermia, tachypnea, and tachycardia. Other findings may include abnormal vital signs, diaphoresis, pupillary abnormalities, gait disturbances or focal neurologic deficits, weight loss, systemic signs and symptoms, and incontinence. A patient with a fluctuating level of consciousness or a disturbance of attention, orientation, and recent memory is also more likely to have an organic etiology. Nonauditory hallucinations and delusions (e.g., visual, olfactory, tactile) are specific but insensitive for organic disease. Auditory hallucinations that are egosyntonic (patient is concerned about the content of the voices but not that they are occurring) are classically described for schizophrenia and other psychiatric disorders.

A careful history for previous diseases including HIV, SLE, or other inflammatory conditions, endocrinologic disorders, and cancer is essential to the evaluation. A history of drug dependence, intravenous drug abuse, or detoxification is frequently comorbid with a functional cause of agitation or psychosis, and it is often impossible to establish a firm diagnosis for chronic abusers. A full accounting of any medications or herbal supplements must be sought, with concentration on new medication, change in dosage of existing medications, or drug interactions.

Other crucial information to obtain during the evaluation is the patient's age, family history, premorbid function, and the time course of the illness. Patients who are older than 40 years and have no previous psychiatric history, productive premorbid function, and an acute onset of symptoms most likely have an organic cause of their illness. Conversely, a slowly progressive decline in a younger patient or a patient with a family history of schizophrenia is more likely to have a functional cause.

Treatment for agitated psychosis usually includes a neuroleptic, benzodiazepine, or both while addressing any organic cause that is identified. The goal is to provide for the safety of patient and staff while alleviating the patient's distress and agitation to allow an appropriate evaluation. Haloperidol (adults: 2.0 to 5.0 mg IV/IM, may repeat) and lorazepam (adults: 1 to 2 mg IV/IM, may repeat; watch for respiratory depression) are among the many medication alternatives. When using neuroleptics without benzodiazepines, one should consider concomitant use of benztropine or diphenhydramine to reduce the risk of acute dystonia and akathisia.

LEGAL ISSUES

Although laws differ between states, some general principles govern treatment of psychotic patients and their ability to participate in or refuse medical care. In general, for medical therapy to be delivered against their will, psychotic patients must have a profound lack of insight and understanding of their illness, be considered a danger to themselves or others, or be gravely disabled.

 SELECTED ORGANIC CAUSES

This chapter addresses common psychiatric causes of psychoses. Medical conditions are addressed in other chapters. The box on pp. 26 and 27 lists selected organic causes to consider when evaluating psychotic patients.

SELECTED ORGANIC CAUSES OF PSYCHOSES

Drug Intoxications
Alcohol
Cocaine
Designer drugs
LSD
Opiates
PCP

Drug Withdrawal
Alcohol
Benzodiazepines
GHB
Tricyclic antidepressants

Medications (Increased in Elderly)
Antiarrhythmics
Antibiotics
Anticholinergics
Antiparkinsonians
Cimetidine
Insulin and hypoglycemics
Isoniazid
Levetiracetam
Neuroleptics (neuroleptic malignant syndrome)
Serotonin reuptake inhibitors (serotonin syndrome)
Steroids
Sympathomimetics

Infections
Encephalitis
HIV
Meningitis
Neurosyphilis
Sepsis

Seizures
Postictal states
Temporal lobe

Neoplasm
Hemispheric
Posterior fossa
Temporal lobe

Cerebrovascular Disease
CNS vasculitis
Intracranial hemorrhage
Multiple sclerosis
SLE
Stroke
TTP

Continued

SELECTED ORGANIC CAUSES OF PSYCHOSES—CONT'D

CNS (Other)
Dementia
Jakob-Creutzfeldt disease
Parkinson's disease
Pick's disease
Pseudobulbar palsy
Wilson's disease

Endocrine
Addison's disease (adrenal insufficiency)
Carcinoid
Cushing's disease (adrenal excess)
Hyperparathyroidism
Hyperthyroidism, hypothyroidism
Pheochromocytoma

Other
Acute intermittent porphyria
Nutritional disorders
Obstructive sleep apnea

Entries in *italics* are the most common causes.

REFERENCES

Allen, MH: Managing the agitated psychotic patient: a reappraisal of the evidence, *J Clin Psychiatry* 61S14:11, 2000.

Anderson WH, Kuehnle JC: Diagnoses and early management of acute psychosis, *N Engl J Med* 305:1128, 1981.

Battaglia J, Moss S, Rush J, et al: Haloperidol, lorazepam, or both for psychotic agitation? A multicenter, prospective, double-blind, emergency department study, *Am J Emerg Med* 15:335, 1997.

Biddinger PD, Isselbacher EM, Fan D, Shepard JA: Case records of the Massachusetts General Hospital. Weekly clinicopathological exercises. Case 5-2005. A 53-year-old man with depression and sudden shortness of breath, *N Engl J Med* 352:709, 2005.

Drugs that may cause psychiatric symptoms, *Med Lett Drugs Ther* 44:59, 2002.

Dubin WR, Weese KJ, Zeezardia JA: Organic brain syndrome, the quiet impostor, *JAMA* 249:60, 1983.

Ellison JM, Jacobs D: Emergency psychopharmacology: a review and update, *Ann Emerg Med* 15:962, 1986.

Frame DS, Kercher E: Acute psychosis: functional versus organic, *Emerg Med Clin North Am* 9:123, 1992.

Hall RCW, Gardner ER, Popkin MK, et al: Unrecognized physical illness prompting psychiatric admission: a prospective study, *Am J Psychiatry* 138:629, 1981.

Lipowski ZL: Delirium (acute confusional state), *JAMA* 258:1789, 1997.

Pine DS, Douglas CJ, Charles E, et al: Patients with multiple sclerosis presenting to psychiatric hospitals, *J Clin Psychiatry* 56:297, 1995.

Rosenthal RN, Miner CR: Differential diagnosis of substance-induced psychosis and schizophrenia in patients with substance abuse disorders, *Schizophr Bull* 23:187, 1997.

Sorrentino A: Chemical restraints for the agitated, violent, or psychotic pediatric patient in the emergency department: controversy and recommendations, *Curr Opin Pediatr* 16:201, 2004.

 PSYCHIATRIC CAUSES

As listed subsequently, psychiatric diagnoses in general are defined by criteria published in DSM-IV, the manual of psychiatric disorders. These diagnoses are based on consensus among leaders in the field. Limited information is available in the medical and psychiatric literature suggesting the prevalence of particular signs and symptoms of the diagnoses.

Schizophrenia

Schizophrenia is a common and heterogeneous disorder that currently has no known cure. There is often a combination of positive symptoms, which are the production of abnormal actions and thoughts, and negative symptoms, which are the absence of usual occurring interests, thoughts, gestures, and actions. According to the DSM-IV, six major criteria must be present to establish the diagnosis, including the provision that symptoms must be present for at least 6 months. The prevalence of schizophrenia in the general population is approximately 1.0 %.

Schizophrenia has five subtypes—paranoid, disorganized, catatonic, undifferentiated, and residual—that are defined by the prominent symptomatology and signs at the time of evaluation. Prodromal symptoms of depression, perplexity, and fear are often present before onset. As the diagnosis is partially dependent on a time course of symptoms, it is not unusual (>70%) to fail to achieve a definitive diagnosis on initial presentation.

To establish the diagnosis, the patient must fit six DSM-IV diagnostic criteria. (DSM criteria are noted in the following in italics, *A* to *F*.)

SYMPTOMS

Characteristic, or type *A*, symptoms define the illness. Two or more of the following need be present for 1 month (or less if treated):

• Delusions
• Hallucinations

- Disorganized speech
- Grossly disorganized or catatonic behavior
- Negative symptoms: (e.g., anhedonia, avolition)

One or more major areas of functioning including work, relationships, or self-care are significantly diminished *(B)*, with continuity for at least 6 months of this worsening *(C)*.

Other mood or schizoaffective disorders are not concurrently diagnosed *(D)*, and a substance abuse or medical condition is not the direct cause *(E)*.

If the patient has an underlying developmental disorder, there must be a development of prominent hallucinations or delusions *(F)*.

SIGNS
- Positive signs: disorganized speech, disorganized or catatonic behavior, excessive motor activity that is apparently purposeless, echolalia or echopraxia
- Negative signs: flat affect, motor immobility, mutism, and maintenance of a rigid posture

WORKUP
- History is the most important clue toward establishing the diagnosis.
- Detailed neurologic examination
- Serum glucose, if indicated
- Oxygen saturation, if indicated
- Evaluation for possible medical etiologies as indicated
- CT, if evidence of focal neurologic process, advanced age, or other suggestion of organic cause
- Lumbar puncture, if fever or evidence of meningeal irritation
- ESR, if concern about collagen vascular or rheumatologic disorder
- EEG, if consideration of underlying ongoing seizure or prolonged postictal state
- MRI, if consideration of demyelinating disease

COMMENTS AND TREATMENT CONSIDERATIONS
Acute psychosis secondary to schizophrenia requires ED psychiatric consultation and generally hospital admission.

REFERENCES
American Psychiatric Association: *Diagnostic and statistical manual of mental disorders*, 4th ed. (DSM-IV), Washington, DC, 1994, The Association.

Schizophreniform Disorder
Schizophreniform disorder is diagnosed using criteria similar to those for schizophrenia, where the episode lasts between 1 and 6 months.

CHAPTER 2

Schizoaffective Disorder

Schizoaffective disorder is defined by DSM-IV as an uninterrupted period of illness during which a major depressive episode, a manic episode, or mixed manic-depressive episode coexists with type A symptoms of schizophrenia.

Brief Psychotic Disorder

A brief psychotic disorder is a time-limited disorder that may occur in response to a significant life stressor (e.g., death in family), may be seen postpartum, or may occur without a stressor. The duration is at least 1 day with a maximum duration of 1 month. The patient eventually returns to his or her previous level of functioning.

Shared Psychotic Disorder

Shared psychotic disorder is a delusional development that exists in a patient with a close relationship to another individual with similar symptoms. Symptoms and signs are similar to those of schizophrenia.

Psychotic Disorder—Not Otherwise Specified

Because of the nature of emergency medicine, the time course of the patient's illness often cannot be followed. This category takes into account the lack of available information to make a specific diagnosis. The diagnosis applies to psychotic patients whose problems cannot be clearly defined as organic or functional. A definitive diagnosis of psychiatric disease is not made until medical conditions have been fully considered.

Major Depression with Psychotic Symptoms

The patient must meet criteria for a major depressive episode and have the following diagnostic symptoms:
- *Mood-congruent psychotic features*—delusions or hallucinations that are consistent with the depressive's ideation (e.g., death, deserved punishment, nihilism)
- *Mood-incongruent psychotic features*—delusions or hallucinations whose themes may not involve typical depressive ideation, including such themes as persecution and thought broadcasting

Anxiety Disorder

Patients with anxiety disorder manifest excessive anxiety and worry about a number of events and activities for at least 6 months. They find it difficult to control, and the anxiety is associated with at least three symptoms (see the following symptoms). The diagnosis may be modified if combined with specific concerns (e.g., social phobias, separation anxiety, and somatization disorder).

Acutely, patients may have panic attacks notable for somatic complaints and signs of adrenergic hyperactivity.

SYMPTOMS
- Restlessness
- Fatigability
- Difficulty with concentration
- Irritability
- Muscle tension
- Sleep disturbance
- Somatic medical complaints

SIGNS
- Tachycardia
- Hypertension
- Diaphoresis (It is imperative to rule out concomitant medical illness that can also cause autonomic changes.)

COMMENTS AND TREATMENT CONSIDERATIONS
Patients with an anxiety disorder or panic attack may have acute chest pain or other somatic complaints that are difficult to distinguish from organic disease in the ED. In general, an organic cause is presumed with appropriate evaluation for possible psychiatric etiology. Treatment of anxiety may be indicated whether the symptom is caused by a medical or psychiatric condition.

REFERENCES
American Psychiatric Association: *Diagnostic and statistical manual of mental disorders*, 4th ed. (DSM-IV), Washington, DC, 1994, The Association.

CHAPTER 2

The Alcoholic Patient

Daniel Grossman

Alcohol-intoxicated patients frequently receive treatment in the (emergency department) ED. Although they generally need only a period of observation until reaching clinical sobriety, alcohol-intoxicated patients, and in particular recurrently intoxicated (alcoholic) patients, are at risk for occult trauma, infection, coingestion, suicide attempts, and other pathologic conditions that may be mistakenly attributed to alcohol intoxication. Unfortunately, the history and physical examination often yields limited information in alcoholic patients; a high index of suspicion and appropriate diagnostic testing are necessary. Determination of alcohol level is generally unnecessary unless coingestion is a possibility or if needed to verify significant ethanol ingestion. Administration of thiamine (100 mg IV) and a bedside blood glucose check should be considered for all patients with alteration in mental status (see Chapter 27, Mental Status Change and Coma).

 ## INTRACRANIAL HEMORRHAGE

Head trauma and coagulopathy are common among alcoholic patients. Between 8% and 18% of alcohol-intoxicated ED patients who have what appears to be minor head injuries show positive computed tomography (CT) scans, and up to 5% need a craniotomy. Alcohol plays a role in many head injuries and often contributes to unfavorable outcomes. Some patients who appear to have alcohol withdrawal seizures actually have structural lesions demonstrated on CT scans.

Patient management generally consists of serial neurologic examinations to determine the mental status of the patient. A neurologic examination must be normal before patients can be discharged. CT scanning of the head is indicated in the following situations: when the patient has a focal neurologic examination or evidence of head trauma; when alcohol does not explain initial findings; or when the patient's mental status does not improve during ED observation.

See Chapter 18, Headache.

REFERENCES

Brickley MR, Shepherd JP: The relationship between alcohol intoxication, injury severity, and Glasgow coma score in assault patients, *Injury* 26:311, 1995.

Cook LS, Levitt MA, Simon B, Williams VL: Identification of ethanol-intoxicated patients with minor head trauma requiring computed tomography scans, *Acad Emerg Med* 1:227, 1994.

Koivumaa-Honkanen H, Honkanen R, Viinamaki H, et al: Life satisfaction and suicide: a 20-year follow-up study, *Am J Psychiatry* 158:433, 2001.

Reeves RR, Pendarvis EJ, Kimble R: Unrecognized medical emergencies admitted to psychiatric units, *Am J Emerg Med* 18:390, 2000.

 COINTOXICATION WITH ETHYLENE GLYCOL, METHANOL, AND ISOPROPYL ALCOHOL

Diagnosing an ingestion of nonethanol alcohols without a reliable history can be difficult. Although rare, ingestion of nonethanol alcohols is potentially lethal and should always be considered. The patient may appear intoxicated but not have an odor of ethanol on the breath. Classically, patients ingesting methanol or ethylene glycol appear ill, have an osmolal gap and an anion gap metabolic acidosis. Isopropyl alcohol can cause hypoglycemia and ketosis without acidosis.

See Chapter 37, Toxic Exposure, Approach to.

 INFECTION

Alcoholics can occasionally have elevated temperatures for reasons unrelated to an acute infection (e.g., delirium tremens). However, when fever is present, a source of infection must be sought and admission should be considered. In one study, 58% of alcoholics had an infectious cause of fever. Alcoholics are susceptible to pneumonia, meningitis, tuberculosis, spontaneous bacterial peritonitis (if cirrhosis and ascites are present), spontaneous bacteremia, endocarditis, and salmonellosis.

REFERENCES

Adams HG, Jordan C: Infections in the alcoholic, *Med Clin North Am* 68:179, 1984.

MacGregor RR, Louria DB: Alcohol and infection, *Curr Clin Top Infect Dis* 17:291, 1997.

Wrenn KD, Larson S: The febrile alcoholic in the emergency department, *Am J Emerg Med* 9:57, 1991.

 GASTROINTESTINAL BLEEDING

Gastrointestinal bleeding (GIB) can be occult or acutely life threatening. Coagulopathy is common among chronic alcoholics as a result of thrombocytopenia and decreased production of clotting factors by the liver. Furthermore, if the liver is cirrhotic, esophageal and gastric varices are often present and may rupture.

See Chapter 6, Bleeding.

 ALCOHOLIC KETOACIDOSIS

Alcoholic ketoacidosis (AKA) occurs after the cessation of a drinking binge by a malnourished, chronic alcoholic resulting in an elevated anion gap acidosis. The diagnosis of AKA is established by the findings of an elevated anion gap acidosis with concurrent ketosis in the absence of a history of diabetes mellitus and with a normal or near-normal serum glucose. Comorbidities such as alcoholic pancreatitis, liver disease, and gastritis that share symptoms and signs with AKA should also be considered.

SYMPTOMS
- Anorexia
- Nausea
- Vomiting
- Abdominal pain
- Orthostatic dizziness

SIGNS
- Odor of ketones on the breath
- Tachycardia
- Orthostatic hypotension
- Tachypnea, particularly with Kussmaul respirations
- Diaphoresis
- The abdomen usually reveals only mild to moderate diffuse tenderness. Marked distention, the absence of bowel sounds, or the presence of peritoneal signs should raise concern for other concomitant intraabdominal pathologic conditions.
- Abnormalities in orientation or level of consciousness ++ (may also indicate other pathologic conditions)

WORKUP

- Glucose (may be normal, low, or mildly elevated +)
- Electrolytes, magnesium, blood urea nitrogen (BUN), creatinine
- Serum ketones
- Artierial blood gas (ABG): generally not necessary. Mixed acid-base disorders are very common, as are electrolyte disorders including hypokalemia, hypomagnesemia, hyponatremia, and hypocalcemia.

COMMENTS AND TREATMENT CONSIDERATIONS

Volume repletion with glucose administration (after thiamine 100 mg IV) and electrolyte repletion (K, Mg) are generally curative. Bicarbonate administration is unnecessary. Comorbidities must be treated. If diagnosed and treated appropriately, AKA is associated with low mortality.

REFERENCES

Braden GL, Strayhorn CH, Germain MJ, et al: Increased osmolal gap in alcoholic acidosis, *Arch Intern Med* 153:2377, 1993.

Hojer J: Severe metabolic acidosis in the alcoholic: differential diagnosis and management, *Hum Exp Toxicol* 15:482, 1996.

Palmer JP: Alcoholic ketoacidosis: clinical and laboratory presentation, pathophysiology, and treatment, *J Clin Endocrinol Metab* 12:381, 1983.

Wrenn KD, Slovis CM, Minion GE, Rutowski R: The syndrome of alcoholic ketoacidosis, *Am J Med* 91:119, 1991.

CHAPTER 3

 HYPOTHERMIA

Hypothermia, defined as a core temperature less than 35° C, may occur in healthy patients after acute cold exposure, or in patients with medical or social conditions that limit adaptive mechanisms or temperature perception. Alcohol blunts temperature sensation in intoxicated patients and increases heat loss through vasodilation, thereby increasing the risk of severe hypothermia. The brain and the heart are sensitive to hypothermia, with signs and symptoms progressively becoming more severe with the severity of hypothermia. In severe hypothermia the patient may appear dead with fixed and dilated pupils and cardiac asystole. Resuscitative measures, including establishment of airway control, in addition to rapid rewarming, are necessary for severe hypothermia. Arrhythmia treatment may be ineffective until core temperature is >32° C. Evaluation and treatment for possible infection or other conditions leading to hypothermia are required.

SYMPTOMS

Vary with degree of hypothermia and underlying medical condition.
Patients may complain of

- Cold or lack awareness of being cold
- Nausea
- Dizziness
- Dyspnea
- Confusion
- Incoordination

SIGNS

Vary with degree of hypothermia and underlying medical condition

- Patient cool to touch
- Shivering (mild hypothermia)
- Apathy (mild hypothermia)
- Paradoxic undressing (mild hypothermia)
- Dysarthria
- Altered mental status (mild to moderate hypothermia)
- Decreased level of consciousness (moderate to severe hypothermia)
- Dysrhythmia (moderate to severe hypothermia)
- Hypotension (moderate to severe hypothermia)
- Respiratory depression (severe hypothermia)
- Decreased or absent bowel sounds (severe hypothermia)
- Muscle rigidity, including abdominal wall rigidity (severe hypothermia)
- Cold-induced tissue injury, including frostbite

WORKUP

- Core temperature evaluation with a rectal or urinary catheter probe because many oral and rectal thermometers do not read below 35° C
- Rapid blood glucose determination
- Thorough physical examination to exclude a primary medical or surgical condition
- Chest x-rays, urinalysis, blood and urine cultures (41% of hypothermic patients in one study were infected)
- Serum electrolytes
- Hematocrit
- CT scanning: consider in particular head CT if altered mental status
- DIC panel
- Serum creatine kinase (CK) to rule out rhabdomyolysis
- Blood alcohol level and directed toxicologic screen
- ECG may show Osborne (J) waves
- Thyroid function tests (for later confirmation of myxedema)

COMMENTS AND TREATMENT CONSIDERATIONS

Passive rewarming with blankets in a warm room is indicated for patients with mild hypothermia. Consider antibiotic treatment pending cultures in appropriate patients including those without a clear exposure history. After securing the airway and initiating advanced cardiac life support (ACLS) procedures, the treatment for severe hypothermia (T < 32.2° C, cardiovascular instability, failure to rewarm using other methods, endocrinologic dysfunction, peripheral dilation caused by trauma or toxic materials, impaired thermoregulation) is active rewarming. Controversy surrounds the effectiveness of active external rewarming methods (e.g., heat lamps, warm baths, or warm blankets). Severe hypothermia should be treated with active core rewarming methods that may include warmed humidified oxygen, warmed intravenous fluids, peritoneal or left thoracic cavity warm fluid lavage, or cardiopulmonary bypass. Patients should receive intravenous fluids during rewarming. In the setting of cardiopulmonary arrest, CPR and positive-pressure ventilation should be performed in concert with maximally aggressive rewarming. Resuscitation is rarely successful until a temperature of 28° C to 30° C is achieved, and many experts recommend withholding attempts at electrical defibrillation and use of drug therapy until the core temperature is at least 28° C.

CHAPTER 3

REFERENCES

Danzl DF, Pozos RS, Auerbach PS, et al: Multicenter hypothermia study, *Ann Emerg Med* 16:1042, 1987.

Lewin S, Brettman LR, Holzman RS, et al: Infections in hypothermic patients, *Arch Intern Med* 141:920, 1981.

McCullough L, Arora S: Diagnosis and treatment of hypothermia, *Am Fam Physician* 70:2325, 2004.

Weyman AE, Greenbaum DM, Grace WJ: Accidental hypothermia in an alcoholic population, *Am J Med* 56:13, 1974.

White JD: Hypothermia: the Bellevue experience, *Ann Emerg Med* 11:417, 1982.

 DELIRIUM TREMENS

See Chapter 27, Mental Status Change and Coma.

Back Pain, Lower
Michael Weitz and Scott W. Rodi

Lower back pain is the most common complaint in the ambulatory setting and is second only to the common cold in resultant missed days of work. The emergency physician must distinguish emergent conditions presenting as back pain (see the box on page 39) from self-limited, musculoskeletal problems. This is facilitated by the identification of "red flags" that should prompt further diagnostic workup.

Ancillary testing is of limited value in the majority of cases. In the absence of trauma, indications for plain films may include age older than 50; pain worst at rest; a history of cancer, osteoporosis, or unexplained weight loss; symptoms present longer than 6 weeks; and prolonged steroid use. In one large study, 1 in 2500 x-ray studies demonstrated a clinically unsuspected finding. A lumbar spine series delivers a gonadal dose equivalent to a daily chest x-ray for 6 years. Oblique and coned lateral views add little information and add radiation exposure.

Advanced imaging should be considered for patients with abnormal vital signs or physical examination findings that may indicate infection or vascular emergency. A history of collagen vascular disease (e.g., Marfan syndrome) predisposing to aortic abnormalities, intravenous drug abuse (IVDA), neurologic complaints, or risk factors for atherosclerosis may indicate a need for imaging studies.

Although the lifetime incidence of sciatica is 40%, only a minority of patients with acute back pain have signs and symptoms clearly caused by nerve root compression. Musculoskeletal back pain is typically self-limited, with significant resolution, regardless of therapy, in one third of patients by week 1 and two thirds by week 7. Recurrence is common, however, affecting up to 40% of patients at 6 months. Sciatica resolves by 6 weeks in more than

50% of patients. The role of surgery for back pain is controversial. The natural history of disc herniation with radiculopathy is that 90% to 95% improve with conservative treatment. A stable neurologic deficit due to nerve root compression from a herniated disc is generally *not* an indication for early surgery. An evolving motor neurologic deficit or bowel or bladder dysfunction requires urgent surgical evaluation and treatment.

REFERENCES

Agency for Health Care Policy and Research: Practice guideline: *Acute low back problems in adults—assessment and treatment*, pub no 95-0643, Dec 1994.

Carragee E, Hannibal M: Diagnostic evaluation of low back pain, *Orthop Clin North Am* 35:7, 2004.

Deyo R, Weinstein J: Low back pain, *N Engl J Med* 344:363, 2001.

Hadler NM: Regional back pain, *N Engl J Med* 315:1090, 1986.

Rodgers K, Jones J: Back pain. In Marx J, Hockberger R, Walls R (eds): *Rosen's emergency medicine concepts and clinical practice*, ed 5. St Louis, 2002, Mosby.

CHAPTER 4

"RED FLAGS" FOR POTENTIALLY SERIOUS DISEASE

Tumor or Infection
Age older than 50 or younger than 20 years
History of cancer
Constitutional symptoms such as fever, chills, or weight loss
Risk factors for spinal infection (recent UTI or pyelonephritis, IVDA, immunosuppression)
Pain that worsens when supine or severe nighttime pain

Cauda Equina Syndrome
Recent onset of bladder dysfunction (e.g., urinary retention, increased frequency, or overflow incontinence)
Bowel dysfunction may occur but usually is seen later, if at all.
Saddle anesthesia or decreased rectal tone
Severe or progressive neurologic deficit in lower extremity not clearly due to pain only

Fracture
Major trauma; minor trauma in older or osteoporotic patients

Abdominal Aortic Aneurysm or Dissection
Abdominal pain
Pulsatile abdominal mass
Atherosclerotic disease
Pulse deficits or asymmetry
Syncope

ABDOMINAL AORTIC ANEURYSM AND DISSECTION

See Chapter 1, Abdominal Pain and Chapter 7, Chest Pain.

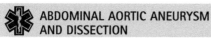 ## CAUDA EQUINA SYNDROME

Cauda equina syndrome is caused by compression of the cauda equina (the thecal sac containing the group of nerve roots remaining after termination of the spinal cord at approximately the L1-L2 level). Symptoms of cauda equina syndrome are dominated by bladder (and possibly bowel) complaints as well as motor and sensory deficits. In a patient with back or leg pain or caudal anesthesia with incontinence or urinary retention, the possibility of cauda equina syndrome should be evaluated immediately because it represents a surgical emergency regardless of etiology. Cauda equina compression is most typically the result of massive central disc herniation but can also be caused by an epidural abscess, hemorrhage, or tumor.

SYMPTOMS
- Low back pain ++++
- Urinary retention or incontinence ++++
- Sciatica may be bilateral.
- Lower extremity weakness, hyperreflexia or both
- Fecal retention or incontinence
- Saddle anesthesia

SIGNS
- Urinary retention ++++
- Decreased rectal tone or perianal sensation (anal wink)
- Motor deficit
- Sensory deficit

WORKUP
- Urinary catheter or bladder ultrasound to determine the "postvoid residual" (the volume of urine remaining in the bladder after the patient voids).
- Emergent MRI
- CT myelogram may be substituted if MRI is not available.

COMMENTS AND TREATMENT CONSIDERATIONS
Emergent assessment and treatment are necessary since the outcome is time dependent; neurosurgical or orthopedic consultation must be arranged immediately.

REFERENCES

Buchner M, Schiltenwolf M: Cauda equina syndrome caused by intervertebral lumbar disk prolapse: mid-term results of 22 patients and literature review, *Orthopedics* 25:727, 2002.

Orendacova J, Cizkova D, Kafka J, et al: Cauda equina syndrome, *Prog Neurobiol* 64:613, 2001.

 TUMOR

A tumor, most commonly a metastatic lesion of the bony spine, should be considered as a possible cause of lower back pain in patients older than 50 years and patients with a history of cancer, unexplained weight loss, or failure of conservative therapy.

SYMPTOMS

- Back pain without a significant identifiable precipitant
- Back pain not relieved with bed rest
- Constitutional symptoms
- Sensory or motor deficits that involve the spinal cord or cauda equina

SIGNS

- Spinous process tenderness
- Sensory or motor deficit if the spinal cord or cauda equina is involved

WORKUP

- Lumbosacral spine films have limited sensitivity.
- ESR sensitivity ++++, but poor specificity
- Bone scan sensitivity ++++, but nonspecific
- MRI ++++
- CT scan if MRI is not available
- CBC is neither sensitive nor specific.

COMMENTS AND TREATMENT CONSIDERATIONS

If tumor is diagnosed, prompt radiation therapy is generally required. Emergent neurosurgical or orthopedic consultation is appropriate.

REFERENCES

Deyo RA, Diehl AK: Cancer as a cause of back pain, *J Gen Intern Med* 3:230, 1988.

Liang M: Roentgenograms in primary care patients with acute low back pain: a cost-effective analysis, *Arch Intern Med* 142:1108, 1982.

CHAPTER 4

Lurie J: What diagnostic tests are useful for low back pain?
Best Pract Res Clin Rheumatol 19:4, 2005.

 SPINAL INFECTIONS

Infections involving the spine include osteomyelitis, epidural abscess, and discitis. The first two conditions can coexist because vertebral osteomyelitis is a major risk factor for the development of an epidural abscess. The incidence of spinal infections in the United States has increased since the 1980s and is greatest in people 60 to 70 years old. These conditions are more common in the setting of chronic renal failure, diabetes, alcoholism, IVDA, and immunosuppression; in patients with a history of prior spinal column abnormality, trauma, or invasive procedure; and in patients with prior urinary tract or pelvic infections. About 20% of patients with an epidural abscess may have no systemic or local predisposing factor. Osteomyelitis is often not diagnosed until 8 to 10 weeks after initial presentation, which consequently leads to significant morbidity. Discitis or disc space infection is typically diagnosed 6 months after the onset of symptoms but may be more acute following disc excision.

SYMPTOMS
- Unrelenting back pain +++++
- Fever +++ (but 50% of patients with vertebral osteomyelitis are *afebrile* at presentation)
- Patients with epidural abscess may also have radicular pain, leg weakness, sensory deficit, neck pain or stiffness, or bladder dysfunction.

SIGNS
- Midline bone and percussion tenderness +++
- Discitis manifests as well-localized midline pain featuring limited motion and exquisite discomfort produced by any jarring movement. Most patients have referred to pain of femoral or sciatic distribution.

WORKUP
- MRI is the "gold standard" +++++ and also differentiates acute transverse myelopathy from spinal cord ischemia.
- ESR is sensitive in advanced disease but is nonspecific.
- Bone scan ++++, but low specificity
- CT scan +++, but misses 50% of epidural abscesses
- CT myelogram can be performed if MRI is not available, contraindicated, or nondiagnostic.

- Lumbosacral spine films are neither sensitive nor specific for infection. Discitis may be demonstrated radiographically by disc space narrowing, sclerosis of subchondral bone, and irregularity of the bone end plates.
- Blood cultures may help to direct antibiotic therapy ++.
- WBC is neither adequately sensitive +++ nor adequately specific to be diagnostically useful.

COMMENTS AND TREATMENT CONSIDERATIONS

An epidural abscess is an orthopedic and neurosurgical emergency requiring rapid evaluation and treatment. Treatment for epidural abscess generally consists of decompressive laminectomy with abscess drainage and a prolonged course of antibiotics. Osteomyelitis is generally treated with extended administration of intravenous antibiotics. *Staphylococcus aureus* is the most common causative organism in both osteomyelitis and epidural abscess, although other agents such as *Escherichia coli*, *Pseudomonas aeruginosa*, or tuberculosis may be causative. An antibiotic course is begun in the ED after cultures are obtained and may include a penicillinase-resistant penicillin in combination with either a third-generation cephalosporin or an aminoglycoside.

Treatment of discitis ranges from conservative therapy with antibiotics and spinal immobilization to surgical débridement and decompression of the disc space.

REFERENCES

Chao D, Nanda A: Spinal epidural abscess: a diagnostic challenge, *Am Fam Physician* 65:7, 2002.

Hlavin ML, Kaminski HJ, Ross JS, Ganz E: Spinal epidural abscess: a ten-year perspective, *Neurosurgery* 27:177, 1990.

Smith AS, Blaser SI: Infectious and inflammatory processes of the spine, *Radiol Clin North Am* 29:809, 1991.

 PYELONEPHRITIS

Urinary tract infections (UTI), including both cystitis and pyelonephritis, may present with back pain. Cystitis typically causes a low lumbar or sacral aching pain, whereas the pain of pyelonephritis typically localizes to the costovertebral angle on the side of the infected kidney. Patients with cystitis usually have dysuria and the other classic symptoms of UTI.

Pyelonephritis can present without urinary symptoms, and back pain is occasionally the chief complaint. Although many risk factors for pyelonephritis are the same as those for cystitis (urinary retention, instrumentation or indwelling catheter, pregnancy, immunosuppression), additional risk factors for pyelonephritis include anatomic abnormalities of the kidney (bifid ureter, ureteral valves, renal scarring from prior infections, and renal calculi). Pyelonephritis is more common in women than men, although men are more likely to have predisposing anatomic abnormalities. Chronic prostatitis also predisposes men to cystitis and pyelonephritis.

SYMPTOMS
- Fever and chills, occasionally rigors
- Nausea or vomiting
- Flank pain
- Dysuria, frequency and urgency may be present whenever cystitis coexists with pyelonephritis.

SIGNS
- Unilateral costovertebral angle tenderness usually present
- Fever
- Malaise
- Unlike musculoskeletal back pain, the back pain of pyelonephritis does not radiate, nor is it exacerbated by movement.
- Flank tenderness to percussion should be elicited.

WORKUP
- In men, examination of the genitalia and prostate is warranted if UTI is a diagnostic concern.
- Urinalysis: pyuria, bacteriuria, and occasionally hematuria
- CBC leukocytosis with neutrophil predominance
- Blood urea nitrogen (BUN) and creatinine are useful if renal insufficiency is suspected.
- Urine cultures are indicated when urinalysis is abnormal and the clinical scenario suggests pyelonephritis.
- Blood cultures are rarely useful because urine cultures yield the causative organism.

COMMENTS AND TREATMENT CONSIDERATIONS
Gram-negative organisms, particularly *E. coli* (90%), are the predominant causative organisms. Many patients, especially otherwise healthy young women, can be treated with oral antibiotics on an outpatient basis. A fluoroquinolone is appropriate except in pregnancy and children, in which case a cephalosporin is often used. Trimethoprim-sulfamethoxazole is no longer first-line therapy in many parts of the United States because resistance continues to emerge. Patients who appear toxic, are immunocompromised, are elderly or otherwise debilitated, are unable to take oral fluids or medications, or have failed oral antibiotics require hospitalization.

Men with pyelonephritis should be strongly considered for hospitalization for parenteral antibiotic therapy. Pyelonephritis requires a more extended course of antibiotic therapy than cystitis, commonly 10 to 14 days.

REFERENCES

David R, DeBlieux PM, Press R: Rational antibiotic treatment of outpatient genitourinary infections in a changing environment, *Am J Med* 118(Suppl 7A):7S, 2005.

Liu H, Mulholland SG: Appropriate antibiotic treatment of genitourinary infections in hospitalized patients, *Am J Med* 118(Suppl 7A):14S, 2005.

 VERTEBRAL COMPRESSION FRACTURES

See Chapter 5, Back Pain, Upper.

CHAPTER 4

Back Pain, Upper
Gerianne E. Dudley and Scott Lundberg

Upper (thoracic) back pain is an unusual presenting complaint in the emergency department compared with the much more common complaints of low back pain and anterior chest pain. Musculoskeletal disease is often the underlying cause, and conservative treatment is frequently successful. However, several more serious disease processes may arise with upper back pain as a chief complaint, and consideration must be given to each of those to avoid potentially disastrous missed diagnoses. Visceral afferents from thoracic nerve roots supply sensation to internal structures such as the heart, lungs, great vessels, retroperitoneum, and abdominal organs. Therefore pain in any area supplied by those dermatomes, including the upper back, must be taken as a potential sign of derangement of one of those vital organs.

 ## AORTIC DISSECTION

See Chapter 7, Chest Pain.

Aortic dissection is characterized by the entrance of blood into the aortic media and is associated with a mortality rate of 1% per hour in the first 48 hours if untreated. The International Registry of Aortic Dissection enrolled 464 patients with documented aortic dissection, of whom 36% had upper back pain, including 33% of type A dissections and 41% of type B dissections. Overall, only 73% (++++) of patients reported chest pain, 23% (++) of patients presented with only upper or lower back pain, and 4% did not report pain.

Underlying conditions associated with dissection include:
- Hypertension ++++
- Atherosclerosis +++
- Known prior aortic aneurysm ++

SYMPTOMS
- Abrupt onset of pain ++++
- Severity of pain rated as worst ever ++++
- Sharp pain +++
- Tearing or ripping pain +++

SIGNS
- Systolic BP >150 +++
- Aortic insufficiency murmur +++
- Pulse deficit ++

WORKUP
- Abnormal chest radiograph ++++, widened mediastinum +++, abnormal aortic contour +++
- Newer generation CT scanning is increasingly used by many centers in the initial evaluation to rule out aortic dissection. MRI and transesophageal echocardiography have demonstrated excellent sensitivity; that of transthoracic echocardiography is poor.

REFERENCES
Hagan PG, Nienaber CA, Isselbacher EM, et al: The International Registry of Acute Aortic Dissection (IRAD): new insights into an old disease, *JAMA* 283:897, 2000.

Khan IA, Nair CK: Clinical, diagnostic, and management perspectives of aortic dissection, *Chest* 122:1, 2002.

Rogers RL: Aortic disasters, *Emerg Med Clin North Am* 22:4, 2004.

ACUTE CORONARY SYNDROME AND MYOCARDIAL INFARCTION

Although acute coronary syndrome (ACS) and acute myocardial infarction (AMI) typically arise with chest pain, radiation to other anatomic sites is common. In addition, evidence is mounting that the "typical" presentation of myocardial ischemia is not typical for many patients, including women, diabetics, and elderly patients. Several case series of patients with proven ACS or AMI, or both, have shown that although men and women had similar rates of chest pain at the time of presentation (~80% for ACS and >95% for AMI), women were much more likely to present with thoracic back pain than men (pooled results: ACS: women 40% versus men 12%; AMI: women 42% versus men 22%). Significant back pain associated with electrocardiographic evidence of ACS/AMI should also arouse suspicion for proximal aortic dissection flap occluding a coronary artery, particularly if thrombolysis is considered. In the International Registry of Aortic Dissection data, 15% of aortic dissections had ischemic ECG change and 3% had ST elevation.

CHAPTER 5

REFERENCES

Goldberg R, Goff D, Cooper L, et al: Age and sex differences in presentation of symptoms among patients with acute coronary disease: the REACT trial, *Coron Artery Dis* 11:399, 2000.

Gupta M, Tabas JA, Kohn MA: Presenting complaint among patients with myocardial infarction who present to an urban, public hospital emergency department, *Ann Emerg Med* 40:2, 2002.

Patel H, Rosengren A, Ekman I: Symptoms in acute coronary syndromes: does sex make a difference? *Am Heart J* 148:1, 2004.

 ## PULMONARY EMBOLISM, PNEUMOTHORAX, AND PNEUMONIA

See Chapter 7, Chest Pain.

 ## PERFORATED ULCER, ABDOMINAL AORTIC ANEURYSM, GALLBLADDER DISEASE, AND PANCREATITIS

See Chapter 1, Abdominal Pain.

 ## VERTEBRAL OSTEOMYELITIS, SPINAL EPIDURAL ABSCESS, HERNIATED DISC, AND TUMOR

See Chapter 4, Back Pain, Lower.

Disc herniation is much less common in the thoracic spine than in the lumbosacral spine; and symptomatic thoracic disc disease is rare. Metastatic disease, on the other hand, is more common in the thoracic spine, with 70% of all spinal metastases found there. Spinal epidural abscess is also most commonly found in the thoracic spine (50% to 80% of cases), followed by lumbosacral (17% to 38%) and cervical (10% to 25%). Vertebral osteomyelitis has no obvious predilection for the thoracic spine, with 45% of cases reported in lumbosacral spine, 35% in thoracic spine, and 20% in cervical spine.

 ## VERTEBRAL COMPRESSION FRACTURE

Vertebral compression fracture, defined as a 15% to 20% reduction of anterior, posterior, or central vertebral body height, occurs in 25% of women older than 50, often after trivial injury such as incurred in bending, lifting, coughing, or sneezing. Risk factors are the same as for osteoporosis: positive family history, prolonged postmenopausal state, glucocorticosteroid use, smoking, alcohol abuse, and medical conditions known to affect calcium or bone metabolism (e.g., renal failure, anticonvulsant use). In younger patients, trauma with axial loading of the spine can also result in thoracic vertebral compression fracture despite normal bone density.

SYMPTOMS
- Acute, severe pain at the fracture site is typical; however, minor fractures in elderly or postmenopausal patients may result in minimal pain or even an asymptomatic patient.
- Pain may radiate anteriorly to the flank or abdomen and increase with movement or Valsalva.
- Radicular pain or symptoms of spinal cord compression (bilateral leg pain, paresthesias, and incontinence) are rare.
- Pain is typically worse with axial loading (i.e., upright posture).

SIGNS
- Spinal tenderness over fracture site
- Paravertebral muscle spasm
- Ileus (abdominal distention and decreased bowel sounds)
- Kyphosis and loss of height
- Inability to touch occiput to wall with patient standing with heels against the wall
- Weakness, sensory deficits, incontinence, or diminished deep tendon reflexes (spinal cord compression) +

WORKUP
- Anteroposterior and lateral spine films. If available, comparison with previous x-rays is helpful to determine age of fracture
- CT scanning may be helpful in defining the severity of the fracture and determining stability
- MRI, if evidence of neurologic deficits

COMMENTS AND TREATMENT CONSIDERATIONS
Treatment is based on the stability of the fracture. More than 90% of compression fractures are stable. If compression is greater than 25% to 50%, angulation is greater than 20 degrees, or there is a fracture at more than one level, the fracture may be unstable. Patients with stable fractures and with no evidence of ileus or spinal cord compression can be discharged home with adequate analgesia, bed rest, and early medical follow-up. Early use of intranasal or subcutaneous calcitonin reduces the pain of osteoporotic vertebral compression fracture. Patients with unstable fractures, intractable pain, inability to care for themselves, or a new neurologic deficit should be admitted and receive medical and orthopedic or neurosurgical consultation.

REFERENCES

Knopp JA, Diner BM, Blitz M, et al: Calcitonin for treating acute pain of osteoporotic vertebral compression fractures: a systematic review of randomized, controlled trials, *Osteoporos Int* 16:1281, 2005.

Patel H, Rosengren A, Ekman I: Symptoms in acute coronary syndromes: does sex make a difference? *Am Heart J* 148:27, 2004.

Santavirta S, Konttinen YT, Heliovaara M, et al: Determinants of osteoporotic thoracic vertebral fracture: screening of 57,000 Finnish women and men, *Acta Orthop Scand* 63:198, 1992.

Bleeding
Lynne McCullough and Carolyn J. Sachs

Bleeding is a common presentation in the emergency department. In most cases, the cause of the bleeding is readily identifiable (e.g., as a result of trauma or originating from the gastrointestinal tract). Evaluation and treatment are directed at the specific cause.

Rarely, bleeding is caused or exacerbated by an underlying blood element defect including platelet abnormalities (in either number or function), problems with coagulation factors, or vascular disorders. Systemic bleeding disorders should be suspected when patients have unusually severe bleeding, spontaneous hemorrhage without trauma, or bleeding from multiple sites.

In general, patients with abnormalities of platelet number (thrombocytopenia) or function (thrombocytopathia) and those with vascular disorders (e.g., capillary fragility) have gingival bleeding, petechiae or easy bruising, gastrointestinal bleeding, excessive menses, hematuria, or prolonged bleeding after dental work. Once controlled, bleeding does not ordinarily recur. Coagulation factor deficiencies typically lead to delayed or recurrent bleeding because, although initial hemostasis is normal, an inadequate fibrin clot forms. This process leads to the formation of deep muscular hematomas, hemarthroses, and, rarely, retroperitoneal bleeding.

See Chapter 39, Trauma, Approach to.

REFERENCES
Bick RL: Vascular thrombohemorrhagic disorders: hereditary and acquired, *Clin Appl Thromb Hemost* 7:178, 2001.
Rick ME, Walsh CE, Key NS: Congenital bleeding disorders, *Hematology (Am Soc Hematol Educ Program)* 559, 2003.

GASTROINTESTINAL BLEEDING

The goal when evaluating gastrointestinal bleeding in the ED is to resuscitate and stabilize patients with an acute GI bleed. In addition, attempts are made to determine the nature and extent of the bleeding, whether it is acute or chronic, and to identify the 10% to 20% of patients who may rebleed. Upper gastrointestinal bleeding (UGIB) is bleeding occurring proximal to the ligament of Treitz; lower gastrointestinal bleeding (LGIB), the less frequent of the two, is distal and is usually due to colonic bleeding.

The five most common causes of nonvariceal UGIB are duodenal and gastric ulcers (50%), gastric erosions (30%), Mallory-Weiss syndrome (10%), and esophagitis. Duodenal ulcers are more common than gastric ulcers. Gastric ulcers are more often associated with the use of nonsteroidal anti-inflammatory drugs and aspirin. Esophageal varices account for a significant minority of UGIB admissions. Many patients with known esophageal varices have GI bleeding originating from other locations.

Perirectal disease, diverticulosis, angiodysplasia, cancer, and inflammatory bowel disease account for the majority of significant LGIB. In patients with a history of abdominal aortic aneurysm (AAA) grafts or occlusive aortoiliac disease, aortoenteric fistulas, a condition with high mortality, should be considered. A decreased hematocrit can lead to cardiac ischemia, particularly in elderly patients with coronary artery disease.

SYMPTOMS

- Red or coffee-ground hematemesis with or without melena indicates UGIB.
- Bright red rectal bleeding usually occurs with LGIB but can be seen with a vigorous UGIB.
- Hematochezia can be associated with either UGIB or LGIB.
- Patients with UGIB may have no symptoms other than hematemesis or melena +++.
- The volume of hematemesis is a poor guide for estimating volume loss.
- For Mallory-Weiss tears, patients have a history of hematemesis ++++ and repetitive vomiting +++. They may also report alcohol consumption ++, aspirin use, coughing, heavy lifting, or pregnancy +.
- Patients with simultaneous UGIB and acute myocardial infarction may report only dizziness, syncope, or acute confusion +++ and not chest pain.

SIGNS

- Hematemesis
- Gross or occult blood in stool
- Hypotension occurs late (typically with about 1500 ml blood loss).
- Tachycardia may appear earlier.
- Cool, clammy extremities and altered mental status occur late (after significant volume loss).
- Ascites, palmar erythema, and spider nevi are suggestive of chronic liver disease, the principal cause of esophageal varices.

WORKUP

- Two large-bore intravenous lines, type and crossmatch blood.
- Nasogastric aspirate with nasogastric tube (NGT) is sensitive ++++ but has low specificity because many foods and medications can give false-positive results on Hemoccult testing. Duodenal bleeds and an acidic stomach can cause false-negative results. In many cases, an NGT need not be placed, particularly if the patient is stable.
- CBC: immediate hematocrit values may not reflect blood loss. Serial values after repletion of the intravascular volume are required.
- Upper endoscopy: use for diagnosis and treatment of UGIB with active bleeding is controversial but is a standard practice in many institutions.
- Sigmoidoscopy or colonoscopy can be used in patients with stable LGIB.
- Arteriography or radionuclide scanning may be considered if endoscopy fails to locate the source despite ongoing bleeding.
- Abdominal films have very low sensitivity and are of little value except when perforation is suspected (see Chapter 1, Abdominal Pain).
- An elevated BUN: creatinine ratio (>25:1) may suggest a UGI source; in rapid bleeds, the BUN can be very high (40 mg/dl). Although interesting, this observation is not useful in diagnosis or treatment.
- ECG in patients at risk for coronary artery disease.

COMMENTS AND TREATMENT CONSIDERATIONS

Nasogastric tubes are often used for diagnosis of possible UGIB but not for treatment. Iced lavage is not beneficial and can cause hypothermia and arrhythmias as well as prolong bleeding; it should not be done. Many clinicians perform room temperature lavage to remove clots and determine cessation of bleeding, although this has not been shown to improve the outcome. Endoscopy and medical therapies are frequently used for unstable patients, with some of the literature reporting efficacy of both methods.

CHAPTER 6

Endoscopy may allow cautery or injection sclerosis in ongoing bleeds. Octreotide, a longer acting somatostatin analogue, appears to control active peptic ulcer bleeding in some patients. The majority of Mallory-Weiss tears stop bleeding spontaneously.

Variceal bleeding should be ruled out in patients with known or suspected liver disease. Sclerotherapy has an immediate effect in many patients; octreotide is also effective when used alone or in combination with endoscopy. Pharmacologic control of variceal bleeding may be attempted with the use of vasopressin or terlipressin (a vasopressin derivative); however, this has the potential to cause peripheral necrosis from systemic vasoconstriction.

In chronic and subacute UGIB, proton pump inhibitors appear more effective than H2 blockers in preventing rebleeding; however, they have not yet been shown to help control bleeding in the acute emergency department setting. Antacid therapy has no role in treating acute bleeds. Rarely used today, esophageal tube tamponade controls 85% of acute variceal bleeds but has the potential to cause aspiration and esophageal perforation and does not confer additional benefit over the use of somatostatin alone.

High-risk patients who may be considered for admission to the ICU include those with any of the following: ongoing bleeding, hypotension, prolonged prothrombin time, altered mental status, more than 8% drop in hematocrit, age younger than 75, or unstable comorbid disease. Independent predictors of an adverse outcome include an initial hematocrit less than 30%, initial systolic blood pressure below 100 mm Hg, red blood in nasogastric lavage, history of cirrhosis or ascites on examination, or history of vomiting red blood. Surgical consultation should be obtained because surgery may be necessary if medical management is ineffective.

Less acutely ill patients at risk for rebleeding may be admitted to a non-ICU setting. The American Society for Gastrointestinal Endoscopy identified four clinical predictors of rebleeding: old age, shock, comorbid diseases, and coagulopathy. Some low-risk patients with GIB can be safely evaluated as outpatients. However, patients with significant UGIB are generally admitted for observation and additional testing such as endoscopy. All discharged patients should be referred for timely follow-up. In particular, most patients with a presumptive diagnosis of bleeding related to hemorrhoids or anal fissure require outpatient sigmoidoscopy or colonoscopy to rule out other pathologic conditions.

REFERENCES

Avgerinos A, Nevens F, Raptis S, et al: Early administration of somatostatin and efficacy of sclerotherapy in acute oesophageal variceal bleeds: the European Acute Bleeding

Oesophageal Variceal Episodes (ABOVE) randomized trial, *Lancet* 350:1495, 1997.

Banares R, Albillos A, Rincon D, et al: Endoscopic treatment versus endoscopic plus pharmacologic treatment for acute variceal bleeding: a meta-analysis. *Hepatology* 35:609, 2002.

Blatchford O, Murray WR, Blatchford M: A risk score to predict need for treatment for upper-gastrointestinal haemorrhage, *Lancet* 356:1318, 2000.

Cales P, Masliah C, Bernard B, et al: Early administration of vapreotide for variceal bleeding in patients with cirrhosis. French Club for the Study of Portal Hypertension, *N Engl J Med* 344:23, 2001.

Collins R, Langman M: Treatment with histamine H2 antagonists in acute upper gastrointestinal hemorrhage: implications of randomized trials, *N Engl J Med* 313:660, 1985.

Eisen GM, Dominitz JA, Faigel DO, et al: An annotated algorithmic approach to upper gastrointestinal bleeding, *Gastrointest Endosc* 53:853, 2001.

Imperiale TF, Teran JC, McCullough AJ: A meta-analysis of somatostatin versus vasopressin in the management of acute esophageal variceal hemorrhage, *Gastroenterology* 109:1289, 1995.

Lee KK, You JH, Wong IC, et al: Cost-effectiveness analysis of high-dose omeprazole infusion as adjuvant therapy to endoscopic treatment of bleeding peptic ulcer, *Gastrointest Endosc* 57:160, 2003.

Lin HJ, Tseng GY, Lo WC, et al: Predictive factors for rebleeding in patients with peptic ulcer bleeding after multipolar electrocoagulation: a retrospective analysis, *J Clin Gastroenterol* 26:113, 1998.

Longstreth GF, Feitelberg SP: Outpatient care of selected patients with acute non-variceal upper gastrointestinal haemorrhage, *Lancet* 345:108, 1995.

Zed PJ, Loewen PS, Slavik RS, et al: Meta-analysis of proton pump inhibitors in treatment of bleeding peptic ulcers, *Ann Pharmacother* 35:1528, 2001.

CHAPTER 6

 THROMBOCYTOPENIA

A low platelet count can result from decreased production, increased utilization, or destruction as well as from splenic sequestration of platelets. Thrombocytopenia should be considered, especially in patients with mucous membrane bleeding or petechial hemorrhages.

Causes of failed platelet production include aplastic and megaloblastic anemia, infection (including HIV), alcohol-induced bone marrow suppression, and bone marrow infiltration with leukemia or with myelodysplastic cells.

Causes of increased platelet destruction or utilization include idiopathic thrombocytopenic purpura, thrombotic thrombocytopenic purpura, and hemolytic-uremic syndrome; drugs, including heparin, quinidine, gold salts, rifampin, sulfa, oral diabetic agents, and ticlopidine; and states of intravascular coagulation (sepsis, metastatic cancer, traumatic brain damage, and obstetric complications such as HELLP and ARDS).

Causes of splenic sequestration should also be considered, including cirrhosis and mononucleosis with secondary splenomegaly, Gaucher's disease, and myelofibrosis with myeloid dysplasia.

SYMPTOMS
- Gingival bleeding
- Prolonged bleeding after dental work
- Epistaxis
- Easy bruising
- Excessive menses
- Hematuria
- GI bleeding

SIGNS
- Multiple scattered petechiae, purpura, or ecchymosis
- Epistaxis
- Other bleeding

WORKUP
- CBC with platelets
- Evaluation of a peripheral blood smear
- Urinalysis (hematuria)
- LFTs and rheumatologic tests, as clinically indicated
- Platelet function studies and bone marrow analysis, although important in the evaluation of otherwise unexplained thrombocytopenia, are not indicated in the emergency setting.

COMMENTS AND TREATMENT CONSIDERATIONS
No treatment is indicated for the majority of cases of thrombocytopenia. Patients with a platelet count below 10,000/mm^3 are thought to be at risk for spontaneous intracranial hemorrhage, and thus replacement is generally recommended at that level. Platelet transfusion may be considered even with a level as high as 50,000/mm^3 in the presence of severe ongoing bleeding. One unit of random donor platelets usually raises the platelet count by 10,000/mm^3. The same precautions taken to prevent allergic

reactions when transfusing other blood products should be followed when transfusing platelets (i.e., pretreatment with acetaminophen and diphenhydramine). For patients who have ongoing heavy bleeding, single-donor platelet units can be transfused to minimize antigenic exposure with multiple transfusions. One unit of single-donor platelets provides the equivalent of 5 to 6 units of random-donor platelets. If TTP or DIC has not been ruled out, platelets should generally not be transfused because it can worsen the thrombotic process.

REFERENCES

Glatt AE, Anand A: Thrombocytopenia in patients infected with human immunodeficiency virus: treatment update, *Clin Infect Dis* 21:415, 1995.

Goebel RA: Thrombocytopenia, *Emerg Med Clin North Am* 11:445, 1993.

McCrae KR, Bussel JB, Mannucci PM, et al: DB: Platelets: an update on diagnosis and management of thrombocytopenic disorders, *Hematology (Am Soc Hematol Educ Program)* 282, 2001.

 IMMUNE THROMBOCYTOPENIC PURPURA

Immune thrombocytopenic purpura (ITP) can be either an acute or chronic condition. The acute form is caused by immune complexes binding to or cross-reacting with platelets, often as the result of a viral infection. Acute ITP occurs predominantly in children, usually younger than 6 years, and is self-limited. Chronic ITP has an insidious onset, occurs three times more commonly in females than in males, and is seen most commonly between the ages of 20 and 40.

SYMPTOMS
- Acute: see Thrombocytopenia
- Chronic: see Thrombocytopenia
- Menometrorrhagia may occur

SIGNS
- See Thrombocytopenia

WORKUP
- The physical examination and laboratory evaluation should focus on the elimination of other causes of thrombocytopenia.
- See Thrombocytopenia
- Bone marrow biopsy is routinely performed during admission or on an outpatient basis to rule out an atypical presentation of aplastic anemia, acute leukemia, or a metastatic tumor.

COMMENTS AND TREATMENT CONSIDERATIONS

Expectant management is often all that is indicated. With the acute childhood form, intravenous immunoglobulin or corticosteroids can be used for symptomatic patients with platelet counts in the 10,000 to 20,000/mm³ range. In cases of severe bleeding from ITP, plasmapheresis may be performed.

Platelet transfusion is of transient benefit and is considered a heroic measure reserved for life-threatening hemorrhage despite conventional treatment. Consultation with a hematologist and follow-up are required.

REFERENCES

Adams JR, Nathan DP, Bennett CL: Pharmacoeconomics of therapy for ITP: steroids, i.v. Ig, anti-D, and splenectomy, *Blood Rev* 16:65, 2002.

George JN, Woolf SH, Raskob GE, et al: Idiopathic thrombocytopenic purpura: a practice guideline developed by explicit methods for the American Society of Hematology, *Blood* 88:3, 1996.

Imbach P: Immune thrombocytopenic purpura and intravenous immunoglobulin, *Cancer* 68(Suppl):1422, 1991.

Stasi R, Provan D: Management of immune thrombocytopenic purpura in adults, *Mayo Clin Proc* 79:504, 2004.

 THROMBOTIC THROMBOCYTOPENIC PURPURA

Classically, thrombotic thrombocytopenic purpura (TTP) is diagnosed when at least four of the following five elements are present, in the absence of another explanation: microangiopathic hemolytic anemia (MAHA), thrombocytopenia, decreased renal function, fever, and neurologic abnormalities. The cause of this disease process is uncertain, but it is characterized by microthrombi (deposits composed of platelets and fibrin) within the lumina of capillaries and arterioles in various locations, creating a variable clinical presentation.

SYMPTOMS

- Neurologic abnormalities are seen most commonly (headache, altered mentation, cranial nerve palsies, hemiparesis, or coma).
- Other symptoms (dependent on organ system involved)
- See Thrombocytopenia

SIGNS

- See Thrombocytopenia

WORKUP
- CBC with platelets
- Urinalysis (may suggest a hemolytic anemia or proteinuria)
- Peripheral blood smear (schistocytes, reticulocytosis)
- Fibrin degradation products and D-dimer
- Bilirubin (indirect)
- LDH
- Electrolytes (elevated BUN, creatinine)

COMMENTS AND TREATMENT CONSIDERATIONS
Once recognized, this disease process constitutes an emergency and should prompt emergency consultation with a hematologist. The primary treatment is plasma exchange transfusion. While waiting for this to be arranged, the emergency physician may consider glucocorticoids and antiplatelet therapy (dipyridamole or aspirin) in patients with acute life-threatening presentations. Platelets should not be transfused unless the patient has an uncontrollable, life-threatening hemorrhage because this can exacerbate the thrombotic process.

REFERENCES
George JN, Sadler JE, Lammle B: Platelets: thrombotic thrombocytopenic purpura, *Hematology (Am Soc Hematol Educ Program)* 315, 2002.

Harkness DR, Byrnes JJ, Lian ECY, et al: Hazard of platelet transfusion in thrombotic thrombocytopenic purpura, *JAMA* 246:1931, 1981.

Lammle B, Kremer Hovinga J, Studt JD, et al: Thrombotic thrombocytopenic purpura, *Hematol J* 5(Suppl 3):S6, 2004.

McCarthy LJ, Dlott JS, Orazi A, et al: Thrombotic thrombocytopenic purpura: yesterday, today, tomorrow, *Ther Apher Dial* 8:80, 2004.

 RENAL DISEASE AND UREMIA
Patients dependent on hemodialysis often report bleeding, which reflects the multifactorial nature of hemostatic abnormalities in renal failure. Their bleeding tendency results from a qualitative and a mild quantitative platelet problem as well as from frequent coagulation factor deficiencies acquired as a result of a nephrotic state, the anticoagulant properties of retained uremic toxins, chronic anemia, and the fact that they receive anticoagulation with dialysis.

WORKUP
- CBC with platelets
- Bleeding time is not generally performed in the ED, although it is the hemostatic test most consistently abnormal with uremia.

COMMENTS AND TREATMENT CONSIDERATIONS

It is important to establish the adequacy and timing of recent dialysis, as dialysis may transiently improve platelet function. Correcting the anemia associated with renal failure (by transfusion of packed red blood cells to an optimum hematocrit of 26% to 30%) also improves platelet function. Platelet replacement has minimal efficacy because the transfused platelets rapidly acquire the uremic deficiency. Nonetheless, in life-threatening hemorrhage, both platelet and cryoprecipitate transfusions are indicated. Desmopressin (DDAVP), a synthetic analogue of vasopressin, increases platelet adhesion through stimulation of the release of von Willebrand factor and factor VIII, resulting in a shortening of the bleeding time in many uremic patients. The drawbacks associated with the use of DDAVP include tachyphylaxis after three or four doses and the side effects of headache, flushing, nausea, and abdominal cramps. Conjugated estrogens are also effective in reducing bleeding, although the mechanism is unclear.

REFERENCES

Dember LM: Critical care issues in the patient with chronic renal failure, *Crit Care Clin* 18:421, 2002.

Eberst ME, Berkowitz LR: Hemostasis in renal disease: pathophysiology and management, *Am J Med* 96:168, 1994.

Hodde LA, Sandroni S: Emergency department evaluation and management of dialysis patient complications, *Am J Emerg Med* 10:317, 1992.

Sagripanti A, Barsotti G: Bleeding and thrombosis in chronic uremia, *Nephron* 75:125, 1997.

 HEMOLYTIC–UREMIC SYNDROME

Hemolytic-uremic syndrome (HUS) is a serious multisystem disease usually affecting young children, with a peak incidence between 6 months and 4 years of age. It usually follows a prodromal infectious illness (well described following diarrhea caused by *Escherichia coli* serotype O157:H7). HUS is both clinically and pathologically similar to TTP, with a predominance of renal symptomatology. Important abnormalities include hemolytic anemia, azotemia, thrombocytopenia, and, frequently, encephalopathy.

SYMPTOMS

- Similar to TTP, although neurologic manifestations less common
- Abdominal pain (may be severe)
- Bloody diarrhea
- Symptoms of circulatory fluid overload including fatigue and generalized weakness, shortness of breath, and swelling

SIGNS
- Pale, weak, ill appearing
- Petechiae or purpura
- Neurologic abnormalities (irritable, obtunded, or focal defects possible), somnolent
- Abdominal tenderness, possibly as a result of hepatic and splenic enlargement
- Hypertension

WORKUP
- CBC with platelets (anemia and thrombocytopenia secondary to destruction or consumption)
- Urinalysis: red and white blood cells, cellular casts, and a significant amount of protein
- Electrolytes, calcium, phosphate—acute renal failure pattern (elevated BUN and creatinine, hyperkalemia, hyponatremia, hyperphosphatemia, hyperuricemia, hypocalcemia)
- Liver function tests
- PT and PTT

COMMENTS AND TREATMENT CONSIDERATIONS
Treatment is generally supportive and focuses on renal failure and its complications. This is an area of active investigation.

REFERENCES
Garg AX, Suri RS, Barrowman N, et al: Long-term renal prognosis of diarrhea-associated hemolytic uremic syndrome: a systematic review, meta-analysis, and meta-regression, *JAMA* 290:1360, 2003.

Liu J, Hutzler M, Li C, Pechet L: Thrombotic thrombocytopenic purpura (TTP) and hemolytic uremic syndrome (HUS): the new thinking, *J Thromb Thrombolysis* 11:261, 2001.

 DISSEMINATED INTRAVASCULAR COAGULATION

Disseminated intravascular coagulation (DIC) is a severe blood clotting abnormality that affects multiple organ systems and occurs in patients with a serious preexisting medical or surgical problem. Many conditions have been associated with the development of DIC including infection, acid-base disturbances, malignancies, burns, traumatic injuries, vascular disorders, transfusion reactions, massive transfusions, and obstetric complications. The emergency physician must initiate the treatment for DIC as well as diagnose and treat the underlying condition.

DIC is characterized by an imbalance in the system of coagulation and fibrinolysis. It is thought to occur as a result of the release of

CHAPTER 6

tissue factor that triggers the coagulation cascade. Small fibrin clots are formed and deposited at the same time fibrinolysis is stimulated, and the process results in the consumption of both coagulation factors and platelets.

SYMPTOMS
- Bleeding and/or thrombosis
- Bleeding from multiple sites, including areas of venipuncture, into the urine, from the gastrointestinal tract, and, most commonly, from the skin and mucous membranes

SIGNS
- See Thrombocytopenia
- Bleeding
- Purpura
- Signs of microthrombi formation and subsequent tissue ischemia (e.g., gangrene, purpura fulminans, renal cortical necrosis, ARDS) can be seen in any organ system.
- CNS findings stemming from an intracerebral hemorrhage

WORKUP
- CBC with platelets (thrombocytopenia)
- PT and PTT (may be prolonged)
- Fibrinogen level (decreased)
- Fibrin degradation products and D-dimer (elevated)
- Blood smear (fragmented RBCs)

COMMENTS AND TREATMENT CONSIDERATIONS
Initially, management should be focused on establishing hemodynamic stability while assessing and treating the underlying condition. Further management then focuses on the replacement of depleted coagulation factors. Usually, fibrinogen is deficient, and this can be replaced with cryoprecipitate. The PT and INR are the best indicators of factor depletion; when they are two to three times greater than normal, fresh frozen plasma (FFP) should be given. Each unit of FFP contains 200 to 250 units of each factor and is usually given 2 units at a time. More than 2 units are generally required to reverse bleeding associated with the coagulopathy. It is also prudent to administer folate and vitamin K (use phytonadione because it has a more rapid onset of action; maximum IV rate is 1 mg/minute).

Heparin is a highly controversial treatment for thromboses and is rarely used in the ED. It does not reliably reverse abnormal coagulation and can exacerbate a bleeding diathesis. Likewise, antifibrinolytic agents are used only with extreme caution. Platelet replacement is effective only transiently and should be given according to the guidelines for general thrombocytopenia, outlined earlier.

REFERENCES

Contreras M, Ala FA, Greaves M, et al: Guidelines for the use of fresh frozen plasma. British Committee for Standards in Haematology, Working Party of the Blood Transfusion Task Force, *Transfus Med* 2:57, 1992.

Franchini M, Manzato F: Update on the treatment of disseminated intravascular coagulation, *Hematology* 9:81, 2004.

Toh CH, Dennis M: Current clinical practice. DIC 2002: a review of disseminated intravascular coagulation, *Hematology* 8:65, 2003.

 LIVER DISEASE AND HEPATIC FAILURE

The pathophysiologic abnormalities associated with liver disease result in hemostatic problems that range from subclinical coagulopathy, unmasked by the performance of a procedure, to brisk, active hemorrhage that can be life threatening. If the patient has liver disease as a result of alcoholism, thrombocytopenia results not only from splenic sequestration but also from decreased production.

CHAPTER 6

SYMPTOMS
- Fatigue
- Anorexia
- Pruritus
- Gastrointestinal bleeding
- Increasing abdominal girth

SIGNS
- Jaundice
- Hematemesis
- Melena or bright red blood from rectum
- Ascites
- Spider nevi
- Asterixis
- Altered mental status
    See Hepatic Encephalopathy in Chapter 27, Mental Status Change and Coma.

WORKUP
- CBC with platelets
- PT and PTT
- Liver enzymes: ALT, AST, alkaline phosphatase
- Tests to rule out infections when indicated (aspiration of ascites, chest x-ray, urinalysis, blood and urine cultures)

COMMENTS AND TREATMENT CONSIDERATIONS

Intervention is indicated for active bleeding or when preparing for an invasive procedure. Packed red blood cells should be replaced as needed to maintain hemodynamic stability. FFP (generally begin with 2 units) immediately supplies missing coagulation factors. The effects of vitamin K are delayed. If vitamin K is administered in the ED, the subcutaneous and intramuscular routes should be avoided because they can cause significant bleeding or hematoma. Platelets are transfused only when bleeding is severe because the transfused platelets rapidly acquire a qualitative defect.

Desmopressin (DDAVP) can also be helpful in reducing the bleeding time in patients with liver disease, as it does with renal failure, and should be considered in the treatment of the bleeding patient with significant liver disease.

REFERENCES

Bosch J, Abraldes JG: Management of gastrointestinal bleeding in patients with cirrhosis of the liver, *Semin Hematol* 41(1, Suppl 1): 8, 2004.

Mammen EF: Coagulopathies of liver disease, *Clin Lab Med* 14:769, 1994.

Paramo JA, Rocha E: Hemostasis in advanced liver disease, *Semin Thromb Hemost* 19:184, 1993.

 ## HEMOPHILIAS AND VON WILLEBRAND'S DISEASE

Hemophilia A (factor VIII) and B (factor IX) are both X-linked recessive, coagulation factor disorders. In both hemophilia A and B a normal level of factor is present, but its coagulant activity is diminished. Hemophilia A is far more common. The clinical presentation varies according to the degree of coagulant activity present. In addition to coagulant activity, factor VIII stimulates platelet adhesion. When this function is diminished, von Willebrand's disease results.

SYMPTOMS AND SIGNS

HEMOPHILIA A AND B

- Hemarthrosis or muscle hematoma is most common. Chronic joint destruction can occur because of repetitive hemarthrosis often caused by minimal trauma.
- Bleeding can also occur elsewhere, including the CNS, and may indicate more severe factor dysfunction. In severe cases (when factor activity is less than 1%), spontaneous hemorrhage is more common.

VON WILLEBRAND'S DISEASE
- Generally less symptomatic than hemophilia
- Epistaxis, excessive bruising, or prolonged bleeding after minor surgery (e.g., dental extractions). Hemarthroses or soft tissue bleeding, as seen with hemophilia, is less common.

WORKUP
- Platelet count (to exclude a quantitative platelet disorder)
- PT/INR and PTT

HEMOPHILIA A AND B
Coagulation screening tests typically show a normal PT and a prolonged PTT, demonstrating a defect in the intrinsic pathway. All screening tests can be normal in hemophilia, however, if the factor activity is greater than 30%. The type of factor deficiency (VIII versus IX) can be established only by specific assay.

VON WILLEBRAND'S DISEASE
Factor activity can be assessed by performing a ristocetin cofactor assay. (This is not routinely performed in the ED.) The bleeding time is typically prolonged.

COMMENTS AND TREATMENT CONSIDERATIONS
Patients with hemophilia should not receive intramuscular injections, have arterial blood gases drawn, or have central venous access attempted without prior and continued factor replacement because life-threatening hemorrhage may occur.

Prompt hemostasis is the goal of therapy. Specific treatment varies with the site and severity of hemorrhage.

Mild to moderate hemophilia may respond to treatment with DDAVP, and it is helpful to know whether the patient has responded to this treatment in the past. When efficacious, DDAVP can produce a threefold increase in factor VIII activity. The usual dose is 0.3 μg/kg IV over 15 to 30 minutes. A response is typically seen within 1 hour. Tachyphylaxis often occurs after three or four doses.

Severe hemophilia or any severity with serious bleeding (determined by either location or amount) requires treatment with specific factor concentrates. Dosing of factor concentrates varies according to the site and degree of hemorrhage. In general, a patient factor activity level of less than 1% should be assumed, and treatment should ensure 50% activity after treatment for most bleeds and 100% activity after treatment for central nervous system or other life-threatening bleeding.

Hemophilia A: Doses range from 15 to 30 U/kg of factor VIII as an initial dose for minor hemorrhage (epistaxis, after dental

CHAPTER 6

extraction, into joints or muscles) to 50 U/kg for life-threatening bleeding (CNS, retropharynx/pharynx, retroperitoneum, or for patients who need emergent surgery).

Hemophilia B: Initial doses range from 25 U/kg of factor IX for minor bleeding to 50-80 U/kg for major hemorrhage.

Circulating antibodies may be formed to infused factor precipitates; this occurs in approximately 15% of patients with severe hemophilia A and 10% of patients with hemophilia B. If a patient is unresponsive to usual therapy, antibodies may be present and can be assayed by the Bethesda inhibitor assay (BIA). The level present can be used as a guide for choosing the most efficacious type of factor replacement therapy.

If the bleeding is life threatening and factor concentrates are not readily available, cryoprecipitate (one bag contains approximately 100 U of factor VIII) or FFP (1 unit of FFP raises factor IX activity by 3%) can be used.

REFERENCES

Brettler DB, Levine PH: Factor concentrates for treatment of hemophilia: which one to choose? *Blood* 73:2067, 1989.

Hoyer LW: Hemophilia A, *N Engl J Med* 330:38, 1994.

Lee JW: Von Willebrand disease, hemophilia A and B, and other factor deficiencies, *Int Anesthesiol Clin* 42:59, 2004.

Logan LJ: Treatment of von Willebrand's disease, *Hematol Oncol Clin North Am* 6:1079, 1992.

Manucci PM, Cattaneo M: Desmopressin: a nontransfusional treatment of hemophilia and von Willebrand disease, *Haemostasis* 22:276, 1992.

 PATIENTS TAKING WARFARIN

Warfarin inhibits hepatic synthesis of the vitamin K–dependent coagulation factors II, VII, IX, and X and the anticoagulant proteins C and S.

SYMPTOMS
- Epistaxis
- Hematemesis
- Hematuria
- Hematochezia or melena
- Change in behavior (particularly after a fall or head trauma)

SIGNS
- Melena or bright red blood in rectum
- Altered mental status
- Ecchymoses

- Bleeding gums
- Hematuria

WORKUP
- CBC with platelets
- INR, PT, and PTT
- Type and screen when significant or ongoing blood loss is evident
- CT of the brain for any (even very minor) head trauma or altered mental status

COMMENTS AND TREATMENT CONSIDERATIONS
Intervention is indicated for active bleeding with high potential morbidity (e.g., intracranial bleeding or significant gastrointestinal bleeding [Table 6–1]). Packed red blood cells should be transfused to maintain hemodynamic stability. For patients with life-threatening bleeding who take warfarin, their iatrogenic coagulopathy should immediately be reversed with FFP or, if available, prothrombin complex concentrate (PCC) and vitamin K. The amount of FFP to replace adequately the vitamin K–dependent clotting factors to a level of 25% is equivalent to approximately 5 to 10 mL/kg (generally begin with 2 units). Although vitamin K can be administered orally, intramuscularly, subcutaneously, and intradermally, the intravenous route has the most rapid onset of action. In general, vitamin K (2 to 10 mg) in the form of intravenous phytonadione is indicated for severe hemorrhage. Although not conclusively demonstrated, administering intravenous vitamin K very slowly and pretreating with antihistamines may decrease the possibility of an anaphylactoid reaction (Table 6–2).

REFERENCES
Ansell J, Hirsh J, Poller L, et al: The pharmacology and management of the vitamin K antagonists: the Seventh ACCP Conference on

TABLE 6–1 CLASSIFICATION OF WARFARIN–ASSOCIATED BLEEDING	
CLASSIFICATION	CHARACTERISTICS
Major	Intracranial Retroperitoneal Intraocular Muscle compartment syndrome Invasive procedure required to stop bleeding Active bleeding from any orifice + BP <90 mm Hg systolic, oliguria, or >2 g fall in hemoglobin
Minor	Any other bleeding

From Makris and Watson

CHAPTER 6

TABLE 6–2

UK GUIDELINES FOR WARFARIN REVERSAL

CLINICAL SITUATION	ACTION
Major bleeding	Stop warfarin Vitamin K (5 mg IV or oral) PCC (50 U/kg) or FFP (15 ml/kg) Caution: FFP may not fully reverse the effect of warfarin—for example, factor IX does not rise >20% after FFP (not reflected in INR)

Nonmajor bleeding
  INR <6.0
  INR >6.0 to <8.0
	
	Omit warfarin
	Omit warfarin

No/minor bleeding
  INR >8.0
  INR >8.0 + other risk factors for bleeding
	
	Omit warfarin
	Omit warfarin + 0.5 to 2.5 mg vitamin K (IV or oral)

FFP, fresh frozen plasma; INR, international normalized ratio; IV, intravenous; PCC, prothrombin complex concentrate.

From British Committee for Standards in Haematology: Guidelines on oral anticoagulation: third edition, *Br J Haematol* 101:374, 1998.

Antithrombotic and Thrombolytic Therapy, *Chest* 126(3 Suppl):204S, 2004.

Fiore LD, Scola MA, Cantillon CE, Brophy MT: Anaphylactoid reactions to vitamin K, *J Thromb Thrombolysis* 11:175, 2001.

Hanley JP: Warfarin reversal, *J Clin Pathol* 57:1132, 2004.

Makris M: Management of excessive anticoagulation or bleeding, *Semin Vasc Med* 3:279, 2003.

Makris M, Watson HG: The management of coumarin-induced over-anticoagulation, *Br J Haematol* 114:271, 2001.

Chest Pain
Mark S. Louden

Chest pain is one of the most frequent presenting complaints in the ED. The patient's history is the single most important source of information for distinguishing between emergent, urgent, and benign conditions. Timely ECG and chest x-rays are often invaluable, whereas blood tests are rarely helpful in the initial evaluation.

 ## PNEUMOTHORAX, TENSION PNEUMOTHORAX, AND PNEUMOMEDIASTINUM

A pneumothorax may occur spontaneously, following trauma, or as an iatrogenic complication (e.g., with central line insertion or aspiration of pleural effusion). Spontaneous pneumothoraces are somewhat more common in patients who are tall and thin and who smoke cigarettes. Spontaneous pneumothoraces are also associated with Marfan's syndrome, smoking crack cocaine, and *Pneumocystis carinii* pneumonia. In trauma, severe injuries outside the chest may mask respiratory symptoms.

Pneumomediastinum may arise in the same way as pneumothorax (spontaneous or traumatic), but it is sometimes accompanied by throat pain or dysphagia.

Tension pneumothorax is caused by buildup of pressure outside the lung, compressing the mediastinum and limiting venous return and cardiac output. Tension pneumothorax should be suspected in trauma patients who are hypoxic or hypotensive and those receiving mechanical ventilation who deteriorate clinically. Clinicians should also have a low threshold for considering the diagnosis in patients who have a known pneumothorax or who are undergoing a procedure that may cause one.

SYMPTOMS
- Acute onset of chest pain or discomfort (often pleuritic) ++++
- Dyspnea with +++ or without chest pain ++

SIGNS
PNEUMOTHORAX
- A healthy patient with a small pneumothorax (usually less than 15% to 20% volume) may have no physical signs.
- Tachypnea
- Tachycardia
- Decreased breath sounds
- Hyperresonance to percussion (may be masked by hemothorax)
- Subcutaneous emphysema
- Patients with preexisting cardiopulmonary disease or other associated injuries may be cyanotic or in shock.

TENSION PNEUMOTHORAX
- Hypotension
- Tracheal deviation (later finding)
- Distended neck veins (later finding)

PNEUMOMEDIASTINUM
- Hamman's sign (crepitance heard over the heart during systole) +++
- Subcutaneous emphysema +++

WORKUP
- Needle thoracostomy followed by tube thoracostomy *before* chest x-ray for patients with a strong suspicion of pneumothorax who are in shock or without a pulse.
- Chest x-rays (Figs. 7–1 and 7–2): Moderate (15% to 60% volume) or large (>60%) pneumothoraces are usually evident. If pneumothorax is suspected, an additional film taken during maximal expiration may increase sensitivity.
- ECG is used primarily to evaluate for other potential causes of chest pain; continuous ECG monitoring determines the presence of a cardiac rhythm in the pulseless patient.
- CT scanning is more sensitive than chest x-ray, but because small pneumothoraces are of little clinical significance, CT is not warranted for this diagnosis alone.
- Contrast-enhanced esophagography is indicated in patients with pneumomediastinum if a spontaneous esophageal rupture is suspected (Boerhaave's syndrome) or if trauma has caused penetration of the esophagus (see Esophageal Rupture).

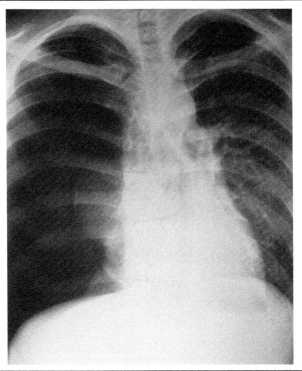

Fig. 7-1 Tension pneumothorax. Anteroposterior chest radiograph demonstrates shift of the mediastinal structures to the left, indicating tension. (Courtesy of Michael Zucker, MD, Los Angeles.)

COMMENTS AND TREATMENT CONSIDERATIONS

Patients with a very small spontaneous pneumothorax (<15%) can be given 100% O_2 in the ED and be observed because spontaneous reabsorption is expected at a rate of 1% of the hemithorax per day. Simple pneumothoraces (<25%) can be aspirated through a small catheter (with 45% to 87% success rate) and observed for 4 to 6 hours (for recurrence or reexpansion pulmonary edema). For some patients, placement of a small-diameter catheter attached to a one-way valve (Heimlich valve) may allow ED discharge with daily follow-up.

Although some large pneumothoraces (particularly after otherwise minor trauma) also do well with the preceding approach, most experts recommend that they, as well as pneumothoraces associated with underlying lung disease, empyema, hemothorax,

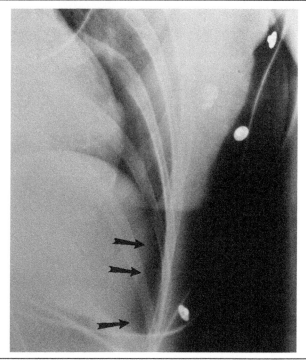

Fig. 7-2 Nontension pneumothorax. Anteroposterior supine chest radiograph shows left deep sulcus sign *(arrows)*. (Courtesy of Michael Zucker, MD, Los Angeles.)

or trauma, should be treated with tube thoracostomy and hospital admission. The same is true for a pneumothorax in a patient with severe cardiopulmonary disease and one who requires air transport.

Management of pneumomediastinum is conservative if the esophagus or bronchi have not been injured.

REFERENCES

Aitchison F, Bleetman A, Munro P, et al: Detection of pneumothorax by accident and emergency officers and radiologists on single chest films, *Arch Emerg Med* 10:343, 1993.

Baumann MH, Noppen M: Pneumothorax, *Respirology* 9:157, 2004.

Delius RE, Obeid FN, Horst HM, et al: Catheter aspiration for simple pneumothorax: experience with 114 patients, *Arch Surg* 124:833, 1989.

Markos J, McGonigle P, Phillips MJ: Pneumothorax: treatment by small-lumen catheter aspiration, *Aust NZ J Med* 20:775, 1990.

Noppen M: Management of primary spontaneous pneumothorax, *Curr Opin Pulm Med* 9:272, 2003.

Panacek EA, Singer AJ, Sherman BW, et al: Spontaneous pneumo-mediastinum: clinical and natural history, *Ann Emerg Med* 21:1222, 1992.

Seow A, Kazerooni EA, Pernicano PG, Neary M: Comparison of upright inspiratory and expiratory chest radiographs for detecting pneumothoraces, *AJR Am J Roentgenol* 166:313, 1996.

PERICARDIAL EFFUSION AND TAMPONADE

Pericardial tamponade is caused by elevated pressure in the pericardial space resulting in equilibration of pericardial, left ventricular, and right ventricular diastolic pressures, which leads to a decrease in preload and cardiac output. An effusion is usually present in pericarditis, but it does not result in tamponade in most cases. The rate at which an effusion develops may determine whether tamponade results. Rapid accumulation of fluid is most likely to develop from a penetrating injury, such as a stab or missile wound; as a complication of central line insertion; or following myocardial rupture after myocardial infarction. It may also follow retrograde aortic dissection. Tamponade from a medical cause of pericarditis is more likely when the underlying cause is a malignancy and when a patient with an existing effusion becomes acutely, severely dehydrated (see also Pericarditis).

SYMPTOMS
- Chest pain and tightness
- Shortness of breath
- Peripheral edema
- Dyspnea on exertion
- Altered mental status

SIGNS
- Tachycardia
- Narrow pulse pressure
- Pulsus paradoxus
- Kussmaul's sign (distention of neck veins with inspiration)
- Pericardial friction rub
- Beck's triad—hypotension, muffled heart sounds, and neck vein distention—is a very late event.

WORKUP
- Pericardiocentesis should be performed immediately for patients in severe shock.

CHAPTER 7

- Echocardiography is the study of choice.
- Central venous pressure or pulmonary artery pressure monitoring may be useful but should not delay echocardiography.
- If the etiology is traumatic or associated with aortic dissection, a thoracic surgeon should be consulted. Preparations should be made for pericardiocentesis, pericardial window, or thoracotomy.
- Patients with penetrating trauma resulting in tamponade, with loss of vital signs in or en route to the ED, are among the few who may benefit from thoracotomy in the ED.

REFERENCES

Maisch B, Seferovic PM, Ristic AD, et al: Guidelines on the diagnosis and management of pericardial diseases executive summary; the task force on the diagnosis and management of pericardial diseases of the European society of cardiology, *Eur Heart J* 25:587, 2004.

McGregor M: Pulsus paradoxus, *N Engl J Med* 301:480, 1979.

Whye D, Barish R, Almquist T, et al: Echocardiographic diagnosis of acute pericardial effusion in penetrating chest trauma, *Am J Emerg Med* 6:21, 1988.

ACUTE CORONARY SYNDROMES (ACUTE MYOCARDIAL INFARCTION AND UNSTABLE ANGINA)

Acute coronary syndrome (ACS), including acute myocardial infarction (AMI), accounts for 650,000 hospital admissions each year and is one of the leading causes of death in the United States. A missed diagnosis of AMI can have fatal or debilitating consequences. Furthermore, a missed diagnosis of AMI is the most common and most costly cause of malpractice litigation in emergency medicine. Reasons for a missed diagnosis of AMI include failure to consider the diagnosis in an atypical presentation; inappropriately relying on a single, normal ECG or serum marker for AMI to rule out infarction; and (perhaps) misinterpreting or not ordering appropriate tests (such as an ECG).

Epidemiologic risk factors for coronary artery disease include history of hypertension, diabetes, smoking, elevated serum cholesterol, male sex, age older than 40, and family history of premature coronary artery disease. However, these do not effectively predict acute ischemia in the ED. The most important diagnostic factors in the ED are (1) symptoms consistent with AMI, (2) past history of ischemic heart disease, and (3) an abnormal ECG (see later). Up to one half of patients have unstable angina before AMI. Cocaine abuse can induce myocardial ischemia in younger individuals who have no other risk factors.

SYMPTOMS

- Chest pain ++++ in acute coronary syndromes (AMI or ischemia) is typically heavy, squeezing, tight, or pressure-like in quality but may be sharp ++, burning, or indigestion-like ++, pleuritic +, or even absent.
- Painless AMI is more common in elderly people and patients with diabetes. The frequency of chest pain decreases steadily after age 65 to 70 and it is present in only 50% at age 80, after which dyspnea is the most common symptom. Pain is typically localized to the retrosternal area or, less often, the left chest. It may localize to the epigastrium or back. It may radiate to, or even primarily localize to, the arm, shoulder(s), jaw, or neck +++. The pain is usually not positional +. The upper limit of constant pain duration is difficult to define but is usually measured in hours, not days.
- Dyspnea
- Diaphoresis +++
- Nausea +++
- Dizziness
- Palpitations
- Apprehension
- Syncope
- Sudden death

SIGNS

- Tachycardia (+++ anterior MIs)
- Bradycardia (+++ inferior MIs)
- Diaphoresis ++
- Premature beats
- Hypertension or hypotension
- Vomiting
- Murmurs; a new murmur with pathologic qualities may indicate papillary muscle dysfunction or rupture (producing mitral regurgitation) or perforation of the interventricular septum.
- Gallops
- Rales
- Altered mental status
- Evidence of peripheral vascular disease (e.g., diminished pedal pulses, femoral bruits, or claudication) also increases the likelihood of coronary artery disease.
- Signs of cerebral ischemia may coexist in 10% of elderly patients.

WORKUP

- A 12-lead ECG should be performed without delay. The ECG may be normal ++ or reveal nondiagnostic or nonspecific ST segment

CHAPTER 7

or T wave changes ++. An abnormal ECG places the patient at high risk for AMI and other complications.

- ST segment elevation of more than 1 mm in two contiguous leads along with chest pain suggests acute infarction +++.
- ST depression (also of more than 1 mm) may indicate ischemia or a non–Q wave MI (a non–Q wave MI evolves in one third of patients with chest pain and ST depression).
- New bundle branch block in a clinical setting consistent with ACS should also be regarded as evidence of ischemia. Ischemia is difficult to identify in the presence of preexisting left bundle branch block (LBBB) or paced ventricular rhythm, both of which produce ST elevations. Criteria that, if present with LBBB, may aid in the detection of ischemia or infarction but, if absent, do not rule these out include (1) ST segment elevation of more than 1 mm concordant with the QRS complex (sensitivity ++, specificity 92% to 94%), (2) ST segment depression of more than 1 mm in lead V1, V2, or V3 (sensitivity ++, specificity 82% to 96%), and (3) ST segment elevation of more than 5 mm discordant with the QRS complex (sensitivity +++, specificity 88% to 92%).
- If the initial ECG is nondiagnostic and the patient remains symptomatic, the ECG should be repeated to assess for dynamic changes. Additional tracings should also be considered after therapeutic interventions as well as after changes in clinical condition.
- Right-sided chest leads can be useful in identifying acute ischemia in the right ventricle and are particularly warranted in patients with inferior MI or a hypotensive response to nitrates.
- Continuous ECG or ST segment trend monitoring is a new technology with potential for detecting changes without repetition of the 12-lead ECG.
- Chest x-ray is useful, especially for identifying CHF or another potential cause of chest pain such as pneumonia, pneumothorax, and aortic dissection.
- Serum markers of myocardial infarction such as troponins I and T and creatine kinase, myocardial bound (CKMB), are useful for diagnosis and prognosis but are not adequately sensitive when measured on a single occasion +++ to rule out AMI or ACS. Troponin and CK show similar sensitivities and timing from onset of ischemia to release; however, troponin remains elevated for several days after an event. An elevated troponin is associated with increased risk of complications.
- CBC, INR, PTT, electrolytes including magnesium, BUN, creatinine, and glucose are typically determined, but results rarely affect ED treatment and they are not necessary before initiation of therapy.
- Serum basic natriuretic peptide (BNP) measurement may be useful for confirming the presence of CHF in patients with respiratory symptoms.

- Markers of inflammation such as myeloperoxidase, CRP, and ESR have no current role in the ED management of chest pain.
- Echocardiography may occasionally provide evidence of ischemia in patients who show no other diagnostic evidence. Sensitivity and specificity, however, are inadequate to warrant generalized use.
- Early stress testing may expedite risk stratification and enable early (8 to 12 hours) discharge for some low-risk patients.
- Radionuclide scanning (such as technetium sestamibi, which irreversibly binds ischemic tissue) may be useful in evaluating low-risk ED patients presenting with clinically atypical chest pain ++++.

COMMENTS AND TREATMENT CONSIDERATIONS
CAUTIONS
1. Never use either nitroglycerin or "GI cocktail" as a *diagnostic* test because they are neither sensitive nor specific for myocardial or GI disease. (They can, of course, be used where appropriate as *treatment*.)
2. Patients with panic disorder, histrionic traits, or psychosis may also have AMI.
3. Overall, many presentations of AMI are atypical, especially in diabetic, elderly, or female patients.
4. Beware of the patient who minimizes significant symptoms.
5. Chest wall tenderness or partial or full reproducibility of chest pain (with pressure applied to the chest) can be present in patients with AMI ++.

Physicians managing patients with an ACS in the ED should be well acquainted with the prevailing therapeutic protocols in their facility in order to coordinate care appropriately with the admitting physician. Barring contraindications, all patients with suspected ACS should receive aspirin (325 mg) and beta-blockers (e.g., metoprolol 5 mg every 5 minutes to a total of 15 mg if heart rate and blood pressure tolerate). Low-flow oxygen is indicated for hypoxia. Nitrates (sublingual nitroglycerin, nitroglycerin paste to skin, or intravenous nitroglycerin) are indicated for control of symptoms. Morphine sulfate may also be used for control of pain. Patients with cocaine-associated chest pain should also be treated with benzodiazepines and may in rare circumstances require an alpha-adrenergic blocker.

Immediate thrombolysis or a percutaneous coronary intervention (PCI) should be considered for the following: (1) chest pain that lasts more than 30 minutes and less than 12 hours and (2) ST elevation greater than 1 mm in two contiguous limb leads, ST elevation greater than 2 mm in two contiguous precordial leads, or new bundle branch block. Choice of revascularization method depends

CHAPTER 7

on availability and experience at the institution and on the presence or absence of contraindications to individual methods. Patients treated with a thrombolytic or angioplasty should be anticoagulated with either enoxaparin or heparin (depending on age and renal function). Although use of a platelet glycoprotein IIb/IIIa inhibitor is recommended by some, their role in ACS patients who are not undergoing PCI is unsupported by current evidence. The use of clopidogrel (Plavix) is also controversial; it may have some role in high-acuity patients.

A diagnosis of AMI is eventually rejected in 5% to 10% of patients who meet the criteria for thrombolysis. The majority of these have unstable angina +++ or other diagnoses, including pericarditis, pancreatitis, esophagitis, and aortic dissection.

REFERENCES

American Heart Association/American College of Cardiology: Guidelines for the diagnosis of ST-elevation acute myocardial infarction, www.acc.org/clinical/guidelines/stemi/index.pdf.

Andersen HR, Nielsen TT, Rasmussen K, et al: A comparison of coronary angioplasty with fibrinolytic therapy in acute myocardial infarction, *N Engl J Med* 349:733, 2003.

Antman EM, Anbe DT, Armstrong PW, et al: ACC/AHA guidelines for the management of patients with ST-elevation myocardial infarction, *J Am Coll Cardiol* 44:671, 2004.

Bayer AJ, Chadha JS, Farag RR, Pathy MS: Changing presentation of myocardial infarction with increasing old age, *J Am Geriatr Soc* 34:263, 1986.

Braunwald E: Application of current guidelines to the management of unstable angina and non-ST elevation myocardial infarction, *Circulation* 108(SIII):28, 2003.

Gitter MJ, Goldsmith SR, Dunbar DN, Sharkey SW: Cocaine and chest pain: clinical features and outcome of patients hospitalized to rule out myocardial infarction, *Ann Intern Med* 115:277, 1991.

GUSTO Angiographic Investigators: The effects of tissue plasminogen activator, streptokinase, or both on coronary artery patency, ventricular function, and survival after acute myocardial infarction, *N Engl J Med* 329:1615, 1993.

ISIS-2: Randomized trial of intravenous atenolol among 16,027 cases of suspected acute myocardial infarction, *Lancet* 2:57, 1986.

Ohman EM, Armstrong PW, Christenson RH, et al: Cardiac troponin T levels for risk stratification in acute myocardial ischemia, *N Engl J Med* 335:1333, 1996.

Schriger DL, Herbert ME: Platelet glycoprotein inhibitors in patients with medically managed acute coronary syndrome: does the enthusiasm exceed the science? *Ann Emerg Med* 38:249, 2001.

Sgarbossa EB, Pinski SL, Barbagelata A, et al: Electrocardiographic diagnosis of evolving acute myocardial infarction in the presence of left bundle-branch block, *N Engl J Med* 334:481, 1996.

 PULMONARY EMBOLUS

Pulmonary embolus (PE) is caused by an obstruction of flow in the pulmonary arteries because of arterial occlusion. It results most commonly from the embolization of a blood clot from the deep veins of the legs (the subject of the following discussion). Fat (after a long bone fracture), air, amniotic fluid, blood clots from another location, and other substances are rare causes of PE. At least one of the following risk factors is present in 90% of patients with PE: immobility, heart disease, cancer, estrogen therapy, previous deep venous thrombosis (DVT) or PE, hypercoagulability, or abnormal thrombolysis. Not all patients with cancer or hypercoagulability are known at the time of presentation.

SYMPTOMS
- Chest pain +++ (two thirds of patients with chest pain describe pleuritic pain)
- Dyspnea ++++
- Cough ++
- Hemoptysis ++
- The entire classic triad of dyspnea, pleuritic chest pain, and hemoptysis is uncommon ++.
- Syncope ++

SIGNS
- Tachypnea >16/min ++++
- Rales +++
- P2 >A2 +++
- Tachycardia +++
- Fever (low grade) +++
- Diaphoresis +++
- Hypotension (in massive PE)
- Hypoxia (by pulse oximetry)
- Pleural friction rub
- Evidence of DVT (calf swelling—one calf with circumference 2 cm greater than opposite calf) ++

WORKUP
- The chest x-ray is abnormal in most patients with PE, but findings are typically nonspecific. The chest x-ray may show atelectasis +++, pleural effusion +++, pleural-based opacities ++,

CHAPTER 7

elevated hemidiaphragm, decreased vascularity ++, or prominent central artery ++.

- ECG pattern of S1-Q3-T3 is present in a small minority of patients. Most ECGs are abnormal in PE, but nearly half reveal only non-specific ST-T wave changes. ECG may, however, occasionally be helpful in diagnosing other pathologic conditions such as MI or pericarditis.

- A normal ABG (and, by extrapolation, a normal pulse oximetry reading) does not exclude the possibility of PE. Although the ABG may reveal hypoxia [Pao_2 <60 (++)] or an increased A-aDo_2, patients with even a massive PE can have a Pao_2 >80 (++) and even a normal A-a gradient (++).

- Plasma D-dimer levels measured by ELISA are useful when interpreted in the context of a protocol that includes an assessment of pretest probability, using either clinical judgment or a formal scale such as the Wells or Geneva criteria. A normal D-dimer alone is insufficiently sensitive to rule out PE in a patient with a moderate or (especially) high prior clinical probability. However, a normal D-dimer by ELISA in the presence of a low clinical probability of PE has an excellent negative predictive value and can rule out PE in such a patient. The D-dimer should thus be measured only in patients with a low prior probability. Only the D-dimer by ELISA should be used in this manner. The lower sensitivities of the latex and whole blood agglutination assays make their use inadvisable. It is important that clinicians be aware which assay technique is used in their hospital. Because of its poor specificity, an abnormal D-dimer should never be considered *diagnostic* of thromboembolism and always requires further workup.

- A ventilation-perfusion (V/Q) scan, which is most likely to be helpful in ruling out disease, should be interpreted in Bayesian fashion. A completely "normal" V/Q scan essentially rules out PE (except perhaps in a patient with a high prior probability), and a "low-probability" V/Q scan is generally sufficient only in the context of a low pretest probability. A low-probability scan without consideration of pretest probability is falsely negative in 10% to 15% of patients. A low-probability or intermediate-probability scan does not rule out PE in a patient with a moderate or high pretest probability.

- Spiral CT angiography, which is increasingly being used in place of V/Q scintigraphy, is most likely to be helpful in ruling in PE (or occasionally in identifying an alternative explanation for a patient's presentation). A clearly positive CT, in the hands of an experienced reader, is generally true positive, and a negative CT can exclude PE in a patient with a low pretest probability. Its use in ruling out PE in the setting of moderate prior probability is controversial, and many experts believe that it is not sufficiently sensitive to rule out disease in a patient with high prior probability.

- Pulmonary angiography remains the "gold standard" for diagnosis of PE—at least in theory—but it is not commonly used in most practices because it is time and labor intensive; entails risk, especially to patients with significant baseline cardiopulmonary disease (up to 0.5% mortality, 6% complications); and is inconclusive in up to 3%.

- Doppler flow and duplex scanning are currently the standard tests for establishing DVT, although contrast venography remains the theoretical gold standard. In a patient with symptoms or signs of DVT, the results of these tests may indicate the need for anticoagulation, thus obviating the need for other (specific) workup of PE.

COMMENTS AND TREATMENT CONSIDERATIONS

Standard therapy for PE includes early anticoagulation (consider before diagnosis is confirmed if suspicion is high and likelihood of complications low) with intravenous unfractionated heparin (UH). Ideally, heparin should be dosed by a weight-based protocol; this is followed by oral anticoagulation, which can be begun on day 1. Low-molecular-weight heparin (LMWH) is as safe and effective as UH, easier to administer (no intravenous line required) and monitor (no PT or PTT necessary), and therefore can allow earlier hospital discharge. Although the acquisition cost of LMWH is far higher, the cost can be more than offset if it results in fewer days of hospitalization.

Thrombolytic therapy or surgical embolectomy is reserved for severe PE (cardiogenic shock, pulmonary hypertension, and right ventricular strain) because of high complication rates. Thrombolytics should generally be administered either before heparin or after heparin is discontinued and PTT is less than 80. Surgical consultation for a vena cava filter may be considered when medical treatment is contraindicated.

REFERENCES

The PISA-PED Investigators: Invasive and noninvasive diagnosis of pulmonary embolus. Preliminary results of the Prospective Investigative Study of Acute Pulmonary Embolism Diagnosis (PISA-PED), *Chest* 107(Suppl):33, 1995.

Goodman LR, Curtin JJ, Mewissen MW, et al: Detection of pulmonary embolism in patients with unresolved clinical and scintigraphic diagnosis: helical CT versus angiography, *AJR Am J Roentgenol* 164:1369, 1995.

Kline JA, Johns KL, Coluciello SA, Israel EG: New diagnostic tests for pulmonary embolism, *Ann Emerg Med* 35:168, 2000.

CHAPTER 7

Perrier A, Desmarais S, Goehring C, et al: D-dimer testing for suspected pulmonary embolism in outpatients, *Am J Respir Crit Care Med* 156:492, 1997.

PIOPED Investigators: Value of the ventilation perfusion scan in the diagnosis of pulmonary embolism, *JAMA* 263:2753, 1990.

Rathbun SW, Raskob GE, Whitsett TL: Sensitivity and specificity of helical computed tomography in the diagnosis of pulmonary embolism: a systematic review, *Ann Intern Med* 132:227, 2000.

Roy PM, Colombet I, Durieux P, et al: Systematic review and meta-analysis of strategies for the diagnosis of suspected pulmonary embolism, *BMJ* 331:259, 2005.

Stein PD, Goldhaber SZ, Henry JW, Miller AC: Arterial blood gas analysis in the assessment of suspected acute pulmonary embolism, *Chest* 109:78, 1996.

Stein PD, Saltzman HA, Weg JG: Clinical characteristics of patients with acute pulmonary embolism, *Am J Cardiol* 68:1723, 1991.

Wolf SJ, McCubbin TR, Feldhaus KM, et al: Prospective validation of Wells criteria in the evaluation of patients with suspected pulmonary embolism, *Ann Emerg Med* 44:503, 2004.

 TRAUMATIC AORTIC RUPTURE

Aortic rupture is usually caused by a sudden impact or deceleration (e.g., a high-speed motor vehicle collision, a fall from a height, or a pedestrian struck by an automobile). Most of the victims of aortic rupture die in the field before transport. The majority of those who reach the ED may survive if they are diagnosed and treated promptly. Many patients are unconscious or have other serious injuries that can mask symptoms of great vessel injury. Great vessel injury should be considered particularly for an injured passenger who struck the steering wheel or who was thrown from the vehicle.

SYMPTOMS
- Chest pain +++
- Dyspnea ++
- Back pain ++
- Hoarseness
- Dysphagia
- Painful extremity

SIGNS
- Abrasions
- Ecchymosis
- Tenderness of the chest wall

- Pseudo-coarctation—elevated blood pressure in the upper extremities with absent femoral pulses ++
- Harsh precordial or interscapular murmur ++

WORKUP

- Supine chest x-ray—wide mediastinum (>8 cm at the level of the aortic knob +++, nonspecific)
- Supine chest x-ray—blurred, indistinct, or wide aortic arch ++++, nonspecific
- Supine chest x-ray—absent aortopulmonary window, wide right paratracheal stripe (>5 mm), abnormal or absent left paratracheal stripe, tracheal deviation to the right, nasogastric tube deviation to the right, apical pleural cap, or downward displacement of the left main stem bronchus
- Fractures of the first two ribs may be a sign of trauma to the upper chest; however, this finding in isolation does not predict aortic trauma.
- None of these signs, or any combination of them, is 100% sensitive or specific. If any are present in the proper clinical setting, further imaging is necessary, although a completely normal upright chest x-ray suggests that aortic rupture is very unlikely.
- Available methods for determining the presence or absence of aortic disruption include helical thoracic CT, MRI, transesophageal echocardiography (TEE), and aortography (the gold standard).
- In stable patients, a helical CT or an MRI scan is almost always sufficient.
- Aortography may be necessary for patients with an indeterminate CT or MRI scan, high clinical concern despite a negative CT, or possibly for definition of the anatomy of lesions identified on positive CT or MRI.
- TEE may be useful (where available and feasible) in unstable patients, especially those requiring immediate operative intervention for other injuries.

COMMENTS AND TREATMENT CONSIDERATIONS

Treatment for traumatic aortic rupture is surgical repair without delay.

REFERENCES

Alkadhi H, Wildermuth S, Desbiolles L, et al: Vascular emergencies of the thorax after blunt and iatrogenic trauma: multi-detector row CT and three-dimensional imaging, *Radiographics* 24:1239, 2004.

Gavant ML, Flick P, Menke P, Gold RE: CT aortography of thoracic aortic rupture, *Am J Roentgenol* 166:955, 1996.

CHAPTER 7

O'Conor CE: Diagnosing traumatic rupture of the thoracic aorta in the emergency department, *Emerg Med J* 21:414, 2004.

Smith MD, Cassidy M, Souther S, et al: Transesophageal echocardiography in the diagnosis of traumatic rupture of the aorta, *N Engl J Med* 332:356, 1995.

Sturm JT, Hankins DG, Young G: Thoracic aortography following blunt chest trauma, *Am J Emerg Med* 8:92, 1990.

Warren RL, Akins CW, Conn AK, et al: Acute traumatic disruption of the thoracic aorta: emergency department management, *Ann Emerg Med* 21:391, 1992.

Woodring JH, Loh FK, Kryscio RJ: Mediastinal hemorrhage: an evaluation of radiographic manifestations, *Radiology* 151:15, 1984.

 ACUTE AORTIC DISSECTION

Acute aortic dissection (AAD) is dissection of the media of the aortic wall by a column of blood. It occurs most commonly in the thoracic aorta, and the age of onset is usually at least 50 years. A history of hypertension is usually (80%) present. Aortic dissection is rare in those younger than 40 years unless other predisposing conditions are present, such as Marfan's syndrome, Ehlers-Danlos syndrome, congenital heart disease, iatrogenic trauma (e.g., cardiac catheterization), bicuspid aortic valve, or pregnancy. AAD should also be considered when acute dysfunction of more than one organ system is observed.

SYMPTOMS
- Chest pain is the most common symptom ++++ and is classically sudden in onset and ripping or tearing in quality.
- Anterior chest pain is more common in ascending aortic dissection ++++; back pain is more common in descending aortic dissection ++++. Coexisting anterior chest pain and back pain are seen less frequently.
- Pain may migrate as the dissection progresses and may also involve the limbs, particularly if the dissection obstructs the origin of a limb vessel.
- Neurologic deficits ++
- Syncope +
- Nausea
- Diaphoresis
- Lightheadedness

SIGNS
- Hypertension (early)
- Hypotension (late)

- Tachycardia
- Blood pressure differentials between extremities or pulse deficits in extremities +++
- Aortic insufficiency (+++ in patients with ascending aorta involvement)
- Murmur over the thoracic inlet
- Tamponade
- Acute stroke + to ++
- Hemoptysis, hematemesis, Horner's syndrome, and SVC syndrome (rare)

WORKUP
- Laboratory tests are of little value except for a type and cross-match and a baseline hemoglobin or hematocrit.
- Chest x-rays are abnormal in most patients, but findings may be subtle. Mediastinal widening +++ and an indistinct aortic knob +++ are the two features most useful for predicting dissection. Tracheal or esophageal deviation, irregular aortic contour +++, change in aortic diameter compared with previous films, and left pleural effusion ++ have been reported. The calcium sign, or displacement of calcified intima (calcium ring > 6 mm from outer border of the aorta), is infrequent +.
- The best choice for establishing a definitive diagnosis is contro-versial. Because mortality is high and occurs quickly (50% within 48 hours of onset), the choice may be dictated by which test is most rapidly available (Table 7–1). The preference of the surgeon who would provide definitive care for proximal dissections is also important.

COMMENTS AND TREATMENT CONSIDERATIONS
Treatment should begin before confirmation of the diagnosis where clinically indicated. The goal is to minimize further progression of the dissection through reduction of the shear forces on the aortic wall, which are a function of the blood pressure and its rate of change (dP/dt). The agents of choice are a combination of the titratable vasodilator sodium nitroprusside and the intravenous beta-antagonist esmolol. Alternative agents include labetalol. The target systolic blood pressure is 100 to 110 mm Hg, with a heart rate of 60. Early consultation with a cardiothoracic surgeon is essential. The definitive management of proximal dissection is generally surgical, whereas for distal dissection it is often medical. Even proximal dissections require aggressive medical management in the first few hours; however, some patients with distal dissection need operative repair. Caution: anticoagulation or thrombolysis following a misdiagnosis as MI or PE can lead to death.

CHAPTER 7

TABLE 7–1
DIAGNOSTIC TESTS FOR AORTIC DISSECTION

TEST	COMMENTS
Aortography +++++	Gold standard Also evaluates valves and branches 95% accurate Invasive, time consuming; may miss thrombosed false channel
Spiral chest CT +++++	Generally rapidly available and often the first test of choice
Transesophageal echocardiography +++++	Can be done at bedside for unstable patients Accuracy operator dependent
MRI +++++	May be preferable for stable patients Sensitivity 90% to 100%; specificity 94% to 99% Visualizes origins of branches Time consuming; difficult to monitor patient Availability varies, may result in delay

REFERENCES

Hagan PG, Nienaber CA, Isselbacher EM: The International Registry of Acute Aortic Dissection (IRAD): new insights into an old disease, *JAMA* 283:897, 2000.

Mukherjee D, Eagle KA: Aortic dissection—an update, *Curr Probl Cardiol* 30:287, 2005.

Sarasin FP, Louis-Simonet M, Gaspoz JM, Junod AF: Detecting acute thoracic aortic dissection in the emergency department: time constraints and choice of the optimal diagnostic test, *Ann Emerg Med* 28:278, 1996.

Sommer T, Fehske W, Holzknecht N, et al: Aortic dissection: a comparative study of diagnosis with spiral CT, multiplanar transesophageal echocardiography, and MR imaging, *Radiology* 199:347, 1996.

 ESOPHAGEAL RUPTURE

Esophageal rupture is a rare but highly life-threatening condition. Because early symptoms can be nonspecific, less than half are correctly diagnosed within the first 12 hours, after which mortality is 25%. Mortality exceeds 60% after 24 hours.

Spontaneous esophageal rupture, or Boerhaave's syndrome, occurs when esophageal pressure is significantly increased (e.g., vomiting against a closed glottis). This usually creates a small, vertical tear of the lower esophagus (90%) on the left side (90%).

Other phenomena reported to induce an esophageal tear include hiccups, childbirth, weight lifting, forceful swallowing, and blunt trauma. The causes of esophageal rupture include Boerhaave's syndrome (15%), trauma (20%), foreign bodies (15%), and iatrogenic causes (50%).

Symptoms may mimic those of (and often lead to misdiagnosis as) perforated ulcer, acute MI, dissecting aortic aneurysm, pulmonary embolism, acute pancreatitis, spontaneous pneumothorax, lung abscess, biliary colic, mesenteric vascular occlusion, incarcerated diaphragmatic hernia, and other entities. Although esophageal rupture is most common after age 50 and is rare in children, it can occur at any age.

SYMPTOMS
- Chest pain +++++, commonly severe, acute, and pleuritic that is generally left sided and preceded by vomiting
- Abdominal or back pain
- Dyspnea
- Dysphagia
- Nausea

SIGNS
- Vital signs may be normal early in the course of this disease but progress to shock.
- Tachypnea
- Fever
- Hamman's sign ++
- Chest examination provides evidence of pleural effusion.
- Subcutaneous emphysema +++
- Meckler's triad of vomiting, lower chest pain, and subcutaneous emphysema may be present.

WORKUP
- Chest x-ray ++++. The most common findings are effusion and infiltrate. Although effusion is more common in this entity, a patient with chest pain, dyspnea, and an effusion is more likely to have a PE (based on the prevalence of the two diseases). "V sign of Naclerio," a V-shaped hypodense area outlining fascial planes behind the heart, may be an early radiographic sign ++. Mediastinal emphysema (pneumomediastinum) may be present +++.
- Esophagography using a water-soluble contrast agent (e.g., Gastrografin) may be diagnostic ++++. If it is negative and concern for the diagnosis persists, proceed to a second study.
- Esophagoscopy
- CT (with or without oral contrast)

- ECG is helpful only to screen for myocardial ischemia as an alternative diagnosis.
- Pleurocentesis may yield the diagnosis when performed. For pleural fluid studies, a pH less than 6.0 is an indicator of esophageal rupture; when esophagography findings are negative, methylene blue given orally may be detected in pleural drainage.
- Routine laboratory tests are of no value in making this diagnosis.

COMMENTS AND TREATMENT CONSIDERATIONS

Treatment of esophageal rupture requires aggressive supportive care, including drainage of gastric and pleural contents and intravenous antibiotics. Early thoracotomy with primary surgical closure of the esophageal defect is usually necessary in spontaneous or traumatic esophageal rupture. Conservative therapy is employed in some cases associated with iatrogenic or foreign body causes and in very late presentations of spontaneous rupture, in which operative mortality approaches that of supportive care.

REFERENCES

Hill AG, Tiu AT, Martin IG: Boerhaave's syndrome: 10 years experience and review of the literature, *ANZ J Surg* 73:1008, 2003.

Vial CM, Whyte RI: Boerhaave's syndrome: diagnosis and treatment, *Surg Clin North Am* 85:515, 2005.

Younes Z, Johnson DA: The spectrum of spontaneous and iatrogenic esophageal injury: perforations, Mallory-Weiss tears, and hematomas, *J Clin Gastroenterol* 29:306, 1999.

 PNEUMONIA

Pneumonia is common and can range from mild to life threatening; depending on the etiology and general health of the patient, it may be treatable with outpatient antibiotics or require admission to the ICU. Patients with asthma, COPD, diabetes, CHF, renal failure, asplenic state (splenectomy or sickle cell patients), chronic liver disease, predilection for aspiration, malnutrition, recent hospitalization (<1 year), and age older than 65 are at particular risk. In winter, influenza pneumonia (potentially severe and complicated by staphylococcal infection) and respiratory syncytial virus (RSV) should be considered in adults and children, respectively. A history of occupational exposure to animals may suggest unusual but potentially severe forms of pneumonia, such as hantavirus (rodent droppings), plague (rodents), tularemia (rabbits), Q fever, psittacosis (pet birds), or avian flu (poultry). History of recent travel to Asia may suggest the possibility of severe acute respiratory syndrome (SARS), and exposure to altitude may cause high-altitude pulmonary edema (HAPE), which may be mistaken for pneumonia. Foreign body aspiration is particularly prevalent in patients younger than 3 and involves food in 61%. Tuberculosis (and respiratory isolation) should be considered in patients at risk for this disease. Pneumonia caused by a bioterrorism agent may also need to be considered in the appropriate context.

SYMPTOMS
- Cough
- Sputum production
- Pleuritic chest pain
- Fever
- Dyspnea/shortness of breath (less frequent in elderly patients)
- Altered mental status

SIGNS
- Fever
- Tachypnea
- Tachycardia
- Diaphoresis
- Crackles
- Egophony
- Dullness to percussion
- Pleural friction rub
- Wasting
- Cyanosis
- Altered mental status
- Hypotension
- Decreased urine output
- Abdominal signs in elderly and very young patients

WORKUP
- Chest x-ray: Standard posteroanterior and lateral (if possible) chest films should be obtained in patients whose symptoms and signs suggest the possibility of pneumonia. When only an antero-posterior film can be obtained, special attention should be paid to the heart shadow, behind which an infiltrate may hide. Plain films of children with a history of foreign body aspiration are normal in 33%; abnormal x-rays findings reveal obstructive emphysema (66%), mediastinal shift (55%), pneumonia (26%), atelectasis (18%), or radiopaque objects (only 3%).
- Arterial blood gases are not useful for diagnosis but may aid in assessing ventilatory status.
- Complete blood count is not generally useful unless there is risk of neutropenia (neutrophil count <1000/ml).

- Creatinine is indicated for sick patients in whom antibiotics may cause renal toxicity or require renal clearance.
- Blood cultures have a low yield in patients who are likely to be treated as outpatients. Cultures are usually negative and seldom alter therapy for admitted patients. Higher yields are seen in severely ill patients, although this infrequently influences management.
- Skin tests for tuberculosis should be obtained in patients at risk (homeless, alcoholic, immigrant, HIV infected). Patients who have been vaccinated with BCG may have a false-positive test. Patients with symptoms and x-ray findings consistent with active tuberculosis should be isolated while awaiting skin test and microbiologic results.
- Sputum cultures are seldom useful because of the difficulty in obtaining an adequate (uncontaminated) specimen and the high incidence of false positives. Sputum induction for AFB or PCP should be done in a negative-pressure room approved for such procedures.
- Thoracentesis should be considered when effusion accompanies pneumonia so that the need for drainage can be determined. The most important test to obtain on the pleural fluid is the pH (pH < 7.0 suggests need for chest tube drainage). Also important are cell count with differential, LDH, protein, glucose, Gram's stain, culture, and AFB and fungal stains and cultures.

COMMENTS AND TREATMENT CONSIDERATIONS

Multiple severity scoring systems, including the Multiple Pneumonia Outcome Research Trial (PORT) and British Thoracic Society (BTS) scoring systems, have been devised and evaluated in community-acquired pneumonia (CAP) in an attempt to facilitate decisions regarding outpatient versus inpatient management and general ward or ICU care. Findings that suggest the need for admission include a pulse >100 to 125 (in adults), respiratory rate (RR) > 20 to 30 (in adults), temperature >38.3° C, hypotension, evidence of extrapulmonary involvement, or acutely altered mental status. Severe pneumonia, suggesting the need for ICU admission, is indicated by a respiratory rate (in adults) >30, shock, and urine output less than 20 ml/hr. Radiographic features that predict increased mortality include multilobar involvement, cavitation, rapid spreading if >50% increase in 48 hours, and effusion.

An apical infiltrate requires consideration of reactivation tuberculosis; cavitation suggests anaerobic abscess, staphylococcus, or *Pseudomonas* infection. Lymphadenopathy on chest x-ray suggests tuberculosis, fungal disease, or neoplasm. Tuberculosis may have an atypical appearance in HIV patients. Although possibly suggestive, the pattern of infiltrate does not reliably distinguish between etiologies for pneumonia.

Choice of therapy should be directed toward pathogens suspected primarily on the basis of epidemiology and the patient's clinical status and should not be delayed in a seriously ill patient. Early administration of antibiotics (less than 8 hours from hospital arrival) has been shown to reduce mortality by 20% to 30% in patients 65 years of age or older.

The increasing prevalence of resistant strains of pneumococcus (and others) makes penicillin and amoxicillin obsolete. A macrolide antibiotic is generally adequate for outpatient therapy in an otherwise healthy patient. For hospitalized, nonimmunosuppressed patients, initial therapy with a combination of a macrolide (erythromycin or azithromycin) and a second- or third-generation cephalosporin is usually adequate. Single coverage with a fluoro-quinolone is an alternative. Consider the addition of vancomycin to cover resistant species of *Streptococcus pneumoniae*. ICU patients should be administered an extended-coverage third-generation cephalosporin (or beta-lactam/lactamase inhibitor) plus a macrolide or fluoroquinolone. Patients with suspected aspiration should receive additional coverage for anaerobic infection with clindamycin or metronidazole.

Patients with known or suspected *Pneumocystis* and a PaO$_2$ <70 should be treated with corticosteroids (prednisone 40 mg by mouth, then twice a day, then taper) 15 to 30 minutes before spe-cific antimicrobial therapy (e.g., trimethoprim/sulfamethoxazole, 15 mg of trimethoprim component/kg/day IV divided q6-8h).

CHAPTER 7

REFERENCES

American College of Emergency Physicians: Clinical policy for the management and risk stratification of community-acquired pneumonia in adults in the emergency department, *Ann Emerg Med* 38:107, 2001.

American Thoracic Society: Guidelines for the initial management of adults with community-acquired pneumonia: diagnosis, assessment of severity, and initial antimicrobial therapy, *Am Rev Respir Dis* 148:1418, 1993.

Bartlett JG, Dowell SF, Mandell LA: Practice guidelines for the man-agement of community-acquired pneumonia in adults, *Clin Infect Dis J* 31:347, 2000.

Bartlett JG, Mundy LM: Community-acquired pneumonia, *N Engl J Med* 333:1618, 1995.

Burton EM, Brick WG, Hall JD, et al: Tracheobronchial foreign body aspiration in children, *South Med J* 89:195, 1996.

Chalasani NP, Valdecanas MA, Gopal AK, et al: Clinical utility of blood cultures in adult patients with community-acquired pneumonia without defined underlying risks, *Chest* 108:932, 1995.

Fine MJ, Auble TE, Yealy DM, et al: A prediction rule to identify low-risk patients with community acquired pneumonia, *N Engl J Med* 336:243, 1997.

Marie TJ, Lau CY, Wheeler, SL, et al: A controlled trial of a critical pathway for treatment of community-acquired pneumonia, *JAMA* 283:749, 2000.

Meehan TP, Fine MJ, Krumholz HM, et al: Quality of care, process, and outcomes in elderly patients with pneumonia, *JAMA* 278:2080, 1997.

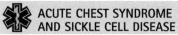

ACUTE CHEST SYNDROME AND SICKLE CELL DISEASE

Acute chest syndrome is a clinical syndrome found in sickle cell patients that may lead to death.

SYMPTOMS
- Severe chest pain ++++
- Fever ++++
- Shortness of breath +++
- Bone pain +++

SIGNS
- Tachypnea
- Rhonchi +++
- Hypoxia
- Elevated temperature

WORKUP
- Chest x-ray may show pulmonary infiltrates +++.
- ABG, if needed, to assess ventilatory status (Pao$_2$ <80 +++)
- Hematocrit shows anemia; reticulocyte count should be elevated.

COMMENTS AND TREATMENT CONSIDERATIONS
The cause of acute chest syndrome is uncertain; it may represent pulmonary infarction, fat embolism, or infection. Cultures of blood and sputum are positive only in a small percentage of patients. Treatment may include intravenous hydration; oxygen; broad-spectrum antibiotics covering *Staphylococcus aureus*, *Mycoplasma*, *Streptococcus pneumoniae*, *and Haemophilus influenzae* (particularly if questionable vaccination history); heparin; and transfusion. Because the effect of treatment on outcome is not clear, patients may need to be admitted to an ICU.

REFERENCES

Stuart MJ, Setty BN: Acute chest syndrome of sickle cell disease: new light on an old problem, *Curr Opin Hematol* 8:111, 2001.

van Agtmael MA, Cheng JD, Nossent HC: Acute chest syndrome in adult Afro-Caribbean patients with sickle cell disease, *Arch Intern Med* 154:557, 1994.

Vichinsky EP, Neumayr LD, Earles AN, et al: Causes and outcomes of acute chest syndrome in sickle cell disease, *N Engl J Med* 342:1855, 2000.

 PERICARDITIS

SYMPTOMS

- Chest pain is the most common presenting symptom +++.
  The pain is usually pleuritic but is sometimes dull; it may radiate to the left trapezius, is exacerbated by supine posture, and is often alleviated by sitting up. The pain may last hours or days and is usually constant but may be intermittent.
- Dyspnea ++
- Fever
- Fatigue
- Malaise
- Abdominal pain
- Syncope

SIGNS

- Pericardial friction rub +++, classically of three components, is best heard over the left sternal border and is usually accentuated by sitting up and leaning forward. Only one or two components may be present, and it may be audible only intermittently or over a limited area. When only a single component is present, it can be confused with a murmur.

WORKUP

- ECG may be abnormal ++++. Changes may evolve in four stages (Table 7–2).
- Ratio of the ST segment elevation to T wave amplitude (ST/T) of 0.25 or greater suggests pericarditis.
- Echocardiography is useful for demonstrating pericardial fluid (effusion, blood) and for determining whether tamponade is present or imminent (see Pericardial Effusion and Tamponade).
- Erythrocyte sedimentation rate (Westergren) may be elevated (over 50 mm/hr) +++ but is nonspecific.
- Chest x-rays are normal unless there is an effusion of 250 ml or other conditions coexist.

CHAPTER 7

TABLE 7-2
ECG EVOLUTION OF ACUTE PERICARDITIS (LEADS I, II, aVL, aVF, V3–6)

STAGE	PR SEGMENT	ST SEGMENT	T WAVES
I	Depressed or baseline	Elevated	Upright
II	Baseline or depressed	Baseline	Upright
III	Baseline	Baseline	Inverted
IV	Baseline	Baseline	Upright or inverted

COMMENTS AND TREATMENT CONSIDERATIONS

The majority of cases are idiopathic (40% to 60%) or viral (20%). Other causes include lupus and other collagen vascular diseases, malignancy (especially lymphoma, melanoma, and breast and lung carcinomas), uremia, bacterial infection or tuberculosis, rheumatic fever, trauma, myocardial infarction (Dressler's syndrome), cardiac surgery, radiation therapy, and certain medications.

Pericarditis usually follows viral symptoms by 2 to 4 weeks but may be concurrent. Pericardial hemorrhage leading to tamponade and death, although rare, has been reported after thrombolysis when pericarditis was misdiagnosed as myocardial infarction.

REFERENCES

Ginzton LE, Laks MM: The differential diagnosis of acute pericarditis from the normal variant: new electrocardiographic criteria, *Circulation* 65:1004, 1982.

Lange RA, Hillis LD: Acute pericarditis, *N Engl J Med* 351:2195, 2004.

Ross AM, Grauer SE: Acute pericarditis: evaluation and treatment of infectious and other causes, *Postgrad Med* 115:67, 2004.

Spodick DH: ECG in acute pericarditis; distributions of morphologic and axial changes by stages, *Am J Cardiol* 33:470, 1974.

Spodick DH: Pericardial rubs: prospective, multiple observer investigation of pericardial friction in 100 patients, *Am J Cardiol* 35:357, 1975.

 ESOPHAGEAL FOREIGN BODIES

Esophageal foreign bodies take many forms; they may be smooth or blunt, food or nonorganic objects, and ingestion may be intentional or accidental. History may be absent, and symptoms vary; the diagnosis and management largely depend on a high index of suspicion, the nature of the object ingested, and the symptoms and signs present. Although less than 1% of foreign body ingestions result in perforation or other serious complications, they account for 15% of esophageal perforations. Once past the esophagus, most foreign bodies pass through the GI tract without complication.

SYMPTOMS
- Suspected ingestion in small children +++, but more than half of children with an esophageal foreign body have no such history; up to 18% are asymptomatic.
- Choking, gagging, or coughing that has resolved on arrival to the ED is a common presentation.
- Poor feeding
- Drooling
- Vomiting
- Difficulty swallowing
- Older children and adults usually report chest, throat, or neck pain; dysphagia; or foreign body sensation.

SIGNS
- Physical signs are absent in most of childhood ingestions +++.
- Drooling
- For delayed cases, see Esophageal Rupture.

WORKUP
- Oropharyngeal examination or indirect laryngoscopy may reveal a foreign object lodged high in the aerodigestive tract.
- Soft tissue neck x-rays may identify a foreign body, soft tissue swelling (especially in delayed cases, suggesting infection), or retropharyngeal air (suggesting perforation).
- X-rays of the chest and abdomen are useful for localizing and identifying some objects, such as coins, button batteries, and other highly radiopaque objects. Coins in the esophagus are generally oriented parallel to the esophagus, as opposed to tracheal coins, which are generally transverse. Diagnostic yield for ingested organic objects, such as fish or chicken bones (representing 60% of adult presentations), is low (false negative in up to 71%). Plastic and aluminum are also not generally visualized.
- Esophagoscopy is the ideal procedure when an object is obstructive, is sharp or irregular, or has a high risk of causing perforation. It can be both diagnostic and therapeutic. Negative findings, or presence only of abrasions or esophagitis, are common.
- CT scan, with or without contrast, may be useful in the diagnosis of perforation (see Esophageal Rupture).
- Esophagography may be useful for identifying obstructive objects or demonstrating perforation, but it carries the risk of

vomiting and aspiration and may delay definitive diagnosis and therapy.

COMMENTS AND TREATMENT CONSIDERATIONS

Ingestions of button batteries pose particular problems. They may contain high concentrations of caustic potassium hydroxide or various potentially toxic metals (e.g., mercury). If lodged in the esophagus, they should be *immediately* removed (endoscopically if available). Once they are past the esophagus, observation while awaiting spontaneous passage may be employed.

Spasmolytic drugs such as glucagon (0.5 to 2.0 mg IM or slow IVP) are reported to aid in the passage of lower esophageal foreign bodies (usually food), but the success rate may not differ from that for placebo. Carbonated beverages might also assist passage. Smooth objects, such as coins, lodged in the distal esophagus pass spontaneously in 60% and may be observed.

Esophageal foreign bodies present for prolonged periods (from 12 to 24 hours) and those in the proximal and middle thirds of the esophagus should be removed. The standard method for removal is endoscopy, but Foley catheter retrograde removal and bougienage (using a dilator to advance the object into the stomach) have been described. Any object, smooth or not, that is present for a prolonged period may cause perforation of the esophagus. Refer adults for further evaluation to rule out obstructing esophageal lesions.

REFERENCES

Chaves DM, Ishioka S, Felix VN, et al: Removal of a foreign body from the upper gastrointestinal tract with a flexible endoscope: a prospective study, *Endoscopy* 36:887, 2004.

Conners GP: A literature-based comparison of three methods of pediatric esophageal coin removal, *Pediatr Emerg Care* 13:154, 1997.

Harned RK II, Strain JD, Hay TC, Douglas MR: Esophageal foreign bodies: safety and efficacy of Foley catheter extraction of coins, *AJR Am J Roentgenol* 168:443, 1997.

Kay M, Wyllie R: Pediatric foreign bodies and their management, *Curr Gastroenterol Rep* 7:212, 2005.

Rimell FL, Thome A Jr, Stool S, et al: Characteristics of objects that cause choking in children, *JAMA* 274:1763, 1995.

Tibbling L, Bjorkhoel A, Jansson E, Stenkvist M: Effect of spasmolytic drugs on esophageal foreign bodies, *Dysphagia* 10:126, 1995.

 PANIC DISORDER

Panic disorder (PD) may be present in a subset of ED patients with chest pain. The quality of pain is often indistinguishable from that of ischemic pain. Because patients with PD often have coexistent CAD, a diagnosis of panic disorder is infrequently made in the ED. Many patients with panic disorder have coexisting symptoms of depression, including suicidal ideation (10%).

SYMPTOMS
- Chest pain
- Dyspnea
- Palpitations
- Dizziness
- Sweating
- Trembling
- Fear of losing control
- Fear of dying
- Perioral (acral) paresthesias
- Prior history of similar events
- Fear of additional attacks

SIGNS
- Tachycardia
- Tachypnea
- Normal examination

WORKUP
- ECG
- Chest x-rays are useful for ruling out other diagnoses.

COMMENTS AND TREATMENT CONSIDERATIONS
ED physicians must be careful not to miss possible myocardial infarction in patients with panic disorder who are at risk as well as not to overlook the potential for suicide in patients with chest pain and other psychiatric symptoms.

REFERENCES
Carter SC, Servan-Schreiber D, Perlstein WM: Anxiety disorders and the syndrome of chest pain with normal coronary arteries: prevalence and pathophysiology, *J Clin Psychiatry* 58(Suppl 3):70, 1997.

Fleet RP, Dupuis G, Kaczorowski J, et al: Suicidal ideation in emergency department chest pain patients: panic disorder a risk factor, *Am J Emerg Med* 15:345, 1997.

Fleet RP, Dupuis G, Marchand A, et al: Panic disorder in emergency department chest pain patients: prevalence, co-morbidity, suicidal ideation, and physician recognition, *Am J Med* 101:371, 1996.

CHAPTER 7

Huffman JC, Pollack MH: Predicting panic disorder among patients with chest pain: an analysis of the literature, *Psychosomatics* 44:222, 2003.

 CHEST PAIN IN CHILDREN

Chest pain is a common presenting complaint in children, accounting for an estimated 650,000 ED visits annually and 0.6% of all visits. Most are due to non–life-threatening conditions, and only 2% require hospital admission. Causes include chest wall pains (24% to 41%), idiopathic (12% to 21%), pulmonary disease (cough, pneumonia, and asthma combine for 21%), minor trauma (5%), and psychogenic (5% to 9%). Cardiac causes (including SVT and brady-cardia, among others) constitute less than 5%. The vast majority of cases require only a history and physical for diagnosis. Family history of MI is actually associated with a decreased likelihood of an organic cause of pain.

SYMPTOMS
- Chest pain of acute onset and pain awakening a child from sleep are associated with organic disease (3- and 3.6-fold increased likelihood, respectively).
- Features or past medical history suggestive of one of the entities discussed in the previous sections (especially pneumonia, pneu-mothorax, pericarditis or pericardial tamponade, traumatic aortic rupture, or esophageal foreign body—the others being very uncom-mon in children) should also elicit further clinical investigation.
- Kawasaki's disease is a rare cause of pain and one of the few causes of ischemic cardiac disease in children.

SIGNS
- Fever (12-fold increased likelihood of organic disease), tachycardia, and other abnormal physical findings may warrant additional testing in the ED.

WORKUP
- Laboratory tests are rarely useful.
- Chest x-rays in children selected on the basis of history and physical are positive in 11% of children with chest pain. If pneu-monia is excluded, positive findings are present in only 2%.
- ECGs are positive in 10% but are commonly misread in the ED (normal conduction intervals, size of the QRS complex, and fea-tures of the ST segment and T wave vary with age and may differ greatly from those in adults), and only 2% to 3% of abnormalities found are clinically relevant.

REFERENCES

Berezin S, Medow MS, Glassman MS, Newman LJ: Chest pain of gastrointestinal origin, *Arch Dis Child* 63:1457, 1988.

Kaden GG, Shenker IR, Gootman N: Chest pain in adolescents, *J Adolesc Health* 12:251, 1991.

Rowe BH, Dulberg CS, Peterson RG, et al: Characteristics of children presenting with chest pain to a pediatric emergency department, *Can Med Assoc J* 143:388, 1990.

Selbst SM: Chest pain in children, *Pediatr Rev* 18:169, 1997.

Selbst SM, Ruddy RM, Clark BJ, et al: Pediatric chest pain: a prospective study, *Pediatrics* 82:319, 1988.

Dental Pain
Steven Go

Physicians typically spend little time learning about dental pathology during their training. However, dental pain is a remarkably common complaint in the ED, and in one study 2% of all dental-related ED visits resulted in hospital admission. It is important to diagnose and manage these emergencies correctly to prevent rare but potentially life-threatening complications, effectively relieve pain, and communicate accurately with the consultants who will be providing definitive care.

 ANATOMY

The Universal/National numbering system is used in the United States to identify the individual teeth (Fig. 8–1). This identification system should be used to convey accurately the location of tooth pathology to consultants. For landmarks in patients with incomplete dentition, it is helpful to remember that the upper central incisors are numbered 8 and 9, whereas the lower central incisors are numbered 24 and 25. Alternatively, the formal names of the teeth may be used.

REFERENCES

American Dental Association: www.ada.org.

Cohen LA, Magder LS, Manski RJ, Mullins CD: Hospital admissions associated with nontraumatic dental emergencies in a Medicaid population, *Am J Emerg Med* 21:540, 2003.

Douglass AB, Douglass JM: Common dental emergencies, *Am Fam Physician* 67:511, 2003.

Go S: Oral and dental emergencies. In Ma OJ, Cline DM (eds): *Emergency medicine manual*, ed 6. New York, 2004, McGraw-Hill, pp 734-739.

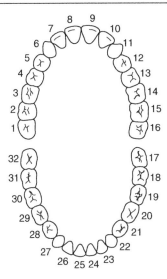

1. 3rd molar (wisdom tooth)
2. 2nd molar (12-yr molar)
3. 1st molar (6-yr molar)
4. 2nd bicuspid (2nd premolar)
5. 1st bicuspid (1st premolar)
6. Cuspid (canine/eye tooth)
7. Lateral incisor
8. Central incisor
9. Central incisor
10. Lateral incisor
11. Cuspid (canine/eye tooth)
12. 1st bicuspid (1st premolar)
13. 2nd bicuspid (2nd premolar)
14. 1st molar (6-yr molar)
15. 2nd molar (12-yr molar)
16. 3rd molar (wisdom tooth)

17. 3rd molar (wisdom tooth)
18. 2nd molar (12-yr molar)
19. 1st molar (6-yr molar)
20. 2nd bicuspid (2nd premolar)
21. 1st bicuspid (1st premolar)
22. Cuspid (canine/eye tooth)
23. Lateral incisor
24. Central incisor
25. Central incisor
26. Lateral incisor
27. Cuspid (canine/eye tooth)
28. 1st bicuspid (1st premolar)
29. 2nd bicuspid (2nd premolar)
30. 1st molar (6-yr molar)
31. 2nd molar (12-yr molar)
32. 3rd molar (wisdom tooth)

Fig. 8–1 Universal/National numbering system. (Adapted with permission from: http://www.ada.org/public/topics/tooth_number.asp. Source: American Dental Association Current Dental Terminology Third Edition (CDT-3), downloaded November 10, 2004.)

DENTAL CARIES AND ABSCESSES

These are perhaps the most common etiologies for dental pain in the ED. Carious pain results from tooth decay that extends into the pulp. It is important to identify the presence of an abscess and distinguish between those that need to be drained and those that

do not. If left untreated, some abscesses may progress to
life/airway-threatening deep space abscesses.

SYMPTOMS
- Pain +++++
- Tooth sensitivity to hot, cold, and sweet stimuli that resolves
  spontaneously within seconds (reversible pulpitis)
- Persistent, spontaneous, poorly localized pain (irreversible
  pulpitis)
- Inability to bite down on tooth because of intense pain
- Neck swelling ++++, neck pain, drooling, muffled voice, dysphagia,
  or trismus +++ may indicate an infection that has spread into the
  neck spaces.

SIGNS
- Normal tooth appearance or opaque white areas in enamel with
  gray undertone (early)
- Visible, discolored cavity (late)
- Failed filling in the painful tooth
- Pain with percussion of the tooth with a metal object
- Localized, fluctuant mass, erythema, and swelling at the gum
  line, buccal sulcus, or palatal tissue indicates the presence of
  an abscess.
- Obvious cellulitis or mass of the buccal tissues indicates a more
  extensive infection.
- Fever may indicate extensive infection.
- Cervical adenopathy
- Fever ++++, pain in the floor of the mouth, protruding tongue,
  and bilateral submandibular swelling may indicate Ludwig's
  angina.

WORKUP
- Determine the status of the patient's airway. For deep space
  neck infections, airway stabilization should be considered and
  emergent bedside evaluation by an oromaxillofacial surgeon or
  otolaryngologist is indicated. Any patient with a potential airway
  complication should be managed in a monitored location with
  ready access to emergency airway equipment.
- Determine whether a drainable abscess is present. Manual
  palpation should be performed along the gum line and the buccal,
  lingual, and palatal surfaces to feel for fluctuance, as visual
  inspection alone can be misleading. If an abscess is found, it may
  be drained in the ED by the emergency physician. Good anesthesia
  is a must, and an inferior alveolar nerve block is particularly useful
  for lower tooth lesions. For extensive abscesses, consultation with
  a dentist is indicated.

- Plain x-rays (unless trauma or deep space abscess is suspected) and laboratory tests are generally of little value in diagnosis.
- Contrast-enhanced computed tomography (CT) may be required to assess for deep neck abscesses; however, no unstable patient or airway-threatened patient should be sent to CT without adequate stabilization. In patients who cannot have CT, plain radiographs (with the same caveat) should be obtained if the diagnosis is not obvious.

COMMENTS AND TREATMENT CONSIDERATIONS

For patients with clinical reversible pulpitis (tooth sensitivity brought on by certain stimuli that resolves in a few seconds), oral analgesia is indicated. If the patient has irreversible pulpitis (persistent, spontaneous severe pain), many practitioners prescribe antibiotics that cover oral flora; however, this is controversial because the literature does not provide definitive evidence to support this practice.

Penicillin and amoxicillin have long been the antibiotics of choice; however, with the rise of beta-lactamase–producing organisms, clindamycin is now commonly prescribed. More recently, azithromycin has been suggested as being efficacious in these settings.

NSAIDs generally suffice for all but the most painful of lesions, although oral narcotics may be necessary in some patients. Pain control in the ED can be achieved with local nerve blocks or oral analgesics, or both.

Although the treatment of abscesses is incision and drainage, they typically arise from infected teeth; therefore, antibiotics and pain medications are still indicated.

Patients should be counseled that treatment with oral medications results only in temporary relief if the damaged tooth is not treated definitively. Therefore, all patients should be referred to an appropriate specialist within 24 to 48 hours, and long courses of antibiotics or analgesics should not be prescribed.

Not all patients who have extensive abscesses appear ill, and those with deep space infections can decompensate rapidly. Therefore, a high index of suspicion should be maintained, and specific signs and symptoms should be elicited to look for these infections. A thorough medical history to detect immunocompromised patients should also be obtained. Facial cellulitis or neck abscesses generally warrant admission and broad-spectrum antibiotics. Any potential airway-threatening or complex abscess requires emergent surgical evaluation.

With the growing popularity of oral piercing, it is important to recognize the increased prevalence of infections that occur in individuals with piercings. Tongue piercing is particularly likely to lead to infectious complications such as permanent ornament embedding, transmission of bloodborne viruses, and lingual infections that can spread to deep spaces.

REFERENCES

ADA Council on Scientific Affairs: Combating antibiotic resistance, *JADA* 135:484, 2004.

Addy LD, Martin MV: Azithromycin and dentistry—a useful agent? *Br Dent J* 197:141, 2004.

Bansal A, Miskoff J, Lis RJ: Otolaryngologic critical care, *Crit Care Clin* 19:55, 2003.

Bibler JT: Oral piercing: the hole story, *Northwest Dent* 82:13, 2003.

Nagle D, Reader A, Beck M, Weaver J: Effect of systemic penicillin on pain in untreated irreversible pulpitis, *Oral Surg Oral Med Oral Pathol Oral Radiol Endod* 70:636, 2000.

Palmer NAO: Revisiting the role of dentists in prescribing antibiotics, *Dent Update* 30:570, 2003.

Rupp T, Surdam D, Touchstone D: ENT emergencies: history, controversy, and management. From http://www.emedhome.com/features_archive-detail.cfm?FID=1825 (accessed November 12, 2004)

Shacham R, Zaguri A, Librus HZ, et al: Tongue piercing and its adverse effects, *Surg Oral Med Oral Pathol Oral Radiol Endod* 95:274, 2003.

 DENTOALVEOLAR TRAUMA

Tooth fractures can occur from even minor trauma if the tooth is carious. Avulsions and luxations require specific maneuvers to save the tooth. All patients with dental trauma should be screened for associated facial injuries.

SYMPTOMS
- Pain +++++
- Loose tooth
- Foreign body sensation in the mouth

SIGNS
- Deformation of the tooth
- Loose tooth (luxation) or completely avulsed tooth
- Discolored tooth (concussion) is a late finding.

WORKUP
- Associated injuries: intraoral lacerations, facial trauma, associated fractures, and adjacent loose or missing teeth must be excluded.

COMMENTS AND TREATMENT CONSIDERATIONS

Fractures are categorized by the Ellis system depending on the deepest level of tissue that is violated, and treatment varies by class (Table 8–1).

Luxated teeth should be gently repositioned and splinted in place with periodontal dressing, with dental follow-up within 24 hours. Avulsed teeth should be immediately rinsed with sterile saline, the socket irrigated, and the tooth reimplanted by the ED physician as soon as possible, taking care to handle the tooth only by the crown. Permanent teeth avulsed less than 3 hours require an emergent dental consultation, but reimplantation should not be delayed for the arrival of the specialist. If the tooth cannot be immediately reimplanted, it should be placed in a balanced pH solution in a commercial tooth saver kit (Hanks' Balanced Salt Solution) or sterile normal saline. If the patient arrives with a history of a recently avulsed tooth but the tooth cannot be located, a careful search of the oral cavity is warranted. Radiographs may be necessary to exclude teeth hidden in associated lacerations. Concussed teeth require nonemergent dental follow-up as pulp damage may have occurred. It is important to remember that all dental trauma, especially in children, requires prompt evaluation and proper handling of damaged teeth in order to minimize future complications. In addition, a sports-related episode of dental trauma may provide an opportunity for the emergency physician to reemphasize the importance of mouth guards to reduce the chance of dental injuries.

CHAPTER 8

REFERENCES

Al-Jundi SH: Type of treatment, prognosis, and estimation of time spent to manage dental trauma in late presentation cases at a dental teaching hospital: a longitudinal and retrospective study, *Dent Traumatol* 20:1, 2004.

TABLE 8–1
ELLIS FRACTURE CLASSIFICATION AND TREATMENT

ELLIS CLASS	DEEPEST TISSUE INVOLVED	TREATMENT
I	Enamel	Pain control. Dental follow-up within 7 days.
II	Dentin	Dry dentin and cover with calcium hydroxide paste. Pain control. Dental follow-up in 24 hours. (In children, treat as class III)
III	Pulp	Ideally, immediate dental evaluation. If no dentist available, treat as in class II.

Labella CR, Smith BW, Sigurdsson A: Effect of mouthguards on dental injuries and concussions in college basketball, *Med Sci Sports Exerc* 34:41, 2002.

Pileggi R, Dumsha TC: The management of traumatic dental injuries, *Tex Dent J* 120:270, 2003.

 SOFT TISSUE TRAUMA

Lacerations are usually evident but must be vigorously sought whenever there is trauma to the lower face.

SYMPTOMS
- Pain +++++
- History of trauma
- Bleeding, swelling

SIGNS
- Laceration in oral cavity
- Posible associated dentoalveolar trauma

WORKUP
- Lacerations should be carefully explored to detect foreign bodies, damage to underlying structures, and extent of the wound.
- If dental trauma is present, radiographs may be necessary to exclude teeth hidden in associated lacerations.
- A very careful neurologic and vascular examination should be done
- A soft tissue lateral neck radiograph, chest radiograph, and/or CT scan with contrast may be necessary to detect extension of wounds or infection into the deep spaces.

COMMENTS AND TREATMENT CONSIDERATIONS
Many nongaping wounds heal with supportive care. However, gaping wounds can serve as "food traps" and therefore potential loci of infections. These wounds should be thoroughly searched for tooth fragments (radiographs may be required), copiously irrigated, and closed with buried, absorbable sutures. Repair of both sides of a through-and-through laceration is controversial; some experts repair only the exterior surface, and others repair the interior laceration first, irrigate the wound with chlorhexidine gluconate (preferred) or saline, and then repair the exterior surface. The routine use of antibiotics is not indicated, but adequate oral analgesia should be provided as well as a prescription for

chlorhexidine gluconate rinses three times a day. Tetanus status should be ascertained and updated as needed. Dental follow-up is essential.

Although many intraoral lacerations are benign, children in particular are at risk for trauma to deeper structures, with occasionally life-threatening complications such as neurovascular injury, deep space abscesses, and mediastinitis. Such trauma usually results from a fall with a sharp object in the mouth but can also occur with even the most seemingly benign of instruments such as toothbrushes. The indicated workup and management of such cases are controversial, but experts agree that an initially benign appearance of a wound does not rule out potentially devastating injuries that can sometimes take several days (or even weeks) to become apparent. Therefore, extra care should be taken in the evaluation of these patients with particular attention to the neurologic examination, and a low threshold for specialist consultation and possible imaging studies should be maintained. If these patients are to be discharged, they must have scheduled, close follow-up, a responsible adult to observe and transport them, and a list of specific symptoms to trigger an earlier return to the ED (e.g., fever, poor oral intake > 24 hours, drooling, difficulty breathing, neck pain or restricted mobility, vomiting, irritability, altered mental status, lethargy, or vision changes).

CHAPTER 8

REFERENCES

Hellmann JR, Shott SR, Gootee MJ: Impalement injuries of the palate in children: review of 131 cases, *Int J Pediatr Otorhinolaryngol* 26:157, 1993.

Kosaki H, Nakamura N, Toriyama Y: Penetrating injuries to the oropharynx, *J Laryngol Otol* 106:813, 1992.

Law RC, Fouque CA, Waddell A, Cusick E: Lesson of the week: penetrating intra-oral trauma in children, *BMJ* 314:50, 1997.

Radkowski D, McGill TJ, Healy GB, Jones DT: Penetrating trauma of the oropharynx in children, *Laryngoscope* 103:991, 1993.

Rayatt SS, Hamlyn P, Magennis P: Penetrating intraoral trauma may occur in adults as well as children, *BMJ* 314:1043, 1997.

Schoem SR, Choi SS, Zalzal GH, Grundfast KM: Management of oropharyngeal trauma in children, *Arch Otolaryngol Head Neck Surg* 123:1267, 1997.

 ## POSTEXTRACTION ALVEOLAR OSTEITIS ("DRY SOCKET SYNDROME")

After most extractions, a clot forms. However, sometimes the clot becomes dislodged (often in smokers) and the exposed tissue becomes painful.

SYMPTOMS

- Pain +++++
- Foul odor
- Foul taste

SIGNS

- Absence of clot in socket
- Fluctuance, swelling, erythema may represent abscess formation.

WORKUP

- Radiographs should be taken to exclude a foreign body or retained root.

COMMENTS AND TREATMENT CONSIDERATIONS

Currently, there is a paucity of well-designed randomized controlled trials in the literature to direct management of this disease entity. However, in an uncomplicated alveolar osteitis, the standard treatment is to irrigate the socket with chlorhexidine gluconate or saline and then pack it with eugenol-impregnated gauze (to be changed daily). Chlorhexidine gluconate for rinses three times a day should be prescribed. Antibiotics against oral flora are given in severe cases, with dental follow-up in 24 hours.

REFERENCES

Blum IR: Contemporary views on dry socket (alveolar osteitis): a clinical appraisal of standardization, aetiopathogenesis and management: a critical review, *Int J Oral Maxillofac Surg* 31:309, 2003.

Delilbasi C, Saracoglu U, Keskin A: Effects of 0.2% chlorhexidine gluconate and amoxicillin plus clavulanic acid on the prevention of alveolar osteitis following mandibular third molar extractions, *Oral Surg Oral Med Oral Pathol Oral Radiol Endod* 94:301, 2002.

Houston JP, McCollum J, Pietz D, Schneck D: Alveolar osteitis: a review of its etiology, prevention, and treatment modalities, *Gen Dent* 50:457, 2002.

Dizziness (Vertigo)
Stephen K. Epstein

Dizziness is one of the more difficult diagnostic dilemmas an emergency physician faces. In particular, vertigo, the illusory sense of motion, must be distinguished from syncope or near-syncope (see Chapter 36, Syncope and Near-Syncope). Vertigo is most often caused by an inner ear process but can be caused by CNS dysfunction. Central (CNS) causes of vertigo may be only minimally symptomatic, in contrast to the generally severe symptoms attributable to peripheral causes. Particular attention must be given to elderly patients, who more frequently have a serious cause of their dizziness.

In addition to a thorough examination, including a detailed neurologic examination (with particular attention to cranial nerve and cerebellar function), attention should be paid to the features of nystagmus, which tend to have characteristic patterns when vertigo is attributable to central or peripheral causes. If not already present at rest, nystagmus can generally be induced by moving a patient quickly from a seated to a lying position and then turning the head gently to the side (Dix-Hallpike test).

 CENTRAL VERTIGO
Cerebellar Hemorrhage and Infarction
Vertigo can be the initial symptom of a CNS process including cerebellar bleeding or infarction. An intracranial process should be suspected in older patients, particularly those at risk for vertebrobasilar artery disease. Neurologic findings should further this suspicion because their presence is specific, but not sensitive, for a CNS process. In contrast to peripheral vertigo, in which there is often dramatic exacerbation of symptoms with head movement, a central CNS lesion may be minimally symptomatic.

109

A complete neurologic examination that includes gait testing is essential.

SYMPTOMS
- Vertigo may be minimal and be the only symptom ++; generally not significantly positional.
- Symptoms associated with pathologic conditions of the posterior circulation (clumsiness, weakness, change in speech) are variably present.
- Altered level of consciousness is uncommon.

SIGNS
- Neurologic findings are variably present and may indicate neurologic dysfunction in vertebrobasilar arterial distribution (e.g., dysmetria, dysarthria, facial palsy, severe ataxia).
- Nystagmus associated with central lesions may be in any direction, but nystagmus that is vertical, multidirectional, or changes direction depending upon the direction of gaze strongly suggests a central process. Nystagmus from peripheral lesions is usually horizontal or rotatory, is worsened by head movement, has a latency period, fatigue, suppresses with visual fixation, and is exacerbated by gaze toward the side of the fast component.

WORKUP
- MRI is the test of choice for imaging the posterior fossa.
- CT demonstrates most bleeding and large lesions.

COMMENTS AND TREATMENT CONSIDERATIONS
One study found a 25% rate of cerebellar infarction in elderly patients who had nystagmus and had been dizzy for more than 2 days. ED consultation with a neurologist or neurosurgeon should be arranged for patients with a central cause of vertigo.

 PERIPHERAL VERTIGO

Peripheral vertigo is generally very symptomatic, with prominent nausea and vomiting. Positioning may dramatically increase the severity of symptoms. History or physical examination may reveal otitis media, recent upper respiratory tract infection, previous exposure to ototoxic drugs, or recurrent episodes with progressive tinnitus and deafness (Ménière's disease). Often a precipitant cannot be found, and a diagnosis of benign positional vertigo is made. Most cases are thought to be caused by free-floating debris (otoliths) in the semicircular canals of the inner ear.

SYMPTOMS
- Profound vertigo ++++
- Nausea and vomiting

SIGNS
- Neurologic examination is normal.
- Nystagmus is typically horizontal or rotary, not vertical, and typically brought about by changes in head position. Generally, there is latency (after the patient looks in a given direction, a few seconds elapse before nystagmus occurs). The nystagmus should fatigue (decrease with prolonged gaze in a given direction). Nystagmus is suppressed by visual fixation.

WORKUP
No ancillary tests are required in the ED if peripheral vertigo is diagnosed.

COMMENTS AND TREATMENT CONSIDERATIONS
Treatment of peripheral vertigo consists of maneuvers to reposition otoliths from the semicircular canals to the utriculus on the inner ear, where they lodge. The Epley maneuver (http://www.dizziness-and-balance.com/disorders/bppv/epley/first.html) remains the most well-known treatment, although other maneuvers exist.

Vestibular suppressant drugs, such as meclizine (25 mg po q6-8h), phenothiazines (prochlorperazine), benzodiazepines (diazepam [Valium]), and scopolamine, may reduce the severity of symptoms. These drugs can cause significant side effects and do not resolve the underlying cause of the symptoms. Spontaneous improvement over the course of several days is the norm, although symptoms are occasionally persistent. Patients should be referred for follow-up because rarely a cranial nerve VIII lesion or other condition requiring treatment is the cause of persistent peripheral vertigo.

REFERENCES
Baloh RW: Vestibular neuronitis, *N Engl J Med* 348:1027, 2003.

Cohen NL: The dizzy patient: update on vestibular disorders, *Med Clin North Am* 75:6, 1991.

Froehling DA, Silverstein MD, Mohr DN, Beatty CW: Does this dizzy patient have a serious form of vertigo? *JAMA* 271:385, 1994.

Furman JM, Cass SP: Benign paroxysmal positional vertigo, *N Engl J Med* 341:1590, 1999.

Herr RD, Zun L, Matthews JJ: A directed approach to the dizzy patient, *Ann Emerg Med* 18:664,1989.

CHAPTER 9

Hotson JR, Baloh RW: Acute vestibular syndrome, *N Engl J Med* 339:680, 1999.

Norrving B, Magnusson M, Holtas S: Isolated acute vertigo in the elderly: vestibular or vascular disease? *Acta Neurol Scand* 91:43, 1995.

Ear Pain
Stephen K. Epstein

Ear pain is a frequent complaint of patients in the ambulatory setting. Although the cause of ear pain is most commonly otitis media (OM) or otitis externa (OE), a number of other conditions can also cause ear pain. Primary causes of ear pain include other infectious processes (e.g., mastoiditis, abscesses, and Ramsay Hunt syndrome) as well as inflammatory processes, eustachian tube dysfunction, trauma, and neoplasms. Referred ear pain may result from neuralgias, neoplasms, and odontogenic causes, among others.

REFERENCES
Shah RK, Blevins NH: Otalgia, *Otolaryngol Clin North Am* 36:1137, 2003.

 OTITIS EXTERNA

OE is an inflammation of the auditory canal resulting in edema, pain, and drainage. It is sometimes referred to as swimmer's ear as recent water exposure is often noted in the patient's history.

SYMPTOMS
- Edema
- Discharge
- Pain
- Recent water exposure or instrumentation of the auditory canal

SIGNS
- Exacerbation of pain with movement of the pinna
- Erythema and edema of the external auditory canal
- Debris in and drainage from the external auditory canal

WORKUP
OE is a clinical diagnosis without need for laboratory studies.

COMMENTS AND TREATMENT CONSIDERATIONS
Treatment consists of removing any debris and treating with antibiotic (and sometimes steroid) ear drops. Fluoroquinolones are effective but expensive; polymyxin B-neomycin-hydrocortisone is an excellent alternative. To ensure that the drops reach into the canal, place a wick in the auditory canal if edema is present. Patients should be instructed to keep the ear dry otherwise.

Consider malignancy in persistent cases or when otalgia is out of proportion to the physical findings (CT/MR imaging).

 MALIGNANT OTITIS EXTERNA

Malignant OE is a rare extension of OE to surrounding tissue of the external auditory canal and bone of the skull base. It is most commonly seen in diabetics and other immunocompromised patients. The usual pathogen is *Pseudomonas aeruginosa*.

SYMPTOMS
- Severe unrelenting pain +++++
- Discharge ++++
- Prior history of OE unresponsive to topical treatment
- Fever and trismus (less common)
- Pain worse with chewing (extension to the TMJ)

SIGNS
- Erythema and edema of the pinna and periauricular tissues
- Exacerbation of pain with movement of the pinna
- Headache
- Cranial nerve palsies (most frequently VII) in advanced cases ++

WORKUP
- CT or bone scan to rule out osteomyelitis of the skull
- CBC is not generally helpful.
- Glucose to rule out diabetes

COMMENTS AND TREATMENT CONSIDERATIONS
Patients who are immunocompromised or have significant infection should be admitted for intravenous antibiotics (e.g., imipenem, meropenem, or a fluoroquinolone). *Pseudomonas* is the most common pathogen, but *Streptococcus*, *Staphylococcus*, and *Proteus* are also seen. Otolaryngologic consultation is required.

REFERENCES

Grandis J, Branstetter BF, Yu VL: The changing face of malignant (necrotising) external otitis: clinical, radiological, and anatomic correlations, *Lancet Infect Dis* 4:34, 2004.

Rubin J, Yu VL: Malignant external otitis: insights into pathogenesis, clinical manifestations, diagnosis, and therapy, *Am J Med* 85:391, 1988.

Santamaria JP, Abrunzo TJ: Ear and nose emergencies. In American College of Emergency Physicians: *Pediatric emergency medicine: a comprehensive study guide*. New York, 1995, McGraw-Hill.

 OTITIS MEDIA

Acute OM is an entity distinct from OM with effusion. The former represents an acute infection characterized by the recent, usually abrupt onset of middle ear inflammation with effusion. There is at least one of erythema of the tympanic membrane (TM), otalgia, or distinct fullness or bulging of the TM. OM with effusion is defined as a TM that has an air/fluid level, and at least two of abnormal color (white, yellow, amber, or bluish), opacification not due to scarring, and decreased or absent mobility.

CHAPTER 10

SYMPTOMS
- Ear pain
- Diminished hearing
- Irritability
- Recent or concurrent URI

SIGNS
- TM bulging, air/fluid level, decreased mobility, erythema
- TM perforation

COMMENTS AND TREATMENT CONSIDERATIONS
There remains considerable controversy over the treatment of acute OM. Not all children with acute OM need to be treated with antibiotics initially, if at all. Low-risk patients (age older than 2, mild pain, temperature less than 39°C, close follow-up ensured, nonimmunosuppressed) may be observed and antibiotics instituted only if there is no improvement within 48 to 72 hours. Amoxicillin remains the first-line drug for the treatment of acute OM. In 1999, the CDC recommended the use of high-dose amoxicillin when there is a high likelihood of resistance to pneumococcus (children in day care, relapses, and younger than 2 years).

Pain should be treated with acetaminophen or ibuprofen. Benzocaine otic drops may also be effective.

REFERENCES

American Academy of Pediatrics/American Academy of Family Physicians Clinical Practice Guideline: *Diagnosis and management of acute otitis media*, March 2004.

Garbutt J, St Geme JW 3rd, May A, et al: Developing community-specific recommendations for first-line treatment of acute otitis media: is high-dose amoxicillin necessary? *Pediatrics* 114:342, 2004.

Glasziou PP: Antibiotics for acute otitis media in children, Cochrane Database Syst Rev CD000219, 2004.

Rothman R, Owens T, Simel DL: Does this child have acute otitis media? *JAMA* 290:1633, 2003.

 MASTOIDITIS

Mastoiditis is an uncommon condition usually seen in children. It is defined as an infection of the mastoid bone and usually is a consequence of acute OM. The diagnosis is made on clinical examination and occasionally may be subtle in patients being treated with antibiotics. Other coexisting or complicating conditions include neck abscess (Bezold abscess), facial nerve palsy, cavernous sinus thrombosis, meningitis, and intracranial abscess.

SYMPTOMS
- Ear pain +++++
- Fever ++++
- Pain and fever lasting more than 4 days ++++
- Discharge +++
- Headache
- Irritability or gastrointestinal upset may be the only symptoms in infants.

SIGNS
- Postauricular swelling with erythema and tenderness +++++
- Mastoid tenderness, especially posterior and superior to the level of the external canal
- Pinna may be displaced outward and forward by the swelling ++++.
- Signs of OM

WORKUP
- Clinical diagnosis without need for laboratory studies
- CT scan is indicated if abscess is a concern.
- Blood cultures are generally low yield.

COMMENTS AND TREATMENT CONSIDERATIONS

Patients with mastoiditis should be admitted for intravenous antibiotics (e.g., ceftriaxone). Otolaryngology should be consulted because mastoidectomy or surgical drainage of a subperiosteal abscess may be indicated. Approximately 90% resolve with conservative therapy alone.

REFERENCES

Harley E, Sdralis T, Berkowitz RG: Acute mastoiditis in children: a 12-year retrospective study, *Otolaryngol Head Neck Surg* 116:29, 1997.

Hawkins DB, Dru D, House JW, Clark RW: Acute mastoiditis in children: a review of 54 cases, *Laryngoscope* 93:568, 1983.

Khafif A, Halperin D, Hochman I, et al: Acute mastoiditis: a 10-year review, *Am J Otol* 19:170, 1998.

CHAPTER 10

Emerging Infections
Sukhjit S. Takhar and Gregory J. Moran

Emergency physicians should be aware of new and unusual infections that may be seen in the emergency department. Infectious diseases may emerge as a result of crossover from animal species, global travel, or development of new antimicrobial resistance. Often these highly contagious and life-threatening infections may appear clinically as a typical viral or bacterial infection. Illnesses such as severe acute respiratory syndrome (SARS), West Nile virus, and avian influenza must be suspected on the basis of the appropriate exposure or travel history and the clinical manifestations. Respiratory isolation should be initiated immediately for suspected SARS or avian influenza, prior to laboratory confirmation. Community-associated methicillin-resistant *Staphylococcus aureus* (MRSA) is now one of the most common causes of skin and soft tissue infections.

 SEVERE ACUTE RESPIRATORY SYNDROME

SARS is a rapidly progressive respiratory illness caused by a novel coronavirus that originated in the Guandong Province of China and subsequently spread to 29 countries in 2003. SARS generally has an incubation period of less then 10 days. The diagnosis is suspected with an appropriate history of exposure with a febrile respiratory illness and confirmed with laboratory testing.

SYMPTOMS
- Dyspnea ++++
- Fever ++++
- Cough +++
- Malaise +++
- Headache +++
- Diarrhea

SIGNS
- Temperature >100.4 ++++
- Hypoxia +++
- Tachypnea +++

WORKUP
- Query about travel to SARS area or close contact with SARS patients within 10 days.
- ELISA testing for IgG antibody may not be positive in early stages of illness.
- CXR findings range from normal to ARDS changes.
- Lymphopenia

COMMENTS AND TREATMENT CONSIDERATIONS
Many SARS cases in 2003 were diagnosed in health care workers. Patients with suspected SARS should be immediately placed in respiratory isolation. Triage protocols should be implemented if SARS transmission is occurring anywhere in the world. Patients should be treated with usual antibiotics for pneumonia. Methylprednisolone may benefit those with severe or progressing disease. Ribavirin has not been shown to be effective but may be useful when combined with interferon alpha.

REFERENCES
Holmes KV: SARS-associated coronavirus, *N Engl J Med* 348:1948, 2003.

http://www.cdc.gov/ncidod/sars/

Peiris JSM, Yuen KY, Osterhuis ADME, Stöhr K: The severe acute respiratory syndrome, *N Engl J Med* 349:2431, 2003.

 AVIAN INFLUENZA

There have been several outbreaks of avian influenza caused by the H5N1 strain among poultry in Asia. There have been sporadic human cases resulting from contact with infected birds as well as cases of suspected human-to-human transmission. If these strains of influenza undergo genetic changes to achieve efficient human-to-human transmission, there is a potential for a severe pandemic. Because these strains are markedly different antigenically from the strains that commonly infect humans, they are highly virulent and associated with a case mortality of up to 70%

SYMPTOMS
- Fever +++++
- Shortness of breath ++++

CHAPTER 11

- Cough ++++
- Diarrhea +++

SIGNS
- Fever ++++
- Tachypnea +++

WORKUP
- Abnormal CXR
- Proximity to Asian poultry farms
- Thrombocytopenia
- Lymphocytopenia
- Rapid antigen test for influenza A
- Confirmation of H5N1 requires specialized testing through the CDC or other agency.

COMMENTS AND TREATMENT CONSIDERATIONS
A pandemic of avian influenza could be devastating globally. Avian influenza requires laboratory biosafety level 3 precautions if isolated. The local health department should be notified immediately. Patients with severe illness should be treated with antibiotics for pneumonia. Oseltamivir is an antiviral agent that may reduce the duration and severity of symptoms if started early in the course. These strains appear to have resistance to amantadine and rimantadine. Methylprednisolone is sometimes used, but it is of unclear benefit.

REFERENCES
Hien T, Liem N, Dung N, et al: Avian influenza A (H5N1) in 10 patients in Vietnam, *N Engl J Med* 350:1179, 2004.
Ungchusak K, Auewarakul P, Dowell S, et al: Probable person-to-person transmission of avian influenza A (H5N1), *N Engl J Med* 352:333, 2005.

 WEST NILE VIRUS

West Nile virus emerged in the United States in New York in 1999 and has spread throughout the country, becoming a major clinical and public health concern. It is a mosquito-borne virus for which birds are the primary host. The majority of West Nile virus infections are asymptomatic or cause a mild self-limited influenza-like illness. Approximately 1 in 150 patients develop neuroinvasive disease. Mortality from meningoencephalitis is about 10% overall. Serious illness is more common in elderly and immunocompromised persons. West Nile virus is suspected in patients who have an unexplained febrile illness or encephalitis, and the diagnosis is confirmed with serology. Transmission is usually by mosquito bite, but there have been reports of the virus being transmitted through blood transfusion and organ donation. There is an increased incidence of West Nile virus in the summer and early fall, when the mosquito population is high.

SYMPTOMS
West Nile fever
- Fatigue ++++
- Fever ++++
- Eye pain ++
- Diarrhea +++
- Arthralgia ++
- Headache ++++

West Nile encephalitis/meningitis
- Muscle weakness +++
- Flaccid paralysis ++
- Confusion ++

SIGNS
West Nile fever
- Maculopapular rash +++
- Fever ++++

West Nile encephalitis/meningitis
- Meningismus ++
- Delirium ++
- Weakness ++

WORKUP
- Consider the disease in patients with viral encephalitis, aseptic meningitis, or other unexplained neurologic disease or febrile illness. There may be an increase in the number of dead birds in the area as well.
- CSF IgM ELISA to West Nile virus. IgM does not cross the blood-brain barrier, so it suggests CNS disease. There may be a cross-reaction with other flavivirus encephalopathies in this test.
- Serum ELISA can confirm infection with West Nile virus.
- CSF pleocytosis and increased protein
- Normal CT scan
- MRI may show evidence of encephalitis.
- EEG with generalized slowing

CHAPTER 11

COMMENTS AND TREATMENT CONSIDERATION

Mosquito repellent with DEET is the best measure to prevent infection. Currently, the treatment for West Nile virus is supportive. The long-term prognosis is unclear, although there appear to be long-lasting sequelae in some cases. IVIG with anti–West Nile virus antibody and interferon alpha show promise in current trials. Blood screening for West Nile virus has reduced the risk of transfusion transmission.

REFERENCES

Nash D, Mostashari F, Fine A, et al: The outbreak of West Nile virus infection in the New York City area in 1999, *N Engl J Med* 344:1807, 2001.

Solomon T: Flavivirus encephalitis, *N Engl J Med* 351:370, 2004.

 COMMUNITY-ASSOCIATED MRSA

Historically, MRSA was an organism found only in nosocomial infections. More recently, MRSA has emerged as a common cause of community-acquired skin and soft tissue infections. Community-associated MRSA was first noted in outbreaks in jails, gyms, and in men who have sex with men. Now it appears that in many areas MRSA is the most common strain of *S. aureus* involved in community-acquired infections, and there are no clear epidemiologic risk factors. Transmission usually occurs through close physical contact or sharing personal items. Because these strains commonly cause spontaneous furunculosis without a precipitating event, many patients suspect the infection is due to a "spider bite." The diagnosis is presumed in patients who have a new abscess with surrounding cellulitis and confirmed with cultures. Occasionally, community-associated MRSA can also be associated with severe pneumonia or sepsis.

SYMPTOMS

- Pain ++++
- Fever ++
- Complaining of "spider bite" ++ in the absence of seeing the spider or the bite occur

SIGNS

- Induration ++++
- Fluctuance +++
- Erythema ++++
- Warmth ++++

WORKUP
- Incision and drainage of abscess
- Wound culture

COMMENTS AND TREATMENT CONSIDERATIONS
Incision and drainage of the abscess are both diagnostic and therapeutic. It is now more important to culture skin infections to rule out MRSA where indicated by history, clinical findings, or local epidemiologic considerations. When there is significant surrounding cellulitis, antibiotics should be prescribed.

Vancomycin is the treatment of choice for severe infections. Oral regimens for community-associated MRSA include clindamycin, doxycycline, or trimethoprim/sulfamethoxazole (TMP/SMX) plus rifampin. Some of these agents, such as TMP/SMX, have poor activity for streptococcal cellulitis. Consider the use of mupirocin ointment in the nares and chlorhexidine body wash for 5 days to prevent recurrence.

CHAPTER 11

REFERENCES
Centers for Disease Control and Prevention: Outbreaks of community-associated methicillin-resistant *Staphylococcus aureus* skin infections—Los Angeles County, California, 2002-2003, *MMWR Morb Mortal Wkly Rep* 52(5):88, 2003.

Moran GJ, Talan DA: Methicillin-resistant *Staphylococcus aureus*: is it in your community and should it change practice? *Ann Emerg Med* 45:321, 2005.

Naimi TS, LeDell KH, Como-Sabetti K, et al: Comparison of community- and health care-associated methicillin-resistant *Staphylococcus aureus* infection, *JAMA* 290:2976, 2003.

Envenomation
Thomas P. Graham and Jacob Cobi Assaf

In the United States, 98,585 bites and envenomations from scorpions, snakes, and spiders were reported to the American Association of Poison Control Centers (AAPCC) in 2002. Fortunately, most bites and envenomations require only conservative management. Nevertheless, because patients are usually unable to identify reliably the animal that inflicted the wound, a careful history and physical examination are required to identify the envenomation, anticipate its expected clinical sequelae, and manage the patient appropriately.

REFERENCE
Watson WA, Litovitz TL, Rodgers GC Jr, et al: 2002 annual report of the American Association of Poison Control Centers Toxic Exposure Surveillance System, *Am J Emerg Med* 21:353, 2003.

ARTHROPOD ENVENOMATION

 SPIDER BITES

Spider bites are a common presenting complaint in the emergency department. In fact, many dermatologic lesions are misdiagnosed as spider envenomations by both the lay public and physicians. Physicians should be aware of the envenomations caused by clinically relevant spiders in their area of practice. In North America, these spiders are the black widow (*Latrodectus* spp), the brown recluse (*Loxosceles* spp), and the hobo spider (*Tegenaria agrestis*). Some other spiders, such as the much feared tarantula, cause localized pain or minor local reactions only. The vast majority of North American spiders are incapable of causing significant local or systemic injury.

Black Widow Spider Bites (Latrodectism)

Latrodectus spiders (Fig. 12–1) are widely distributed throughout North America and worldwide. They produce potent neurotoxic venom, causing predominantly systemic symptoms. Symptoms and signs are minimal or absent at the bite site. Because of this lack of a local reaction, bites may go unnoticed, making the diagnosis challenging. Mortality is rare but can occur in patients with severe coronary artery disease or other serious comorbidities. Black widow bites can precipitate premature labor.

SYMPTOMS

Symptom onset is usually within 1 to 2 hours, ranging from a few minutes to 12 hours. Symptoms peak within 12 hours but may persist for days.

- Generalized abdominal and back pain predominates +++ with or without generalized chest pain. Isolated abdominal, back, or chest pain is unusual.
- Muscle spasms and rigidity +++
- Fasciculations +++
- Local or extremity pain +++
- Nausea/vomiting ++
- Headache +
- Hyperesthesias or paresthesias (uncommon)
- Local pain or pruritus (uncommon and mild if present)

CHAPTER 12

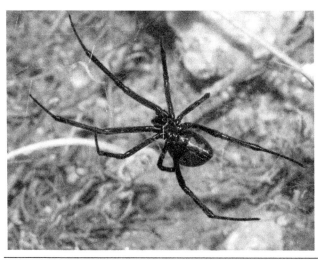

Fig. 12–1 Black widow spider, *Latrodectus mactans*. (Courtesy of Richard Seaman, Palm Springs, CA).

125

SIGNS

- Abdominal tenderness and rigidity (which may mimic peritonitis) +++
- Back muscle tenderness and rigidity +++
- Hypertension ++, may be severe, especially in previously hypertensive patients
- Diaphoresis ++
- Local reactions to the bite are mild or absent. Papules, mild induration, urticaria, or perspiration localized to the site of the bite may be present. Fang marks are tiny, 1 to 2 mm apart, and difficult to see without magnification.
- Seizures (rare)

WORKUP

- The history of a bite by a large, shiny black spider or simply a needle prick sensation while reaching into an undisturbed area (such as a woodpile) is sometimes obtained.
- Laboratory studies are generally not helpful except to exclude other disease processes when the diagnosis is unclear. Leukocytosis is frequently present but is nonspecific.
- The severity of *Latrodectus* envenomation can be graded (Table 12–1).

COMMENTS AND TREATMENT CONSIDERATIONS

Symptomatic treatment is all that is necessary for most patients. Opiates (e.g., morphine sulfate) are indicated for analgesia. Benzodiazepines (e.g., diazepam [Valium]) are effective for treating muscle spasms. Opiates and benzodiazepines can cause respiratory depression when given together, so patients should be monitored closely. Calcium gluconate (10% IV) may also help to alleviate

TABLE 12–1 GUIDELINES FOR GRADING THE SEVERITY OF *LATRODECTUS* ENVENOMATION	
GRADE	DESCRIPTION
1	Asymptomatic, or local pain at envenomation site Normal vital signs
2	Muscular pain at envenomated extremity, or extension of muscular pain to the abdomen or chest Local diaphoresis of envenomation site or involved extremity Normal vital signs
3	Generalized muscular pain in back, abdomen or chest, headache Diaphoresis remote from envenomation site Abnormal vital signs: hypertension, tachycardia

symptoms, but beneficial effects are short lived. Consideration may be given to use of antivenom (1 or 2 vials IV) for patients with clinically severe (grade 3) reactions or serious complications (e.g., acute cardiac ischemia, seizures, preterm labor). Most patients can be discharged after several hours of observation if symptoms are controlled.

REFERENCES

Boye, LV, McNally JT, Binford GJ: Spider bites. In Auerbach PS (ed): *Wilderness medicine*, ed 4. St. Louis, 2001, Mosby, pp 807-838.

Clark RF, Wethern-Kestner S, Vance MV, et al: Clinical presentation and treatment of black widow spider envenomations: a review of 163 cases, *Ann Emerg Med* 21:782, 1992.

Isbister GK, Graudins A, White J, et al: Antivenom treatment in arachnidism, *J Toxicol Clin Toxicol* 41:291, 2003.

Saucier JR: Arachnid envenomations, *Emerg Med Clin North Am* 22:405, 2004.

Ushkaryov YA, Volynski KE, Ashton AC: The multiple actions of black widow spider toxins and their selective use in neuro-secretion studies, *Toxicon* 43:527, 2004.

Necrotic Arachnidism (Recluse Spider and Hobo Spider Bites)

Envenomation by a brown recluse or related spider can result in a poorly healing necrotic ulcer at the site of the bite (necrotic arachnidism or loxoscelism) and rarely a severe systemic illness. Victims rarely present to the ED immediately after a bite because initial symptoms are absent or mild. Over days to weeks, a poorly healing ulcer develops at the bite site. True brown recluse spiders (*Loxosceles reclusa*, also known as the "violin spider" or "fiddleback spider") are found only in the southern and midwestern United States. Other *Loxosceles* species may be found in the southwestern United States and Mexico and are also capable of causing necrotic lesions (Fig. 12–2). *Loxosceles* spiders are reclusive and rarely bite. Hobo spiders (*Tegenaria agrestis*) are native to the northwestern United States and many parts of Europe. Although not well studied, they are thought to cause severe necrotic reactions very similar to *Loxosceles* bites. Necrotic arachnidism is grossly overdiagnosed by physicians. The differential diagnosis of a non-healing cutaneous ulcer is extensive, and the diagnosis of necrotic arachnidism should not be made without supporting evidence.

SYMPTOMS
LOCAL
• Early local symptoms are minimal; pain at the site of the bite may be minimal or absent.

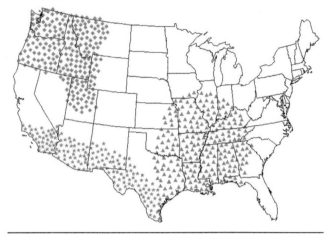

Fig. 12-2 Distribution of spiders causing necrotic wounds in the United States. *Loxosceles reclusa,* brown recluse *(triangles),* other *Loxosceles* species *(stars), Tegenaria agrestis,* hobo spider *(diamonds).*

- Pruritus
- Swelling
- Erythema

SYSTEMIC
Systemic symptoms are rare but may be severe and delayed up to 72 hours.
- Fevers, chills
- Malaise
- Headache
- Anorexia, nausea, vomiting
- Chest and abdominal pain
- Arthralgias and myalgias

SIGNS
LOCAL
- Immediate local signs are generally unimpressive.
- Edema may surround the bite site and angioedema may occur.
- Progression to necrotic lesion may begin within several hours of the bite; the first sign is a purpuric or a hemorrhagic lesion at the site. This may be surrounded by erythema, a ring of pallor, or both.
- A hemorrhagic bulla with a necrotic center develops by day 2 to 3.

- Several days to 2 weeks later an eschar forms, which then sloughs, leaving a persistent ulcer. The ulcer is commonly 7 cm or smaller with an irregular borders and a dry base.
- Healing is slow and results in scarring.

SYSTEMIC

Systemic symptoms manifest before the necrotic lesion develops, generally within hours, progress over 24 to 48 hours, and resolve by 72 to 96 hours. In rare cases multiorgan failure develops.
- Maculopapular or other rash
- Clinical evidence of DIC, hepatic or renal failure, or shock
- Altered mental status, seizures, or coma

WORKUP
- Laboratory studies are not helpful unless systemic symptoms are present. In these cases CBC, coagulation studies, renal and liver function tests, and urinalysis are indicated.
- An ELISA assay for brown recluse venom has been developed but is not widely available.

COMMENTS AND TREATMENT CONSIDERATIONS
Misdiagnosis is common. Consider other causes of ulcerated lesions, including cellulitis, cancer, fungal infections, pyoderma gangrenosum, and cutaneous anthrax. The cosmetic outcome of necrotic spider bites is often very poor. Dapsone therapy is advocated by some experts for brown recluse bites if initiated within 72 hours. However, potential side effects of this agent along with inconclusive data on effectiveness make its use controversial. Unfortunately, no other treatment has yet been established to be effective. Specific antivenom is not commercially available. Surgical excision of the wound, steroid injections, cyproheptadine, and topical nitroglycerin have been advocated but have no proven benefit. Hyperbaric oxygen is a promising treatment option for necrotic spider bites but requires further study. Education of the patient and close follow-up for wound care are important.

REFERENCES
Bryant SM, Pittman LM: Dapsone use in *Loxosceles reclusa* envenomation: is there an indication? *Am J Emerg Med* 21:89, 2003.

Hogan CJ, Barbaro KC, Winkel K: Loxoscelism: old obstacles, new directions, *Ann Emerg Med* 44:608, 2004.

Swanson DL, Vetter RS: Bites of brown recluse spiders and suspected necrotic arachnidism, *N Engl J Med* 352:700, 2005.

CHAPTER 12

Vetter RS, Cushing PE, Crawford RL, et al: Diagnoses of brown
recluse spider bites (loxoscelism) greatly outnumber actual
verifications of the spider in four western American states,
Toxicon 42:413, 2003.

Wright SW, Wrenn KD, Murray L, et al: Clinical presentation and
outcome of brown recluse spider bite, *Ann Emerg Med* 30:28,
1997.

 BITES AND STINGS BY HYMENOPTERA

Many insects of the order Hymenoptera (ants, bees, and wasps)
sting and inject venom defensively. Stings by bees account for the
majority of Hymenoptera-related ED visits. Although Hymenoptera
venom from a single sting does not generally cause serious direct
toxicity, it can precipitate anaphylaxis in sensitized individuals
leading to airway compromise, circulatory collapse, and death
(see Chapter 34, Shortness of Breath). Local hypersensitivity
reactions are much more common.

Multiple stings due to swarming can cause serious morbidity
or even death (Fig. 12–3). In the southern and southwestern
United States, Africanized honeybees ("killer bees") have become
a concern. Although their venom is no more toxic than that of
native bees, they swarm more easily and are more likely to result
in multiple stings. Multiple stings by fire ants (*Solenopsis invicta*),
distributed throughout the southern United States, can also cause
significant morbidity.

SYMPTOMS
- Localized intense pain (very common)
- Localized pruritus (common)
- Nausea (uncommon)
- Dyspnea, throat tightness, or chest tightness may indicate
  anaphylaxis.

SIGNS
- Stinger embedded in wound (uncommon)
- Local erythema and warmth, which may mimic cellulitis
- Local or generalized urticaria
- Vomiting: common with multiple stings
- Renal failure: rare, often a delayed complication of multiple
  stings
- Fire ant stings result in multiple sterile pustules.
- Airway obstruction
- Hypotension

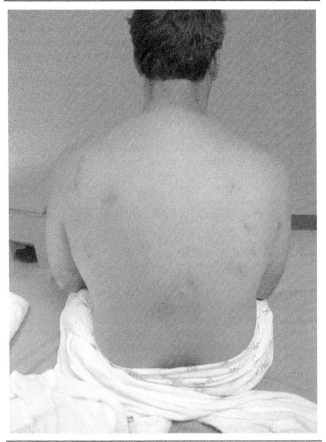

Fig. 12-3 Multiple bee stings after a honeybee swarm.

WORKUP
- A history of sting or bite is usually present.
- Laboratory studies are generally not helpful unless renal failure is suspected.
- Carefully evaluate victims for signs of anaphylaxis or other systemic reaction.

COMMENTS AND TREATMENT CONSIDERATIONS
If present, the stinger should be removed. Anaphylaxis and related syndromes, although uncommon, may occur immediately or soon

after a sting and are life-threatening emergencies. The history of a previous (sensitizing) sting is not always present in cases of severe systemic reactions. Patients who have experienced anaphylactic reactions to Hymenoptera stings should carry an epinephrine autoinjector (EpiPen) when they are outdoors.

Local hypersensitivity reactions result in redness, swelling, and pruritus. Such reactions are often confused with cellulitis (which is uncommon after Hymenoptera bites or sting) and treated inappropriately with antibiotics. The rapid onset of signs (within 24 hours) and presence of pruritus are characteristic of hypersensitivity reactions and can help differentiate them from cellulitis. Antihistamines are indicated for local reactions, with the addition of oral glucocorticosteroids for more extensive reactions. Patients with local hypersensitivity reactions are not necessarily at risk for severe systemic reactions.

Multiple stings can cause vomiting, dyspnea, hypotension, or renal failure. Very large numbers of stings (usually 1000 or more) can be fatal as a result of the toxin, even in the absence of an anaphylactic reaction.

REFERENCES

Bircher AJ: Systemic immediate allergic reactions to arthropod stings and bites, *Dermatology* 210:119, 2005.

Minto SA, Bechtel HB, Erickson TB: North American arthropod envenomation and parasitism. In Auerbach PS (ed): *Wilderness medicine*, ed 4. St. Louis, 2001, Mosby, pp 863-887.

Steen CJ, Janniger CK, Schutzer SE, et al: Insect sting reactions to bees, wasps, and ants, *Int J Dermatol* 44:91, 2005.

Yates AB, Moffitt JE, de Shazo RD: Anaphylaxis to arthropod bites and stings: consensus and controversies, *Immunol Allergy Clin North Am* 21:635, 2001.

 SCORPION STINGS

There are approximately 30 species of scorpions in the United States, but the only native species with a potentially lethal sting is *Centruroides exilicauda*, the bark scorpion. The bark scorpion is native to Arizona and portions of adjacent states. Scorpion venom is complex but is principally neurotoxic, affecting both somatic and autonomic neurons. Scorpions deliver venom from a stinger at the end of the tail.

SYMPTOMS

LOCAL

- Pain at the site of the sting +++++ is often very severe.
- Local paresthesias +++; remote paresthesias are less common.
- Muscle cramping +++

- Hyperesthesia +++
- Pruritus +++

SYSTEMIC
- Apprehension +++
- Headache +++
- Dizziness ++
- Nausea ++
- Palpitations ++
- Shortness of breath ++
- Dyspnea ++

SIGNS
LOCAL
- Hyperesthesia to touch or pain on movement of the envenomated body part ++++
- Erythema +++
- Puncture site visible +++
- Edema +++
- Induration ++

SYSTEMIC
Systemic findings reflect the neurotoxic nature of the venom.
- Tachycardia (>100) ++++ and hypertension (>130/90) +++ from sympathetic autonomic nervous system stimulation
- Occasionally parasympathetic autonomic findings predominate with bradycardia (<60) ++, hypotension (<90/60) +, salivation ++, lacrimation ++, urination, defecation.
- Diaphoresis +++
- Wheezing ++ or stridor
- Rales ++
- Vomiting ++
- Cranial nerve dysfunction: mydriasis ++, roving eye movement ++, nystagmus, blurred vision, dysphagia, dysphonia
- Priapism +
- Altered mental status: restlessness or agitation, seizures (rare)
- Skeletal muscle dysfunction: fasciculations, involuntary muscle jerks (may be mistaken for seizure activity)

WORKUP
Diagnosis and treatment are primarily determined by clinical signs. Laboratory studies are rarely useful following stings by North American scorpions and should be reserved for patients who are systemically ill. Stings from other species around the world may require additional testing.
- ECG and troponins for patients experiencing chest pain

CHAPTER 12

133

- Creatine kinase (CK) and urine myoglobin for patients with severe sustained muscle activity

GRADES OF SCORPION ENVENOMATION
- Grade I—Local pain and/or paresthesias
- Grade II—Remote pain and/or paresthesias
- Grade III—Cranial nerve, autonomic, or somatic skeletal dysfunction: blurred vision, roving eye movement, salivation, tongue fasciculations, dysphagia, dysphonia, and involuntary jerking
- Grade IV—Combined cranial nerve, autonomic, and somatic skeletal dysfunction

COMMENTS AND TREATMENT CONSIDERATIONS
Analgesia and local wound care including tetanus prophylaxis are the only treatments needed for most patients suffering scorpion stings in the United States. Pain may be severe and parenteral opiates may be necessary.

Children are especially at risk for severe systemic reactions to envenomation. Morbidity and mortality are also higher among the elderly and those with comorbid conditions such as severe coronary disease. Patients experiencing systemic reactions should be hospitalized and may need antivenom. Antivenom for *Centruroides* envenomations is effective for severe envenomations and recommended to all patients with grade III and IV envenomations. The antivenom (1 vial [5 ml] IV in 50 ml saline over 30 minutes) resolves systemic symptoms but has no effect on pain and paresthesias. If symptoms persist or progress, the dose may be repeated once. Antivenom has been associated with immediate and delayed hypersensitivity reactions. Severe systemic reactions may require airway management, treatment with vasodilators (e.g., nitroprusside), anticholinergic agents (atropine), beta-blockers, anticonvulsants, and antiemetics.

REFERENCES
Bond GR: Antivenom administration for *Centruroides* scorpion stings: risks and benefits, *Ann Emerg Med* 21:788, 1992.

Forrester MB, Stanley SK: Epidemiology of scorpion envenomations in Texas, *Vet Hum Toxicol* 46:219, 2004.

LoVecchio F, McBride C: Scorpion envenomations in young children in central Arizona, *J Toxicol Clin Toxicol* 41:937, 2003.

LoVecchio F, Welch S, Klemens J, et al: Incidence of immediate and delayed hypersensitivity to Centruroides antivenom, *Ann Emerg Med* 34:615, 1999.

Osnaya-Romero N, deJesus Medina-Hernandez T, Flores-Hernandez SS, et al: Clinical symptoms observed in children envenomated by scorpion stings, at the children's hospital from the State of Morelos, Mexico, *Toxicon* 39:781, 2001.

Suchard JR, Connor DA: Scorpion envenomation. In Auerbach PS (ed): *Wilderness medicine*, ed 4. St. Louis, 2001, Mosby, pp 839-862.

MARINE ENVENOMATIONS

 ### VERTEBRATES (FISH)

Stingrays and multiple species of scorpionfish (lionfish, zebrafish, stonefish, and many others) can cause serious envenomations in humans. Stingrays envenomate through a stinger at their tail, whereas most others envenomate through direct contact with their spines. Virtually all fish venom is heat labile, in contrast to invertebrate venom. Anaphylactic reactions can occur after envenomations but are rare.

SYMPTOMS
- Severe pain at the site of envenomation
- Localized pruritus
- Foreign body sensation if there are retained spines or stinger parts

SIGNS
- Punctate erythematous lesions (fish with spines)
- Puncture (stingrays)
- Vesicles
- Retained foreign body palpable or visible
- Signs of anaphylaxis: bronchospasm, stridor, rash, hypotension (see Anaphylaxis in Chapter 34, Shortness of Breath)

WORKUP
- A history of contact or a sting is usually present.
- Laboratory studies are not helpful.

COMMENTS AND TREATMENT CONSIDERATIONS
The venom is heat labile and inactivated by immersion in water as warm as the victim tolerates. Local wound care and tetanus prophylaxis should be provided. Foreign bodies should be considered, especially with stingrays.

 ### INVERTEBRATES (JELLYFISH AND SEA URCHINS)

Jellyfish (man of war, box jellyfish, and many others) are members of the phylum Coelenterata, marine invertebrates that include the corals, sea anemones, and jellyfish. Jellyfish inject venom into the

CHAPTER 12

skin of human victims using a multitude of tiny nematocysts, or "stinging cells." Although envenomations by the Australian box jellyfish can result in death, mortality is extremely rare in North America. Anaphylaxis can occur but is also rare.

Sea urchin envenomation usually occurs when the victim inadvertently touches or steps on an urchin.

SYMPTOMS
- Localized pain and pruritus +++++, which may be severe
- Systemic symptoms (nausea, malaise, and headache) are uncommon following North American envenomations.

SIGNS
- "Tentacle prints": erythematous curvilinear, raised lesions where tentacles have brushed across skin
- Local urticaria or edema
- Vesicles or bullae are uncommon.
- Signs of anaphylaxis: bronchospasm, stridor, rash, hypotension (see Anaphylaxis in Chapter 34, Shortness of Breath)

WORKUP
- A history of contact with a spine or a stinger is usually present.
- Laboratory studies are not helpful.

COMMENTS AND TREATMENT CONSIDERATIONS
Tentacles, if present, should be carefully removed from the skin as soon as possible. Affected areas should initially be flushed with sea water (NOT fresh water, which causes further firing of nematocyst cells). Avoid rubbing the area, which can also activate firing. Nematocysts should be inactivated with 5% acetic acid (vinegar), aluminum sulfate (Stingose), or a similar solution. Urine or isopropyl alcohol may be effective when no other treatment is available. The inactivated nematocysts can then be scraped off with the edge of a sharp instrument.

Sea urchin envenomations are treated differently than those of other invertebrates. Treatment is immersion of the affected part in hot water and wound care with prompt removal of embedded spines.

REFERENCES
Auerbach PS: Envenomation by aquatic vertebrates. In Auerbach PS (ed): *Wilderness medicine*, ed 4. St. Louis, 2001, Mosby, pp 1488-1506.
Auerbach PS: Envenomation by aquatic invertebrates. In Auerbach PS (ed): *Wilderness medicine*, ed 4. St. Louis, 2001, Mosby, pp 1450-1487.

Church JE, Hodgson WC: The pharmacological activity of fish venoms, *Toxicon* 40:1083, 2002.

Currie BJ: Marine antivenoms, *J Toxicol Clin Toxicol* 41:301-308, 2003.

Fenner PJ: Dangers in the ocean: the traveler and marine envenomation I. Jellyfish, *J Travel Med* 5:135, 1998.

Fenner PJ: Dangers in the ocean: the traveler and marine envenomation II. Marine vertebrates, *J Travel Med* 5:213, 1998.

Perkins RA, Morgan SS: Poisoning, envenomation, and trauma from marine creatures, *Am Fam Physician* 69:885, 2004.

SNAKE BITES

Although snake bites create anxiety and sometimes excruciating pain, mortality is rare, with 1 to 15 deaths annually in the United States. Deaths most often occur in children or the elderly and in most cases are a result of delayed or insufficient antivenom therapy or immediate hypersensitivity to the venom.

There are two families of venomous snakes in North America: the Viperidae (pit vipers) and the Elapidae (coral snakes). At least 96% of venomous snake bites by native U.S. snakes are caused by pit vipers, with coral snakes accounting for no more than 4%. Pit vipers are characterized by:

- A triangular head
- A pair of heat-sensing pits located between each eye and the nostril
- Elliptical pupils
- A pair of long hollow erectile fangs attached to the maxilla that are folded back along the roof of the mouth until the snake is ready to strike

In contrast, coral snakes and nonvenomous snakes have a rounded head, no pits, round pupils, and small fixed fangs.

North American coral snakes can be identified by their color pattern, which differentiates them from the nonvenomous kingsnake and other mimics. The red and yellow bands of the coral snake are adjacent, whereas on the kingsnake the colored bands are separated by a black band. North American coral snakes also have a black head, whereas most mimics have a red or other colored head. Recognition of this distinction has given rise to the well-known rhyme "Red on yellow, kill the fellow. Red on black, venom lack."

The two most important prehospital actions after snake bite are immobilization of the victim and the injured body part and rapid transport to the nearest medical facility where appropriate therapy, including antivenom treatment as necessary, can be given.

CHAPTER 12

FAMILY VIPIRIDAE, SUBFAMILY CROTALINAE

The subfamily Crotalinae includes the rattlesnakes (genus *Crotalus*), copperhead and cottonmouth (water moccasin) (*Agkistrodon*), and Pygmy rattler and Massasauga (*Sistrurus*). Crotaline venom is a complex mixture of digestive enzymes, peptides, low-molecular-weight substances, and minerals. Although the effects of envenomation vary between species, the venom generally causes local tissue necrosis and systemic consumption coagulopathy and vascular damage. There may be neuromuscular dysfunction, especially following bites by the Mojave rattlesnake. In severe cases these processes result in hypovolemic shock, metabolic acidosis, renal failure, and death. The clinical signs and symptoms of Crotaline envenomation generally begin within 30 to 60 minutes of the bite. Up to 25% of bites do not result in envenomation ("dry bite"), in which case the only symptoms are those of a puncture wound.

SYMPTOMS AND SIGNS
See Tables 12–2 and 12–3.

TABLE 12–2

SYMPTOMS AND SIGNS OF CROTALINE ENVENOMATION

EARLY		LATE	
Local	Systemic	Local	Systemic
Severe pain*	Nausea, vomiting	Progressive swelling	Coagulopathy
Puncture wounds with bloody drainage†	Diarrhea	Ecchymosis and bullae	Dyspnea
Swelling	Salivation	Compartment syndrome	Cardiovascular collapse
Erythema	Perioral paresthesia	Necrosis	Seizures
Paresthesia	Generalized weakness Tachycardia Tachypnea Anxiety Altered mental status Hypotension Anaphylaxis (rare)	Ulceration Wound infection (uncommon)	Coma GI and pulmonary bleeding

*Pain is present in over 90% of viper bites except bites from the Mojave rattlesnake.
†Fang marks can vary from scratches to paired or multiple puncture wounds.

TABLE 12-3

GUIDELINES FOR ASSESSING THE SEVERITY OF NORTH AMERICAN PIT VIPER ENVENOMATION

TYPES OF SIGNS OR SYMPTOMS	SEVERITY OF ENVENOMATION		
	Minimal	Moderate	Severe
Local	Swelling, erythema, or ecchymosis confined to the site of the bite	Progression of swelling, erythema, or ecchymosis beyond the site of the bite	Rapid swelling, erythema, or ecchymosis on the entire body part
Systemic	No systemic signs or symptoms	Non–life-threatening signs and symptoms (nausea, vomiting, perioral paresthesias, myokymia, and mild hypotension)	Markedly severe signs and symptoms (hypotension, altered sensorium, tachycardia, tachypnea, and respiratory distress)
Coagulation	No coagulation abnormalities or other important laboratory abnormalities	Mildly abnormal coagulation profile without clinical bleeding; mild abnormalities on other laboratory tests	Markedly abnormal coagulation profile with evidence of bleeding or threat of spontaneous hemorrhage (immeasurable INR, APTT, and thrombocytopenia with platelet count <20,000/ml); other laboratory tests may be severely abnormal

12

CHAPTER

WORKUP

- Complete blood count
- PT, PTT, fibrinogen, and D-dimer
- Electrolytes, urea, creatinine, and creatine kinase
- Urinalysis
- Blood typing and crossmatch

- Chest x-ray if respiratory symptoms
- ECG

COMMENTS AND TREATMENT CONSIDERATIONS

Following a bite, the limb should be immobilized in a neutral position. Constricting clothing and jewelry should be removed. Evidence does not support the use of constricting bands or wide-area pressure dressings for pit viper envenomations, and these interventions can worsen local ischemia. If they have already been applied, venous constricting bands should generally not be removed until after an IV has been established and the patient has arrived at a medical facility. There is no convincing evidence in support of incision with or without suction. Acute systemic allergic reactions, including anaphylaxis, are uncommon but can be immediately life threatening and should be treated aggressively (see Anaphylaxis in Chapter 34, Shortness of Breath).

Repeated measurement of the envenomated limb and marking of the leading edge of the swelling assist in monitoring progression of local effects. Generally accepted indications for the use of antivenom are progression of local signs, systemic symptoms or signs, and development of coagulation abnormalities. Two commercial antivenoms are currently in production. Wyeth Wyeth-ESI Lederle, which had halted production of the equine Antivenom Crotalidae Polyvalent (ACP), has resumed manufacture, but this antivenom remains in short supply. Savage Laboratories produces the ovine Crotalidae Polyvalent Immune Fab (CroFab) antivenom. The recommended initial treatment is Crotaline Polyvalent Immune Fab antivenom 4 to 6 vials IV. Allergic reaction to the antivenom can occur. A history of allergies and previous bites should be obtained and risk versus benefit analyzed prior to treatment. Continuous monitoring is essential, and resuscitation equipment and medications, including epinephrine, should be immediately available. If the patient fails to improve, the initial dose should be repeated. Recurrence either locally with renewed swelling or systemically with coagulopathy is common. Consultation with a poison center or individual with experience in management of snake bites is strongly recommended.

Tetanus prophylaxis should be administered as needed. Traditional measures that are not currently recommended include cryotherapy, electric shock, and excision. Fasciotomy is indicated only for documented compartment syndrome unresponsive to limb elevation and antivenom.

 FAMILY ELAPIDAE

The family Elapidae includes the cobras, coral snakes, and sea snakes. In North America, the elapid of interest is the coral snake, of which there are three species: Eastern coral snake, Texas coral snake, and the Western (Sonoran) coral snake. The major components of coral snake venom are alpha neurotoxins, which block acetylcholine nicotinic receptors, causing weakness and paralysis. The coral snake is small and nonaggressive. The mouth is small and has fixed anterior fangs. When biting, the coral snake has to hold on briefly and chew in order to envenomate. This makes effective envenomation of humans difficult. About 50% of coral snake bites never result in symptoms or signs of envenomation; these are thought to be dry bites.

Coral snake envenomation results in minimal early signs and symptoms that include minor pain and fang marks without swelling. Even minimal redness or edema is present in only about half of envenomations, and bullae are seen in only 5%. The onset of neurotoxic symptoms may take hours to develop.

SYMPTOMS
- Paresthesia +++
- Nausea, vomiting ++
- Dizziness ++
- Euphoria ++
- Weakness ++
- Diplopia ++
- Dyspnea ++
- Diaphoresis ++
- Muscle tenderness ++

SIGNS
- Fang marks ++++ are present but can be easily overlooked unless the site of the bite is known.
- Local swelling ++ is often minimal or absent.
- Fasciculations +
- Drowsiness, weakness, apprehension
- Weakness
- Dysphagia
- Dyspnea
- Salivation, nausea, and vomiting
- Weakness of extraocular muscles, miotic pupils, bulbar paralysis
- Respiratory depression
- Confusion
- Seizures

COMMENTS AND TREATMENT CONSIDERATIONS
A wide-area pressure dressing (Sutherland wrap) applied proximally within minutes of the time of the bite may improve the outcome of coral snake bites. If a pressure dressing has been applied, it

CHAPTER 12

141

should be removed at a health care facility after an IV has been started.

Administration of antivenom (*M. fulvius* antivenom 5 vials IV) is appropriate for all patients who are known to have been bitten by a coral snake without regard to symptoms. Minimal early signs and symptoms should not dissuade the physician from giving antivenom because it is less effective if delayed until major symptoms develop. The dose may be repeated if symptoms progress. Tetanus prophylaxis should be administered as needed.

REFERENCES

Alberts MB, Shalit M, LoGalbo F: Suction for venomous snakebite: a study of "mock venom" extraction in a human model, *Ann Emerg Med* 43:181, 2004.

Bush SP: Snakebite suction devices don't remove venom: they just suck, *Ann Emerg Med* 43:187, 2004.

Gold BS, Barish RA, Dart RC: North American snake envenomation: diagnosis, treatment and management, *Emerg Med Clin North Am* 22:423, 2004.

Gold BS, Dart RC, Barish RA: Current concepts: bites of venomous snakes, *N Engl J Med* 347:347, 2002.

Hals GD, Brittain E: Bites and stings: an overview of close encounters with nature Part I, *Emerg Med* 26:95, 2005.

Hals GD, Brittain E: Bites and stings: an overview of close encounters with nature Part II, *Emerg Med* 26:112, 2005.

Lavonas EJ, Gerardo CJ, O'Malley G, et al: Initial experience with Crotalidae polyvalent immune Fab (ovine) antivenom in the treatment of copperhead snakebite, *Ann Emerg Med* 43:200, 2004.

LoVecchio F, Klemens J, Welch S, Rodriguez R: Antibiotics after rattlesnake envenomation, *J Emerg Med* 23:327, 2002.

Ruha A-M, Curry SC, Beuhler M, et al: Initial postmarketing experience with crotalidae polyvalent immune fab for treatment of rattlesnake envenomation, *Ann Emerg Med* 39:609, 2002.

Extremity Pain and Numbness
Steven Go

Nontraumatic extremity pain is not a particularly common or dangerous-sounding complaint. However, this symptom may arise in several disorders such as vascular, spinal, and infectious emergencies that are virtually impossible to diagnose unless the emergency physician's clinical suspicion for them is high. Severe, unexplained pain should cause the emergency physician to consider serious conditions even when the physical examination is initially unimpressive.

 NECROTIZING FASCIITIS

Patients with necrotizing fasciitis, if seen early in the course of the disease, may present with severe pain without obvious signs of infection. Severe, unexplained pain should lead the emergency physician to consider this diagnosis because early surgical intervention is required to prevent death.

See Chapter 30, Rash.

 ACUTE ARTERIAL OCCLUSION

Peripheral arterial disease results in significant morbidity and mortality. Its most immediately limb-threatening manifestation, acute arterial occlusion (AAO), generally arises with an abrupt onset of pain and can result in significant mortality, especially in elderly persons (as high as 42%). Classic findings—the five Ps of pain, pallor, paresthesia, pulselessness, and paralysis—generally occur late, and their absence does not exclude an acute event. Ischemic tissue death can begin within 4 hours. Chronic arterial insufficiency can also cause ischemic changes. Worsening claudication or rest

143

claudication may be the presenting symptom in the lower extremities that have collateral flow.

It is important to determine the cause of the obstruction because treatment can vary on the basis of whether the obstruction is due to in situ thrombosis or an embolus. Thrombosis is likely in the presence of preexisting peripheral vascular disease as a result of local stasis. Embolic disease frequently occurs in patients without preexisting symptoms of peripheral arterial occlusive disease and is associated with atrial fibrillation or recent cardioversion. Cocaine use has also been associated with acute arterial thrombosis.

SYMPTOMS
Severity of symptoms depends on the location of the occlusion and on the level of collateral flow that developed previously.
- Pain +++++
- Coldness
- Paresthesia
- Numbness
- Paralysis
- Patients with acute embolic occlusion in digits may complain only of sudden pain and coldness

SIGNS
- Ischemic pain (typically worsens with passive stretch of ischemic muscles)
- Coldness
- Tenderness
- Pallor and/or cyanosis, livedo reticularis (a fishnet appearance of the skin)
- Sensory deficit
- Paralysis (late)
- Pulse deficit
- Ulceration and gangrene (in late stages of hypoperfusion)
- Bruits may be heard in the presence of fistulas or aneurysms.

WORKUP
- Bedside Doppler examination should be used to determine the presence or absence of pulses. Studies have demonstrated that physicians are inaccurate in determining the presence of pulses by palpation alone.
- The ankle-brachial index (ABI), defined as the highest Doppler-derived systolic ankle blood pressure in either the dorsalis pedis or posterior tibial artery in each leg divided by the highest brachial artery systolic pressure, may indicate severity of disease (<50% indicates severe insufficiency). ABIs may be falsely elevated

in patients with calcified lower extremity vessels (diabetics and renal failure patients). In those cases, the toe-brachial index (TBI) may be of use; however, this measurement requires a special small blood pressure cuff for the toe.

- Allen's test (measuring the number of seconds of capillary refill in the hand by the ulnar and radial arteries) should be done if upper extremity occlusion is suspected.
- ECG (and/or echocardiography) should be obtained if an embolic cause is suspected.

COMMENTS AND TREATMENT CONSIDERATIONS

The clinician should take care not to confuse AAO with low flow due to diminished cardiac output superimposed on preexisting chronic occlusive disease or ischemic signs caused by massive deep venous thrombosis (*phlegmasia cerulea dolens*).

After arterial occlusion has occurred, loss of muscle viability soon follows. Therefore, when an AAO is suspected, an emergent vascular surgical consultation is warranted before other investigative studies are begun. These may include color flow Doppler studies or arteriography. Magnetic resonance angiography has been shown to be very highly accurate for assessment of lower extremity ischemia but can introduce long delays before definitive treatment.

Depending on the location of the occlusion, treatment may involve catheter-directed thrombolysis, stenting, or surgery. Several randomized comparisons of thrombolysis and surgery have been published, and at least three have shown similar limb salvage with decreased morbidity and mortality in the patients treated with catheter-directed thrombolysis. Finally, the etiology of the occlusive lesion should be determined and aggressively treated.

REFERENCES

Ascher E, Hingorani A, Markevich N, et al: Acute lower limb ischemia: the value of duplex ultrasound arterial mapping (DUAM) as the sole preoperative imaging technique, *Ann Vasc Surg* 17:284, 2003.

Clagett GP, Sobel M, Jackson MR, et al: Antithrombotic therapy in peripheral arterial occlusive disease: the seventh AACP conference on antithrombotic and thrombolytic therapy: evidence-based guidelines, *Chest* 126:609S, 2004.

Criqui MH, Frorek A, Klauber MR, et al: The sensitivity, specificity, and predictive value of traditional clinical evaluation of peripheral arterial disease: results from noninvasive testing in a defined population, *Circulation* 71:516, 1985.

Katzen BT: Clinical diagnosis and prognosis of acute limb ischemia, *Rev Cardiovasc Med* 3(S2):S2, 2002.

CHAPTER 13

Koelemay MJW, Lijimer JG, Stoker J, et al: Magnetic resonance angiography for the evaluation of lower extremity arterial disease: a meta-analysis, *JAMA* 285:1338, 2001.

Mohler ER: Peripheral arterial disease: identification and implications, *Arch Intern Med* 163:2306, 2003.

Ouriel K: Comparison of thrombolytic treatment of peripheral arterial disease, *Rev Cardiovasc Med* 3(S2):S7, 2002.

Richards T, Pittathankal AA, Magree TR, Galland RB: The current role of intra-arterial thrombolysis, *Eur J Vasc Endovasc Surg* 16:166, 2003.

Zhou W, Lin PH, Bush RL, et al: Acute arterial thrombosis associated with cocaine abuse, *J Vasc Surg* 20:291, 2004.

 COMPARTMENT SYNDROME

Compartment syndrome (CS) occurs when the intracompartmental pressure compresses the neurovascular structures in an osseofascial space. It can occur in the leg (most common), foot, hand, forearm, arm, shoulder, thigh, and buttocks, with or without fractures. Some conditions predispose to CS, including hemophilia, sickle cell disease, and anticoagulant use. The majority of cases occur after trauma (acute or repetitive, including exercise), but CS can also occur as the result of less obvious etiologies such as intraoperative lithotomy positioning. The clinical diagnosis of CS is often difficult, and a high level of suspicion is mandatory to prevent untoward outcomes.

SYMPTOMS
- Pain +++++ (may be out of proportion to the injury)
- Tightness and swelling
- Throbbing
- Paresthesias
- Weakness (late)
- Numbness (late)

SIGNS
- Swollen, tense compartment +++++
- Pain ++++ is exacerbated by passive stress of the compartment in question, although the severity of pain on passive stretch or palpation does not predict the amount of pressure.
- Diminished two-point discrimination +++
- Hyperesthesia
- Anesthesia
- Skin may be shiny and warm.
- Weakness (late)
- Loss of pulse (late)

146

WORKUP

- Compartment pressure measurement +++++. Traditionally, hand-held needle manometers were used to measure these pressures, but modern transducer-tipped probes have been shown to be more accurate and easier to use. More recently, less invasive ultrasonic devices have been proposed for this indication as well.
- Serial measurements should be performed by the same operator using the same method when possible.
- Nerve stimulation studies, arteriography, and Doppler studies have been described as diagnostic adjuncts but have limited use in an emergent setting.
- Laboratory testing is not useful.
- The limb in question should not be elevated to avoid reducing perfusion further.
- Patients should be kept fasting in preparation for possible emergent fasciotomy.

COMMENTS AND TREATMENT CONSIDERATIONS

Fasciotomy, done to relieve the increased pressure, is the treatment of CS. The level of pressure at which fasciotomy is indicated is controversial. Many cite a threshold from 30 to 45 mm Hg. Alternatively, compartment pressure as a percentage of diastolic pressure has been used as a threshold. In general, elevated compartment pressures (30 mm Hg or greater) or a strong clinical suspicion of neurovascular compromise should prompt emergency orthopedic or surgical bedside evaluation. Quick action is important as delayed fasciotomy has been associated with poor outcomes, most commonly related to infection that follows tissue necrosis. Failure to diagnose CS can have devastating consequences, and serial measurements may be required; the patient may need to be admitted for reevaluation if the diagnosis is unclear. CS should always be suspected in extremity injuries.

CHAPTER 13

REFERENCES

Bankes MJK, Dowd GSE, Lewis AAM: Compartment syndrome following pelvic surgery in the lithotomy position, *Ann R Coll Surg Engl* 84:170, 2002.

Bertoldo U, Nicodemo A, Pallavicini J, Masse A: Acute bilateral compartment syndrome of the thigh induced by spinning training, *Injury* 34:791, 2003.

Burns BJ, Sproule J, Smyth H: Acute compartment syndrome of the anterior thigh following quadriceps strain in a footballer, *Br J Sports Med* 38:218, 2004.

Ehsan O, Darwish A, Edmundson C, et al: Non-traumatic lower limb vascular complications in endurance athletes: review of the literature, *Eur J Vasc Endovasc Surg* 28:1, 2004.

Elliott KGB, Johnstone A: Diagnosing acute compartment syndrome, *J Bone Joint Surg Br* 85:625, 2003.

Heemskerk J, Kitslaar P: Acute compartment syndrome of the lower leg: retrospective study on prevalence, technique and outcome of fasciotomies, *World J Surg* 27:744, 2003.

Hope MJ, McQueen MM: Acute compartment syndrome in the absence of fracture, *J Orthop Trauma* 18:220, 2004.

Jawed S, Jawad ASM, Padhiar N, Perry JD: Chronic exertional compartment syndrome of the forearms secondary to weight training, *Rheumatology* 40:344, 2001.

Lynch JE, Heyman JS, Hargens AR: Ultrasonic device for the noninvasive diagnosis of compartment syndrome, *Physiol Meas* 25:N1, 2004.

Mithofer K, Lhowe DW, Vrahas MS: Clinical spectrum of acute compartment syndrome of the thigh and its relation to associated injuries, *Clin Orthop* 425:223, 2004.

Pease MF, Harry L, Nanchahal J: Acute compartment syndrome of the leg, *BMJ* 325:557, 2002.

Tiwari A, Haq AI, Myint F, Hamilton G: Acute compartment syndrome, *Br J Surg* 89:397, 2002.

DEEP VENOUS THROMBOSIS

Risk factors for deep venous thrombosis (DVT) include active malignancy, paralysis, paresis or immobilization of an extremity, recent bedridden state, advanced age, pregnancy and postpartum state, premenopausal estrogen use, obesity, hypercoagulable states, congestive heart failure, trauma, long bone fractures, dehydration, and polycythemia. This section focuses primarily on lower extremity DVT. It is important to note that clinical diagnosis of DVT is *unreliable*, and classic signs and symptoms are often misleading or absent. A scoring system, commonly known as the Wells criteria (in addition to several variants), is now in widespread use to characterize the pretest probability of lower extremity DVT in conjunction with diagnostic tests (Table 13–1).

SYMPTOMS
- Pain
- Swelling
- Erythema

SIGNS
- Normal examination +++
- Swelling (measured difference between lower extremities)
- Warmth
- Erythema

TABLE 13–1

MODIFIED WELLS CRITERIA FOR PREDICTING THE PRETEST PROBABILITY OF DVT

CLINICAL CHARACTERISTIC	SCORE
Active cancer (patient receiving treatment for cancer within the previous 6 months or currently receiving palliative treatment)	1
Paralysis, paresis, or recent plaster immobilization of the lower extremities	1
Recently bedridden for 3 days or more or major surgery within the previous 12 weeks requiring general or regional anesthesia	1
Localized tenderness along the distribution of the deep venous system	1
Entire leg swollen	1
Calf swelling at least 3 cm larger than that on the asymptomatic side (measured 10 cm below tibial tuberosity)	1
Pitting edema confined to the symptomatic leg	1
Collateral superficial veins (nonvaricose)	1
Previously documented deep vein thrombosis	1
Alternative diagnosis at least as likely as deep vein thrombosis	−2

Score: ≥2, DVT likely; <2, DVT unlikely. In patients with bilateral symptoms, the more symptomatic leg is used. Prevalence of DVT or PE within 3 months: "likely" 27.9% (95% CI: 23.9-31.8); "unlikely" 5.5% (95% CI: 3.8-7.6)
Adapted with permission from Wells PS, Anderson DR, Rodger M, et al: Evaluation of D-dimer in the diagnosis of suspected deep-vein thrombosis, *N Engl J Med* 349:1227, 2003.

- Tenderness of the thigh or calf
- Fever
- Homans' sign (frequently mentioned, but unreliable)
- Palpable venous "cord" in the popliteal fossa

WORKUP

- D-dimer. This is a cross-linked derivative of fibrin that is frequently elevated in patients with thromboembolic diseases. Several different types of D-dimer assays exist. Overall, ELISA and quantitative rapid ELISA-based assays are more sensitive (96%) than quantitative latex and whole blood methods (85% and 87%, respectively). However, whole blood methods are more specific (93%) than either quantitative latex (66%) or ELISA assays (38% to 44%) in all patients. Therefore, D-dimer should be

CHAPTER 13

used only in the context of an evidence-based protocol. *Advantages*: Noninvasive; rapid; can be very sensitive. *Disadvantages*: Test profile varies with specific assay used at each institution. D-dimer can be falsely negative in high-risk patients (i.e., patients who have a high pretest probability of disease). Assays that are very sensitive are less specific.

- Ultrasonography. Includes duplex ultrasonography (compression plus pulsed Doppler signal) and color flow duplex imaging (duplex plus color pulsed Doppler signal). *Advantages*: Noninvasive; average sensitivity and specificity for proximal DVT is 97%; can diagnose conditions other than DVT; relatively inexpensive. *Disadvantages*: Operator dependent; inaccurate for DVT below the knee (sensitivity as low as 75%); frequently negative in patients with proven PE; not available after hours in many institutions.

- Contrast venography. Formerly the "gold standard," is now used infrequently because of potential complications and availability and quality of noninvasive studies. *Advantages*: Considered the gold standard; can view entire deep system of lower extremity. *Disadvantages*: Invasive; contrast dye load; can rarely cause DVT; cannot be done in 10% of patients (inability to acquire venous access, infection, renal insufficiency, previous allergy); interobserver disagreement (10%).

- Impedance plethysmography. Seldom used in the United States. *Advantages*: Noninvasive; may be useful for serial examinations for propagation of calf vein thrombosis. *Disadvantages*: Poor performance below the knee; cannot distinguish between thrombotic and nonthrombotic obstruction of venous flow (e.g., CHF can lead to a positive result); poor in obese or uncooperative patients; variable sensitivity and specificity for proximal DVT have been reported.

- Spiral CT and MRI. *Advantages*: High accuracy reported in small trials to date. *Disadvantages*: High cost, limited data. Currently, a second-line diagnostic strategy in light of the rise of D-dimer/ ultrasound protocols

COMMENTS AND TREATMENT CONSIDERATIONS

The diagnosis of DVT has been extensively researched with hundreds of studies published in the last several years alone. Despite this, the optimal diagnostic strategy to detect DVT remains controversial, primarily because of questions regarding the objectivity and reproducibility of the Wells criteria, the gradual downward trend in the literature of the prevalence of thromboembolic events in the Wells "low-risk" groups, and the widely differing test characteristics of the various D-dimer assays.

Currently, the literature supports using a systematic scoring system to assess pretest probability and then performing a

D-dimer test to stratify risk further. Depending on the results, this is followed by ultrasonography. However, in light of the variability of the test characteristics of currently available D-dimer assays, it is prudent for clinicians to do the following:

1. Determine a pretest probability of disease and understand the test characteristics of the D-dimer assay at their institution before ordering the D-dimer test.

2. Use the D-dimer only to help confirm decisions in low-risk groups (as opposed to no-risk or high-risk groups).

3. Use only a negative D-dimer result to make clinical decisions. For example, a positive result in a population with virtually no risk of a thromboembolic event should not prompt ordering of further (unnecessary) studies.

Alternatively, some centers simply perform ultrasonography routinely, sometimes repeating the study in 7 days for high-risk patients who have a normal initial study. Currently, no one protocol has emerged as the definitive standard of care. It is up to the clinician to determine what specific diagnostic tests (including the specific D-dimer assay) are available at his or her institution and then to select the appropriate evidence-based protocol to use.

Traditionally, proximal DVT required admission for anticoagulation to prevent pulmonary embolism. Although this is still a reasonable strategy for high-risk, complicated, or noncompliant patients, the advent of low-molecular-weight heparin (LMWH) has made outpatient treatment for selected patients a viable alternative. If LMWH or outpatient therapy is contraindicated (e.g., creatinine >2.5 mg/dl, pregnancy, pulmonary embolus, multiple DVTs), admission is required. Inpatient anticoagulation with LMWH or unfractionated heparin (UFH) dosed in a weight-based protocol may be used, along with a vitamin K antagonist. Catheter-directed thrombolytics rarely play a role in the management of DVT unless it is in the upper extremity, where several case series have shown excellent outcomes. In contrast, systemic thrombolytics are not indicated for DVT. Some investigators have reported encouraging results for surgical management of selected DVT; however, these results are preliminary.

Management of calf DVT is controversial. Treatment options include admission for UFH and outpatient treatment with LMWH or nonsteroidal antiinflammatory drug treatments. Many centers perform serial ultrasonography to monitor the calf DVT for signs of progression. If outpatient management is elected, close follow-up is essential.

Emergency physicians may consider prescribing compression stockings to patients with known DVT to help prevent the pain, edema, skin discoloration, and ulceration that commonly occur in these patients (postthrombotic syndrome). They should also

151

consider administering anticoagulation to prevent DVT in all admitted patients.

REFERENCES

Buller HR, Agnelli G, Hull RD, et al: Antithrombotic therapy for venous thromboembolic disease: the seventh AACP conference on antithrombotic and thrombolytic therapy, *Chest* 125:401S, 2004.

Joffe HV, Goldhaber SZ: Upper-extremity deep vein thrombosis, *Circulation* 106:1874, 2002.

Kahn SR, Ginsberg JS: Relationship between deep venous thrombosis and the postthrombotic syndrome, *Arch Intern Med* 154:17, 2004.

Stein PD, Russell DH, Patel KC, et al: D-dimer for the exclusion of acute venous thrombosis and pulmonary embolism: a systematic review, *Ann Intern Med* 140:589, 2004.

Tovey C, Wyatt S: Diagnosis, investigation, and management of deep vein thrombosis, *BMJ* 326:1180, 2003.

Wells PS, Anderson DR, Bormanis J, et al: Value of assessment of pretest probability of deep-vein thrombosis in clinical management, *Lancet* 350:1795, 1997.

Wells PS, Anderson DR, Rodger M, et al: Evaluation of D-dimer in the diagnosis of suspected deep-vein thrombosis, *N Engl J Med* 349:1227, 2003.

 SUPERIOR VENA CAVA SYNDROME

Superior vena cava syndrome (SVCS) is a process characterized by obstruction of venous return in the thoracic portion of the SVC and is associated with facial or upper extremity swelling. This condition is most commonly seen in patients with malignancy because of a hypercoagulable state or in patients with intrathoracic neoplasms that compress the SVC. The diagnosis is established clinically, with imaging studies performed to identify the causal lesion. In an immunocompromised host, tuberculosis or histoplasmosis should be considered. Less common causes include goiter, fibrosis, and aortic valve replacement. Iatrogenic causes include pacer wires, catheters, and central lines. Although symptoms may have a gradual onset, they may rapidly progress to become life threatening.

SYMPTOMS
- Swelling of face, upper extremities, upper chest
- Dyspnea
- Cough
- Chest pain

- Difficulty swallowing
- Hoarseness
- Stridor
- Headache
- Nasal stuffiness
- Tongue swelling
- Nausea
- Lightheadedness
- Can be occult

SIGNS
- Facial edema ++++
- Jugular venous distention +++
- Distention of thoracic veins +++
- Dyspnea +++
- Facial plethora ++
- Upper extremity edema ++
- Cyanosis ++
- Paralysis of true vocal cords
- Papilledema
- Syncope
- Horner's syndrome (rare)

WORKUP
- Chest x-rays ++++
- Computed tomography +++++
- MRI +++++
- Venography not generally required
- Nuclear flow studies (using nonthrombogenic tracers) recommended by some authors

COMMENTS AND TREATMENT CONSIDERATIONS
Early consultation is important. If SVCS is due to a neoplasm, the most common treatment is radiation therapy, chemotherapy, or a combination thereof. Endovascular stenting has been proposed to relieve the obstruction in a more rapid fashion. Emergent stabilization measures may include elevation of the head of bed, oxygen, steroids, and occasionally diuretics.

REFERENCES
Abner A: Approach to the patient who presents with superior vena cava obstruction, *Chest* 103(Suppl):394, 1993.

Baker GL, Barnes HJ: Superior vena cava syndrome: etiology, diagnosis, and treatment, *Am J Crit Care* 1:54, 1992.

Courtheoux P, Alkofer B, Al Refai M: Stent placement in superior vena cava syndrome, *Ann Thorac Surg* 75:158, 2003.

CHAPTER 13

Kim Y, Kim K, Ko Y: Endovascular stenting as a first choice for the palliation of superior vena cava syndrome, *J Korean Med Sci* 19:519, 2004.

Lanciego C, Chacon JL, Julian A, et al: Stenting as a first option for endovascular treatment of malignant superior vena cava syndrome, *Am J Roentgenol* 177:585-593, 2001.

Otten TR, Stein PD, Patel CK, et al: Thromboembolic disease involving the superior vena cava and brachiocephalic veins, *Chest* 123:809, 2003.

 SPINAL CORD COMPRESSION (NONTRAUMATIC)

See Chapter 4, Back Pain, Lower.

Eye Pain and Redness
Joseph S. Englanoff

A chief complaint of an irritated, red eye is a common occurrence in the ED. The majority of cases typically involve viral or bacterial conjunctivitis, but other infections and noninfectious causes must always be considered. Global conjunctival injection should be distinguished from perilimbic injection, which is commonly seen in iritis.

True eye pain is a concerning symptom, as conjunctival irritation alone generally causes itching or a gritty sensation but not pain. Pain is caused by pathologic conditions of other structures, such as the cornea, iris, and deeper eye tissues, or by inflammation of tissues surrounding the eye.

If topical anesthesia (used only for diagnostic and not prescribed for therapeutic purposes) does not provide pain relief, pathologic conditions deep to the cornea should be suspected. Consensual pain (eye pain elicited by shining a light in the opposite, unaffected eye) suggests iritis. Pain with eye movement is suggestive of bulbar or retrobulbar neuritis in the absence of orbital cellulitis, which causes similar symptoms. Eye pain with systemic symptoms raises the concern of glaucoma.

A complete ophthalmologic examination, including visual acuity, lid eversion to rule out foreign body, and pupillary, slit-lamp, and funduscopic examinations, is necessary in most cases in which typical conjunctivitis is not obvious. Measurement of intraocular pressure (IOP) and indirect ophthalmoscopy should also be performed when indicated.

 ## ACUTE ANGLE-CLOSURE GLAUCOMA

In acute angle-closure glaucoma, onset of symptoms is usually sudden and is often secondary to rapid pupillary dilation (e.g., after entering a darkened room or after use of anticholinergic or sympathomimetic [mydriatic] ophthalmic medications). Patients may appear systemically ill and report nausea and vomiting as well as headache and eye pain. Most patients with angle-closure glaucoma are older than 50 years.

SYMPTOMS
- Monocular eye pain and/or frontal headache usually of sudden onset
- Diffuse blurred vision (almost always)
- Colored halos around bright objects
- Systemic symptoms including nausea and vomiting secondary to vagal stimulation

SIGNS
- Closed angle or a shallow anterior chamber that may be seen by illuminating the iris temporally and failing to see the light reflection on the nasal aspect of the iris
- Corneal haziness or cloudiness almost always seen secondary to corneal edema
- Conjunctival injection
- Fixed mid-dilated pupil (very common)

WORKUP
- IOP measurement is necessary to rule out glaucoma. Pressure can be measured by Schiøtz tonometer, applanation method, Tono-Pen, or air-puff tonometer.
- Slit-lamp examination may show a shallow anterior chamber; glycerin eye drops may be needed to rid the cornea temporarily of edema and allow visualization of the anterior chamber.
- Palpation of the globe is a crude and unreliable method for assessing increased IOP.
- Funduscopic examination may be difficult, but mydriatic drops should not be used.

COMMENTS AND TREATMENT CONSIDERATIONS
Acute angle-closure glaucoma is an emergency that requires immediate ophthalmologic consultation. Outcome depends on the duration of the attack as opposed to the level of IOP, with total and permanent loss of vision usually occurring in about 12 hours. The goal of therapy is to decrease IOP as quickly as possible by instituting measures to both decrease production and increase removal of aqueous humor. While awaiting emergent ophthalmologic consultation, consider administering pilocarpine 2% every 15 minutes until pupillary constriction, then every 4 hours as needed

(treat opposite eye prophylactically every 6 hours); topical timolol maleate 0.5% one drop; acetazolamide (carbonic anhydrase inhibitor) 500 mg po/IV; isosorbide or glycerin 1 ml/kg po (if no nausea or vomiting) or mannitol 20% IV (2.5 to 10 ml/kg) over 30 to 60 minutes. Antiemetics are also useful. In skilled hands, immediate anterior chamber paracentesis has been shown to be very safe and effective in controlling the IOP and eliminating symptoms in acute angle-closure glaucoma. Trials with latanoprost 0.005%, a topical prostaglandin F_2 analogue, have shown some benefit as well in reducing IOP. Definitive treatment is a peripheral iridotomy.

REFERENCES

Fingeret M: Glaucoma medications, glaucoma therapy, and the evolving paradigm, *J Am Optom Assoc* 69:115, 1998.

Hillman JS: Acute closed-angle glaucoma: an investigation into the effects of delay in treatment, *Br J Ophthalmol* 63:817, 1979.

Lam DS: Efficacy and safety of immediate anterior chamber paracentesis in the treatment of acute primary angle-closure glaucoma: a pilot study, *Ophthalmology* 109:64, 2002.

Saw SM: Interventions for angle-closure glaucoma: an evidence-based update, *Ophthalmology* 110:1869, 2003.

Sivalingam E: Glaucoma: an overview, *J Ophthalmic Nurs Technol* 15:15, 1996.

 ORBITAL CELLULITIS

Orbital cellulitis must be distinguished from less severe infections including periorbital (preseptal) cellulitis. Orbital cellulitis must always be considered in any case of eyelid inflammation because of the devastating sequelae of brain abscess, cranial nerve palsies, and possibly blindness or death from sepsis. Orbital cellulitis may complicate ethmoid sinusitis.

SYMPTOMS

- Eye pain
- Pain with eye movement
- Intense eyelid swelling
- Vision may be normal but blurred.
- Diplopia (common)
- Fever
- Headaches

SIGNS

- Eyelid inflammation with edema, erythema, and tenderness (Fig. 14–1)

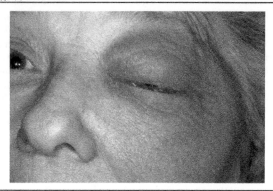

Fig. 14-1   Orbital cellulitis. Deep orbital infection is more commonly seen in children. (From Palay DA, Krachmer JH: *Ophthalmology for the primary care physician.* St Louis, 1997, Mosby.)

- Proptosis and restricted eye movement or pain with movement (very common)
- Conjunctival injection, chemosis, and subconjunctival hemorrhages (common)
- APD, with or without papilledema, possible with orbital apex involvement (uncommon)
- Fifth cranial nerve sensory deficits (uncommon)

WORKUP
- CT scan of the orbits and sinuses rules out orbital cellulitis in equivocal cases and delineates infection margins if positive.
- Complete ophthalmologic evaluation is essential, checking for restrictive eye movement, afferent pupillary defect, proptosis, and papilledema.
- CBC and ESR are not useful.
- Blood cultures may be helpful in patients who appear toxic.

COMMENTS AND TREATMENT CONSIDERATIONS
The most common causative organisms are *Staphylococcus aureus* (methicillin resistance is emerging gradually) and *Streptococcus pyogenes*, with *S. pneumoniae* and *Haemophilus influenzae* becoming increasingly rare because of immunization. In post-traumatic orbital cellulitis, gram-negative bacilli are occasionally involved. Treatment for orbital cellulitis begins with broad-spectrum intravenous antibiotics (e.g., an antistaphylococcal agent and a third-generation cephalosporin). ED consultation, followed by hospital admission, is required.

REFERENCES

Buckingham SC: Emergence of community-associated methicillin-resistant *Staphylococcus aureus* at a Memphis, Tennessee Children's Hospital, *Pediatr Infect Dis J* 23:619, 2004.

Seah LL, Fu ER: Acute orbital cellulitis—a review of 17 cases, *Ann Acad Med Singapore* 26:409, 1997.

Starkey CR: Medical management of orbital cellulitis, *Pediatr Infect Dis J* 20:1002, 2001.

Tole DM, Anderton LC, Hayward JM: Orbital cellulitis demands early recognition, urgent admission, and aggressive management, *J Accid Emerg Med* 12:151, 1995.

Uzcategui N, Warman R, Smith A, Howard CW: Clinical practice guidelines for the management of orbital cellulitis, *J Pediatr Ophthalmol Strabismus* 35:73, 1998.

 ANTERIOR UVEITIS AND IRITIS

CHAPTER 14

Anterior uveitis and iritis can be caused by a number of systemic and local processes including juvenile rheumatoid arthritis, ulcerative colitis, ankylosing spondylitis, Reiter's syndrome, tuberculosis, syphilis, herpes, leukemia, lymphoma, and ocular trauma.

SYMPTOMS
- Photophobia (almost always)
- Unilateral gradual onset of eye pain
- Red eye without discharge
- Blurred vision (common)
- Excessive tearing
- Other symptoms of primary medical condition

SIGNS
- Perilimbal injection
- Consensual photophobia—pain in the involved eye when light is shined in the uninvolved eye (very common)
- Miosis may be present.
- Cornea may be normal.

WORKUP
- Slit-lamp examination: cells and flare (WBC and RBC) in the anterior chamber are the hallmark signs. Posterior synechiae (iris adherent to the lens) may be seen.
- IOP may be low.
- Evaluation for possible primary disorder may include CBC, ESR, RPR, ANA, HLA-B27, FTA-ABS, PPD, Lyme titer, and chest radiograph.

COMMENTS AND TREATMENT CONSIDERATIONS

Anterior uveitis and iritis are ophthalmologic urgencies that, when diagnosed, need very close follow-up with an ophthalmologist. The initial treatment consists of topical cycloplegic agents and topical steroids (e.g., prednisolone [Pred Forte] 1% q4-6h or loteprednol etabonate 0.5% [Lotemax]). This regimen rids the patient of the photophobia and suppresses the inflammatory response. The majority of cases resolve in 2 to 4 weeks, with long-term complications being permanent synechiae and glaucoma.

REFERENCES

Nishimoto JY: Iritis: how to recognize and manage potentially sight-threatening disease, *Postgrad Med* 99:255, 1996.

Rothova A: Corticosteroids in uveitis, *Ophthalmol Clin North Am* 15:389, 2002.

Samudre SS: Comparison of topical steroids for acute anterior uveitis, *J Ocul Pharmacol Ther* 20:533, 2004.

Suttorp-Schulten MS, Rothova A: The possible impact of uveitis in blindness: a literature survey, *Br J Ophthalmol* 80:844, 1996.

Talley DK: Traumatic anterior uveitis, *Optom Clin* 3:21, 1993.

 RUPTURED GLOBE AND INTRAOCULAR FOREIGN BODY

A ruptured globe is caused by a penetrating or blunt blow to the eye that results in a full-thickness scleral or corneal disruption. The patient's history may include exposure to a high-velocity projectile (including hammering metal) or blunt trauma (including air bag). A high index of suspicion is paramount because up to 50% of ruptures are occult.

SYMPTOMS

- Decreased vision
- Nausea and vomiting
- Eye pain

SIGNS

Examine *both* eyes for comparison.

- Decreased visual acuity ++++
- No obvious evidence of rupture +++
- Decreased IOP ++++, although in obvious rupture it is prudent to *avoid* tonometry.
- Hyphema ++++, limited specificity. Ruptured globe must be ruled out when hyphema is present.
- Hemorrhagic chemosis ++++, if subconjunctival hemorrhage of > 180 degrees

- Afferent pupillary defect ++++, limited specificity
- Oval or pear-shaped tenting of the pupil is a subtle but specific sign.
- Fluorescein streaming indicates a full-thickness corneal laceration.
- Increased or decreased depth of anterior chamber ++++
- Vitreal hemorrhage ++++, specificity limited

WORKUP
- Orbital x-ray to rule out metallic foreign body
- Orbital CT, with coronal, sagittal, and axial cuts of 1.5 mm, is best for localizing rupture site and foreign body and for evaluating other associated injuries, such as orbital fractures and hemorrhage.
- MRI can help in identifying low-density, nonmagnetic intraocular foreign bodies but provides little added benefit to orbital CT.

COMMENTS AND TREATMENT CONSIDERATIONS
Place a metallic protective shield over the eye and keep the patient NPO while awaiting ED ophthalmologic consultation. Avoid manipulation of the globe; do not perform tonometry or patching.

Because of the high risk of rebleeding, avoid salicylates and nonsteroidal antiinflammatory drugs (NSAIDs) in hyphemas. Consider prophylactic antibiotics (e.g., IV vancomycin and either gentamicin or a second- or third-generation cephalosporin) to prevent endophthalmitis. Avoid topical antibiotics. Administer tetanus prophylaxis if indicated.

REFERENCES
Brady SM: The diagnosis and management of orbital blowout fractures: update 2001, *Am J Emerg Med* 19:147, 2001.

Coles WH: Indirect global ruptures and sharp scleral injuries. In Fraunfelder FT, Roy FH (eds): *Current ocular therapy*, ed 4. Philadelphia, 1995, WB Saunders.

Lee HJ: CT of orbital trauma, *Emerg Radiol* 10:168, 2004.

Navon SE: Management of the ruptured globe, *Int Ophthalmol Clin* 35:71, 1995.

Shingleton BJ: Eye injuries, *N Engl J Med* 325:408, 1991.

Zhu Y: Combining diagnosis of IOFB and complications with multiple image-related methods, *Chin J Ophthalmol* 39:520, 2003.

CONJUNCTIVITIS, KERATITIS, AND OPHTHALMIA NEONATORUM

Most cases of conjunctivitis have bacterial, viral, or allergic etiologies and are easily treated. Allergic conjunctivitis is usually seasonal, recurrent, and bilateral and results in pruritus and watery discharge.

CHAPTER 14

Bacterial conjunctivitis is neither pruritic nor seasonal and arises with a purulent discharge, early morning crusting of the eyelid, and a beefy red conjunctiva. *Staphylococcus* spp, *Streptococcus pneumoniae*, and *Haemophilus influenzae*, the most common causes of bacterial conjunctivitis, rarely bring about significant sequelae and are treated with topical antibiotics. However, infections with *Pseudomonas aeruginosa* and *Neisseria gonorrhoeae* are considered medical emergencies because both can penetrate and perforate the cornea within 24 hours. Contact lens wearers are susceptible to *Acanthamoeba* and *P. aeruginosa*.

Viral conjunctivitis causes a watery discharge and follicular hypertrophy. Although adenovirus remains the leading viral cause of viral conjunctivitis, herpes simplex 1 and 2 and herpes zoster can lead to scarring and blindness with recurrence. In elderly persons, ocular complications occur in 50% with recurrent V_1 distribution herpes zoster (always consider with vesicular rash around the eye or tip of nose).

N. gonorrhoeae, Chlamydia trachomatis, and herpes simplex 1 and 2 must be considered as a cause of ophthalmia neonatorum. *N. gonorrhoeae* generally occurs within 2 to 4 days of life and *Chlamydia* within 5 to 13 days. Neonatal *C. trachomatis* is associated with a 50% risk of pneumonia over the ensuing 2 to 3 months. Herpetic infections develop in half of neonates exposed to genital herpes during birth, and ocular herpes develops in 20% of these.

A fungal cause should be considered in patients who are immunocompromised and those with a history of trauma involving organic matter.

SYMPTOMS
Patients with bacterial and viral etiologies present similarly.
- Ocular pain and redness
- Photophobia (with keratitis)
- Foreign body sensation
- Crusting, discharge
- Decreased vision

N. gonorrhoeae
- Initially unilateral +++++
- Thick discharge

C. trachomatis
- Watery discharge +++
- Mucopurulent discharge +++

HERPES SIMPLEX
- Unilateral +++++
- Watery discharge, less with recurrence
- Risk factors: immunosuppression, sunlight, local trauma, stress

SIGNS

N. gonorrhoeae
- Hyperpurulent discharge
- Severe chemosis

C. trachomatis
- Lid edema ++++
- Conjunctival hyperemia
- Hypertrophic papillae without follicles

PRIMARY HERPES SIMPLEX KERATITIS
- Punctate lesions (more common in primary infection) on fluorescein staining, often *not* typical dendritic pattern (Fig. 14–2)
- Lid lesions, periocular dermatitis ++++
- Decreased corneal sensitivity +++
- Uveitis (very rare)
- Isolated ocular involvement in neonates (rare); search for disseminated disease.

HERPES ZOSTER OPHTHALMICUS
- Punctate lesions or dendritic ulcers on fluorescein staining ++++
- Lesions along nasociliary branch of trigeminal nerve (tip of the nose) +++

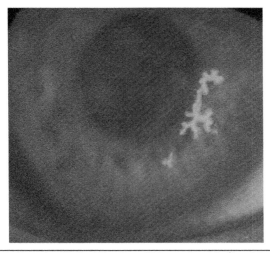

Fig. 14–2 Herpes keratitis. Dendritic pattern with fluorescein uptake. (From Palay DA, Krachmer JH: *Ophthalmology for the primary care physician.* St Louis, 1997, Mosby.)

WORKUP
- Full ophthalmologic examination including search for foreign bodies and slit-lamp examination with fluorescein staining of cornea
- Gram stain and culture: patients younger than 1 month; *or* if older than 1 month, or adult, and systemic evidence of STD (usually adolescents and older), immunocompromised, thick purulent discharge, or no improvement after 48 hours of antibiotic therapy

SPECIAL CONSIDERATIONS

CORNEAL ULCER
- Gram stain and culture (may require débridement by ophthalmologist)

N. gonorrhea
- Gram stain and culture
- Genital and pharyngeal cultures

C. trachomatis
- ELISA and immunofluorescent studies for *C. trachomatis* ++++ (very high specificity)
- Gram stain has poor sensitivity.
- Genital culture
- PCR more sensitive than culture for *C. trachomatis*

HERPES SIMPLEX, HERPES ZOSTER
- Serologies not helpful

COMMENTS AND TREATMENT CONSIDERATIONS
All routine cases of bacterial keratitis should be treated with broad-spectrum topical antibiotics and referred for ophthalmologic follow-up. Patients with corneal ulcers (especially if contact lens wearers) or those infected with *N. gonorrhoeae, C. trachomatis*, and herpes need aggressive care and generally an ED ophthalmologic consultation. Patients with suspected *N. gonorrhoeae* and *C. trachomatis* conjunctivitis may have concomitant oral or genital infections that are often asymptomatic +++.

N. gonorrhoeae
If younger than 1 month with mild disease, treat with single-dose ceftriaxone 125 mg IM or cefotaxime 100 mg IM in close consultation and follow-up with an ophthalmologist. In adults with mild infection, use ceftriaxone 125 mg IM/IV. The presence of a hypopyon (a layered infiltrate in the anterior chamber suggesting

endophthalmitis), severe purulent conjunctivitis with corneal involvement, or large or multiple ulcers suggests more serious disease that requires ED ophthalmologic consultation and possible hospital admission.

C. trachomatis
In pediatric or pregnant patients, treat with erythromycin 50 mg/kg/day, divided in four doses, po for 2 to 3 weeks. In other adults, treat with doxycycline 100 mg po bid for 2 weeks.

HERPETIC KERATITIS
HERPES SIMPLEX
Consider ED ophthalmologic consultation. Treatment often includes topical antivirals (e.g., trifluridine 1% 1 drop 9 times/day). Cycloplegics to reduce pain and topical antibiotics for secondary bacterial infection may also be prescribed. Consider admission for neonates with herpes because of the risk of disseminated disease.

HERPES ZOSTER
Consider ED ophthalmologic consultation. Famciclovir 500 mg tid po for 10 days early in the course of herpes zoster may lessen the severity of the disease.

IN GENERAL
Avoid topical steroids and topical anesthetics until ophthalmologic consultation. Avoid atropine for cycloplegia because of its long-lasting effect.

REFERENCES
Liesegang TJ: Bacterial keratitis, *Infect Dis Clin North Am* 6:815, 1992.
Mader TH, Stulting RD: Viral keratitis, *Infect Dis Clin North Am* 6:831, 1992.
Ng EW, Golledge CL: The management of ocular infections, *Aust Fam Physician* 25:1831, 1996.
Stonecipher KG, Jensen H: Diagnosis, laboratory analysis, and treatment of bacterial corneal ulcers, *Optom Clin* 4:53, 1995.

 ## OCULAR CHEMICAL BURNS
Both acidic and alkaline substances can cause serious corneal and conjunctival damage. Although all but the most trivial of exposures require copious (liters of) irrigation, alkaline substances are

particularly notable for causing deep burns. Ammonia (fertilizer and household cleaners) is one of the most aggressive alkaline substances, followed by lye (drain cleaners), lime (plaster, cement), and magnesium hydroxide. A detailed ophthalmologic examination is generally deferred until after irrigation has normalized the eye pH.

SYMPTOMS
- Pain following history of exposure
- Decreased vision (depending on extent of injury)

SIGNS
- Conjunctival erythema, edema
- Decreased visual acuity
- Corneal clouding in severe burns
- Stromal whitening in severe burns
- Increased IOP in alkali burns

WORKUP
- Baseline and postirrigation eye pH measurements (pH of normal tears approximately 7.3 to 7.6)

COMMENTS AND TREATMENT CONSIDERATIONS
There are no specific antidotes. Any solid or particulate matter should be removed. After topical anesthesia, copious lavage using normal saline or lactated Ringer should be started immediately until eye pH is approximately 7.4. (Consider use of specialized lenses attached to IV fluid bags and deliver several liters of fluid.) Patients are generally given topical antibiotics following irrigation and a full examination. Cycloplegics and systemic analgesics may be necessary to relieve pain; avoid atropine for cycloplegia because of its long-lasting effects. Obtain ophthalmologic consultation for significant alkali exposure and deep corneal acid burns. Administer tetanus prophylaxis if indicated.

REFERENCES
Mead M: Evaluation and initial management of patients with ocular and adnexal trauma. In Albert DM, Jakobiec FA (eds): *Principles and practice of ophthalmology*, Philadelphia, 1994, WB Saunders.

Pfister RR: Alkaline injury. In Fraunfelder FT, Roy FH (eds): *Current ocular therapy*, ed 4, Philadelphia, 1995, WB Saunders.

Slansky HH: Acid burns. In Fraunfelder FT, Roy FH, editors: *Current ocular therapy*, ed 4. Philadelphia, 1995, WB Saunders.

Wagoner MD: Chemical injuries of the eye: current concepts in pathophysiology and therapy, *Surv Ophthalmol* 41:275, 1997.

CORNEAL ABRASION

SYMPTOMS
- Significant eye pain +++++
- Foreign body sensation
- Photophobia
- Tearing
- Irritable infant without other condition

SIGNS
- Eyelid edema
- Conjunctival injection may be present

WORKUP
- Slit-lamp examination: hallmark sign is an epithelial defect noted with fluorescein +++++ (if a surrounding infiltrate is seen, it is infected and by definition is now a corneal ulcer).
- Eversion of the eyelids for evaluation of any possible foreign body (suspect a foreign body especially if vertical linear abrasions are noted on the cornea.)

COMMENTS AND TREATMENT CONSIDERATIONS
Corneal abrasions are extremely painful but if treated properly heal in 24 to 72 hours. Treatment consists of topical antibiotics, topical cycloplegic medications with oral analgesics, and daily follow-up until the epithelial defect resolves. Topical NSAIDs have also been shown to be of benefit in reducing pain. Patching is no longer recommended except to provide comfort or for very large abrasions. No contact lenses should be worn until complete resolution.

REFERENCES
Alberti MM: Combined indomethacin/gentamicin eyedrops to reduce pain after traumatic corneal abrasion, *Eur J Ophthalmol* 11:233, 2001.

Kaiser PK: A comparison of pressure patching versus no patching for corneal abrasions due to trauma or foreign body removal, *Ophthalmology* 102:1936, 1995.

Michael JG: Management of corneal abrasion in children: a randomized clinical trial, *Ann Emerg Med* 40:67, 2002.

Patterson J, Fetzer D, Krall J, et al: Eye patch treatment for the pain of corneal abrasion, *South Med J* 89:227, 1996.

Poole SR: Corneal abrasion in infants, *Pediatr Emerg Care* 11:25, 1995.

14

CHAPTER

Fever (Elevated Temperature)
Virginia M. Ribeiro

Temperature elevation can occur through two general mechanisms: (1) the hypothalamic set point (typically 37° C) can be adjusted upward because of infections, toxins, or drugs (defined as "fever") or (2) the body's mechanisms to compensate adequately for heat stress can be overwhelmed by an exogenous or endogenous heat load or decreased heat dissipation (defined as "hyperthermia"). Important historical clues to the cause of an elevated temperature include associated symptoms, duration and magnitude of temperature elevation, occupational exposures, travel, recreational history, and presence of an immunocompromised state. Any suggestion of an infectious cause for elevated temperature should lead to evaluation for a source and, when appropriate, antibiotic therapy. Important physical examination clues suggesting a possible infectious source of fever include altered mental status, stiff neck, rash, lymphadenopathy, abnormal lung examination findings, joint effusions, heart murmurs, or other localizing findings. *This chapter focuses on hyperthermia.* Causes of fever are addressed in other chapters.

 DRUG-INDUCED HYPERTHERMIA

Drug-induced hyperthermia can be classified into five clinical syndromes:
1. Malignant hyperthermia (MH): A genetic disorder of skeletal muscle metabolism characterized by hyperthermia and muscle rigidity. MH most often results from use of succinylcholine alone or in combination with inhalational anesthetics (i.e., halothane, enflurane, isoflurane).
2. Anticholinergic toxicity: Anticholinergics are associated with hyperthermia in both therapeutic and toxic doses.

Hyperthermia results from muscular hyperactivity combined with decreased sweating. Dry axillae help differentiate it from sympathomimetic toxicity. Other symptoms include altered mental status, seizures, confusion, agitation, coma, dry mouth, tachycardia, mydriasis, urinary retention, and decreased bowel sounds. Treatment is primarily supportive and includes cooling and sedation. The role of physostigmine is unclear; it can relieve central nervous system effects, but there is a risk of severe adverse effects.

3. Sympathomimetic toxicity: All sympathomimetics can cause hyperthermia, which is idiosyncratic. Symptoms include agitation, coma, hallucinations, seizures, and altered mental status. Treatment is supportive and consists of aggressive cooling, benzodiazepines, and chemical paralysis and intubation if necessary.

4. Neuroleptic malignant syndrome (NMS)

5. Serotonin syndrome

Signs and symptoms of drug-induced hyperthermia depend on the activity of the drug. The following drugs and classes of drugs, listed by mechanism, should be considered.

CHAPTER 15

Drugs That Cause Muscular Hyperactivity

- Antipsychotics
- Halothane, succinylcholine (malignant hyperthermia)
- Hallucinogens: lysergic acid diethylamide (LSD), phencyclidine (PCP)
- Isoniazid (INH)
- Lithium
- Methaqualone
- Monoamine oxidase inhibitors
- Serotonin syndrome
- Strychnine
- Sympathomimetics including amphetamines and "designer" amphetamines, cocaine, theophylline, ephedrine, pseudoephedrine
- Tricyclic antidepressants

Drugs That Cause Hypermetabolism

- Salicylates
- Sympathomimetics
- Thyroid hormone
- Withdrawal: ethanol and sedative-hypnotics

Drugs That Impair Thermoregulation

- Antipsychotics (phenothiazines)
- Ethanol

Drugs That Impair Heat Dissipation

- Anticholinergics
- Antipsychotics
- Skeletal muscle relaxants
- Sympathomimetics

Symptoms, signs, and workup vary with intoxication. See Chapter 37, Toxic Ingestion, Approach to.

REFERENCES

Callaway CW, Clark RF: Hyperthermia in psychostimulant overdose, *Ann Emerg Med* 24:68, 1994.

Chan TC, Evans SD, Clark RF: Drug-induced hyperthermia, *Crit Care Clin* 13:785, 1997.

Halloran LL, Bernard DW: Management of drug-induced hyperthermia, *Curr Opin Pediatr* 16:211, 2004.

Rosenberg J, Pentel P, Pond S, et al: Hyperthermia associated with drug intoxication, *Crit Care Med* 14:964, 1986.

 NEUROLEPTIC MALIGNANT SYNDROME

The pathophysiology of NMS has not been clearly established, although it is thought to result from dopaminergic blockade in the hypothalamus and basal ganglia. DSM-IV criteria for the diagnosis of NMS include elevated temperature with muscular rigidity accompanied by two or more of the following: diaphoresis, dysphagia, tremor, incontinence, altered consciousness, mutism, tachycardia, blood pressure changes, leukocytosis, or elevated creatinine kinase in association with antipsychotic medication usage. All conventional and atypical antipsychotics have resulted in NMS. Incidence is approximately 1% of treated patients. NMS may present variably. It usually occurs 3 to 9 days after initiation of neuroleptic therapy or addition of second neuroleptic medication, although it can occur at any time during therapy and is not dose related. Symptoms usually develop over 24 to 72 hours.

PRECIPITANTS

- Use of conventional antipsychotics (phenothiazines, butyrophenones, thioxanthenes) or atypical antipsychotics (clozapine [Clozaril], risperidone [Risperdal], olanzapine [Zyprexa], quetiapine [Seroquel], ziprasidone [Geodon], aripiprazole [Abilify])
- Withdrawal of dopaminergic stimulants in Parkinson's disease (amantadine, levodopa/carbidopa, bromocriptine)
- Dopamine antagonist use (metoclopramide, tetrabenazine, promethazine, prochlorperazine, amoxapine, reserpine, droperidol)
- Tetracyclic antidepressants
- Monoamine oxidase inhibitors

SYMPTOMS
- Elevated temperature (+++++)
- Rigidity (+++++)
- Dyspnea (++)
- Tremor (++)
- Urinary incontinence
- Dysphagia
- Diaphoresis
- Drowsiness
- Confusion
- Agitation

SIGNS
- Elevated temperature (usually 38.5° to 42° C)
- Extrapyramidal symptoms (78% in atypical, 95% in conventional antipsychotics): "lead pipe" rigidity, which may be localized, trismus, masked facies ++, dyskinesia, akinesia, dystonia, bradykinesia, mutism, nystagmus
- Altered mental status: from confusion and agitation to lethargy, stupor, and coma ++
- Autonomic dysfunction: tachycardia ++++, labile blood pressure +++, diaphoresis +++, tachypnea +++, hyperreflexia ++, pallor, dysrhythmias, cardiac arrest

WORKUP
- Diagnosis is established clinically and by exclusion (i.e., one must be sure that no infectious or metabolic processes are responsible for the increased temperature; head CT or brain MRI, lumbar puncture, blood and urine cultures, chest x-ray, thyroid function tests may be required).
- Urinalysis (check for myoglobinuria) and creatinine kinase to exclude rhabdomyolysis
- CBC, BUN, creatinine, LFTS, electrolytes, calcium, magnesium, coagulation studies
- Drug levels are typically normal.

COMMENTS AND TREATMENT CONSIDERATIONS
The key to treatment of NMS is recognition of the syndrome, withdrawal of the offending medication, and intensive supportive care. If infection is suspected, antibiotic administration is reasonable pending culture results. Treatment is focused on the alleviation of symptoms and prevention of complications and consists of hydration, cooling, benzodiazepine sedation, and maintenance of appropriate fluid and electrolyte balance. There is no convincing evidence that any specific treatment alters outcome. Among those that have been proposed: bromocriptine 2.5 to 5.0 mg po tid-qid

(up to 40 to 60 mg/day); dantrolene sodium 2.5 mg initially then 10mg/kg/day IV divided tid-qid (if muscle rigidity severe); amantadine 100 to 200 mg bid (preferred for NMS in Parkinson's disease); and electroconvulsive therapy (may be indicated if no response for 2 days). Levodopa with or without carbidopa tid-qid has also been suggested. If NMS is precipitated by abrupt cessation of dopaminergic therapy, restart immediately. One study reported that patients receiving pharmacologic therapy do worse and have more complications.

DIFFERENTIAL DIAGNOSIS
- Anticholinergic toxicity
- CNS infection (encephalitis, meningitis)
- CNS vasculitis
- Drug fever
- Extrapyramidal syndrome
- Heat stroke
- Lethal catatonia
- Sepsis
- Serotonin syndrome
- Strychnine poisoning
- Tetanus
- Thyrotoxicosis
  See also Chapter 37, Toxic Exposure, Approach to.

REFERENCES
Ananth J, Parameswaran S, Gunatilake S, et al: Neuroleptic malignant syndrome and atypical antipsychotic drugs, *J Clin Psychiatry* 65:464, 2004.

Bhanushali MJ, Tuite PJ: The evaluation and management of patients with neuroleptic malignant syndrome, *Neurol Clin* 22:389, 2004.

Carbone JR: The neuroleptic malignant and serotonin syndromes, *Emerg Med Clin North Am* 18:317, 2000.

Caroff SN, Mann SC: Neuroleptic malignant syndrome, *Med Clin North Am* 77:185, 1993.

De la Cour J: Neuroleptic malignant syndrome: do we know enough? *J Adv Nurs* 21:897, 1995.

Farer DK: Neuroleptic malignant syndrome induced by atypical antipsychotics, *Expert Opin Drug Saf* 2:21, 2003.

Rosebush P, Stewart T, Mazurek MF: The treatment of neuroleptic malignant syndrome. Are dantrolene and bromocriptine useful adjuncts to supportive care? *Br J Psychiatry* 159:709, 1991.

Velamoor VR, Swamy GN, Parmar RS, et al: Management of suspected neuroleptic malignant syndrome, *Can J Psychiatry* 40:545, 1995.

SEROTONIN SYNDROME

The hyperstimulation of CNS 5-HT1A and possibly 5-HT2 receptors is believed to cause the serotonin syndrome. Generally, the use of two or more agents that increase serotonin levels is implicated, although use of a single agent can precipitate the disorder. Most cases result from the addition of a new serotonergic medication or increase in the dose of one currently prescribed. Onset is usually within 24 hours of ingestion or overdose (75%).

The syndrome is usually a triad of symptoms involving mental/behavioral changes, autonomic dysfunction, and neuro-muscular abnormalities, although only one group of symptoms may predominate and there can be variable severity. Proposed diagnostic criteria require the presence of three of the following in the setting of a known serotonergic agent: altered mental status, myoclonus, agitation, hyperreflexia, shivering, tremor, ataxia, diar-rhea, or fever. In addition, these symptoms must be without other apparent etiology (infectious, toxic, or metabolic) and without a recent increase or addition of a neuroleptic.

Precipitants include the following:

1. Drug combinations—*serotonin precursors or agonists* (trypto-phan, LSD, lithium, L-dopa, buspirone [BuSpar], trazodone), *serotonin-release agents* (see item 3), *SSRIs* (paroxetine [Paxil], fluoxetine [Prozac, Sarafem], sertraline [Zoloft], fluvoxamine [Luvox], citalopram [Celexa], escitalopram [Lexapro]), *non-selective serotonin reuptake inhibitors* (clomipramine [Anafranil], imipramine, amitriptyline, doxepin, desipramine, dextromethor-phan, meperidine, venlafaxine [Effexor], nefazodone [Serzone], pentazocine [Talwin], tramadol [Ultram], trazodone, fenflu-ramine), *nonspecific inhibitors of serotonin metabolism* (St. John's wort, MAOIs)
2. Increased serotonin precursors or agonists
3. Increased release of serotonin (3,4-methylenedioxymethamphet-amine [Ecstasy], amphetamines and amphetamine derivatives such as phentermine and fenfluramine, cocaine, reserpine) 5-HT1 agonists such as sumatriptan, rizatriptan, naratriptan, and zolmitriptan cannot cross the blood-brain barrier and are considered unlikely to cause serotonin syndrome.

SYMPTOMS

- Cognitive/behavioral dysfunction (+++): altered mental status, mania, hallucinations, and confusion
- Autonomic dysfunction: diaphoresis (+++), diarrhea (++), lacrimation, shivering (++), nausea, vomiting
- Neuromuscular abnormalities: akathisia (+++), fever (+++)

CHAPTER **15**

SIGNS

- Cognitive/behavioral dysfunction: altered mental status (+++), coma, delirium, mutism, agitation, encephalopathy, restlessness
- Autonomic dysfunction: hyperthermia (+++), tachypnea (+++), mydriasis (++), tachycardia, alterations in blood pressure
- Neuromuscular abnormalities (+++): rigidity (+++), myoclonus (+++), hyperreflexia (+++), tremor (++) incoordination (++) (often limited to the legs), clonus, nystagmus, akathisia
- Seizure (++)

DIFFERENTIAL DIAGNOSIS

- Anticholinergic toxicity
- CNS infection
- Delirium tremens
- Heat stroke
- Neuroleptic malignant syndrome
- Sepsis
- Sympathomimetic toxicity

WORKUP

- The diagnosis is made clinically and requires taking an appropriate drug history and excluding other causes (infectious, metabolic, primary neurologic, and other drug-induced syndromes)
- The diagnosis is suggested by recent increase in dose or addition of serotonergic agent with no change or addition of a dopaminergic agent
- Urinalysis and CK if muscle rigidity is present to exclude rhabdomyolysis

COMMENTS AND TREATMENT CONSIDERATIONS

Mild to moderate cases usually resolve in 24 to 72 hours with discontinuation of the inciting drug. Treatment is mostly supportive, involving aggressive cooling, intravenous fluids, sedatives, cardiac monitoring, anticonvulsants, antihypertensives, benzodiazepines (decrease muscular hyperactivity, agitation, and seizure), and rarely paralytics (reduce hyperthermia caused by muscle hyperactivity). If the patient is moderately to severely symptomatic and conventional supportive therapy fails, treatment with nonspecific inhibitors of serotonin has been proposed without clearly established benefit. Cyproheptadine 12 mg po, then 4 mg po q2h for 24 hours, or methysergide 2 mg po bid has been successful in case reports. Studies have shown clinical improvement with chlorpromazine 50 to 100 mg IM in combination with cyproheptadine if NMS is not suspected. Consultation with a toxicologist is recommended. Bromocriptine (increases brain serotonin) and dantrolene (may increase central serotonin metabolism and increase serotonin) are not recommended. Complications include hypertension, arrhythmias, rhabdomyolysis, myoglobinuria, renal failure, hepatic failure, DIC, and ARDS.

REFERENCES

Birmes P, Coppin D, Schmitt L, Lauque D: Serotonin syndrome: a brief review, *CMAJ* 168:1439, 2003.

Brown TM, Skop BP, Mareth TR: Pathophysiology and management of serotonin syndrome, *Ann Pharmacother* 30:527, 1996.

Carbone JR: The neuroleptic malignant and serotonin syndromes, *Emerg Med Clin North Am* 18:317, 2000.

Ener RA, Meglathery SB, Van Decker WA, Gallagher RM: Serotonin syndrome and other serotonergic disorders, *Pain Med* 4:63, 2003.

Gillman PK: The serotonin syndrome and its treatment, *J Psychopharmacol* 13:100, 1999.

Graudins A, Stearman A, Chan B: Treatment of the serotonin syndrome with cyproheptadine, *J Emerg Med* 16:615, 1998.

LoCurto MJ: The serotonin syndrome, *Emerg Med Clin North Am* 15:665, 1997.

Martin TG: Serotonin syndrome, *Ann Emerg Med* 28:520, 1996.

Mills KC: Serotonin syndrome: a clinical update, *Crit Care Clin* 13:763, 1997.

CHAPTER 15

HEATSTROKE

Heatstroke, defined as core temperature above 40° C and CNS dysfunction, is a life-threatening condition in which the patient's thermoregulatory mechanisms are unable to respond adequately to heat stress. This results in an increase in body temperature leading to organ dysfunction and failure. Temperatures are usually very high, ranging from 40° to 47°C. In classic heatstroke there is inadequate dissipation of exogenous heat. Precipitants include exposure to high ambient temperature in a patient with a preexisting disease (cardiopulmonary disease, diabetes, alcohol, chronic mental illness, and obesity) or medication (phenothiazines, anticholinergics, sedatives, diuretics) that limits sweating or disrupts salt/water balance. This may occur, for example, in older patients who are confined to a hot environment. Care must be taken to rule out infectious causes of fever in these patients.

In exertional heatstroke there is excessive production of heat. Precipitants include physical exertion, high temperature, humidity approaching 100% (evaporation ceases), and incomplete acclimatization. Rapid and aggressive cooling measures are imperative in all heatstroke patients.

Heat exhaustion is a less emergent form of heat illness that is treated primarily by cooling and oral or IV fluid replacement. Symptoms include nausea, vomiting, headache, weakness, and muscle cramps. Heat cramps may also occur and seem to be related to salt depletion. Treatment consists of oral or IV fluid and salt repletion.

SYMPTOMS
- Fever +++++
- Altered mental status (agitation, confusion) +++++
- Headache
- Dizziness
- Weakness
- Anorexia
- Stupor
- Diarrhea
- Vomiting

SIGNS
- Elevated temperature +++++
- Altered mental status (coma, stupor, agitation, delirium) +++++
- Hot, dry skin ++++
- Tachycardia
- Tachypnea
- Hypotension ++
- Oliguria (may be sign of rhabdomyolysis in exertional heat stroke)
- ECG changes (ST segment or T wave abnormalities, conduction disturbances)
- Focal neurologic deficits in severe cases

WORKUP
- Rule out other causes of elevated temperature (an infection workup with cultures, CT, and LP is often indicated).
- Urinalysis, CK, creatinine (in anticipation of rhabdomyolysis and acute renal failure)
- Electrolytes, glucose, calcium, CBC
- Evaluate for multiorgan dysfunction (e.g., liver function tests and chest x-ray).
- PT and PTT (in anticipation of DIC, a frequent complication)
- ECG (may show ST depression, T wave changes; sinus tachycardia is the most common rhythm, but arrhythmias have been described)

COMMENTS AND TREATMENT CONSIDERATIONS
Treatment consists of rapid cooling with evaporative methods (water sprayed on disrobed patient along with use of fans).

This is preferred over applying ice packs to axillae and groin, which promotes vasoconstriction peripherally. Cold water or ice immersion is often physically limited by requirements for the patient's care. Internal cooling by nasogastric tube is not recommended because of risk of water intoxication. Cooling should exceed 0.1° to 0.2° C/min with aggressive treatment until temperature reaches 39° C (102° F) to avoid hypothermia. Use continuous core temperature monitoring. Oxygenation, airway, and hemodynamic support are provided as needed. Empirical antibiotics are given when uncertain of infection. Benzodiazepines should be given for shivering (phenothiazines may decrease ability to cool patient). Treat hypokalemia if also acidotic, as it represents a true deficit. Treat hyperkalemia in the setting of rhabdomyolysis. No antipyretics should be given because their effects depend on a normally functioning hypothalamus. Admit the patient to the intensive care unit. If rhabdomyolysis is present, fluids should be alkalinized and furosemide administered to keep urine output at 100 ml/hr.

In classic heatstroke, intravenous fluids are generally indicated but should be used with care to avoid pulmonary edema. Many heatstroke victims are normovolemic and peripherally vasodilated with distributive shock and high output failure; cooling redistributes fluids from periphery to core. In exertional heatstroke, intravenous fluids and electrolyte replacement are required. Complications include cardiovascular dysfunction (including CHF), DIC, acute renal failure (5% classic and 25% to 30% exertional), rhabdomyolysis, seizure, liver injury (very common), ARDS, electrolyte disorders, and death. Up to 20% to 30% of patients have residual neurologic deficits.

REFERENCES

Bouchama A, Knochel JP: Heat stroke, *N Engl J Med* 346:1978, 2002.

Graham BS, Lichtenstein MJ, Hinson JM, Theil GB: Nonexertional heatstroke, *Arch Intern Med* 146:87, 1996.

Khosla R, Guntupalli KK: Heat-related illnesses, *Crit Care Clin* 15:251, 1999.

Lugo-Amador NM, Rothenhaus T, Moyer P: Heat-related illness, *Emerg Med Clin North Am* 22:315, 2004.

Tek D, Olshaker JS: Heat illness, *Emerg Med Clin North Am* 10:299, 1992.

Fever in Children under 2 Years of Age
Maureen McCollough

Most fevers in children are the result of benign viral conditions, but the emergency physician must identify the children whose fever is caused by a life-threatening illness. Meningitis and other serious infections may be occult or produce only nonspecific symptoms in children younger than 2 years.

Febrile infants of any age who are ill appearing (e.g., weak cry, inconsolable by parent, decreased alertness and responsiveness) should receive a full "septic workup," including lumbar puncture (LP), unless another significant source is identified and meningitis is not suspected. Blood and urine cultures should be obtained as part of this evaluation for sepsis. Rapid and limited attempts should be made to obtain cultures before administering antibiotics, but treatment should *never* be substantially delayed in order to accomplish diagnostic procedures (including LP). These patients should be given intravenous antibiotics early in their ED course and be admitted to the hospital after an appropriate evaluation.

Children brought to the ED with a fever should receive a thorough physical examination. All their clothes should be removed to allow a complete examination of the skin for petechiae, purpura, and cellulitis. Their level of alertness and activity should be documented. An 8-month-old who is grabbing for a stethoscope and smiling but has a temperature of 104° F is of less concern than an 8-month-old with a temperature of 101.8° F who is lethargic and ill appearing on the gurney. "Playful," "interactive," "smiling," "cooing," and "consolable" are useful descriptions of children who appear well. Children who are "lethargic," "irritable," "sleepy," and "inconsolable" are more likely to have a serious cause of fever, such as meningitis.

Any child with a fever who has an abnormal mental status should have antibiotics administered and an LP performed. A chest x-ray to screen for pneumonia should be considered in any child who has signs of lower respiratory tract disease, such as tachypnea, grunting, nasal flaring, or retractions. Urinary tract infection, more common in female children, can present with fevers and vomiting. If the cause of the fever cannot be identified, both a urinalysis and urine culture are recommended in male infants under 6 months old and in female infants under 1 year because urinalysis alone may miss an infection in this age group.

This chapter is directed toward the diagnosis and treatment of previously healthy infants. Those who are immunocompromised or have other significant medical problems need special consideration.

REFERENCES
American College of Emergency Physicians: Clinical policy for children younger than three years presenting to the emergency department with fever, _Ann Emerg Med_ 42:530, 2003.

INFANTS UNDER 4 WEEKS OF AGE
Physical examination cannot reliably rule out serious disease in infants younger than 4 weeks. Therefore, most authorities agree that such infants should receive intravenous antibiotics and a full septic workup and be admitted to the hospital.

WORKUP
- Blood culture
- Catheterized or suprapubic tap for urinalysis and urine culture
- Chest x-ray
- LP
- Stool culture, if history of diarrhea

COMMENTS AND TREATMENT CONSIDERATIONS
Intravenous antibiotics (e.g., ampicillin 50 mg/kg IV for infants younger than 7 days, 100 mg/kg for infants older than 7 days, plus gentamicin 2.5 mg/kg for patients in both age groups) should be given. Cefotaxime 50 mg/kg/dose or another equivalent cephalosporin should be used if the CSF is suspicious or positive for meningitis. Vancomycin 15 mg/kg/dose should be considered if the infant is critically ill or the mother has previously been treated for group B streptococcus. Consider acyclovir 20 mg/kg/dose if the infant is critically ill or seizing or the mother has a history of herpes. These patients should be admitted to the hospital and treated with antibiotics pending culture results (see Meningitis).

INFANTS BETWEEN 4 AND 12 WEEKS OF AGE
Until recently, most (in many cases all) febrile infants between 4 and 12 weeks of age were admitted to the hospital because of the

CHAPTER **16**

awareness that such infants may have serious illness with only subtle signs. There is now evidence, however, that with the application of validated criteria, such as the Rochester and Philadelphia criteria, well-appearing term infants with a negative workup in the emergency department and good follow-up can be safely sent home. Obviously, a high index of suspicion for the possibility of meningitis or other serious infection is critical, and LP should be performed in children who do not appear well. Overt signs such as meningismus are frequently absent.

Many experts distinguish between the infant over 8 weeks of age who has a social smile and is interactive with its parent and environment and the very young infant less than 8 weeks of age who does little more than sleep. They feel more comfortable clinically ruling out the possibility of meningitis in a 9- or 10-week-old compared with a 5- or 6-week-old. Therefore, these experts are more conservative with the very young infant, less than 8 weeks old, and more often do a complete septic workup including an LP, especially when a reasonable source for the fever cannot be found on clinical examination. A more conservative approach should also be taken with the very young infant who already has a significant past medical history such as previous urinary tract infections, meningitis, or VP shunts. Significant controversy does exist, however, regarding the need to conduct tests in well-appearing term infants for whom close follow-up is available.

WORKUP
For the evaluation of a well-appearing term infant without significant past medical history between 4 weeks and 12 weeks of age presenting with a fever without a source:
- Full physical examination
- LP, if clinically indicated, especially with infants 4 to 8 weeks old
- Chest x-ray, if clinically indicated
- Urinary catheter or suprapubic tap for urinalysis and urine culture if no source of fever is identified
- Stool for WBC and culture, if history of diarrhea
- Blood culture
- CBC, controversial (see Occult Bacteremia)

COMMENTS AND TREATMENT CONSIDERATIONS
Ill-appearing infants should have a full septic workup for sepsis and be treated with intravenous antibiotics (e.g., ampicillin 100 mg/kg IV divided plus cefotaxime 50 mg/kg or ceftriaxone 50 mg/kg) pending culture results. If the risk of meningitis is high and drug-resistant *Streptococcus pneumoniae* is a concern, vancomycin can be used instead of ampicillin.

INFANTS OLDER THAN 12 WEEKS AND LESS THAN 2 YEARS OF AGE

Fever in children in this age range is common, and serious conditions are generally more clinically apparent. However, early presentations of life-threatening disease processes can be subtle. Older infants and children may show signs of focal diseases, which are addressed in other chapters.

COMMENTS AND TREATMENT CONSIDERATIONS

Treatment should be directed toward underlying conditions when possible. Decisions regarding admission are generally based on clinical appearance and underlying disease process. Ill-appearing children with a fever but without a source of infection should receive a full septic workup and antibiotic treatment without delay (e.g., ceftriaxone 50 to 100 mg/kg IV). If the risk of meningitis is high and drug-resistant *S. pneumoniae* is a concern, vancomycin can be added (see also Meningitis and Occult Bacteremia).

REFERENCES

Chiu CH, Lin TY, Bullard MJ: Identification of febrile neonates unlikely to have bacterial infections, *Pediatr Infect Dis J* 16:59, 1997.

MENINGITIS

See also Chapter 18, Headache.

SYMPTOMS
- May be variable and subtle
- Altered responsiveness ranging from irritability to lethargy
- Vomiting and decreased oral intake
- Fever is common but not universal, especially in the neonate.

SIGNS
- May be irritability alone or nonspecific
- May not have nuchal rigidity (especially in infants under 1 year)
- Seizures
- Altered mental status and signs of circulatory collapse, such as mottling or decreased capillary refill
- Disseminated intravascular coagulation can be a sequela of septic shock.

COMMENTS AND TREATMENT CONSIDERATIONS

Treatment should not be delayed to obtain specimens. Antibiotics should be chosen on the basis of age and underlying disease.

CHAPTER 16

In the few cases in which it may be appropriate to delay LP in order to do CT first, blood should be drawn for blood cultures and antibiotics then given *before* CT. LP should then be performed if not contraindicated by CT findings. This strategy identifies the cause of bacterial meningitis in most cases, even when LP is performed 1 to 2 hours after the initiation of antibiotics. Younger infants, less than 4 to 8 weeks old, should be treated with ampicillin for *Listeria* coverage and either gentamicin or a third-generation cephalosporin, such as cefotaxime. Vancomycin should be added for infants with a positive Gram stain or in whom bacterial meningitis is highly suspected because streptococcal resistance is increasing. Ceftriaxone or cefotaxime (plus vancomycin if indicated) is used in older children. Dexamethasone 0.15 mg/kg IV may be given before antibiotics when meningitis is strongly suspected.

REFERENCES

Barkin R (ed): *Pediatric emergency medicine: concepts and clinical practice*. St Louis, 1992, Mosby.

Talan DA, Hoffman JR, Yoshikawa TT, Overturf GD: Role of empiric parenteral antibiotics prior to lumbar puncture in suspected bacterial meningitis: state of the art, *Rev Infect Dis* 10:365, 1988.

 ## MENINGOCOCCEMIA

Neisseria meningitidis, a gram-negative diplococcus, can cause occult bacteremia, meningitis, and sepsis. Meningococcemia is characterized by a classic petechial rash (see Fig. 30-6). A significant proportion of patients with a fever and petechial rash have a bacterial infection. Of these, half are caused by *N. meningitidis*. Even with antibiotics and supportive care, the mortality rate for meningococcemia is significant. Because meningococcemia is often fulminant in its presentation and patients can deteriorate dramatically over minutes to hours, IV antibiotics should be given immediately when meningococcemia is suspected (fever and petechiae or purpura).

See Chapter 30, Rash.

REFERENCES

Salzman MB, Rubin LG: Meningococcemia, *Infect Dis Clin North Am* 10:709, 1996.

 ## WELL-APPEARING FEBRILE CHILD WITHOUT A SOURCE AND OCCULT BACTEREMIA

The well-appearing child between 12 weeks and 2 years of age with a high fever (>39° C) and no source for that fever has been the subject of much debate over the past two decades. The biggest concern has been whether or not the child had occult bacteremia, for which the usual causative organisms included *Haemophilus influenzae*, *S. pneumoniae*, and *N. meningitidis*. Previously, the concern was that, if left untreated, occult bacteremia could develop into a serious bacterial infection such as meningitis, pneumonia, or septic arthritis. Occult bacteremia was a consideration in any child with a significant fever (usually greater than 39° C with an increased risk as the temperature rose) who did not have an obvious source for the fever on physical examination, chest x-ray, or urinalysis.

The concern over bacteremia has greatly diminished since the widespread use of the *H. influenzae* and *S. pneumoniae* vaccines. Prior to the introduction of these vaccinations, the occult bacteremia rate was approximately 3%. Evidence from the mid-1990s, after the *H. influenzae* vaccine was introduced, demonstrated that the bacteremia rate had declined to 1.5% to 2%. Today, 5 years after the introduction of the *S. pneumoniae* vaccine, the occult bacteremia rate is probably less than 1%. Previously, laboratory tests such as the WBC, absolute neutrophil count (ANC), or C-reactive protein (CRP) were used to determine which children were at increased risk for occult bacteremia. Given the low prevalence of occult bacteremia today, many experts are no longer recommending routine laboratory testing, blood cultures, or empirical antibiotics in the pursuit of occult bacteremia.

CHAPTER 16

SYMPTOMS
- Fever
- Nonspecific symptoms

SIGNS
- Well-appearing child 12 weeks to 2 years old
- Fever
- Nonfocal examination

WORKUP
For the evaluation of a well-appearing child 12 weeks to 2 years of age without significant past medical history presenting with a fever without a source.
- Urinalysis and culture are recommended in any female less than 2 years of age, any uncircumcised male less than 1 year old, or any circumcised male less than 6 months old.
- Chest x-ray is indicated if there are signs of lower respiratory tract disease.
- Lumbar puncture—because meningitis is not considered occult in this age group, LP would be recommended in any ill-appearing child or a child with signs of meningitis.

- CBC, blood cultures: most experts now agree that routine laboratory testing is no longer necessary in well-appearing vaccinated young febrile children. Although they are protected by herd immunity, a more conservative approach is recommended for unvaccinated young children, and a CBC and blood cultures may be indicated in this population. For any child who does have a blood culture, verify the address and phone number so that the family may be reached.

COMMENTS AND TREATMENT CONSIDERATIONS

Until recently, management of febrile but well-appearing young children included empirical antibiotics such as ceftriaxone. With the declining incidence of occult bacteremia and evidence that one may wait for the results of blood cultures before initiating antibiotic therapy without increasing the risk of adverse outcomes, empiric antibiotic therapy is rarely given to previously healthy, vaccinated children. Follow-up within 24 hours (sooner if any changes) is necessary for all these children regardless of the treatment strategy.

REFERENCES

American College of Emergency Physicians: Clinical policy for children younger than three years presenting to the emergency department with fever, *Ann Emerg Med* 42:530, 2003.

Baraff LJ: Clinical policy for children younger than three years presenting to the emergency department with fever, *Ann Emerg Med* 42:546, 2003.

Baraff LJ, Bass JW, Fleisher GR, et al: Practice guideline for the management of infants and children 0 to 36 months of age with fever without source, *Ann Emerg Med* 22:1198, 1993.

Harper MB, Bachur R, Fleisher GR: Effect of antibiotic therapy on the outcome of outpatients with unsuspected bacteremia, *Pediatr Infect Dis J* 14:760, 1995.

Isaacman DJ, Karasic RB, Reynolds EA, Kost SI: Effect of number of blood cultures and volume of blood on detection of bacteremia in children, *J Pediatr* 128:190, 1996.

Kaplan SL, Mason EO Jr, Wald ER, et al: Decrease of invasive pneumococcal infections in children among 8 children's hospitals in the United States after the introduction of the 7-valent pneumococcal conjugate vaccine, *Pediatrics* 113:443, 2004.

Ling PL, Michaels MG, Janosky J, et al: Incidence of invasive pneumococcal disease in children 3 to 36 months of age at a tertiary care pediatric center 2 years after licensure of the pneumococcal conjugate vaccine, *Pediatrics* 111:896, 2003.

Rothrock SG, Harper MB, Green SM, et al: Do oral antibiotics prevent meningitis and serious bacterial infections in children with

Streptococcus pneumoniae occult bacteremia? A meta-analysis, *Pediatrics* 99:438, 1997.

Whitney CG, Farley MM, Hadler J, et al: Decline in invasive pneumococcal disease after the introduction of protein-polysaccharide conjugate vaccine, *N Engl J Med* 348:1737, 2003.

 ## KAWASAKI'S SYNDROME

See Chapter 30, Rash.

CHAPTER 16

Fractures Not to Miss
Scott W. Rodi

Missed fractures are a significant cause of morbidity in ED patients and are the leading cause of malpractice suits against emergency physicians. The subject of this chapter is limited to extremity fractures of clinical significance that may be diagnostically subtle. Some fractures may not be apparent on initial x-ray examination. In some circumstances (such as possible scaphoid fracture of the wrist), patients should be treated as if they have a fracture, even if x-rays are "negative," and should receive appropriate treatment and referral for reexamination.

SIGNS
Most fractures are suggested by clinical examination findings (swelling, deformity, and bone tenderness). Examination should include peripheral pulses, capillary refill, and distal sensation, motor function, and palpation of and range of motion (ROM) of joints proximal and distal to the suspected injury. If on the basis of inspection or palpation a fracture is thought likely, ROM should be deferred until after radiographic assessment to avoid further injury. Assessment of possible rotatory deformity is also important in metacarpal and finger injuries. Any cutaneous disruption in the area of injury should be noted and treated as a possible open fracture. Associated injuries and evidence of a compartment syndrome should also be sought (see Chapter 13, Extremity Pain and Numbness).

WORKUP
Most fractures can be identified on plain radiographs in the ED. The simplest way to identify a fracture is to trace the cortical lines, looking for abnormalities including lucencies, step-offs, acute angulations, buckles, or sclerotic lines. Effusions, soft tissue swelling, and bone fragments should be noted. Patients who sustain traumatic injuries in certain conditions (e.g., osteoporosis) or locations

(e.g., wrist) have notoriously subtle signs, and presumptive treatment or additional imaging techniques may be necessary if clinical suspicion of fracture is sufficient.

At least two perpendicular views should be obtained when assessing any fracture. Additional oblique views should be considered for periarticular fractures. Joints proximal and distal to the suspected injury should also be x-rayed *when clinically indicated.* Comparison views of the contralateral, asymptomatic extremity are sometimes helpful, particularly in children. Groups of bones effectively forming a ring (pelvis, forearm, wrist, tibia-fibula, mandible) typically break at two points, and both lesions should be sought. In some fractures, however, the second "break" is in a ligament or joint, rather than bone, and may not be visible on x-ray.

Accurate fracture description is important for charting and consultation. Fractures are described by anatomic location (intra-articular, proximal, middle or distal third of a long bone, and so forth), direction of fracture line (transverse, oblique, spiral), and degree of comminution (i.e., fragmentation) or impaction (i.e., compression). The relationship of the axes of the distal and proximal fragments is described in degrees of angulation and the amount of contact between fractured ends as opposition. *Dislocation* refers to a total disruption of joint surfaces, with the position of the distal fragment described relative to the proximal one. *Subluxation* refers to partial disruption and diastasis to a disruption of the interosseous membrane. Children may have distinct x-ray presentations of fracture because of their increased bone compliance and growth plate activity. These are described as the following:

- Greenstick: bowing of a bone without distinct fracture line
- Torus: buckling of the bone cortex
- Salter-Harris: scheme for characterization of growth plate fractures (Fig. 17–1)

Have a low threshold to immobilize and seek orthopedic follow-up for any injury near an open physis given the possibility of an occult Salter I or V injury.

COMMENTS AND TREATMENT CONSIDERATIONS

As always, airway, breathing, and circulation should be addressed first. Significant blood loss can occur with many fractures, up to 500 ml with tibial fractures, 1000 ml with femur fractures, and 3000 ml with pelvic fractures. Intravenous access and close observation for hypovolemia should be considered with relevant injuries.

When a fracture or dislocation leads to vascular compromise at the site of or distal to the injury, immediate relocation/reduction should be initiated. This is generally accomplished by applying in-line traction followed by exaggeration of the mechanism of injury and then distraction to reduce the bone deformity. Arterial imaging

CHAPTER **17**

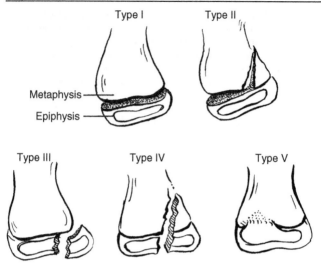

Fig. 17-1 Salter-Harris classification of growth plate fractures in children.

(generally an arteriogram) is necessary for detecting signs of vascular impairment despite reduction, as well as for knee dislocations and perhaps other high-energy injuries near blood vessels.

Patients with open fractures should begin a regimen of broad-spectrum antibiotics (e.g., cefazolin and gentamicin). Wounds should be covered with a moist, sterile dressing; cultures are not indicated. Tetanus prophylaxis should be administered according to standard protocols.

If compartment syndrome is suspected, pressures must be measured in all potentially involved compartments (see Chapter 13, Extremity Pain and Numbness).

Most fractures should be splinted to provide comfort, maintain reduction, and minimize the risk of fat embolization. Bone injuries are painful, and appropriate analgesia is required. Evidence of a pathologic fracture, intra-articular fracture, or physeal injury should prompt orthopedic consultation.

 THE PAINFUL SHOULDER

Evaluation of shoulder pain after trauma should be guided by the mechanism of injury and include consideration of possible thoracic and cervical injuries. In addition to humeral, clavicular, and other more obvious fractures, the possibility of scapular fractures and glenohumeral dislocations must be investigated.

Scapular Fractures

Scapular fractures are uncommon (0.5% to 1% of all fractures, 5% of shoulder fractures) and occur most often in 40- to 60-year-olds as a result of major trauma.

SIGNS
- Local tenderness
- Usually resist abduction, as the first 90 degrees of abduction is largely scapulothoracic

WORKUP
- X-rays: AP shoulder view initially; if not apparent, then add transscapular views
- CT scan if necessary

COMMENTS AND TREATMENT CONSIDERATIONS
The significance of a scapular fracture is primarily as a marker for major injuries (+++ have associated fractures). Head injury (++), hemopneumothorax (++), cervical spine fracture (++), rib fracture (+++), and brachial plexus injury should be sought. Approximately 10% involve the glenoid and are associated with a high rate of osteoarthritis. Mortality is approximately 10%.

Glenohumeral Dislocations

Anterior dislocation is the most common shoulder dislocation and is generally caused by abduction with external rotation. Posterior dislocation is rare and is the most commonly missed major dislocation. It may be caused by a sudden, forceful muscle contraction (e.g., epilepsy or electric shock) or direct blow. Luxatio erecta is a rare dislocation that occurs when the superior aspect of the humeral head lies below the inferior rim of the glenoid fossa.

SIGNS
- Anterior: may feel mass anterior, inferior, or medial to normal glenohumeral joint with posterior sulcus. Internal rotation is restricted.
- Posterior: note a prominent coracoid with an anterior sulcus. External rotation is restricted.
- Luxatio erecta: patient may have arm locked overhead in abduction (Fig. 17–2).

WORKUP
- X-ray: AP and a scapular Y view. Anterior: humeral head may overlap glenoid or be inferior to coracoid on AP and will not lie in center of Y on scapular Y view (Fig. 17–3). Posterior: head may appear more symmetric ("light bulb" sign) and will not be centered on Y.
- Axillary view or CT if suspicious (Figs. 17–4 and 17–5).

CHAPTER 17

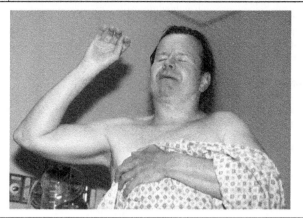

Fig. 17-2 Luxatio erecta, a rare form of shoulder dislocation.

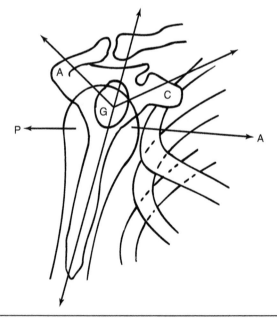

Fig. 17-3 Y, or transscapular, views of the shoulder to identify possible dislocation. *A*, Acromion; *C*, coracoid; *G*, glenoid; *P*, direction of posterior dislocation; *A*, direction of anterior dislocation. (Courtesy of Michael F. Rodi, MD.)

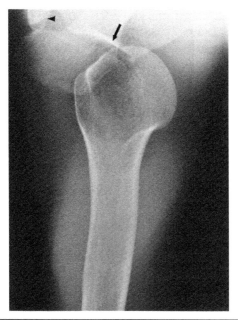

Fig. 17-4 Axillary shoulder view of posterior dislocation of the glenohumeral joint. Coracoid process is anterior *(arrowhead)*. Glenoid fossa *(arrow)*. (Courtesy of Michael Zucker, MD, Los Angeles.)

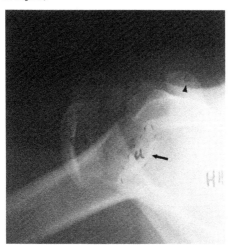

Fig. 17-5 Axillary shoulder view of posterior dislocation of glenohumeral joint. The humeral head is posterior to the glenoid. Coracoid is anterior *(arrowhead)*. Glenoid fossa *(arrow)*. (Courtesy of Michael Zucker, MD, Los Angeles.)

COMMENTS AND TREATMENT CONSIDERATIONS

Treatment consists of early ED reduction with appropriate sedation and analgesia. Associated injuries to the axillary nerve (10% to 15%), cervical spine, and chest wall should be considered. Humeral head fractures should be noted; posterolateral fractures (Hill-Sachs) (Fig. 17–6) are associated with anterior dislocations, and anterolateral (reverse Hill-Sachs) are associated with posterior dislocations. Glenoid lip fractures (Bankart lesions) are noted in 80% of patients with recurrent dislocations. After reduction, patients should be immobilized in sling and swathe and referred to orthopedics for consideration of early arthroscopic repair, especially in first-time dislocations.

 ## THE PAINFUL ELBOW IN CHILDREN

In children, many significant injuries that involve elbow pain are radiographically subtle; "sprain" is a dangerously conservative

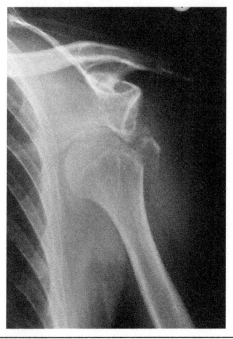

Fig. 17–6 AP view of shoulder demonstrates anterior dislocation of the glenohumeral joint. Hill-Sachs fracture with avulsion of greater tubercle. (Courtesy of Michael Zucker, MD, Los Angeles.)

diagnosis in this setting. If doubt exists, the elbow should be immobilized and an ED orthopedic consultation obtained. Comparison views of the asymptomatic elbow may be helpful but are often not required.

Supracondylar Humeral Fracture

Supracondylar humeral fractures represent 3% of all fractures in children and 85% of elbow fractures in children. They are generally caused by a fall on the outstretched hand (FOOSH), usually with hyperextension of the elbow. The male-to-female ratio is 9:1, with a bimodal age distribution: 2 to 8 and 11 to 15 years old.

SIGNS
• Tenderness at distal humerus and resistant to motion in all planes
• Neurologic deficit ++, most commonly anterior interosseous nerve

WORKUP
• X-ray: AP and lateral views of the elbow. Occult fracture is suggested by fat pad displacement, especially posterior (Fig. 17–7), and displacement of the anterior humeral line (greater than one third of capitellum normally lies anterior to anterior cortex of distal humerus (Fig. 17–8); less than this suggests fracture).

COMMENTS AND TREATMENT CONSIDERATIONS
Supracondylar humeral fractures are associated with significant morbidity including brachial artery and nerve injury and compartment syndrome. Volkmann's contracture and cubitus varus deformity (10%) are possible sequelae. Moderate flexion should be attempted if pulse deficit is noted. Orthopedic consultation is necessary, and patients are generally admitted for observation if there is significant displacement.

MEDIAL EPICONDYLAR AVULSION FRACTURE
Represents 5% to 10% of elbow injuries in children, usually occurring in those 9 to 15 years of age. To diagnose radiographically, if the trochlear ossification center is visible, the medial epicondyle ossification center should appear normal; if not, a displaced fracture should be suspected. This fracture is associated with elbow dislocation and loss of forearm flexor attachment, and the prognosis is guarded.

LATERAL CONDYLE FRACTURE
Usually Salter IV fractures that require operative repair. An orthopedist should be consulted even if the fracture appears

CHAPTER 17

193

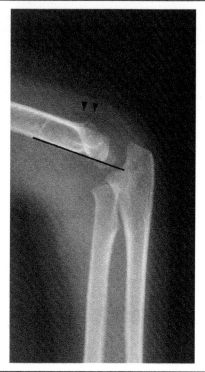

Fig. 17-7 Lateral view of elbow shows supracondylar fracture in a child. The posterior fat pad is displaced *(arrowheads)*, indicating hemarthrosis. The anterior humeral line is abnormal, indicating posterior displacement of the distal humerus *(line)*. (Courtesy of Michael Zucker, MD, Los Angeles.)

radiographically nondisplaced. Complications include nonunion, cubitus valgus, ulnar nerve palsy, and osteonecrosis.

RADIAL HEAD SUBLUXATION (NURSEMAID'S ELBOW)

This elbow injury is common in 2- to 5-year-olds and is usually caused by sudden traction of the hand, pulling the radial head out of the annular ligament. Children with this injury usually hold the elbow stiffly in flexion and pronation. The diagnosis is generally made by a typical history and physical examination. X-rays may be considered in unusual cases to exclude fracture; the radiocapitellar line is inspected for radial head subluxation (Fig. 17–9) and evidence of fracture. Subluxations are reduced by supination and flexion (or extension) of the elbow while applying pressure over the radial head with the thumb.

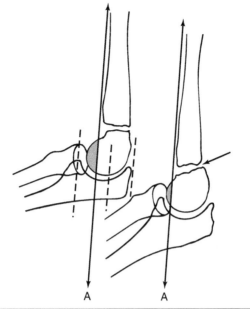

Fig. 17-8 Depiction of "true" lateral view to assess possible supracondylar fracture. A, Normal—one third of capitellum lies anterior to anterior humeral line. B, Less than one third of capitellum lying anterior to anterior humeral line indicates a probable supracondylar fracture *(arrow)*. A, Anterior humeral line. (Courtesy of Michael F. Rodi, MD.)

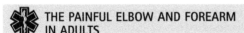 THE PAINFUL ELBOW AND FOREARM IN ADULTS

Even if an obvious forearm fracture is noted, associated elbow and wrist injuries must be suspected and aggressively pursued as missed associated injuries may result in long-term pain and disability.

Galeazzi Fracture

A Galeazzi fracture is fracture of the distal third of the radius with associated dislocation or subluxation of the distal radioulnar joint (DRUJ) caused by an axial load on a pronated forearm.

SIGNS
• Tenderness at DRUJ in addition to fracture site

WORKUP
• X-ray: AP/lateral forearm including elbow and wrist. Widened DRUJ, ulnar styloid fracture, or radius >5 mm shorter than ulna suggests the diagnosis.

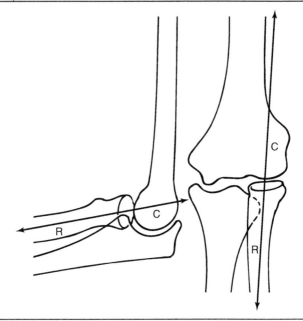

Fig. 17-9   Depiction of "true" AP and lateral views of the elbow to assess possible dislocation of the radial head. *R*, Radius; *C*, capitellum. Arrows represent the radiocapitellar line drawn through the shaft of the radius; if the line does not pass through the capitellum, the radial head is probably dislocated. (Courtesy of Michael F. Rodi, MD.)

COMMENTS AND TREATMENT CONSIDERATIONS
Patients should be observed for compartment syndrome while an orthopedic consultation in the ED is obtained.

Monteggia Fracture
A Monteggia fracture involves the proximal third of the ulna and is associated with radial head dislocation caused by a direct blow to the forearm ("nightstick" injury) or fall on a pronated hand.

SIGNS
• Tenderness at fracture site and radial head
• Decreased ROM

WORKUP
• X-ray: AP lateral forearm (with wrist and elbow). Displacement of the radiocapitellar line should be sought; normally, a line through the proximal radius intersects with the capitellum in all views (see Fig. 17-9).

COMMENTS AND TREATMENT CONSIDERATIONS
An orthopedic consultation in the ED should be obtained because the fracture may require surgical reduction.

Radial Head Fracture
Radial head fracture is generally caused by FOOSH with the elbow extended and the hand pronated or by a fall backward with the hand supinated.

SIGNS
• Pain and swelling over the radial head, which can be elicited by palpation of the elbow laterally with the thumb during supination and pronation. A concomitant wrist injury or mechanical block to supination should be investigated (may need surgery).

WORKUP
• X-ray: Frequently occult. If fracture is not visible, look for signs of effusion including elevated anterior fat pad ("sail sign") or visible posterior fat pad.

COMMENTS AND TREATMENT CONSIDERATIONS
A small minority of patients with radial head fracture have associated elbow dislocation, and a few have DRUJ injury. If <30% of the head is involved and is nondisplaced (Mason I), fracture may be treated with a sling and early ROM (vast majority of cases); if >30% (Mason II) with poor ROM or comminuted (Mason III), surgery may be necessary.

Coronoid Process Fracture
Coronoid fracture is present is 2% to 15% of elbow dislocations.

SIGNS
• Painful elbow
• Possible instability or decreased ROM

WORKUP
• X-ray: AP/lateral radiographs of elbow. Type I: tip avulsion; type II: <50% fractured; type III: >50%. The prognosis is worse and associated injuries greater with increasing grade.

COMMENTS AND TREATMENT CONSIDERATIONS
Significance is as marker of possible elbow dislocation; consider orthopedic consultation.

 THE PAINFUL WRIST
Many wrist injuries are subtle, and a diagnosis of sprain should not be made until a careful evaluation has eliminated other possibilities.

A zone of vulnerability has been described (Fig. 17–10); tenderness or x-ray abnormality in this arc should prompt careful evaluation.

Scaphoid Fractures
Scaphoid fractures are the most commonly missed fractures and represent 60% to 70% of carpal fractures. They typically occur as a result of FOOSH.

SIGNS
- Tenderness with or without swelling in anatomic snuff-box (++++, 40% specific) or at scaphoid tubercle (++++, 57% specific)

WORKUP
- X-ray: four-view series (AP, lateral, and AP in radial and ulnar deviation) with specific scaphoid views. On follow-up films, 2% to 20% reveal a fracture and 2% to 5% remain false negatives (Fig. 17–11).

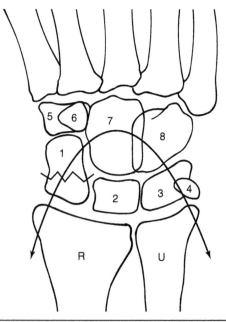

Fig. 17–10 Zone of vulnerability *(arrow)* on AP view of the wrist to evaluate possible combination fractures or injuries. *1,* Scaphoid (navicular); *2,* lunate; *3,* triquetrum; *4,* pisiform; *5,* trapezium (greater multangular); *6,* trapezoid (lesser multangular); *7,* capitate; *8,* hamate; *R,* radius; *U,* ulna. (Courtesy of Michael F. Rodi, MD.)

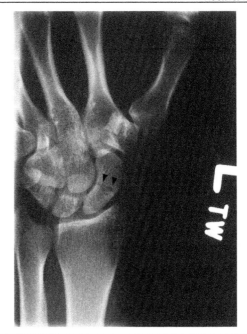

Fig. 17–11 AP view of wrist demonstrates scaphoid fracture *(arrowheads).* (Courtesy of Michael Zucker, MD, Los Angeles.)

COMMENTS AND TREATMENT CONSIDERATIONS

If no fracture is seen but an occult fracture is suspected because of snuff-box tenderness, a thumb-spica splint is applied and x-rays repeated in 14 days. Earlier reexamination by an orthopedist may facilitate earlier discontinuation of the splint if the patient has a normal examination. Alternatively, some studies have shown clear benefit to early definitive diagnosis by MRI at the time of initial ED evaluation. Primary concern is nonunion or avascular necrosis (with subsequent chronic pain) because blood supply may enter through the distal pole only. If fracture is displaced (>1 mm) and angulated, an orthopedic consultation should be obtained for possible early surgery. No associated injuries are present in most cases.

Wrist tenderness can be caused by other carpal bone fractures including a triquetrum fracture, which is often apparent only on a lateral wrist x-ray.

Lunate and Perilunate Dislocations

Lunate dislocation is an uncommon injury in which the lunate alone is dislocated while the rest of the carpals remain in place; perilunate dislocation (also uncommon) occurs when all carpals except the lunate dislocate posteriorly and usually occurs with FOOSH.

SIGNS
• Swollen, tender wrist with decreased ROM and pain with axial compression of third metacarpal. Tenderness of the lunate itself should be examined. This is elicited by compression over the depression present just proximal to the third metacarpal and is exacerbated when the wrist is flexed, which brings the lunate up into the "empty space."

WORKUP
• X-ray: AP/lateral of wrist. On AP, uniform space between carpals (1 to 2 mm) is noted (see Fig. 17–10) in the normal wrist. Widening, or a triangular-appearing lunate, suggests ligamentous disruption or dislocation. On lateral x-rays, the radius, lunate, and capitate should line up, appearing like multiple cups seated in saucers. If the lunate appears empty, a dislocation is suspected. If the capitate and radius are still aligned, a lunate dislocation is most likely; if the radius and capitate are not aligned, a perilunate dislocation is likely (Figs. 17–12 to 17–14).

COMMENTS AND TREATMENT CONSIDERATIONS
An urgent orthopedic consultation for reduction is necessary. The prognosis is guarded and ROM limited. Evidence of median nerve compression should be sought.

 THE PAINFUL HIP

Pelvic fractures from high-energy mechanisms are diagnostically straightforward but are associated with high morbidity and mortality and have a high risk of hemorrhagic shock. In reviewing pelvic films, sacroiliac joints and pubic symphysis should be checked for symmetry and sacral foramina arcuate lines and acetabular lines for irregularities (Fig. 17–15). Hip fractures in elderly people are similarly associated with high morbidity and mortality but may be radiographically occult on plain films and require CT or MRI for diagnosis.

Proximal Femur Fractures
Hip fractures are common (250,000 a year in the United States), particularly among elderly women (74% >65 years old; female to male, 4:1). They occur commonly after falls, and it is important to elicit any antecedent symptoms such as chest pain or dizziness that may indicate a primary medical or surgical condition that caused the fall.

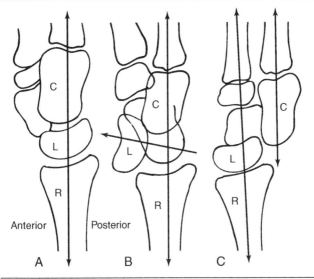

Fig. 17-12   Depiction of "true" lateral view of the wrist to assess lunate and perilunate dislocations. Normal **(A)**, lunate dislocation **(B)**, perilunate dislocation **(C)**. *R*, Radius; *L*, lunate; *C*, capitate. (Courtesy of Michael F. Rodi, MD.)

SIGNS

- Thigh, knee, or groin pain
- Affected extremity may appear shortened and externally rotated if displaced; however, alignment may be normal, and the patient may even be ambulatory if there is no displacement.

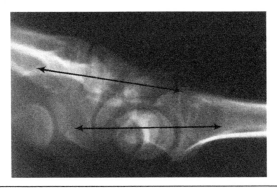

Fig. 17-13   Lateral view of wrist shows perilunate dislocation. The radiolunate line *(bottom arrow)* is intact, but the lunate-capitate relationship is disrupted with dorsal dislocation of the capitate *(top arrow)*. (Courtesy of Michael Zucker, MD, Los Angeles.)

201

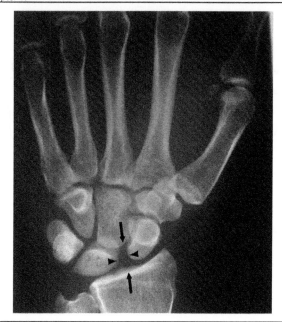

Fig. 17-14 AP view of wrist shows scapholunate dissociation. The gap between the lunate and scaphoid is greater than 4 mm *(arrowheads)*. (Courtesy of Michael Zucker, MD, Los Angeles.)

WORKUP

• X-ray: AP, lateral, and internal rotation views of affected hip and an AP pelvic view to check that cortices are unbroken, trabecular pattern is smooth, and there are no sclerotic lines (Fig. 17-16). Shenton's line and neck-shaft angle (normal, 120 to 130 degrees) are traced (Fig. 17-17). Fractures may be radiographically occult (2% to 9%) and MRI (approaching 100% sensitive and specific) should be strongly considered, especially in the elderly, if there is clinical concern for hip fracture and no fracture is identified. Although less sensitive and specific than MRI, CT may be used if MRI is not available.

COMMENTS AND TREATMENT CONSIDERATIONS

Associated conditions to consider include ipsilateral upper extremity fracture (1% to 2%) and cervical spine injury. Morbidity and mortality are high; less than one half regain prefracture level of function and mortality is 15 times greater than in age-matched controls in the

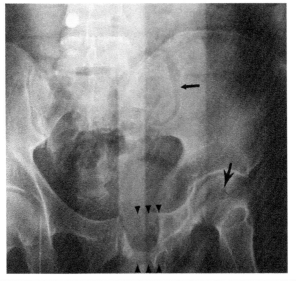

Fig. 17-15 AP view of pelvic fractures. Disruption of symphysis pubis and fractures of left rami *(arrowheads)* and disruption of the anterior ligaments of the left sacroiliac joint *(small arrow)*. Also note left acetabular fracture *(large arrow)*. (Courtesy of Michael Zucker, MD, Los Angeles.)

first month after injury. Medical complications are minimized by early surgery. Consider pathologic fracture in younger patients.

Pediatric Hip Pain

In addition to fractures, considerations in a child complaining of hip (or knee) pain should include transient synovitis, avascular necrosis, slipped capital femoral epiphysis, and septic hip (see Chapter 25, Limping Child/Child Won't Walk). Avulsion fractures should be considered in adolescents, specifically ASIS (sartorius origin), AIIS (rectus femoris origin), and ischial tuberosity (hamstrings origin).

 THE PAINFUL KNEE

Most fractures and dislocations about the knee are radiographically obvious. Clinical criteria have been developed for determining which patients need x-ray examination. The Ottawa Knee Rule is a commonly utilized clinical decision aid. According to the criteria, knee radiographs are required only for patients with knee injuries

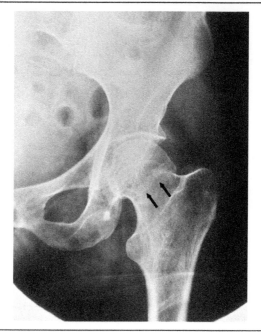

Fig. 17–16 AP hip radiograph shows femoral fracture. Impacted fracture of the neck of the femur, Garden I type *(arrows)*. (Courtesy of Michael Zucker, MD, Los Angeles.)

who have one or more of the following: (1) age 55 years or older, (2) tenderness at the head of the fibula, (3) isolated tenderness of the patella, (4) inability to flex to 90 degrees, and (5) inability to bear weight both immediately and in the ED (four steps).

An apparently isolated fibular fracture should prompt careful evaluation of the ankle, and a fat-fluid level on a lateral radiograph or a lipohemarthrosis on arthrocentesis should prompt an evaluation for an intraarticular fracture. Soft tissue injuries to the knee can generally be managed with a knee immobilizer, crutches, and outpatient follow-up. Nontraumatic knee pain may represent septic arthritis (see Chapter 24, Joint Pain).

Knee Dislocation

Dislocation of the knee is usually caused by motor vehicle accidents, sports injuries, or falls. Dashboard injuries cause posterior dislocations (i.e., posterior translation of tibia), and

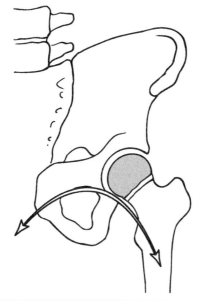

Fig. 17–17 AP view of the pelvis with Shenton's line to assess fracture, dislocation, or subluxation of the acetabulum and femoral head. (Courtesy of Michael F. Rodi, MD.)

CHAPTER 17

hyperextension injuries cause anterior dislocations. Popliteal artery injury is common after knee dislocation and requires emergent vascular surgical consultation for repair.

SIGNS
- May be obviously dislocated or grossly unstable, which may indicate dislocation with spontaneous reduction.
- Popliteal fossa may be full owing to vascular injury or may appear normal if decompressed by capsular tear.
- Diminished pulses or neurologic deficit.

WORKUP
- If appears dislocated on examination, reduce immediately.
- Surgery if diminished pulses
- X-ray and angiography (some centers prefer observation with selective angiography) if dislocation is thought to have occurred

- If grossly unstable, treat as a spontaneously reduced dislocation (angiography).

COMMENTS AND TREATMENT CONSIDERATIONS

Generally, traction-countertraction with conscious sedation effectively reduces knee dislocations. Between 30% and 40% of dislocations are associated with popliteal artery injury, most of which require amputation if surgical repair is delayed >8 hours. It is imperative to have a low threshold for angiography if dislocation is evident or suspected.

Tibial Plateau Fracture

Tibial plateau fracture may occur in younger individuals when valgus stress (e.g., bumper injury) causes lateral plateau fracture. The injury may be more subtle in the elderly, in whom axial compression can cause fracture.

SIGNS

- Local tenderness, usually decreased ROM
- Possible varus or valgus laxity

WORKUP

- X-ray: AP, lateral, and oblique views. Only sclerotic line below articular surface may be seen. Fracture should be suspected if AP view shows that lateral margin of tibia is >5 mm beyond lateral cortex of femur.
- CT or MRI is confirmatory.

COMMENTS AND TREATMENT CONSIDERATIONS

Fractures of the medial plateau (20% of cases) should be treated as high-energy injuries or as possible spontaneous relocations; angiogram to evaluate the integrity of the popliteal artery may be helpful. Patients should be observed for compartment syndrome while an orthopedic consultation in the ED is obtained.

Markers of Anterior Cruciate Injury

Anterior cruciate injury is the most common ligamentous knee injury. A rapid effusion may develop following twist, rapid deceleration, or hyperextension; 35% report an audible "pop."

SIGNS

- Lachman ++++, gentle traction, as it can be falsely negative if patient resists with muscles because of pain
- Laxity with anterior drawer +++

WORKUP
- X-rays: AP and lateral. Note Segond fracture (vertical fracture of lateral plateau), tibial spine avulsion, or "kissing contusion" (fracture of lateral condyle and lateral tibial plateau).

COMMENTS AND TREATMENT CONSIDERATIONS
Orthopedic consultation is necessary. Surgical results are especially favorable with bone avulsions.

 THE PAINFUL ANKLE AND FOOT

Most injuries to the foot and ankle are clinically and radiographically obvious. The mortise view should always be assessed for uniform joint space around the talus and the lateral view to check calcaneus and posterior tibial integrity. The base of the fifth metatarsal should be checked in all patients with tenderness in this area after ankle inversion.

Maisonneuve Fracture
Maisonneuve fracture is a disruption—bony or ligamentous—of the medial ankle and proximal fibula and is usually caused by external rotation of the ankle.

SIGNS
- Tenderness at medial malleolus and proximal fibula

WORKUP
- X-ray: ankle series and AP and lateral views of proximal fibula. Only widening (i.e., no ankle fracture) may be noted if the deltoid ligament is ruptured.

COMMENTS AND TREATMENT CONSIDERATIONS
The instability of fibular fractures often necessitates surgical treatment. Fibular shortening predisposes to early arthritis. Obtain early orthopedic consultation if suspected.

Lisfranc Fracture-Dislocation
Lisfranc fracture-dislocation is a tarsometatarsal dislocation caused by hyperplantar flexion over fixed forefoot; 20% are missed.

SIGNS
- Midfoot pain
- Midfoot swelling
- Difficulty ambulating

CHAPTER 17

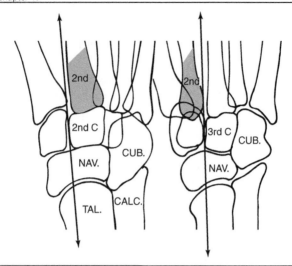

Fig. 17-18 AP and oblique views of the normal foot to assess fractures, dislocations, and subluxations in the foot (note the normal alignment of the tarsometatarsal joints–Lisfranc joints). (Courtesy of Michael F. Rodi, MD.)

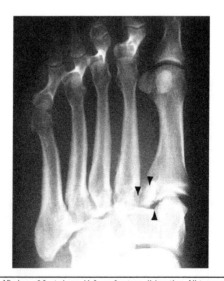

Fig. 17-19 AP view of foot shows Lisfranc fracture-dislocation. All tarsometatarsal joints are involved. Note malalignment of first and second metatarsals *(arrowheads)*. (Courtesy of Michael Zucker, MD, Los Angeles.)

WORKUP
- X-ray: AP, lateral, and oblique. Suspect if bone fragment is seen at any metatarsal base. On normal AP, medial border of second metatarsal (MT) and middle cuneiform are aligned, and on normal oblique, medial border of third MT and lateral cuneiform are aligned (Figs. 17–18 and 17–19). On lateral, no MT should appear dorsal to cuboid. May confirm by CT.

COMMENTS AND TREATMENT CONSIDERATIONS
Orthopedic consultation should be obtained in the ED. Surgery is often necessary. Posttraumatic arthritis is common.

Calcaneus Fracture

A calcaneus fracture is usually caused by a fall or jump but may result from twisting.

SIGNS
- Local swelling and tenderness
- Unable to bear weight

WORKUP
- X-ray: Bohler's angle (Figs. 17–20 and 17–21) <30 degrees suggests a fracture, as do sclerotic lines in the calcaneal body, disruption of trabeculae, increased density (overlapping bone), and cortical lucencies. Also consider axial views or CT.

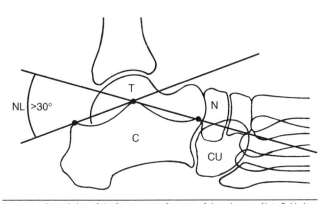

Fig. 17–20   Lateral view of the foot to assess fractures of the calcaneus. Note Bohler's angle; if less than 30 degrees, suspect fracture of the calcaneus. *T*, Talus; *C*, calcaneus; *N*, navicular; *CU*, cuboid. (Courtesy of Michael F. Rodi, MD.)

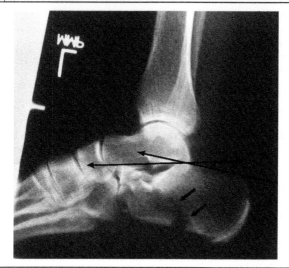

Fig. 17–21   Lateral view of foot shows calcaneus fracture. Intra-articular fracture *(short arrows)*. Bohler's angle is abnormal *(long arrows, arrowhead)*. (Courtesy of Michael Zucker, MD, Los Angeles.)

COMMENTS AND TREATMENT CONSIDERATIONS
Associated injuries should always be considered, especially to the axial skeleton; 10% have dorsolumbar compression fractures and compartment syndrome. The x-ray needs to be inspected closely to rule out talar dome fractures, which may have a similar clinical presentation.

Fifth Metatarsal Fracture
There are three general fracture types of the fifth metatarsal: ankle twist causes avulsion fracture of the tuberosity at the base of the fifth metatarsal by contraction of the plantar fascia (dancer's); landing on the lateral border of the foot causes fracture at the metaphyseal-diaphyseal junction (Jones); and repetitive impact causes fatigue fracture at the diaphyseal base ("stress").

SIGNS
• Local tenderness at base of fifth metatarsal

WORKUP
• X-ray: AP, lateral, oblique
• Bone scan if negative and concern for stress fracture

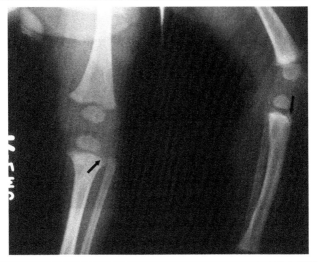

Fig. 17-22 AP and lateral knee radiographs demonstrate corner, or "bucket-handle," fracture of the proximal tibia *(arrows)* as a result of nonaccidental trauma (child abuse). (Courtesy of Michael Zucker, MD, Los Angeles.)

- Normal apophysis in children (long axis parallel to metatarsal) should not be confused with avulsion fracture (usually perpendicular).

COMMENTS AND TREATMENT CONSIDERATIONS
Consider ED orthopedic consultation or close follow-up for patients with intraarticular tuberosity fractures or diaphyseal fractures. Posterior splint and crutches with orthopedic referral are necessary in most other cases.

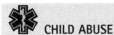 **CHILD ABUSE**

Many fractures are especially associated with abuse. Multiple fractures at different stages of healing are seen in 23% to 85% of abuse cases. Subperiosteal bone formation, "bucket-handle" fractures (i.e., fractures at the metaphyseal corners of long bones, Fig. 17–22), and fractures of the ribs, femur (especially in the nonambulatory), fingers, humerus, pelvis, spine, and skull are all suggestive of possible abuse.

See Chapter 22, The Irritable Child.

REFERENCES

Armstrong CP, Van der Spuy J: The fractured scapula: importance and management based on a series of 62 patients, *Injury* 15:324, 1984.

Browner B, Jupiter J, et al: *Skeletal trauma: fractures, dislocations and ligamentous injuries*. Philadelphia, 20092, WB Saunders.

Bucholz R, Hedman J: *Rockwood and Green's fractures in adults*, ed 5. Philadelphia, 2002, Lippincott Williams & Wilkins.

Calandra JJ, Goldner RD, Hardaker WT Jr: Scaphoid fractures: assessment and treatment, *Orthopedics* 15:931, 1992.

Carty HM: Fractures caused by child abuse, *J Bone Joint Surg Br* 75:849, 1993.

Council on Scientific Affairs: AMA diagnostic and treatment guidelines concerning child abuse and neglect, *JAMA* 254:796, 1985.

Englanoff J, Anglin D, Hutson HR: Lisfranc fracture-dislocation: a frequently missed diagnosis in the emergency department, *Ann Emerg Med* 26:229, 1995.

Freeland P: Scaphoid tubercle tenderness: a better indicator of scaphoid fractures? *Arch Emerg Med* 6:46, 1989.

Hoppenfeld S: *Physical examination of the spine and extremities*. London, 1976, Appleton-Century-Crofts.

Kaufman SL, Martin LG: Arterial injuries associated with complete dislocation of the knee, *Radiology* 184:153, 1992.

Kezdi-Rogus PC, Lomasney LM: Radiologic case study: plain film manifestations of ACL injury, *Orthopedics* 17:967, 1994.

Lawrence SJ, Botte MJ: Jones' fractures and related fractures of the proximal fifth metatarsal, *Foot Ankle* 14:358, 1993.

Leventhal JM, Thomas SA, Rosenfield NS, et al: Fractures in young children: distinguishing child abuse from unintentional injuries, *Am J Dis Child* 147:87, 1993.

Miller MD: Commonly missed orthopedic problems, *Emerg Med Clin North Am* 10:151, 1992.

Raby N, de Lacy G, Berman L: *Accident and emergency radiology—a survival guide*. Philadelphia, 1995, WB Saunders.

Regan W, Morrey BF: Classification and treatment of coronoid process fractures, *Orthopedics* 15:845, 1992.

Rockwood C, Wilkins K, King R: *Fractures in children*. Philadelphia, 1984, JB Lippincott.

Simon R., Koenigsknecht S: *Emergency orthopedics, the extremities*. New York, 2001, McGraw-Hill.

Stiell IG, Greenberg GH, Wells GA, et al: Derivation of a decision rule for the use of radiography in acute knee injuries, *Ann Emerg Med* 26:405, 1995.

Treiman GS, Yellin AE, Weaver FA, et al: Examination of the patient with a knee dislocation: the case for selective arteriography, *Arch Surg* 127:1056, 1992.

Waeckerle JF: A prospective study identifying the sensitivity of radiographic findings and the efficacy of clinical findings in carpal navicular fractures, *Ann Emerg Med* 16:733, 1987.

Waizenegger M, Barton NJ, Davis TR, et al: Clinical signs in scaphoid fractures, *J Hand Surg [Br]* 19:743, 1994.

CHAPTER 17

Headache
Joshua N. Goldstein and Jonathan A. Edlow

Headache is a common complaint of patients seen in the ED. Studies indicate that for only a few percent of these patients can headache be attributed to serious causes (life or vision threatening). Distinguishing these patients from the vast majority is the goal. In pursuing this goal, do not draw unwarranted conclusions from either the degree of pain or its relief. Patients can have a great deal of pain yet suffer from a relatively benign condition; conversely, others complain of mild pain yet have life-threatening illnesses. Nonnarcotic analgesics have been reported to relieve the pain of subarachnoid hemorrhage, pseudotumor cerebri, and brain tumor. Therefore, careful attention must be given to the cornerstone of diagnosis—a careful history and physical examination.

Besides the standard questions asked of any patient with a painful condition (onset, duration, alleviating factors, and so forth), some aspects of the history warrant special emphasis. For example, ask about recent trauma because some patients, especially the elderly, can have a subdural hematoma weeks after a head injury, even a minor one. If the patient suffers from regular headaches, it is important to establish whether the current episode deviates from the normal pattern. Abrupt severe onset suggests subarachnoid hemorrhage. Although vomiting is common with migraines, it also suggests intracranial hemorrhage or elevated intracranial pressure (ICP).

Age is important; up to 15% of patients older than 65 years with new onset of headache have a serious medical condition. Even the season may be significant; during the winter months, carbon monoxide poisoning should be considered as a possible diagnosis.

Prior history of or risks for HIV infection, malignancy, and neurosurgery should be obtained. Record the drug history (both therapeutic and recreational), with anticoagulants, MAO inhibitors, and cocaine being especially important.

With the understanding that a complete physical examination be done, focus on the vital signs, sinuses, tympanic membranes, optic fundi, cornea, temporal arteries, neck, and skin (rash and color). A neurologic examination is essential; components that are commonly omitted are bedside visual field and gait testing. Both of these can be performed quickly and cover a great deal of neuroanatomic territory. It is noteworthy that some patients with intracranial masses have a completely normal examination.

Laboratory tests, neuroimaging studies, and examination of the cerebrospinal fluid (CSF) must be tailored to the individual situation. Routine neuroimaging of unselected patients with headache yields a very low incidence of significant abnormalities. The availability of CT scanners has encouraged physicians to perform a scan routinely before doing a lumbar puncture (LP). This practice is unnecessary in many cases in patients with a normal neurologic examination, and obtaining a CT scan should never delay antibiotic administration in suspected bacterial meningitis. Post–lumbar puncture headache is more common in younger, thinner females and is reduced by using smaller needles that split rather than transect the dural fibers.

Although this section focuses on the diagnosis and treatment of emergent conditions, it is equally important to relieve pain in the vast majority of patients with less serious illnesses. Although some patients are seeking narcotics, most are not. Although one tries to avoid prescribing narcotics to drug-seeking patients, it is more important to provide pain relief to patients with legitimate pain.

REFERENCES

Clinical policy: critical issues in the evaluation and management of patients presenting to the emergency department with acute headache, *Ann Emerg Med* 39:108, 2002.

Hasbun R, Abrahams J, Jekel J, Quargliarello V: CT of the head before lumbar puncture in adults with suspected meningitis, *N Engl J Med* 245:1727, 2001.

 SUBARACHNOID HEMORRHAGE

Subarachnoid hemorrhage (SAH) can be caused by rupture of a cerebral aneurysm or arteriovenous malformation. Although aneurysmal SAH typically has an abrupt onset and is described by patients as the worst headache of their life, a significant minority have less severe symptoms. Early diagnosis of SAH is essential, especially when the patient is still in good clinical condition, because the prognosis is better. Prompt evaluation with CT scan and LP excludes this condition. Physicians should have a low

CHAPTER 18

threshold for performing CT and LP in patients with new or unfamiliar headaches.

SYMPTOMS

- Headache ++++. Characteristically the abrupt onset of severe headache ("worst headache of life" or "thunderclap" headache), usually global; with onset during exercise. Can be associated with nausea, vomiting, and transient loss of consciousness.
- Patients may give a history of a *warning headache* ++, a distinctive headache, also referred to as a sentinel bleed, that preceded the current SAH by days to weeks. This headache is thought to be due to a minor leak of blood or occasionally bleeding or dissection into the wall of the aneurysm. If the patient seeks medical care, and the warning headache is recognized for what it is (a small SAH), critical intervention can occur that prevents subsequent and often more serious SAH.
- Neck pain: from blood irritating the meninges (can be the only presenting complaint but is less commonly present)
- Back and radicular pain: occurs later in some patients from irritation as the blood settles into the lumbar thecal sac. Is far less common than headache.

SIGNS

- Meningismus +++
- Retinal subhyaloid hemorrhage +
- Significant bleeding often with a fluid level seen on funduscopic examination
- Focal or generalized neurologic abnormalities

WORKUP

- CT scan: first-line test; 90% to 95% sensitive in first 24 hours, 80% by day 3, 70% by day 5, continues to decline over time. MRI: has not been as sensitive for acute blood as CT but technology is rapidly improving, and some MR sequences can detect SAH with high sensitivity.
- LP: must be performed after a negative CT. Red blood cells are seen within 2 hours of headache onset. Xanthochromia takes hours to develop; by spectrophotometry it is almost always present from 12 hours to 2 weeks; however, most hospital laboratories use visual inspection, which is less sensitive; spectrophotometry has false positives. The vast majority of patients who have experienced a thunderclap headache but have normal CT and LP results have a benign course.
- Angiography or MR angiography (MRA): Once diagnosed by CT or LP, to identify the source of bleeding.

COMMENTS AND TREATMENT CONSIDERATIONS

Once SAH is diagnosed, obtain rapid neurosurgical consultation for angiography and definitive surgical or endovascular therapy. Nonspecific treatment includes bed rest, isotonic fluids to prevent hyponatremia (which could cause or worsen cerebral edema), and nimodipine within the first 12 hours (to decrease vasospasm).

REFERENCES

Edlow JA, Bruner KS, Horowitz GL: Xanthochromia, *Arch Pathol Lab Med* 126:413, 2002.

Edlow JA, Caplan LR: Avoiding pitfalls in the diagnosis of subarachnoid hemorrhage, *N Engl J Med* 342:29, 2000.

Edlow JA, Wyer PC: How good is a negative cranial CT in excluding subarachnoid hemorrhage? *Ann Emerg Med* 36:507, 2000.

Morgenstern LB, Luna-Gonzales H, Huber JC Jr, et al: Worst headache and subarachnoid hemorrhage: prospective, modern computed tomography and spinal fluid analysis, *Ann Emerg Med* 32:297, 1998.

BACTERIAL MENINGITIS

Patients with bacterial meningitis—inflammation of the tissues around the brain or spinal cord—rarely present with headache without fever. Early administration of antibiotics is imperative and should not be delayed for the performance of diagnostic testing. If bacterial meningitis is strongly suspected, blood should be drawn for blood cultures and antibiotics then given before LP or CT. This strategy identifies the cause of bacterial meningitis in most cases, even when LP is performed 1 to 2 hours after the initiation of antibiotics. Antibiotics should be given after the LP only if the LP can be performed without delay. Nonbacterial meningitides, such as herpes meningoencephalitis, may present without fever. Some nonbacterial meningitides also require emergent treatment.

SYMPTOMS
- Fever ++++
- Headache ++++
- Nausea ++++, vomiting +++
- Neck stiffness ++++
- Altered mental status
- Photophobia
- Rash ++

SIGNS
- Classic triad +++: fever, nuchal rigidity, change in mental status
- Temperature >38° C ++++

- Seizures ++
- Mental status change +++ ranging from lethargy and confusion to coma
- Focal neurologic deficit +++ including cranial nerve deficits
- Aphasia ++
- Papilledema +
- Meningismus +++: nuchal rigidity, Brudzinski's sign, Kernig's sign
- Rash: maculopapular, petechial, purpuric ++

WORKUP

- CT scan before LP for mental status change, focal neurologic deficit, papilledema, AIDS
- Lumbar puncture for CSF analysis: opening pressure (>20 cm water ++++), cell count and differential (WBC >100 cells/mm^3 ++++, WBC >999/mm^3 ++++), glucose, protein, Gram stain, culture. Other tests only as indicated: India ink, latex agglutination (if negative Gram stain) cryptococcal antigen, antibody studies for histoplasmosis, coccidioidomycosis, blastomycosis, VDRL, Lyme serology, cultures for tuberculosis, fungi, anaerobes.
- Blood cultures +++

COMMENTS AND TREATMENT CONSIDERATIONS

Do not unreasonably delay antibiotics for diagnostic evaluation. If the LP cannot be performed immediately, antibiotics should be given before the LP. An LP performed after the administration of antibiotics still reveals the causative organism by Gram stain, culture, or latex agglutination studies in most cases. If the LP can be done immediately, antibiotics may be administered as soon as the fluid is obtained. If the index of suspicion for bacterial meningitis is high, there is no reason to delay antibiotics while awaiting results from an LP. If CT is needed because of a focal neurologic finding, concern regarding HIV, or other conditions, obtain blood cultures first and then start antibiotics that target the most likely organism(s). If there are no contraindications by CT, perform the LP immediately after the imaging study.

Meningismus often does not develop in infants, who may have only fever, irritability, lethargy, poor feeding, and/or vomiting. Elderly patients may present with lethargy or obtundation without fever; meningeal signs may also be absent. Patients (especially children) who have recently been treated with antibiotics may have minimal symptoms.

The current recommendations for initial empiric therapy include either ceftriaxone (infants and children 50 mg/kg or 2 g adults) or cefotaxime (infants and children 50 mg/kg or 2 g adults) and vancomycin (15 mg/kg, max 1 g) to cover resistant *S. pneumoniae*.

This regimen broadly targets the most likely organisms. It is modified in selected populations of patients:

- Age <3 months: Group B streptococcus, *E. coli*, *Listeria monocytogenes* (add ampicillin 50 mg/kg)
- Age 3 months to <18 years: *N. meningitidis*, *S. pneumoniae*, *H. influenzae*
- Age 18 to 50: *S. pneumoniae*, *N. meningitidis*
- Age >50: *S. pneumoniae*, *L. monocytogenes*, gram-negative bacilli (add ampicillin 2 g)
- Immunocompromised: ampicillin, vancomycin 1 g, ceftazidime 2 g
- Head trauma, neurosurgery, or CSF shunt: vancomycin 1 g plus ceftazidime 2 g

Evidence for adjuvant dexamethasone is increasing. It is given 15 minutes before or with the first dose of antibiotic: 10 mg (adults), 0.15 mg/kg (pediatric), intravenously, every 6 hours. Anticonvulsants may be added if necessary.

REFERENCES
de Gans J, van de Beek D; European Dexamethasone in Adulthood Bacterial Meningitis Study: Dexamethasone in adults with bacterial meningitis, *N Engl J Med* 347:1549, 2002.

Tureen, JH: Bacterial meningitis. In Rakel RE, Bope ET: *Conn's current therapy*, ed 56. Philadelphia, 2004, Elsevier.

van de Beek D, de Gans J, Spanjaard L, et al: Clinical features and prognostic factors in adults with bacterial meningitis, *N Engl J Med* 351:1849, 2004.

CHAPTER 18

 ## SUBDURAL AND EPIDURAL HEMATOMA

Intracranial bleeding into either the subdural or epidural space is another cause of headache. Epidural and subdural hematomas (EDH and SDH) manifesting shortly after acute head trauma are relatively easy to recognize. However, these entities can also be delayed (by days to weeks), particularly SDH in elderly patients. In these cases, patients can present with isolated headache and no localizing neurologic findings.

SYMPTOMS
- Decreased level of consciousness (LOC) following head injury
- Headache (common in conscious patients and those with chronic SDH)
- Seizures +
- Focal neurologic symptoms (variable)
- Confusion, personality changes (chronic SDH)

SIGNS
- Diminished LOC including coma
- Focal neurologic signs including dilated pupil and hemiparesis. Classically, the dilated pupil is ipsilateral to the hematoma and the hemiparesis is contralateral; however, the pupil may be contralaterally dilated (+) and the hemiparesis can be ipsilateral (+). This is caused either by direct injury of the third nerve or midbrain or by compression of the contralateral cerebral peduncle. (Patients with dilated pupils from this mechanism have severely diminished LOC; anisocoria in a conscious patient nearly always represents local eye injury, a postsurgical pupil, or presence of mydriatic drops.)
- May have normal examination or very subtle deficits

WORKUP
- Noncontrast brain CT scan should be done promptly to define size, location, and presence of associated injuries (e.g., cerebral contusion). Blood on CT scan in SDH between 10 to 20 days may appear isodense (with brain) and thereafter hypodense.
- Careful evaluation for signs of noncranial trauma

COMMENTS AND TREATMENT CONSIDERATIONS
Most patients with SDH or EDH arrive at the emergency department shortly after trauma. Careful attention must be paid to the airway, breathing, and circulation (ABCs), especially ventilation. Consult neurosurgery early for possible surgical decompression and use of mannitol. Hyperventilation significantly decreases ICP but should be used only as a temporizing measure in patients suspected to be actively herniating. The goal of hyperventilation should be a Pco_2 in the low to middle 30s. The ED placement of burr holes is now rarely indicated.

Rarely, an EDH has a delayed presentation (after an initially normal CT scan), usually within 12 to 24 hours; thus, an initially normal CT scan does not entirely exclude EDH, and caution is appropriate when the pretest probability is high.

Chronic SDHs are far more common, especially in the elderly, in whom they can present acutely or weeks after injury (which may be minor) with headache (+++), focal weakness, confusion, personality changes, anisocoria, seizures, and changes in LOC. These symptoms and signs can be mild or transient. Have a low threshold for CT scanning in the elderly and anticoagulated patients with head trauma.

REFERENCES
Chen JC, Levy ML: Causes, epidemiology and risk factors of chronic subdural hematoma, *Neurosurg Clin North Am* 11:399, 2000.

Jagoda A, Cantril S, Wears R, et al: Clinical policy: neuroimaging and decision-making in adult mild traumatic brain injury in the acute setting, *Ann Emerg Med* 40:231, 2002.

Roberts I, Schierhout G, Wakai A: Mannitol for acute traumatic brain injury, *Cochrane Database Syst Rev* CD00149, 2000.

Springer MFB, Baker FJ: Cranial burr hole decompression in the emergency department, *Am J Emerg Med* 6:640, 1988.

 ## CARBON MONOXIDE POISONING

See Chapter 37, Toxic Exposure, Approach to.

 ## ACUTE CEREBROVASCULAR DISEASE (STROKE AND TRANSIENT ISCHEMIC ATTACK)

See Chapter 44, Weakness and Fatigue.

 ## BENIGN INTRACRANIAL HYPERTENSION (PSEUDOTUMOR CEREBRI)

Pseudotumor cerebri is a rare (~1/100,000) cause of headache that is most commonly seen in overweight women (~20/100,000). Associations with vitamin A, tetracycline, estrogen and steroid use, steroid tapering, and various endocrinologic disorders have been reported, but their absence does not preclude the diagnosis. A brain imaging study followed by an LP is required to establish the diagnosis. The diagnostic criteria are:

- Elevated ICP (>200 mm H_2O)
- Normal neurologic examination except papilledema (and sixth nerve palsy)
- Normal neuroimaging (no mass or ventricular enlargement)
- Normal CSF (except low CSF protein)
- No suspicion of cerebral venous sinus thrombosis or other cause for elevated ICP.

SYMPTOMS
- Headache +++ can be constant or intermittent, often ++ retrobulbar, and sometimes worse with eye movement.
- Transient visual obscurations +++ defined as visual symptoms lasting seconds to minutes
- Visual loss +
- Neck pain +
- Nausea and vomiting (+++ for nausea, ++ for vomiting)
- Diplopia +
- Tinnitus +
- Radicular back and neck pain +
- Diminished sense of smell +

SIGNS

- Papilledema +++, but precise figures are unavailable because the diagnosis may be made less often in its absence. May be asymmetric or even unilateral.
- Sixth nerve palsy (by definition, to make the diagnosis, no other neurologic physical findings are allowed).

WORKUP

- By definition, an imaging study (CT or MRI) and an LP are required to make the diagnosis.
- Evaluation may include MRA or cerebral venography if venous sinus thrombosis is suspected.

COMMENTS AND TREATMENT CONSIDERATIONS

Removing CSF relieves symptoms. When the diagnosis is suspected, more than the usual amount of CSF should be removed when performing the LP. Over time, the patient may require repeated LPs. The inciting drug, if any, should be stopped and any endocrine disorder treated. Acetazolamide, furosemide, and glucocorticoids have been used and may be effective. No controlled trials have shown these to be more effective than surgical therapy. Surgical therapy consists of CSF diversion procedures, the most common of which is lumboperitoneal shunting.

REFERENCES

Friedman DI: Pseudotumor cerebri, *Neurol Clin* 22:99, 2004.

Friedman DI, Jacobson DM: Diagnostic criteria for idiopathic intracranial hypertension, *Neurology* 59:1492, 2002.

Jones JS, Nevai J, Freeman NP, McNinch DE: Emergency department presentation of idiopathic intracranial hypertension, *Am J Emerg Med* 17:517, 1999.

Wall M: The headache profile of idiopathic intracranial hypertension, *Cephalalgia* 10:331, 1990.

 TEMPORAL ARTERITIS

Temporal arteritis (TA), also known as giant cell arteritis (GCA), is a vasculitis of large and medium arteries that commonly, although not exclusively, involves the temporal artery. It should be considered in every patient older than 50 who complains of headache.

SYMPTOMS

- Headache ++++, unilateral temporal headache +++
- Weight loss +++
- Visual disturbance +++, including unilateral vision loss ++ or diplopia ++

- Jaw claudication +++
- Polymyalgia rheumatica +++
- Myalgia +++

SIGNS
- Palpable temporal artery abnormality +++, including tenderness +++, enlargement +++, absent pulse +++, or nodularity ++
- Scalp tenderness +++
- Ischemic optic neuropathy ++ on funduscopic examination
- Fever ++
- Cranial nerve palsy ++ including diplopia, ptosis

WORKUP
- Erythrocyte sedimentation rate (ESR): usually elevated +++++, ESR >50 mm/hr ++++, ESR >100 mm/hr +++
- CBC: anemia +++

COMMENTS AND TREATMENT CONSIDERATIONS
GCA is a clinical diagnosis. The most common symptom is headache, classically temporal. The most specific symptoms are jaw claudication and diplopia. The most common physical finding is an abnormal temporal artery: typically enlarged, nodular, cordlike, tender, and nonpulsatile. The most helpful laboratory study is an ESR; an elevated ESR is extremely sensitive (although not specific) for temporal arteritis. A normal ESR does not exclude the diagnosis, nor does the level correlate with severity of disease. If supported by the clinical evidence, immediate treatment should be initiated to prevent significant morbidity (e.g., blindness and cerebral infarction). Treatment consists of prednisone 40 to 60 mg/day for at least 1 month, followed by a taper guided by symptoms. A temporal artery biopsy should be scheduled within 1 to 2 days to establish a definitive diagnosis.

REFERENCES
Chavin JM: Cranial neuralgias and headaches associated with cranial vascular disorders, *Otolaryngol Clin North Am* 36:1079, 2003.
Smetana GW, Shmerling RH: Does this patient have temporal arteritis? *JAMA* 287:92, 2002.

 ACUTE SINUSITIS

Acute sinusitis is an infection of one of the paranasal sinus cavities of the face. It is one of the most common conditions treated in ambulatory practice, and guidelines on diagnosis and management have been published by the American Academy of Otolaryngology

CHAPTER 18

and the CDC. The physician must distinguish the common maxillary sinusitis from the more severe infections in the frontal, ethmoid, and sphenoid sinuses or a combination of them, which, because of risk of serious complications, may require hospital admission for administration of intravenous antibiotics. At a minimum, close follow-up is necessary for these patients if they are discharged.

SYMPTOMS
- Recent URI ++++ or allergic rhinitis
- Nasal discharge ++++, typically mucopurulent
- Facial pain +++, particularly when bending forward +++
- Initial improvement, then worsening symptoms ++++
- Headache +++
- Maxillary toothache ++

SIGNS
- Fever +++
- Purulent rhinorrhea +++
- Sinus tenderness +++
- Abnormal transillumination of sinuses (frontal or maxillary)

WORKUP
- For routine sinusitis the diagnosis is clinical and no imaging required.
- Sinus CT: especially for possible frontal, sphenoid, or ethmoidal sinusitis, and orbital/cranial complications
- Sinus x-ray: sensitivity +++ and specificity (35% to 75%)

COMMENTS AND TREATMENT CONSIDERATIONS
Most patients presenting with nasal discharge or congestion have a viral URI. The diagnosis of bacterial sinusitis should be considered only in patients who have had symptoms suggestive of sinusitis for at least 7 days. In most cases sinusitis is a clinical diagnosis and sinus radiographs or CT scanning should be reserved for complicated sinusitis. Acute uncomplicated sinusitis may be treated with a 10- to 14-day course of antibiotics directed against common pathogens (*S. pneumoniae* and *H. influenzae*); the CDC recommends amoxicillin for mild disease with no previous antibiotic use (88% efficacy) and amoxicillin/clavulanic acid (Augmentin) or a fluoroquinolone for moderate disease or recent antibiotic use. Decongestants should also be used (oral or nasal; caution against use of nasal preparations >3 days). Patients who do not respond after 72 hours of treatment should undergo imaging and potentially ENT referral. Chronic sinusitis (symptoms lasting more than 3 months) should be treated with broad-spectrum antibiotics to cover other pathogens (*S. aureus* and anaerobes), in addition to usual microbes.

Acute ethmoid, sphenoid, and frontal sinusitis have a higher risk of serious complications than routine maxillary sinusitis and may require intravenous antibiotics and hospital admission. Acute ethmoid sinusitis is more commonly seen in children and is associated with periorbital cellulitis (swelling, erythema, and warmth) and orbital cellulitis (chemosis, proptosis, and gaze disturbance). Acute sphenoid sinusitis is manifested by severe, progressive headache (++++), often increasing with activity or coughing, nausea and vomiting (+++), and fever (+++). Sphenoid sinusitis may be complicated by ophthalmologic (chemosis, proptosis, ptosis, diplopia, or ophthalmoplegia) or neurologic symptoms (particularly hypoesthesia of the first and second divisions of the fifth cranial nerve). Intracranial abscess, meningitis, and osteomyelitis of the frontal bone (Pott's puffy tumor) are complications of frontal sinusitis. For patients with complicated sinusitis who are well enough to be discharged, amoxicillin/clavulanic acid or a fluoroquinolone is appropriate.

REFERENCES

Hickner JM, Bartlett JG, Besser RE, et al: Principles of appropriate antibiotic use for acute rhinosinusitis in adults: background, *Ann Emerg Med* 37:703, 2001.

Kibblewhite DJ, Cleland J, Mintz DR: Acute sphenoid sinusitis: management strategies, *J Otolaryngol* 17:159, 1988.

Scheid DC, Hamm RM: Acute bacterial rhinosinusitis in adults, *Am Fam Physician* 70:1685, 2004.

CEREBRAL VENOUS THROMBOSIS (EXCEPT CAVERNOUS SINUS THROMBOSIS)

Cerebral venous thrombosis (CVT) is a rare entity that can be difficult to diagnose and for which commonly used ED imaging studies can be normal. Consider it when a young patient presents with a stroke that does not follow usual arterial vascular territories. Routine measurement of the opening pressure of spinal fluid is one safeguard against misdiagnosis.

SYMPTOMS
- Headache +++, not location specific
- Thunderclap headache +
- Focal neurologic deficit ++
- Seizures ++: focal or generalized
- Vomiting ++

SIGNS
- Papilledema ++
- Mental status changes +

- Cranial nerve palsies +
- Dysarthria/dysphasia +
- Hemiplegia

WORKUP
- CT with and without contrast; may be normal in up to 20% of CVT
- LP: may see increased opening pressure, increased protein, or increased RBCs
- MRI: useful to distinguish CVT from pseudotumor cerebri
- Angiography: "gold standard"; next modality if MRI is negative; four-vessel study needed; must visualize entire venous phase
- D-dimer: often positive but a negative study does not exclude the diagnosis
- Blood culture
- Coagulation studies

COMMENTS AND TREATMENT CONSIDERATIONS
Approximately 40% of patients have isolated intracranial hypertension (headache and papilledema) that can be confused with pseudotumor cerebri.

The underlying causes of CVT are diverse:
- Septic thrombosis usually from infections of middle third of face and sphenoid or ethmoid sinus; otitis media/mastoiditis; septicemia; endocarditis (especially with dehydration)
- Hypercoagulable states including malignancies, inflammatory diseases, factor V Leiden, and hereditary antithrombin III, protein C, and protein S deficiencies.
- Pregnancy, puerperium, and oral contraceptive use
- Head trauma (open or closed, with or without fracture) and neurosurgical procedures

Treatment is controversial. Anticonvulsants should be used to treat seizures and may be administered prophylactically. Anticoagulation is often used despite the risk of intracranial hemorrhage. Heparin has been shown to decrease morbidity and mortality in one randomized controlled trial. Catheter-delivered thrombolysis has also been used. Other treatments include use of mannitol and repeated LPs to decrease elevated ICP. High-dose broad-spectrum intravenous antibiotics are required for septic CVT.

REFERENCES
Ciccone A, Canhao P, Falcao F, et al: Thrombolysis for cerebral vein and dural sinus thrombosis, *Cochrane Database Syst Rev* CD003693, 2004.

de Bruijn SF, Stam J, Kappelle LJ: Thunderclap headache as first symptom of cerebral venous sinus thrombosis, *Lancet* 348:1623, 1996.

Ferro JM; ISCVT Investigators: Prognosis of cerebral vein and dural sinus thrombosis: results of the International Study on Cerebral Vein and Dural Sinus Thrombosis (ISCVT), *Stroke* 35:664, 2004.

Stam J: Thrombosis of the cerebral veins and sinuses, *N Engl J Med* 352:1791, 2005.

 CAVERNOUS SINUS THROMBOSIS

The most common cause of cavernous sinus thrombosis is sphenoid or ethmoid sinusitis. Careful attention to the HEENT examination often suggests this unusual entity. Rapid treatment with high-dose broad-spectrum intravenous antibiotics and surgical consultation are essential. Surgical drainage of the cavernous sinus itself is rare but may be necessary in management of complicating conditions including sinusitis, brain abscess, orbital abscess, or dental infection.

SYMPTOMS
- Fever ++++
- Headache +++: severe, frontal or retroorbital pain
- Lethargy +++
- Diplopia +
- Vomiting, seizures +, hemiplegia +, and dysarthria are not as commonly seen as with other cerebral venous thromboses.

SIGNS
- Periorbital/orbital edema +++: progressive unilateral or bilateral
- Chemosis ++++, proptosis ++++, and/or ptosis ++++
- Cranial nerve findings: isolated abducens nerve palsy (sixth cranial nerve travels directly through sinus) or involvement of third, fourth, and fifth cranial nerves ++++ and paresthesias in a V1/V2 distribution
- Fever ++++
- Funduscopy: venous engorgement +++, papilledema +++
- Meningismus ++

WORKUP
- CT
- MRI
- Blood culture before starting antibiotics
- ENT (and possible infectious diseases) consultation

REFERENCES
Bhatia K, Jones NS: Septic cavernous sinus thrombosis secondary to sinusitis: are anticoagulants indicated? A review of the literature, *J Laryngol Otol* 116:667, 2002.

CHAPTER 18

Cannon ML, Antonio BL, McCloskey JJ, et al: Cavernous sinus thrombosis complicating sinusitis, *Pediatr Crit Care Med* 5:86, 2004.

Dolan RW, Chowdhury K: Diagnosis and treatment of intracranial complications of paranasal sinus infections, *J Oral Maxillofac Surg* 53:1080, 1995.

Ebright JR, Pace MT, Niazi AF: Septic thrombosis of the cavernous sinuses, *Arch Intern Med* 161:2671, 2001.

 BRAIN OR PARAMENINGEAL ABSCESS

Careful attention to risk factors is crucial in diagnosing brain and parameningeal abscess because patients can have a normal examination, no fever, and no leukocytosis. Predisposing factors include:
- An ENT infection (otitis media, sinusitis, mastoiditis)
- A distant infection (by hematogenous spread): dental infection, skin infection (with bacteremia), endocarditis/congenital heart disease, pulmonary infection
- Prior head injury
- Steroid use/immunosuppression
- Neurosurgical procedure

SYMPTOMS
- Headache +++
- Focal neurologic deficit +++
- Diffuse neurologic symptoms ++:coma, seizures, behavioral disturbances
- Subtle personality changes (with frontal lobe)
- Nausea and vomiting ++

SIGNS
- Fever ++
- Toxic appearing +
- Meningismus +: especially with occipital or temporal lobe
- Papilledema ++
- Focal neurologic deficit +++: mild hemiparesis most common

WORKUP
- CT *with contrast* is very sensitive. Antibiotics should be started before scan if the diagnosis is being considered.
- MRI, if available without significant time delay
- LP: only if signs of meningismus or diffuse neurologic symptoms and if CT scan is negative; even in cases of definite brain abscess, the CSF analysis is usually nonspecific and does not yield the causative organism. Therefore, not only is LP potentially dangerous, but it rarely helps diagnostically.

- CBC: WBC >10,000 ++
- Blood culture before starting antibiotics

COMMENTS AND TREATMENT CONSIDERATIONS
Infection is polymicrobial in approximately half of cases.
Treatment consists of high-dose intravenous antibiotics selected
to cover the likely organisms. If a cutaneous source is likely,
S. aureus coverage is needed. Corticosteroids should be administered
for symptomatic cerebral edema. Neurosurgery should be consulted.
Surgical drainage is sometimes necessary.

REFERENCES
Calfee DP, Wispelwey B: Brain abscess, *Semin Neurol* 20:253, 2000.
Seydoux C, Francioli P: Bacterial brain abscesses: factors influenc-
ing mortality and sequelae, *Clin Infect Dis* 15:394, 1992.

ACUTE NARROW-ANGLE GLAUCOMA

Acute narrow-angle glaucoma (ANAG), also called acute angle-closure
glaucoma, is characterized by an acute increase in intraocular
pressure with progressive damage to the optic nerve. Presentation
usually includes headache and eye pain, and patients typically
appear systemically ill with nausea, vomiting, and abdominal pain.
ANAG can manifest without eye symptoms but can be diagnosed
on eye examination including intraocular pressure. Patients
typically have a red eye with corneal edema.

See Chapter 14, Eye Pain and Redness.

BRAIN TUMOR

To diagnose a brain tumor, the index of suspicion must be high
because there is no characteristic pattern of signs and symptoms.
The classic combination of early morning headache and
papilledema is uncommon.

SYMPTOMS
- Headache: +++ for both primary and metastatic brain tumors;
  the quality of the headache varies broadly.
- Headache worse on bending or with Valsalva's maneuver ++
- Headache with nausea and vomiting +++; in patients with normal
  ICP, headache +++ and vomiting ++; in patients with elevated
  ICP, headache ++++ and vomiting +++.
- Worst headache of life ++; notably, the headache may also be
  mild or be relieved by nonnarcotic analgesia.
- Severe morning headache with vomiting: ++

CHAPTER 18

- At least one neurologic symptom ++++ other than headache; symptoms vary according to the location and size of the tumor.

SIGNS
- Any focal abnormality on neurologic examination depending on location and size of the tumor
- Papilledema: +++ in patients with elevated ICP (not seen in patients with normal ICP)
- Ataxia: +++ in patients with increased ICP (+ in patients with normal ICP)

WORKUP
Workup involves a brain imaging study, ideally an MRI or a contrast-enhanced CT scan. Emergently, a noncontrast CT scan provides enough information to discharge the patient safely, but it does not rule out tumor or abscess with certainty. Early follow-up is required.

COMMENTS AND TREATMENT CONSIDERATIONS
Patients with neuroimaging confirmation of an intracerebral tumor require immediate neurosurgical and/or neurologic consultation. Anticonvulsants should be considered. Intravenous dexamethasone may benefit patients with evidence of edema surrounding the tumor. Dexamethasone and sometimes mannitol are also used if there is evidence of significantly elevated ICP. Hyperventilation should be considered a brief temporizing measure, to be used only in the event of active herniation and while preparing for operative intervention. For patients without clinical signs or imaging evidence of increased ICP, no immediate intervention may be necessary.

REFERENCES
Forsyth PA, Posner JB: Headaches in patients with brain tumors: a study of 111 patients, *Neurology* 43:1678, 1993.
Purdy RA, Kirby S: Headaches and brain tumors, *Neurol Clin North Am* 22:39, 2004.

HIV/AIDS Patient, Approach to the
Michael Menchine

Few diseases have changed the course of medicine and then been changed by the course of medicine within 20 years. Whereas in the late 1980s emergency departments and hospital wards throughout urban America were filled with suffering AIDS patients, currently HIV-related illness is primarily an outpatient phenomenon. Patients are living longer, and the infection has changed from one of progressive disease and certain death to a chronic disease (Fig. 19–1). It is

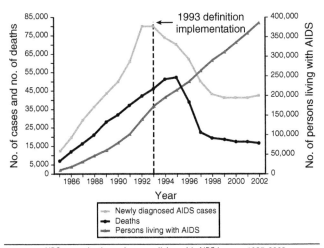

Fig. 19-1 AIDS cases, deaths, and persons living with AIDS by year, 1985-2002, United States. (From the Centers for Disease Control and Prevention: HIV/AIDS Surveillance Report, 2002:14. Also available at http://www.cdc.gov/hiv/stats/hasrlink.htm.)

essential that emergency physicians consider disease processes, particularly infections, that are rare in the general population but are frequent causes of morbidity and mortality in HIV/AIDS patients.

The approach to the AIDS patient is not dissimilar to the approach to other ED patients. Priority is given to rapid identification and resuscitation if signs of shock or respiratory compromise are present. Patients with sepsis syndromes should receive early treatment with broad-spectrum antibiotics in a similar fashion to other patients, but they may require additional antibiotics to cover infections seen more frequently in HIV/AIDS patients (see later). Once the patient has been assessed and stabilized, the examiner should proceed with a focused history and physical. When evaluating the HIV/AIDS patient, additional historical elements should include CD4 count, viral load, use of highly active antiretroviral therapy (HAART), years since diagnosis, and prior AIDS-defining illnesses.

The spectrum of disease in HIV patients with CD4 counts >200/mm^3 is very similar to that in non-HIV patients, whereas those with CD4 counts <50/mm^3 experience illnesses that are unlikely to be encountered in non-HIV patients. Many patients are knowledgeable regarding the status of their HIV-related illness and know exact CD4 counts, viral loads, and comprehensive medical history. However, many disadvantaged, substance-abusing, and otherwise disenfranchised patients may know little about the extent of their HIV-related illness. Further, empirical data suggest that >2% of ED patients are unknowingly infected with HIV. In such cases, the emergency physician must seek all available ancillary data to help stage the disease. Use of prophylactic medications such as trimethoprim/sulfamethoxazole (TMP/SMX) (<200/mm^3), ganciclovir, or azithromycin (<50/mm^3) suggests low CD4 counts. Physical examination revealing thrush, temporal wasting, and oral hairy leukoplakia suggests more advanced disease and enhanced risk for opportunistic infection. Routine blood count can be used to calculate the absolute lymphocyte count. In HIV-infected patients, an absolute lymphocyte count less than 1000 cells/mm^3 correlated with a CD4 count less than 200/mm^3 with 96% specificity. These elements aid the clinician in determining the stage of HIV disease and subsequent risk for associated pathology. Obtaining primary care physician or infectious disease specialist input is prudent and often informative although not always required.

The diagnostic challenge to the emergency physician is that HIV can directly or indirectly affect every organ system with life-threatening diseases. Commonly, patients present with nonspecific complaints such as fatigue or fevers. Further, the time-honored rule "Occam's razor" does not apply in advanced HIV illness, in which multiple diagnoses are common.

The probability of developing an opportunistic infection depends roughly on the following factors: degree of immunosuppression, exposure, virulence of pathogen, and the use of chemoprophylaxis.

REFERENCES

Kelen GD: Emergency department-based HIV screening and counseling: experience with rapid and standard serologic testing, *Ann Emerg Med* 33:147, 1999.

Palella FJ: Declining morbidity and mortality among patients with advanced human immunodeficiency virus infection, *N Engl J Med* 338:853, 1998.

Shapiro NI, Karras DJ, Leech SH, Heilpern KL: Absolute lymphocyte count as a predictor of CD4 count, *Ann Emerg Med* 32:323, 1998.

CLASSIFICATION OF HIV/AIDS

Surprisingly, there is no satisfactory clinical staging system for HIV/AIDS. In 1993 the CDC issued a revised classification system that is used to study the epidemiology of the HIV disease:

Category A—Acute HIV infection, asymptomatic infection, persistent generalized lymphadenopathy.

Category B—Symptomatic HIV disease. This category consists of diseases that are influenced by HIV but might be seen in relatively immunocompetent patients as well. It includes mucocutaneous candidiasis, advanced cervical dysplasia, oral hairy leukoplakia, idiopathic thrombocytopenic purpura, disseminated shingles, pelvic inflammatory disease, particularly if complicated by tuboovarian abscess, peripheral neuropathy, and constitutional symptoms, such as fever (38.5° C) or diarrhea lasting more than 1 month.

Category C—Patients with AIDS-defining illness (defined in CDC 1987) including cryptococcal meningitis, *Pneumocystis carinii* pneumonia, Kaposi sarcoma, and recurrent pneumonia.

This classification system is further subcategorized by CD4 count:

Category 1—CD4 count >500/mm^3

Category 2—CD4 count 200 to 499/mm^3

Category 3—CD4 count <200/mm^3

Thus, a patient with HIV infection, no symptoms, and a CD4 count of 350/mm^3 would be categorized as A2. AIDS is defined as a CD4 count <200mm^3 or category C disease.

According to the CDC definition, patients are classified according to the most advanced disease they have had. Thus, if a patient at one time had a CD4 count of 45/mm^3 with *Pneumocystis carinii* pneumonia (PCP), that patient is considered to have C3 disease even if response to therapy has resulted in a symptom-free life with CD4 counts >500/mm^3. However, new data suggest that the risk of opportunistic infection appears to be very low in patients with replenished CD4 counts (>200/mm^3). HIV specialists now contend that this classification scheme may not accurately characterize an individual patient's level of immunosuppression at a given time. Specific knowledge of the CD4 count and, to a lesser extent, the viral load is more predictive than the CDC classification system.

REFERENCES

CDC: 1993 Revised classification system for HIV infection and expanded surveillance case definition for AIDS among adolescents and adults, *MMWR Recomm Rep* 41(RR-17):1, 1992.

CDC: Revision of the CDC surveillance case definition for acquired immunodeficiency syndrome, *MMWR Morb Mortal Wkly Rep* 36:1S, 1987.

de Quiros, JCLB: A randomized trial of the discontinuation of primary and secondary prophylaxis against *Pneumocystis carinii* pneumonia after highly active antiretroviral therapy in patients with HIV infection, *N Engl J Med* 344:159, 2001.

PULMONARY INFECTIONS

Pulmonary infections are the leading cause of morbidity and mortality in HIV/AIDS patients. Traditionally, PCP has been the most important pulmonary pathogen in AIDS patients in developed countries. However, over the past 10 years, community-acquired pneumonia (CAP) has overtaken *Pneumocystis* to become the leading cause of death in AIDS patients. This is largely due to PCP prophylaxis with TMP/SMX in HIV/AIDS patients with CD4 counts <200/mm^3. Tuberculosis should also be considered in all HIV-positive patients with subacute or chronic pulmonary complaints. Worldwide, *Mycobacterium tuberculosis* (TB) is more common and lethal than PCP or CAP and may occur at higher CD4 counts (>200/mm^3). Indeed, isolating all HIV/AIDS patients admitted with respiratory complaints is prudent while diagnostic testing is performed to exclude TB. Other opportunistic infections including *Coccidioides*, *Histoplasma*, and cytomegalovirus (CMV) generally occur with CD4 counts <50.

See Community-Acquired Pneumonia in Chapter 34, Shortness of Breath.

PNEUMOCYSTIS CARINII **PNEUMONIA**

Pneumocystis is a common pulmonary pathogen in the patient with advanced HIV/AIDS. There is no definitive diagnostic test for PCP that can be applied in the ED. Therefore, a high index of suspicion for this disease in ill-appearing patients commonly leads to empiric therapy for PCP in addition to CAP and other potential causes of pneumonia.

PCP is nearly unique to patients with CD4 count <200/mm^3. Serologic studies indicate that nearly all people have had exposure by age 2, and reactivation of latent infection is thought to be the primary source of the disease in the immunocompromised. Disease is triggered by both the replication of the *Pneumocystis* fungus and the host inflammatory response. In patients with severe disease, the host response may exaggerate the hypoxia and result in respiratory decompensation. Typical symptoms include the subacute (days to weeks) onset of pleuritic chest pain, fever, and dyspnea.

CHAPTER 19

SYMPTOMS
- Fever
- Dyspnea on exertion progressing to shortness of breath at rest
- Pleuritic chest pain
- Fatigue/malaise
- Cough

SIGNS
- Tachypnea
- Fever
- Hypoxemia
- Wheezing
- Wasting

WORKUP
- Pulse oximetry
- Arterial blood gas
- Chest x-ray: the different radiographic patterns suggest specific pathogens (Table 19–1); however, these patterns are insufficiently sensitive and specific to determine initial therapy.
- CBC
- LDH
- Sputum Gram stain and culture for other organisms; currently, *P. carinii* cannot be grown in culture.
- Sputum for silver stain, PCP direct fluorescence antibody
- Sputum for acid-fast bacilli

TABLE 19–1

PREDICTION OF ETIOLOGIC AGENT OF PNEUMONIA IN HIV/AIDS PATIENTS BASED ON CHEST RADIOGRAPH FINDINGS

Diffuse Interstitial Infiltrates

Pneumocystis carinii pneumonia (80% of low-CD4-count HIV-infected patients with diffuse interstitial infiltrates)

Mycobacterium tuberculosis (TB) and other mycobacterial species

Fungal (other than *P. carinii*) pneumonia

Bacterial pneumonia (particularly *H. influenzae*)

Viral pneumonia

Toxoplasmosis

Nonspecific interstitial pneumonitis.

Focal Infiltrates

Community-acquired pneumonia (54% of low-CD4-count HIV patients), predominantly

Pneumococcus

Pneumocystis (34%)

M. tuberculosis (TB) and other mycobacterial species; patients with upper lobe consolidation have a higher rate of *Pneumocystis* and TB.

Cavities Lesions and Pulmonary Abscesses

Mycobacterium tuberculosis (TB) and other mycobacterial species

Aspergillus

Bacterial infections including CAP, septic emboli, and aspiration pneumonias (anaerobic bacteria)

Pneumothorax

Pneumocystis carinii infection causes the formation of thin-walled pulmonary blebs susceptible to spontaneous rupture. Pneumothorax may complicate acute *Pneumocystis* infection, and *Pneumocystis* infection should be sought in any HIV/AIDS patient with spontaneous pneumothorax.

Pleural Effusion

- Bacterial pneumonia
- *M. tuberculosis* (TB)
- Kaposi sarcoma (KS): large and often bloody effusions are seen in TB and KS.
- *Pneumocystis* (34%): occasionally small effusions
- Noninfectious diseases: congestive heart failure, nephropathy, and rheumatologic conditions

Chest Radiograph without Infiltrates

A normal chest x-ray does not exclude significant pulmonary pathology in the AIDS patient with pulmonary symptoms. If significant

dyspnea or hypoxemia is present, high-resolution CT of the chest may help define pulmonary pathology.
- *Pneumocystis carinii* pneumonia: chest x-ray commonly normal or near normal
- *Mycobacterium tuberculosis* (TB)

COMMENTS AND TREATMENT CONSIDERATIONS

In light of the vast and lethal differential diagnosis, the majority of low-CD4-count AIDS patients with acute pulmonary disease should be admitted for workup and treatment. Early fiberoptic bronchoscopy and high-resolution CT of the chest are often indicated to help guide therapy. PCP continues to be the most common AIDS-defining opportunistic infection. However, the risk of *Pneumocystis* infection is markedly altered by the use of TMP/SMX and the CD4 count. PCP is quite rare with CD4 counts >200, with CAP relatively more common.

The choice of empiric antibiotic therapy for the HIV/AIDS patient with respiratory complaints without a definitive diagnosis is complex. In general, an acutely ill patient with purulent sputum production can be treated with antibiotics to cover *Pneumococcus*, *Haemophilus influenzae*, *Mycoplasma*, and *Legionella*. Generally, fluoroquinolones should not be used empirically for CAP in the HIV/AIDS patient because these antibiotics have antimycobacterium properties that may affect the ability to diagnose TB if symptoms do not resolve. Patients with a more gradual onset (over 1 to 3 weeks) of symptoms characterized predominantly by fever and shortness of breath are good candidates for empirical therapy for PCP. Intravenous or oral TMP/SMX is recommended as the first-line agent. Corticosteroids help attenuate the inflammatory response generated by the rapid killing of the *Pneumocystis* protozoa. The administration of prednisone prior to TMP/SMX is recommended if arterial blood gas reveals $pO_2 < 70$ mm Hg.

REFERENCES

DeLorenzo LJ, Huang CT, Maguire GP, et al: Roentgenographic patterns of *Pneumocystis carinii* pneumonia in 104 patients with AIDS, *Chest* 91:323, 1987.

Furman AC, Jacobs J, Sepkowitz KA: Lung abscess in patients with AIDS, *Clin Infect Dis* 22:81, 1999.

Hirschtick RE, Glassroth J, Jordan MC, et al: Bacterial pneumonia in persons infected with the human immunodeficiency virus, *N Engl J Med* 333:845, 1995.

Sattler F, Nichols L, Hirano L, et al: Nonspecific interstitial pneumonitis mimicking *Pneumocystis carinii* pneumonia, *Am J Respir Crit Care Med* 156:912, 1997.

Sepkowitz KA: Effect of HAART on natural history of AIDS-related opportunistic disorder, *Lancet* 351:228, 1998.

CHAPTER 19

Thomas CF: *Pneumocystis* pneumonia, *N Engl J Med* 350:2487, 2004.

Wolff AJ, O'Donnell AE: Pulmonary manifestations of HIV infection in the era of highly active antiretroviral therapy, *Chest* 120:1888, 2001.

NEUROLOGIC MANIFESTATIONS

Neurologic complications of HIV/AIDS are common and include primary HIV infection syndromes, opportunistic infection, and complications from medical therapy. Neurologic disease is the initial illness in 10% to 20% of symptomatic HIV infection.

SYMPTOMS
- Headache
- Numbness
- Weakness/paralysis
- Fever
- Nausea and vomiting
- Neck stiffness
- Visual changes
- Photophobia
- Confusion
- Lethargy
- Personality changes
- Seizures

SIGNS
- Fever
- Meningismus
- Altered mental status
- Coma
- Seizure
- Weakness
- Paralysis

WORKUP
- Contrast-enhanced head CT
- MRI of the brain
- Lumbar puncture with opening spinal pressure and cerebral spinal fluid (CSF) for Gram stain, culture, cell count, differential, glucose, protein, AFB stain and culture, *Cryptococcus* antigen, India ink stain, fungal culture, CSF VDRL
- Serum *Cryptococcus* IgG
- Serum *Toxoplasma gondii* IgG

HEADACHE

See Chapter 18, Headache.

Although the most common cause of headache in the HIV/AIDS patient is a primary headache syndrome (migraine, tension, cluster), the wide and lethal array of opportunistic infections mandates a workup for HIV patients with new headache. Infections of the CNS including toxoplasmosis, *Cryptococcus* meningitis, neurosyphilis, CMV encephalitis, TB meningitis, CNS lymphoma, bacterial meningitis (especially *Listeria monocytogenes* meningitis), and aseptic (viral) meningitis are the most common pathologic diseases seen in AIDS patients with headache. Notably, aside from aseptic meningitis, these diseases are almost exclusively seen in patients having CD4 counts <200/mm³ and most commonly with CD4 counts <100/mm³. Non–HIV-related illness including subarachnoid hemorrhage, vertebral artery dissection, sinusitis, temporal arteritis, and carbon monoxide poisoning should also be considered. In general, HIV/AIDS patients with CD4 counts <200/mm³ should undergo neuroimaging and lumbar puncture to evaluate previously undiagnosed headache.

 ***CRYPTOCOCCUS NEOFORMANS* MENINGITIS**

Cryptococcus neoformans meningitis is the most common systemic fungal infection in the HIV/AIDS patient. Approximately 10% of AIDS patients develop *Cryptococcus* infection during the course of their disease. *Cryptococcus* meningitis typically occurs in HIV-infected patients with CD4 counts <100/mm³. The most common presentation consists of nonspecific complaints including headache, fevers, vomiting, or fatigue. Nuchal rigidity and photophobia are often absent. Half of patients have significantly increased intracranial pressure without hydrocephalus. The diagnosis should be suspected solely on the basis of headache or fever in an HIV/AIDS patient with CD4 count below 200/mm³. The diagnosis is confirmed by the presence of *Cryptococcus* in the CSF demonstrated by India ink stain, a positive CSF cryptococcal antigen, or fungal culture. Patients with HIV infection and neurologic symptoms should have neuroimaging prior to lumbar puncture to exclude mass lesion or noncommunicating hydrocephalus.

FOCAL NEUROLOGIC FINDINGS

Many patients with HIV/AIDS with CD4 counts <200/mm³ presenting with focal neurologic findings have a mass lesion discovered on neuroimaging, most commonly relate to toxoplasmosis or CNS

239

CHAPTER 19

TABLE 19–2
CHARACTERISTICS OF TOXOPLASMOSIS VERSUS CNS LYMPHOMA

	TOXOPLASMOSIS	CNS LYMPHOMA
Epidemiology	More common	Less common
Typical CD4 count	<50/mm³	<100/mm³
Number of lesions	Multiple	Single
Ring enhancement on contrast CT	Yes	Yes
SPECT scan	No uptake	Significant uptake
CSF findings	Pleocytosis	Malignant cells in advanced disease
Serum tests	*Toxoplasma gondii* IgG antibody positive	None
Therapy	Sulfadiazine/pyrimethamine	Chemotherapy/radiation

lymphoma (Table 19–2). Other causes of CNS mass lesions include progressive multifocal leukoencephalopathy (PML), cryptococcoma, tuberculoma, syphilitic gumma, brain abscess, and aspergillosis. HIV patients with new focal neurologic findings and CD4 >200/mm³ most commonly have suffered an ischemic stroke.

 TOXOPLASMOSIS

Toxoplasmosis occurs in the setting of advanced HIV with CD4 counts usually <50/mm³. It is caused by the reactivation of the latent parasite *T. gondii*, whose definitive host is the common household cat. Toxoplasmosis most commonly presents with multiple CNS mass lesions and severe surrounding edema. Diffuse encephalitis caused by *Toxoplasma* may occur and portends a poor prognosis.

 CNS LYMPHOMA

Primary CNS lymphoma also arises in advanced HIV disease with CD4 counts <100/mm³. HIV-associated CNS lymphoma is caused by reactivation of latent CNS EBV infection. Lesions may be single or multiple. Untreated, CNS lymphoma leads to death in 2 to 5 months.

An HIV-positive patient with a low CD4 count and a mass lesion on CT scan should be admitted and treated empirically for toxoplasmosis with a multiagent regimen such as sulfadiazine, pyrimethamine, folinic acid, and possibly systemic corticosteroids while diagnostic studies including serum *T. gondii* antibodies, CSF cytology, and SPECT scanning are undertaken. Patients who worsen clinically despite appropriate therapy for toxoplasmosis are candidates for brain biopsy to determine a definitive diagnosis.

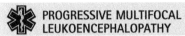

PROGRESSIVE MULTIFOCAL LEUKOENCEPHALOPATHY

PML is characterized by multiple rapidly progressive focal neurologic deficits. The causative etiologic agent is reactivation of the ubiquitous JC virus, which typically lies dormant in the CNS of immunocompetent individuals from childhood to death without sequelae. In contrast to that in toxoplasmosis and CNS lymphoma, the CT scan is normal. MRI, however, reveals multiple foci limited to brain white matter without surrounding edema. PML is most commonly seen in patients with end-stage AIDS and is associated with high 6-month mortality. No specific therapy for PML has proved effective; however, symptoms may recede mildly with HAART.

PERIPHERAL NEUROPATHY

Peripheral neuropathy has been linked to both HIV illness and therapy for HIV illness. Symptoms are predominantly sensory with gradual onset of bilaterally symmetrical numbness first involving the feet and later the hands. Mild weakness may be present, but severe weakness should prompt further workup. The differential diagnosis includes HIV neuropathy, HAART-related neuropathy, nutritional deficiency (B_{12}, folate), alcohol neuropathy, diabetic neuropathy, syphilis, and lumbar disc disease.

CONFUSION

Confusion in the HIV/AIDS patient is a diagnostic challenge. Patients with low CD4 counts are at risk for opportunistic and routine infections, CNS neoplasms, metabolic encephalopathies, medication-induced cognitive impairment, substance abuse and withdrawal, multi-infarct dementia, pseudodementia from depression, and HIV dementia.

CHAPTER 19

HIV DEMENTIA

HIV dementia affects more than 10% of advanced AIDS cases. It is appropriately diagnosed only in patients with slowly progressive cognitive difficulties without focal neurologic deficits who have had neuroimaging and CSF analysis to exclude other etiologies. Currently, there is no treatment.

REFERENCES

Marmidi A: Central nervous system infections in individuals with HIV-1 infection, *J Neurovirol* 8:158, 2002.

Rothman RE: A decision guideline for emergency department utilization of noncontrast head computed tomography in HIV-infected patients, *Acad Emerg Med* 6:1010, 1999.

Sperber K: Neurologic consequences of HIV Infection in the era of HAART, *AIDS Patient Care STDS* 17:509, 2003.

GASTROINTESTINAL MANIFESTATIONS

Gastrointestinal (GI) complications of HIV and treatment of HIV affect nearly all HIV patients at some point in the course of their disease. Common presenting complaints include odynophagia, abdominal pain, and diarrhea. Common diagnoses include oral hairy leukoplakia, *Candida* and CMV esophagitis, AIDS-related biliary disease, pancreatitis, and gastrointestinal bleeding. Pelvic inflammatory disease, although not a GI illness, is an important cause of morbidity in HIV-positive women.

 ORAL HAIRY LEUKOPLAKIA

Oral hairy leukoplakia (OHL) is caused by EBV infection of the keratinized oral epithelium. The diagnosis is confirmed by visual inspection and absence of resolution with antifungal therapy.

SYMPTOMS
- White coating on tongue
- Impaired taste
- Mouth pain

SIGNS
- White coating on the lateral tongue and buccal mucosal that does not scrape off with a tongue blade

COMMENTS AND TREATMENT CONSIDERATIONS

Large, obstructing oral lesions can be treated with acyclovir, ganciclovir, or podophyllin. OHL predicts forthcoming progression to AIDS. Although the mean CD4 count of patients who develop OHL is 486/mm^3, 50% of patients with HIV and OHL develop AIDS within 16 months.

 ESOPHAGITIS (*CANDIDA* AND CMV)

Esophagitis is extremely common in the symptomatic HIV patient. In fact, *Candida albicans* esophagitis is now the most common opportunistic infection in HIV. Other common etiologies are CMV, HSV, varicella-zoster virus, malignancy, and pill esophagitis.

SYMPTOMS
- Odynophagia
- Dysphagia
- Chest pain
- Heartburn
- Anorexia
- Weight loss
- Fever
- Abdominal pain

SIGNS
- White lesions on tongue
- Anorexia
- Fever

WORKUP
- Chest radiograph
- Barium esophagram
- Upper endoscopy

These studies are not indicated in the ED unless complications (e.g., perforation, obstruction, bleeding) are suspected.

COMMENTS AND TREATMENT CONSIDERATIONS
In general, patients with symptoms suggestive of esophagitis should be treated empirically with the antifungal fluconazole for 7 to 10 days. If symptoms subside, the diagnosis of *Candida* esophagitis can be inferred. If symptoms persist, upper endoscopy with biopsy should be performed to determine the etiology. CMV is the most common agent in refractory cases and requires prolonged antiviral therapy with ganciclovir or foscarnet. CMV esophagitis typically occurs in patients with CD4 <50/mm^3. Patients unable to tolerate oral feeding or hydration must be admitted for intravenous therapy and inpatient workup.

CHAPTER 19

ABDOMINAL PAIN

See Chapter 1, Abdominal Pain.

Abdominal pain in the AIDS patient mandates a careful evaluation of common, non–HIV-related illness as well as HIV-associated pathologies. Careful history and physical examination should focus on the onset, duration, location, quality, exacerbating, and ameliorating factors for the pain. CD4 count and complete medication list should be obtained. In general, approximately 10% of AIDS patients presenting to the ED with abdominal pain require surgical intervention. The characteristics of acute abdominal pain in AIDS patients are similar to those of a healthy population. Leukocytosis is even less sensitive in AIDS patients than non-AIDS patients with acute appendicitis and other surgical conditions causing abdominal pain. Nonsurgical causes of abdominal pain in AIDS patients commonly include CMV enterocolitis, pancreatitis, lymphoma, KS, HIV cholangitis, and cryptosporidium enteritis. Bowel obstruction may complicate KS, GI lymphoma, and *Mycobacterium avium* complex (MAC) infection. Intestinal perforation may complicate bowel obstruction or occur independently as a result of CMV colitis. CMV colitis occurs in patients with very low CD4 counts (<50/mm^3) and typically presents with abdominal pain and diarrhea. Endoscopy reveals severe epithelial ulcerations that predispose to perforation. Toxic megacolon may complicate CMV colitis.

 HIV BILIARY DISEASE

Fever and right upper quadrant pain in the AIDS patient suggest cholecystitis (often acalculous) or cholangitis. Typically occurring in patients with a CD4 count <100/mm^3, AIDS-related cholecystitis and cholangitis follow biliary epithelial destruction caused by a variety of opportunistic infections, most commonly *Cryptosporidium* (60%), microsporidia, and CMV. AIDS patients rarely develop jaundice. Workup includes LFTs, lipase, amylase, and abdominal imaging with CT or ultrasound. Imaging of the gallbladder frequently reveals an edematous wall without gallstones. Prompt broad-spectrum antibiotic therapy should be initiated and surgical consultation obtained. ERCP with sphincterotomy and/or cholecystectomy may be indicated.

 PANCREATITIS

Pancreatitis is significantly more common in HIV/AIDS patients than in the general population. In addition to the typical causes seen in the non-HIV patient (gallstones and alcohol), the HIV-infected patient is at risk for developing pancreatitis related to medications and opportunistic infection. The antiretroviral nucleoside revere transcriptase inhibitor didanosine (ddI) causes pancreatitis in 2% to 6% of users. Zalcitabine and systemic pentamidine also cause pancreatitis. Symptoms include epigastric abdominal pain and vomiting. An elevated serum lipase level supports the diagnosis. Treatment includes admission for IV hydration, bowel rest, narcotic analgesics, and antiemetics. Abdominal imaging including the hepatobiliary tree to exclude choledocholithiasis is generally indicated. Mortality from acute pancreatitis is higher in HIV-infected patients than non–HIV-infected patients.

 ## PELVIC INFLAMMATORY DISEASE

Pelvic Inflammatory Disease (PID) is frequent in HIV-infected women. Conversely, 8% of all women hospitalized with PID are found to be HIV infected. The microbiology of PID in HIV-positive women is similar to that in HIV-negative women. Leukocytosis, however, is frequently absent in HIV-infected women with PID.

SYMPTOMS
- Pain in the pelvis, lower abdomen, and low back
- Fever
- Mucopurulent vaginal discharge
- Vaginal bleeding

COMMENTS AND TREATMENT CONSIDERATIONS
HIV-infected women with PID are at higher risk for tuboovarian abscess, treatment failure, and prolonged hospitalization. Accordingly, admission for intravenous antibiotic therapy is commonly recommended for HIV-positive PID patients.

 ## DIARRHEA

Diarrhea is an extremely common symptom in the HIV-infected patient. Treatment in the emergency department is generally directed to rehydration and initiation of an evaluation to determine the etiology. A wide variety of enteric pathogens and HIV medications may be responsible. Generally, acute febrile enterocolitis is caused by *Salmonella*, *Campylobacter*, *Shigella*, *E. coli*, or *Clostridium difficile* and may occur in patients with normal or near-normal CD4 counts. Treatment of acute enterocolitis is generally with an oral fluoroquinolone antibiotic and supportive care. Admission should be considered for severe symptoms and dehydration.

245

Chronic diarrhea occurs in patients with low CD4 counts (often <50/mm³) and is most often due to *Cryptosporidium,* microsporidia, *Isospora, Cyclospora, Giardia, Entamoeba histolytica*, MAC, CMV, and HIV itself and as a complication of HAART. Chronic diarrhea complicates 30% of patients treated with protease inhibitors. Workup includes stool culture for enteric pathogens, *C. difficile* toxin, ova and parasites, cryptosporidia immune assay, acid-fast stain (for MAC and cryptosporidia), and trichrome stain (for microsporidia). Colonoscopy with biopsy is indicated to evaluate for CMV colitis (typical affecting the ascending colon). Unfortunately, one third of AIDS patients with chronic diarrhea have a nondiagnostic workup. CMV colitis usually responds to ganciclovir or foscarnet. MAC enteritis often responds to ethambutol and clarithromycin. Medical treatment for microsporidia, *Cyclospora*, and *Isospora* is often unsuccessful. The most effective therapy is to improve immune function through HAART.

REFERENCES

Barbosa C: Pelvic inflammatory disease and human immunodeficiency virus infection, *Obstet Gynecol* 89:65, 1997.

Edward C, Oldfield EC: Evaluation of chronic diarrhea in patients with human immunodeficiency virus infection, *Rev Gastroenterol Disord* 2:176, 2002.

Leigh JE: Oral opportunistic infections in HIV-positive individuals: review and role of mucosal immunity, *AIDS Patient Care STDS* 18:443, 2004.

Slavin EM: The AIDS patient with abdominal pain: a new challenge for the emergency physician, *Emerg Med Clin North Am* 21:987, 2003.

Sobel JD: Gynecologic infections in human immunodeficiency virus-infected women, *Clin Infect Dis* 31:1225, 2000.

 GASTROINTESTINAL BLEEDING

See Chapter 6, Bleeding.

In HIV-infected patients with CD4 >200/mm³, the etiology of upper gastrointestinal bleeding (UGIB) is similar to that in non–HIV-infected individuals and is dominated by peptic ulcer disease and gastritis. However, UGIB in HIV-infected patients with CD4 <200/mm³ is most commonly caused by intestinal KS, followed by esophageal ulcer, then gastritis and peptic ulcer disease. CMV esophagitis may cause UGIB, and CMV colitis may result in lower gastrointestinal bleeding. All patients with UGIB should have early gastroenterology consultation and be admitted to monitor for early rebleeding. Initial management is the same as for non–HIV-infected patients, that is, at least two large-bore antecubital intravenous catheters, crystalloid fluid resuscitation, and cross-matching of blood.

OCULAR MANIFESTATIONS

Cytomegalovirus is the leading cause of ocular disease in the patient with advanced HIV. Other opportunistic infections such as *T. gondii*, *Pneumocystis*, and varicella-zoster virus can produce vision-threatening retinal disease.

 CMV RETINITIS

Patients with a CD4 count <200/mm³ have a 4% annual risk of developing CMV retinitis, and this risk increases dramatically when CD4 counts fall below 50/mm³. Typically, the disease is characterized by progressive, unilateral, painless vision loss and can be readily diagnosed by characteristic coalescing white exudates in a vascular pattern on funduscopic examination.

SYMPTOMS
- Blurred vision
- Floaters
- Flashes
- Decreased vision
- Eye pain is uncommon.

SIGNS
- Decreased visual acuity
- Exudates and hemorrhage on funduscopic examination
- Retinal detachment

COMMENTS AND TREATMENT CONSIDERATIONS
Untreated, CMV retinitis can result in retinal detachment and complete vision loss. Treatment of CMV retinitis is generally through intravenous systemic antivirals such as ganciclovir. New advances now allow ophthalmologists to insert a ganciclovir-releasing ocular implant (Vitrasert implant) that obviates the need for systemic therapy.

REFERENCES
Whitcup SM: Cytomegalovirus retinitis in the era of highly active antiretroviral therapy, *JAMA* 283:653, 2000.

HIV-RELATED MALIGNANCY

 KAPOSI SARCOMA

KS is the most frequent malignancy associated with HIV disease. The disease is far more common in HIV-infected men who have sex

CHAPTER 19

with men than in intravenous drug (IVD) users. The causative etiologic agent is human herpes virus 8 (HHV-8). Typically, characteristic lesions (1- to 2-cm nonpruritic purple nodules first affect the face, oropharynx, and feet of patients with CD4 count <200/mm^3). Near-simultaneous eruption of KS lesions in multiple skin regions is common. KS may affect internal organs, most commonly the GI tract and pulmonary system, where the lesions may cause bleeding or obstruction.

SYMPTOMS
- Skin lesions
- Abdominal pain
- Hematemesis
- Pulmonary complaints

SIGNS
- 1- to 2-cm nonpruritic purplish nodules often involving more than one area on the skin simultaneously

WORKUP
- Diagnosis suspected on clinical grounds and confirmed with biopsy

COMMENTS AND TREATMENT CONSIDERATIONS
Local radiation therapy has been effective for isolated lesions; systemic chemotherapy is often necessary when the disease is widespread.

REFERENCES
Schwartz RA: Kaposi's sarcoma: an update, *J Surg Oncol* 87:146, 2004.

HIV–RELATED SYSTEMIC ILLNESSES

 ACUTE RETROVIRAL SYNDROME

The acute retroviral syndrome is characterized by a nonspecific viral syndrome occurring 1 to 6 weeks following HIV exposure. Studies suggest that approximately 50% of patients experience the syndrome, although it often goes unrecognized. Symptoms typically last 10 to 14 days and are followed by return to normal health. Rare cases progress to encephalitis, Guillain-Barré syndrome, or peripheral neuropathy. Laboratory evaluation during the acute retroviral syndrome reveals markedly diminished CD4 counts often <200/m^3, high viral load, and elevated ESR and transaminases. The acute retroviral syndrome is difficult to diagnose given the nonspecific signs and symptoms but should be considered in high-risk populations including men who have sex with men, IVD users, and health care workers with recent occupational exposure.

SYMPTOMS
- Fever
- Sweats
- Malaise
- Truncal rash
- Pharyngitis
- Headache
- Neck stiffness
- Mouth pain

SIGNS
- Fever
- Meningismus
- Generalized lymphadenopathy
- Hepatosplenomegaly
- Oral ulcers

COMMENTS AND TREATMENT CONSIDERATIONS
Antiretroviral therapy for the acute retroviral syndrome is controversial because of the lack of data showing long-term clinical benefit. Urgent consultation with an HIV specialist is appropriate to plan evaluation and management.

REFERENCES
Dybul M: Guidelines for using antiretroviral agents among HIV-infected adults and adolescents, *Ann Intern Med* 137:381, 2002.
Perlmutter BL: How to recognize and treat acute HIV syndrome, *Am Fam Physician* 60:535, 1999.

 RECONSTITUTION ILLNESS

A unique set of symptoms and diseases, termed the immune reconstitution inflammatory syndrome (IRIS), may occur in advanced HIV/AIDS patients 1 to 2 months after beginning therapy with HAART. IRIS is caused by a rapid increase in cell-mediated inflammatory response to latent opportunistic infections. A variety of manifestations of IRIS have been described, most prominently including MAC lymphadenitis, exacerbations of pulmonary and CNS *M. tuberculosis* infection, exacerbations of *C. neoformans* meningitis, and CMV uveitis.

REFERENCES

Shelburne SA: The immune reconstitution inflammatory syndrome, *AIDS Rev* 5:67, 2003.

 MYCOBACTERIUM AVIUM COMPLEX

Currently, disseminated MAC is a common bacteriologic infection seen in patients with advanced HIV disease. The risk of developing disseminated MAC is approximately 20% for patients with CD4 counts <50/mm³. Median survival is 6 to 9 months. The incidence of disseminated MAC infection has dropped dramatically with standard chemoprophylaxis in AIDS patients with CD4 <50/mm³ and the effectiveness of HAART therapy. MAC is a ubiquitous acid-fast bacillus that is inhaled and spreads hematogenously. Disseminated MAC is characteristic by infection in the bone marrow and lymphatic system. Typical signs and symptoms include chronic fever, weight loss, diarrhea, malaise, and profound anemia. Diagnosis is confirmed by culture of the MAC organism from blood, biopsy, or bone marrow. MAC may reside in the bronchial tree and GI tract without causing invasive disease; thus, culture from stool and sputum does not confirm disseminated disease.

SYMPTOMS
- Fever
- Weight loss
- Diarrhea
- Malaise

SIGNS
- Fever
- Lymphadenopathy
- Hepatosplenomegaly

WORKUP
- Alkaline phosphatase is elevated
- CBC: severe anemia

COMMENTS AND TREATMENT CONSIDERATIONS
Treatment for disseminated MAC consists of clarithromycin and ethambutol for at least 12 to 18 months.

REFERENCES
Karakousis PC: *Mycobacterium avium* complex in patients with HIV infection in the era of highly active antiretroviral therapy, *Lancet Infect Dis* 4:557, 2004.

Wagner D: Nontuberculous mycobacterial infections: a clinical review, *Infection* 32:257, 2004.

HIGHLY ACTIVE ANTIRETROVIRAL THERAPY

HAART has dramatically changed the severity of HIV disease in the United States and prolonged life expectancy for HIV-infected individuals. However, HAART side effects limit its effectiveness in some patients. As HAART continues to reduce the risk of opportunistic infection and prolong survival, the deleterious effects of the therapy have gained increasing attention. A detailed discussion of HAART side effects is beyond the scope of this chapter. Table 19–3 summarizes the most important adverse effects of the most commonly used HAART medications.

TABLE 19–3
HAART MEDICATIONS AND THEIR IMPORTANT ADVERSE EFFECTS

DRUG	ABBREVIATION	IMPORTANT ADVERSE EFFECTS
Nucleoside Reverse Transcriptase Inhibitors		
Zidovudine	AZT	Nausea, headache, rash, lactic acidosis, elevated LFTs
Lamivudine	3TC	Neutropenia
Didanosine	ddI	Diarrhea, pancreatitis, gout, peripheral neuropathy
Zalcitabine	ddC	Peripheral neuropathy, mouth ulcers, pancreatitis
Stavudine	d4T	Peripheral neuropathy, lactic acidosis
Tenofovir	TDF	Nausea, vomiting, diarrhea, hypophosphatemia
Abacavir	ABC	Rash, fever, myalgias, arthralgias
Nonnucleoside Reverse Transcriptase Inhibitors		
Nevirapine	NVP	Rash, increased LFTs
Delavirdine	DLV	Rash
Efavirenz	EFV	Rash, CNS depression
Protease Inhibitors		
Saquinavir	INV/FTV	Increased LFTs, vomiting, diarrhea, abdominal pain
Ritonavir	RTV	Vomiting, diarrhea, abdominal pain, elevated LFTs, hypertriglyceridemia,
Indinavir	IDV	Elevated LFTs, nephrolithiasis
Amprenavir	APV	Rash, vomiting, diarrhea, abdominal pain
Nelfinavir	NFV	Vomiting, diarrhea, abdominal pain

Modified from Montessori V: Adverse effects of antiretroviral therapy for HIV infection, *CMAJ* 170:229, 2004.

19

CHAPTER

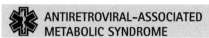 **ANTIRETROVIRAL–ASSOCIATED METABOLIC SYNDROME**

The antiretroviral-associated metabolic syndrome encompasses a set of metabolic derangements commonly seen in patients taking HAART, particularly in those taking protease inhibitors. The syndrome has four components: lipodystrophy, dyslipidemia, insulin resistance, and bone disease. Lipodystrophy affects 50% of patients treated with HAART and is characterized by redistribution of fat from peripheral location to central locations. Limb wasting is seen in conjunction with increased abdominal fat and a dorsocervical fat pad ("buffalo hump"). A lipid profile of low HDL, high LDL, and very high triglycerides is associated with HAART. Insulin resistance ensues, and >5% of HAART patients develop overt type 2 diabetes. As a result, HAART may be associated with an increased risk of myocardial infarction or ischemic stroke. HAART-associated bone disease may lead to premature osteoporosis and fracture.

REFERENCES

Montessori V: Adverse effects of antiretroviral therapy for HIV infection, *CMAJ* 170:229, 2004.

Vella S, Floridia M: Antiviral therapy. In Cohen J, Powderly WG, Steven M, et al (eds): *Infectious diseases*, ed 2. London, 2003, Elsevier.

OCCUPATIONAL EXPOSURE

Exposure to HIV-infected bodily fluids is an occupational hazard for health care workers. In practice, however, HIV seroconversion in health care professionals has been an extremely rare event, with only 56 confirmed cases and another 138 possible cases since the onset of HIV-related illness.

The overall risk of seroconversion after an HIV-contaminated needlestick is 0.3%, or 1 in 300. The risk after mucous membrane exposure is 0.09%, or less than 1 in 1000. Postexposure prophylaxis (PEP) is used to lower the rate of seroconversion, although the exact risk reduction is unknown. PEP should be initiated as soon as possible after exposure because animal models suggest that it is ineffective if given >24 to 36 hours after the exposure. PEP includes two or three antiretrovirals for a period of 4 weeks. Infectious disease consultation is recommended any time PEP is being given. An updated, online guide to help manage treatment and documentation of occupational exposure is available at http://www.needlestick.mednet.ucla.edu.

REFERENCES

CDC: Updated Public Health Service guidelines for the management of health-care worker exposures to HBV, HCV, HIV and recommendations for postexposure prophylaxis, *MMWR Recomm Rep* 50(RR-11):1, 2001.

CHAPTER 19

Hypertension
Mark S. Louden and Atilla Uner

Patients with elevated blood pressure frequently visit the ED. Their "hypertension" may be the result of essential hypertension, the effect of a specific pathologic process, a by-product of the stress of the ED visit, or an erroneous blood pressure reading. Hypertensive emergency is an elevation in blood pressure that causes end-organ dysfunction. True hypertensive emergency develops in only 1% to 2% of patients with hypertension. A good history, physical examination, and a few simple tests are all that are generally required to rule out end-organ damage that requires emergent intervention. In the absence of such a condition, hypertension generally requires only close follow-up.

Severe hypertension associated with acute myocardial ischemia, renal damage, CNS dysfunction, or other end-organ disease should be treated with easily titratable intravenous medications. Neither oral nor sublingual medications should be used in this circumstance. Blood pressure should generally not be lowered to a "normal" pressure because patients with a history of hypertension have elevated cerebral pressure requirements. Nitroprusside is an effective, short-acting, and titratable agent, and it requires moment-to-moment monitoring to prevent hypotension. A newer but more expensive alternative is fenoldopam, which may offer an advantage in patients with renal failure.

In some hypertensive patients, lowering blood pressure can be detrimental. For example, high blood pressure in patients with acute stroke may be "appropriate" as a homeostatic mechanism to maintain blood flow to threatened parts of the CNS. In addition, overly aggressive treatment of asymptomatic blood pressure elevations, without evidence of end-organ dysfunction, is unnecessary and can have deleterious effects, such as stroke, myocardial infarction (MI), or fetal distress.

Initial workup consists of ruling out other causes of the presenting signs and symptoms, such as stroke, infection, or toxicologic emergency (e.g., cocaine overdose), and evaluating for other coexistent end-organ damage or dysfunction.

 AORTIC DISSECTION

See Chapter 7, Chest Pain.

 MYOCARDIAL INFARCTION

See Chapter 7, Chest Pain.

 CONGESTIVE HEART FAILURE

See Chapter 34, Shortness of Breath.

 STROKE

For patients with ischemic stroke or intracerebral hemorrhage, acute pharmacologic reduction of blood pressure should generally be avoided. Initial blood pressure elevations usually resolve spontaneously in 12 to 72 hours (80% with significant improvement in 4 hours), and overly aggressive therapy may worsen ischemia. Active treatment should be employed in cases of persistent, extreme elevation of pressure (SBP >220, DBP >120, mean arterial pressure [MAP] >140). Pressure should then be reduced over 24 hours, with titrated intravenous therapy. If the patient is at risk for MI, congestive heart failure (CHF), or aortic dissection, more rapid reduction of pressure may be required. In subarachnoid hemorrhage, therapy may be needed to lessen the likelihood of rebleeding if analgesics, sedation, and rest do not reduce pressure to near prebleeding levels.

See Chapter 18, Headache, and Chapter 44, Weakness and Fatigue.

CHAPTER 20

REFERENCES

Adams H, Adams R, Del Zoppo G, Goldstein LB: Guidelines for the early management of patients with ischemic stroke: 2005 guidelines update a scientific statement from the Stroke Council of the American Heart Association/American Stroke Association, *Stroke* 36:916, 2005.

Carlberg B, Asplund K, Hägg E: The prognostic value of admission blood pressure in patients with acute stroke, *Stroke* 24:1372, 1993.

Fischberg GM, Lozano E, Rajamani K, et al: Stroke precipitated by moderate blood pressure reduction, *J Emerg Med* 19:339, 2000.

Lisk DR, Grotta JC, Lamki LM, et al: Should hypertension be treated after acute stroke? A randomized controlled trial using single photon emission computed tomography, *Arch Neurol* 50:855, 1993.

Powers WJ: Acute hypertension after stroke: the scientific basis for treatment decisions, *Neurology* 43:461, 1993.

Rodgers A, MacMahon S, Gamble G, et al: Blood pressure and risk of stroke in patients with cerebrovascular disease: the United Kingdom Transient Ischaemic Attack Collaborative Group, *BMJ* 313:147, 1996.

 HYPERTENSIVE ENCEPHALOPATHY

SYMPTOMS
- Severe headache
- Confusion
- Lethargy
- Vomiting

SIGNS
- Markedly elevated blood pressure and abnormal mental status are essential features (mental status may fluctuate).
- Papilledema is usually, if not always, present.
- Fever should suggest another cause, such as meningitis, encephalitis, thyroid storm, or neuroleptic malignant syndrome.

WORKUP
- Evaluate for other possible causes of signs and symptoms.
- Head CT without contrast (or other neurologic imaging; MRI may be useful) is essential for ruling out hemorrhagic CNS lesions or a mass or large stroke with increased intracranial pressure.
- O_2 saturation to rule out hypoxia
- Glucose
- Urinalysis to look for protein or blood, indicating renal involvement
- Electrolytes, BUN, creatinine
- ECG to detect evidence of cardiac ischemia (may be masked or silent)
- Chest x-ray to detect CHF or investigate for evidence of dissection, if suspected
- Blood smear for detection of hemolysis, suggesting thrombotic thrombocytopenic purpura (TTP)

COMMENTS AND TREATMENT CONSIDERATIONS

Nitroprusside has long been the treatment of choice in most situations and should be titrated to produce symptomatic improvement to a maximum diastolic pressure reduction of 20% to 25% or to a diastolic pressure of 100, whichever is higher. Its use requires careful hemodynamic monitoring. Labetalol, fenoldopam, and nicardipine are alternatives.

REFERENCES

Healton EB: Hypertensive encephalopathy and the neurologic manifestations of malignant hypertension, *Neurology* 32:127, 1982.

Katsumata Y, Maehara T, Noda M, et al: Hypertensive encephalopathy: reversible CT and MR appearance, *Radiat Med* 11:160, 1993.

Veron J, Marik PE: The diagnosis and management of hypertensive crises, *Chest* 118:214, 2000.

 HYPERTENSIVE RETINAL HEMORRHAGE OR PAPILLEDEMA

SYMPTOMS
- Headache and visual loss are frequent.
- Patients may be asymptomatic.

SIGNS
- Abnormal funduscopic examination
- The blood pressure must be severely elevated to cause papilledema; if the blood pressure is only moderately elevated, other etiologies should be strongly considered.
- Other signs of other end-organ damage

WORKUP
- Urinalysis to look for protein or blood, indicating renal involvement
- Electrolytes, BUN, creatinine
- ECG to detect evidence of cardiac ischemia
- Chest x-ray to detect CHF or evidence of dissection, if suspected
- CBC to detect hemolysis, suggesting TTP
- Other tests should be tailored to detect evidence of end-organ damage.

COMMENTS AND TREATMENT CONSIDERATIONS

The priority is treatment of the underlying hypertension with ophthalmologic consultation to further evaluate acute versus chronic changes through indirect ophthalmoscopy. In the absence of other conditions (or of a specific cause of the hypertension) requiring different therapy, nitroprusside is the treatment of choice.

REFERENCES

Murphy C: Hypertensive emergencies, *Emerg Med Clin North Am* 13:973, 1995.

Zampaglione B, Pascale C, Marchisio M, Cavallo-Perin P: Hypertensive urgencies and emergencies: prevalence and clinical presentation, *Hypertension* 27:144, 1996.

 PREECLAMPSIA AND ECLAMPSIA

Preeclampsia is a complication of pregnancy characterized by hypertension, edema, and proteinuria. The diagnosis of eclampsia is made when seizures begin. The disease does not occur until after the 20th week of gestation, except with hydatidiform mole. Some patients do not know (or admit) that they are or may be pregnant. Those without adequate prenatal care may not know the gestational age. Approximately 14% of cases occur in the postpartum period (25% of these in the 2- to 14-day range). HELLP syndrome (hemolysis, elevated liver function tests, and low platelets) occurs in up to 10% of cases of severe preeclampsia and carries a high risk of disseminated intravascular coagulation (DIC) (30%).

SYMPTOMS

- Swelling of the hands, face, legs
- Abdominal pain (especially epigastric and right upper quadrant)
- Headache
- Visual disturbances
- Altered mental status
- Seizures may be among presenting complaints and are required for the diagnosis of eclampsia.

SIGNS

- Hypertension is diagnosed at much lower pressures than in other situations. Blood pressure of 140/90, or an increase of 30/15 from baseline, is abnormal.
- Edema, although isolated leg edema may be normal.
- Altered mental status
- Hyperreflexia
- Petechiae
- Bruising

WORKUP

- Urinalysis should be obtained for all patients who are beyond their 20th week of pregnancy; any more than a trace of protein is abnormal.

- CBC with platelets
- Liver function tests
- PT, PTT, fibrin, and fibrin degradation products (DIC panel) should be obtained if HELLP is suspected.
- CT may be performed to assess other potential causes of altered mental status or seizures.
- Workup for possible infection should be considered if seizure might be caused by meningitis.

COMMENTS AND TREATMENT CONSIDERATIONS

Once the diagnosis is made or is strongly suspected, immediate obstetric consultation is essential. Delivery, usually by cesarean section, remains the treatment of choice for eclampsia. Hydralazine (10 mg IV) has been the traditional treatment, but labetalol is equally efficacious and can be given as a titratable IV drip, starting at 2 mg/min. Nicardipine is another alternative and may be started at 5 mg/hr. Patients with end-organ dysfunction or microangiopathy should have their diastolic pressure reduced to less than 90 within 1 hour. Less severe cases may await emergency obstetric consultation. Overly aggressive therapy may cause hypotension, thus worsening uteroplacental ischemia. Seizure prophylaxis (usually with magnesium sulfate 4 g load over 20 minutes, then 2 g/hr; watch for respiratory depression) should generally be instituted in cases of severe preeclampsia, preeclampsia at term, or eclampsia. Seizure treatment may include benzodiazepines. Beware of common misdiagnoses (e.g., cholecystitis and hepatitis) and commonly missed diagnoses (e.g., TTP, hemolytic-uremic syndrome, and sepsis) (see Chapter 32, Seizure, Adult).

REFERENCES

Cunningham FG, Lindheimer MD: Hypertension in pregnancy, *N Engl J Med* 326:927, 1992.

Duldner JE, Emerman CL: Stroke: comprehensive guidelines for clinical assessment and emergency management. II, *Emerg Med Rep* 18:213, 1997.

Magee LA, Cham C, Waterman EJ, et al: Hydralazine for treatment of severe hypertension in pregnancy: meta-analysis, *BMJ* 327:955, 2003.

Miles JF, Martin JN Jr, Blake PG, et al: Postpartum eclampsia: a recurring perinatal dilemma, *Obstet Gynecol* 76:328, 1990.

Schobel HP, Fischer T, Heuszer K, et al: Preeclampsia—a state of sympathetic overactivity, *N Engl J Med* 335:1480, 1996.

Sibai BM: Diagnosis, prevention, and management of eclampsia, *Obstet Gynecol* 105:402, 2005.

Sibai BM, Taslimi MM, el-Nazer A, et al: Maternal-perinatal outcome associated with the syndrome of hemolysis, elevated liver

CHAPTER 20

enzymes, and low platelets in severe preeclampsia-eclampsia, *Am J Obstet Gynecol* 155:501, 1986.

 ## CATECHOLAMINE EXCESS

Catecholamine excess has many causes including pheochromocytoma, sympathomimetic overdose (e.g., cocaine, amphetamines, decongestant or diet pills), withdrawal from alcohol, clonidine or sedative-hypnotics, and monoamine oxidase inhibitor (MAOI) interactions with certain foods.

SYMPTOMS
- Anxiety
- Abdominal discomfort
- Diaphoresis
- Headache
- Nausea
- Palpitations

SIGNS
- Hypertension
- Tachycardia
- Diaphoresis
- Pallor
- Signs of specific end-organ damage

WORKUP
- O_2 saturation to rule out hypoxia
- Glucose check to rule out hypoglycemia
- Urinalysis to look for protein or blood, indicating renal involvement
- Electrolytes, BUN, creatinine
- ECG to detect evidence of cardiac ischemia
- Chest x-ray to detect CHF or evidence of dissection, if suspected
- A drug screen may be informative if the history is considered unreliable, but it does not detect over-the-counter diet pills, some amphetamine derivatives, or MAOIs.
- Other tests should be tailored to detect evidence of end-organ damage.

COMMENTS AND TREATMENT CONSIDERATIONS
Benzodiazepine therapy may be adequate for reduction of blood pressure in cocaine overdose. Rarely, in severe cases, alpha-blockade with phentolamine may be required. Labetalol is, at best, a

second-line choice, and beta-blockade without alpha-blockade is contraindicated as it may worsen the hypertension. Nitroprusside is a reasonable alternative when the others are unavailable or ineffective.

Thyroid storm may mimic this syndrome.

 ## THYROID STORM

See Chapter 29, Palpitations and Tachycardia.

 ## ASYMPTOMATIC HYPERTENSION

Asymptomatic hypertension may be due to situational ("white coat") or undiagnosed hypertension. Coarctation of the aorta should be considered in patients younger than 20 years and upper and lower extremity blood pressures compared.

SYMPTOMS
None; no chest pain, shortness of breath, headache, dizziness, or abdominal pain

SIGNS
None

WORKUP
Diagnostic testing is indicated only if the blood pressure remains severely elevated after repeated measurement and a hypertensive emergency is suspected.
- Urinalysis to look for protein or blood, indicating renal involvement
- Pregnancy test if possibility of pregnancy
- Electrolytes, BUN, creatinine
- Consideration of ECG to rule out silent cardiac ischemia

COMMENTS AND TREATMENT CONSIDERATIONS
Because it is not possible to determine whether a patient's hypertension is situational or undiagnosed chronic hypertension, close follow-up for a recheck is usually all that is required for patients who remain asymptomatic and whose diagnostic evaluation is normal. Acute lowering of asymptomatic blood pressure in the emergency department provides no benefit and carries risk. Specifically, sublingual antihypertensive medication should be avoided, and an asymptomatic elevated blood pressure should not be "chased" with repeated doses of any medicine because this can lead to excessive blood pressure reduction.

CHAPTER 20

REFERENCES

Grossman E, Messerli H, Groczicki T, Kowey P: Should a moratorium be placed on sublingual nifedipine capsules given for hypertensive emergencies and pseudoemergencies? *JAMA* 276:1328, 1996.

Joint National Committee on Prevention, Detection, and Treatment of High Blood Pressure: The sixth report of the Joint National Committee on Prevention, Detection, and Treatment of High Blood Pressure, *Arch Intern Med* 157:2413, 1997.

Kaplan NM, Gifford RW: Choice of initial therapy for hypertension, *JAMA* 275:1577, 1996.

Shayne PH, Pitts SR: Severely increased blood pressure in the emergency department, *Ann Emerg Med* 41:513, 2003.

Tach AM, Schultz PJ: Nonemergent hypertension: new perspectives for the emergency medicine physician, *Emerg Med Clin North Am* 13:1009, 1995.

Zeller KR, Kuhnert LV, Matthews CM: Rapid reduction of severe asymptomatic hypertension: a prospective, controlled trial, *Arch Intern Med* 149:2186, 1989.

Hypotension
Myles D. Greenberg

Low blood pressure is a common finding during initial evaluation of a patient, and the emergency physician must determine whether a life-threatening condition is causing the hypotension. Hypotension should prompt a thorough history and physical examination to search for serious conditions. The approach to hypotensive patients should be initiated in the same way as the approach to all emergency patients: airway and breathing first, then circulation. If patients are hemodynamically unstable, two large-bore peripheral intravenous lines should be started. Most patients should initially receive fluid resuscitation using isotonic crystalloid solutions.

After initial resuscitation, history and physician examination may indicate the need for emergent intervention despite the lack of a definitive diagnosis confirmed by ancillary tests.

Hypovolemia from bleeding (internal or external) or dehydration, limitation of cardiac output (e.g., cardiac tamponade), tension pneumothorax, massive pulmonary embolism, myocardial infarction, arrhythmia, sepsis, toxic ingestion, and metabolic emergencies are general categories to consider in the approach to hypotension.

 ACUTE HYPOVOLEMIA

Acute hypovolemia is a condition of decreased intravascular volume that may be caused by blood loss or dehydration. Hypovolemia is primarily a clinical diagnosis. Initial hematocrit in the setting of blood loss is normal until fluid equilibration has time to dilute the intravascular compartment.

See Chapter 39, Trauma, Approach to.

TENSION PNEUMOTHORAX

Tension pneumothorax is caused by a defect in the lung that allows air to escape and create pressure in the pleural space; this in turn causes compression of the heart or great vessels that limits venous return and cardiac filling, decreasing systemic blood pressure. This diagnosis often must be made clinically because there may not be time for radiologic confirmation. Tension pneumothorax and cardiac tamponade have similar manifestations. Close attention must be paid to the chest, lung, heart, and trachea examinations to differentiate these two entities. Treatment of tension pneumothorax consists of immediate chest decompression. If tube thoracostomy cannot be accomplished immediately, the patient's chest should be decompressed using a large-bore intravenous catheter placed above the rib, in the midclavicular line, at the second intercostal space. Needle thoracostomy should be followed by chest tube placement as soon as possible.

See Chapter 7, Chest Pain.

 ## CARDIAC TAMPONADE

Cardiac tamponade is an increase of fluid within the pericardial space that can occur abruptly or over time. Acute effusions are more likely to cause rapid hemodynamic compromise, and if they are not promptly drained, death may ensue. In the acute setting, tamponade can be difficult to differentiate from tension pneumothorax, which is more common. Immediate ED ultrasound can be diagnostic. Immediate management of tamponade consists of aggressive fluid resuscitation followed by pericardiocentesis, operative pericardial window, or, if caused by penetrating trauma, ED operative thoracotomy.

See Chapter 7, Chest Pain.

REFERENCES

Eisenberg MJ, Munoz de Romeral L, Heidenreich PA, et al: The diagnosis of pericardial effusion and cardiac tamponade by 12-lead ECG: a technology assessment, *Chest* 110:318, 1996.

Lange RL, Botticelli JT, Tsagaris TJ, et al: Diagnostic signs in compressive cardiac disorders: constrictive pericarditis, pericardial effusion, and tamponade, *Circulation* 33:763, 1966.

Symmes JC, Berman ND: Early recognition of cardiac tamponade, *Can Med Assoc J* 116:863, 1977.

GASTROINTESTINAL BLEEDING

See Chapter 6, Bleeding.

 ABDOMINAL AORTIC ANEURYSM AND THORACIC AORTIC DISSECTION

Internal bleeding caused by aortic catastrophe can cause immediately life-threatening hypotension.

See Chapter 1, Abdominal Pain, and Chapter 7, Chest Pain.

 ARRHYTHMIAS

See Chapter 29, Palpitations and Tachycardia.

 SEPSIS

See Chapter 44, Weakness and Fatigue.

 MYOCARDIAL INFARCTION AND PULMONARY EMBOLISM

See Chapter 7, Chest Pain.

 TOXIC INGESTION

See Chapter 37, Toxic Exposure, Approach to.

 ORTHOSTATIC HYPOTENSION

See Chapter 36, Syncope and Near-Syncope.

 ECTOPIC PREGNANCY

See Chapter 41, Vaginal Bleeding.

 NEUROGENIC/SPINAL SHOCK

Acute spinal cord injury can rarely lead to peripheral vasodilation and hypotension. This is a diagnosis of exclusion.

 MYXEDEMA COMA

See Chapter 44, Weakness and Fatigue.

CHAPTER 21

The Irritable Child
Alisa McQueen, Frances McCabe, and Neal Peeples

Few symptoms in medicine are less specific than crying in an infant. All infants cry and at some point seem irritable to their parents. This chapter reviews a number of serious diagnoses that may present with the same nonspecific symptoms of irritability. Vomiting frequently accompanies irritability in infants and must also be recognized as a potentially ominous sign of a more serious disease (see Chapter 43, Vomiting Child).

The most commonly accepted definition of excessive crying in pediatrics is crying that lasts 3 hours a day, 3 days a week, for at least 3 weeks. Repeated episodes of inconsolable crying are often attributable to "colic." The prevalence of colic varies greatly (3.3% to 25%) depending on the method of the study and the definition of colic used. Unfortunately, no reliable method has been developed for diagnosing a child's crying as colic without first excluding a myriad of other potentially serious diagnoses. Colic appears to remit by the age of 3 months, making this diagnosis highly suspect in an infant older than 3 months. Only after all emergent diagnoses have been adequately considered and eliminated can a diagnosis of colic be considered.

REFERENCES

Garrison MM, Christakis DA: A systematic review of treatments for infantile colic, *Pediatrics* 106:184, 2000.

Gatrad AR, Sheikh A: Persistent crying in babies, *BMJ* 328:330, 2004.

Lucassen PL, Assendelft WJ, van Eijk JT, et al: Systematic review of the occurrence of infantile colic in the community, *Arch Dis Child* 84:398, 2001.

INFECTION

Infants with serious infections may have few or nonspecific symptoms, such as irritability.

MENINGITIS

See Chapter 16, Fever in Children under 2 Years of Age.

 SEPTIC ARTHRITIS AND OSTEOMYELITIS

See Chapter 25, Limping Child/Child Won't Walk.

 URINARY TRACT INFECTION

Although not as immediately life or limb threatening, urinary tract infections (UTIs) may be responsible for irritability in infants. UTIs develop in approximately 1% of infants, with premature infants at even higher risk. Because many UTIs are associated with structural urinary tract abnormalities, it is important to diagnose these before permanent renal damage ensues.

SYMPTOMS
- Crying
- Irritability
- Poor feeding

SIGNS
- Fever ++; occasionally present
- Lethargy
- Vomiting
- Jaundice

WORKUP
- Urinalysis; dipstick positive for leukocyte esterase or nitrate has only limited sensitivity (+++). Sensitivity of microscopic analysis for leukocytes and bacteria is better (+++) but is still limited.
- Urine culture +++++, obtained by catheterization or suprapubic tap, is the "gold standard" test and should be obtained even though results will not be available in the ED. Urine specimens obtained by bag collection are too frequently contaminated with surrounding skin flora and should not be sent for culture.
- Urinary tract imaging studies are usually obtained later in the outpatient setting.

COMMENTS AND TREATMENT CONSIDERATIONS
Urosepsis should be considered in all infants younger than 3 months with UTI. Hospitalization and parenteral antibiotics may be necessary, particularly in the first 30 days of life.

CHAPTER 22

REFERENCES

Du J: Colic as the sole symptom of urinary tract infection in infants, *Can Med Assoc J* 115:334, 1976.

Huicho L, Campos-Sanchez M, Alamo C: Metaanalysis of urine screening tests for determining the risk of urinary tract infection in children, *Pediatr Infect Dis J* 21:1, 2002.

SURGICAL EMERGENCIES

 INTUSSUSCEPTION

See Chapter 1, Abdominal Pain.

 TESTICULAR TORSION

See Chapter 31, Scrotal Pain.

INJURIES

Careful physical examination of the irritable infant may reveal an occult injury. Many injuries are accidental, but any injury that is inconsistent with the stated mechanism, or incompatible with the child's developmental ability, should raise suspicion for child abuse.

 CORNEAL ABRASION

Corneal abrasions are usually thought to be caused by an infant inadvertently scratching his or her own cornea.

SYMPTOMS
- Irritability
- Crying
- Eye pain

SIGNS
- Inconsolable crying
- Eye redness
- Excessive tearing (tearing begins after age 4 weeks), particularly unilateral

WORKUP
- Topical corneal anesthesia and fluorescein staining with Wood's lamp examination generally establish the diagnosis of a foreign body or an abrasion.

COMMENTS AND TREATMENT CONSIDERATIONS

Patching of the affected eye has not been shown to speed healing or improve outcome. Topical antibiotic ointment is generally prescribed and may help prevent infection and provide some degree of pain relief. Topical corneal anesthesia should not be prescribed for outpatient use.

REFERENCES

Harkness M: Corneal abrasion in infancy as a cause of inconsolable crying, *Pediatr Emerg Care* 5:242, 1989.

Michael JG, Hug D, Dowd MD: Management of corneal abrasion in children: a randomized clinical trial, *Ann Emerg Med* 40:67, 2002.

 HAIR TOURNIQUET

A hair can become wrapped around a digit or the penis of an infant, causing constriction and potentially resulting in amputation if the hair is not removed.

SYMPTOMS

- Pain in the digit or penis

SIGNS

- Inconsolable crying
- Erythema and swelling of the digit
- Constricting hair can become enveloped in surrounding edematous tissue, thereby obscuring the correct diagnosis.

WORKUP

- Thorough physical examination of digits and genitalia.

REFERENCES

Alpert J, Filler R, Glaser H: Strangulation of an appendage by hair wrapping, *N Engl J Med* 273:866, 1965.

Klusmann A, Hans-Gerd L: Tourniquet syndrome—accident or abuse? *Eur J Pediatr* 163:495, 2004.

 CHILD ABUSE

Physical child abuse is defined as the nonaccidental injury of a child, ranging from minor bruises and lacerations to severe head trauma and death. It is estimated that 1 million children in the United States are seriously abused by parents or caretakers, and between 2000 and 5000 deaths annually are attributable to child abuse. Evidence has shown that without intervention 50% of abused children suffer some escalation of the violence.

Although few injuries are pathognomonic for abuse, certain patterns of injury are associated with nonaccidental injury. Histories that are inadequate, inconsistent with the injury pattern, or incompatible with the developmental ability of the child should raise suspicion. Delay in seeking medical attention for an injury is also associated with abuse. Risk factors for abuse include premature birth, neonatal hospitalization, or other circumstance that might interfere with normal parent-infant bonding; adolescent parents; children with a congenital abnormality or special needs; and irritability and colic. The absence of risk factors, however, does not preclude child abuse: no child is immune. A high index of suspicion is required, and most states mandate reporting for any case of suspected abuse. Many institutions have developed interdisciplinary teams to assist with assessment of potential cases of abuse.

SYMPTOMS
- Symptoms are highly nonspecific.
- Irritability
- Crying
- Poor feeding, failure to thrive
- Inability or reluctance to engage with parent or other adult
- Immediate engagement with strangers

SIGNS
- Bruises +++; combining all age groups, this is the most common sign.
- Welts
- Burns ++; look for small, circular cigarette burns to palms and soles, stocking-glove distribution of immersion burns, geometric shapes from application of electric appliances, linear marks or bruises from belts or cords, and injuries of different ages.
- Fractures ++; over half of fractures may be nonaccidental in infants younger than 1 year of age. Although not pathognomonic, the following fractures are highly suspicious for abuse: femoral in a nonambulatory child, nonsupracondylar humeral, metaphyseal or "bucket handle," rib (++, with 90% of these occurring in infants younger than age 2), and diaphyseal in conjunction with concurrent skeletal or extraskeletal injury.
- Head injury +++ (majority in those <2 years). Seizures, lethargy, and decreased level of consciousness can be signs of intracranial trauma. Subdural hematoma may be precipitated by violent shaking or blunt trauma. Infants less than 12 months of age have the highest incidence of head injuries, which cause the greatest morbidity and mortality of all abuse patterns.

- Retinal hemorrhages (in most severely shaken infants); concurrent intracranial and skeletal injury has higher specificity for abuse.
- Abdominal injuries from blunt trauma remain difficult to detect, and a high index of suspicion is required. Rare signs include bruises on the abdominal wall or manifestations of solid or hollow organ injury.
- Sexual abuse: blood or discharge noted in underwear, bruising on perineum, evidence of a sexually transmitted disease; during examination for physical evidence of sexual abuse, care should be taken to ensure that retraumatization does not occur. In some cases, it may be necessary to perform the examination under anesthesia.
- Signs of child neglect include malnutrition and poor hygiene.

WORKUP
- Plot height, weight, and head circumference for documentation of failure to thrive.
- Radiographic skeletal survey may reveal old healed fractures. The survey includes x-ray of the skull, spine, chest, and extremities.
- CT of head if intracranial trauma suspected
- Ultrasonography may demonstrate subperiosteal hemorrhages in infants.
- Bone scan may identify rib fractures not evident on x-ray.
- Consider platelet count and coagulation studies in patients with significant bruising to rule out alternative diagnoses.

COMMENTS AND TREATMENT CONSIDERATIONS
Any suspected cases of child abuse or neglect must be reported to child protective services in accordance with local statutes. Visible injuries should be photographed. Documentation of the stated history and the observed injuries should be detailed and objective, without subjective interpretation. For example, bruises that appear to be of different ages should be described by their size and color, not by their estimated age, as few physicians are able to assess accurately the age of a bruise.

See Chapter 39, Trauma, Approach to.

REFERENCES
Bariciak ED, Plint AC, Gaboury I, et al: Dating of bruises in children: an assessment of physician accuracy, *Pediatrics* 112:804, 2003.
Council On Scientific Affairs: AMA diagnostic and treatment guidelines concerning child abuse and neglect, *JAMA* 254:796, 1985.
Kellogg N and the Committee on Child Abuse and Neglect: The evaluation of sexual abuse in children, *Pediatrics* 116:506, 2005.

CHAPTER **22**

Leventhal JM, Thomas SA, Rosenfield NS, et al: Fractures in young children. Distinguishing child abuse from unintentional injuries, *Am J Dis Child* 147:87, 1993.

Ng CS, Hall CM, Shaw DG: The range of visceral manifestations of non-accidental injury, *Arch Dis Child* 77:167, 1997.

Peck MD, Priolo-Kapel D: Child abuse by burning: a review of the literature and an algorithm for medical investigations, *J Trauma* 53:1013, 2002.

Sheridan R: Outpatient burn care in the emergency department, *Pediatr Emerg Care* 21:449, 2005.

Additional references can be found on the National Clearinghouse on Child Abuse and Neglect Information website at: http://nccanch.acf.hhs.gov/.

CARDIAC DISEASE

Irritability in infants may be caused by cardiac disease, including structural defects and arrhythmias.

 STRUCTURAL DEFECTS

Congestive heart failure (CHF) as a result of left-to-right shunts and, more rarely, left ventricular dysfunction may present with an insidious onset of symptoms. The structural lesions most often associated with CHF include ventricular septal defect, atrioventricular canal, large patent ductus arteriosus, myocarditis, cardiomyopathy, and anomalous origin of the coronary arteries.

SYMPTOMS
- Poor feeding
- Crying
- Irritability

SIGNS
- Sweating with feeding
- Poor weight gain
- Lethargy
- Tachypnea is often the only lung finding; rales are often absent.
- Pallor
- Diastolic rumble at the apex, murmur, S3 gallop, and hepatomegaly
- Oliguria
- Cardiogenic shock; poor peripheral perfusion may result from excess sympathetic stimulation and cause peripheral vasoconstriction with cool, pale skin. Poor peripheral perfusion can also cause sluggish capillary refill or weak pulses.
- Hypotension is a late sign of shock in infants.

WORKUP
- ECG; increased amplitude in leads reflecting the right heart are normal in the newborn because of elevated pulmonary vascular resistance and decrease in the first 6 to 8 weeks of life.
- Chest x-ray may demonstrate cardiomegaly, or increased pulmonary markings from left-to-right shunting, or certain classic morphologies (e.g., the "boot-shaped" heart of tetralogy of Fallot)
- Cardiac echocardiography by a skilled operator identifies most structural abnormalities.

COMMENTS AND TREATMENT CONSIDERATIONS
In infants with left-to-right shunts the severity of the shunt gradually worsens over the first 2 months of life as pulmonary pressures gradually decrease. This is in contrast to infants with right-to-left shunts—the cyanotic lesions—who may rapidly decompensate in the first few days or weeks of life with closure of the ductus arteriosus. In these infants, use of prostaglandin infusion in consultation with pediatric cardiology can maintain ductus patency and be lifesaving.

 ARRHYTHMIAS

The most common symptomatic arrhythmia in infants is supraventricular tachycardia (SVT); 80% of cases occur in children younger than 12 months, and 60% occur in the first 4 months of life. Ventricular tachycardia is much less common in infants and is usually associated with abnormal myocardium, congenital or acquired myopathies, long QT syndrome, or postsurgical scarring.

SYMPTOMS
- Crying
- Irritability
- Poor feeding
- Arrhythmias may be asymptomatic.

SIGNS
- Heart rates are in excess of 220, often 250 to 300.
- Irritability and feeding intolerance are often the only early signs.
- Tachycardia that is sustained can cause poor peripheral perfusion and CHF seen in the structural lesions noted previously.

WORKUP
- ECG. Once converted to normal sinus rhythm, a widened QRS because of a delta wave indicative of an accessory pathway may be visible in infants with SVT ++.

CHAPTER **22**

273

- Electrolytes, K+, Ca2+, and Mg2+, should also be checked if the patient has a reason for electrolyte abnormality.
- Chest x-ray to look for cardiomegaly
- Cardiac echo, as SVT may be associated with a structural cardiac defect ++ (often done as an outpatient procedure)
- Holter monitor (often done as an outpatient procedure)

COMMENTS AND TREATMENT CONSIDERATIONS

Because of high vasomotor tone and great cardiovascular reserve, newborns can tolerate high heart rates, even exceeding 300, for long periods. Their symptoms can be very subtle for hours before any significant sign of heart failure is evident, making early diagnosis difficult. Vagal maneuvers and adenosine are the preferred therapy for SVT in a hemodynamically stable patient. The patient in shock should be urgently cardioverted. SVT with aberrant conduction is uncommon in children, and, as with adults, wide complex tachycardia should be initially treated as ventricular tachycardia.

REFERENCES

Danford DA: Clinical and basic laboratory assessment of children for possible congenital heart disease, *Curr Opin Pediatr* 12:487, 2000.

Lee C, Mason LJ: Pediatric cardiac emergencies, *Anesthesiol Clin North Am* 18:287, 2001.

Mahle WT: A dangerous case of colic: anomalous left coronary artery presenting with paroxysms of irritability, *Pediatr Emerg Care* 14:24, 1998.

Vos P, Pulles-Heintzberger CF, Delhaas T: Supraventricular tachycardia: an incidental diagnosis in infants and difficult to prove in children, *Acta Paediatr* 92:1058, 2003.

Jaundice
Yi-Mei Chng and David F. M. Brown

Jaundice is a yellowing of the skin, sclera, and mucous membranes caused by increased levels of bilirubin. Clinical jaundice is usually not obvious until the serum bilirubin concentration exceeds 2.5 mg/dl. Causes of jaundice can be divided into three groups: prehepatic, hepatic (either hepatocellular or intrahepatic cholestasis), and posthepatic (extrahepatic obstruction). History and physical examination generally suggest the likely cause of jaundice, which may be confirmed by laboratory tests or imaging studies. Patients with new-onset jaundice should be hospitalized on an individualized basis as warranted by the underlying disease process.

 VIRAL HEPATITIS

Hepatitis A and E are transmitted through the fecal-oral route and have similar incubation periods of 15 to 60 days. Hepatitis A virus (HAV) is more common in the United States, and hepatitis E is more common in Asia, Africa, and Russia. Acute hepatitis A is usually diagnosed by the patient's history (nonspecific symptoms followed by jaundice and abdominal pain), especially because it tends to be associated with epidemics. More than 75% of adults who contract HAV have symptoms, whereas up to 70% of children younger than 6 years who contract HAV are asymptomatic. A two-dose vaccine against HAV is available for persons above the age of 2.

Hepatitis B, C, and D are transmitted parenterally. Hepatitis B is the most common and leads to a chronic carrier state in 10% of adults and 90% of neonates infected with it. The incubation period for hepatitis B is 30 to 90 days. A three-dose vaccine against hepatitis B virus (HBV) is available, and a combination HAV and HBV vaccine has been approved for adults. Hepatitis C virus (HCV) has been associated with posttransfusion hepatitis but is also associated with

IV drug abuse. It has an incubation period of 30 to 90 days. Hepatitis D virus (HDV) can infect only persons who are actively producing surface antigen for hepatitis B (HBsAg).

SYMPTOMS

During incubation phase: none.

During active phase:

- Viral symptoms in early prodrome. Fever ++++, nausea +++, vomiting +++, malaise, fatigue, anorexia, headache, and chills
- Disturbance of taste
- Pruritic rash, arthralgias and arthritis, especially with hepatitis B
- Altered mental status and seizures with hepatic encephalopathy in fulminant disease

SIGNS

- Dark urine
- Clay-colored stools
- Scleral or sublingual icterus
- Jaundice +++
- Tender hepatomegaly +++
- Splenomegaly +
- Lymphadenopathy ++
- Low-grade fever
- Skin excoriations (because of scratching)
- Asterixis, hyperreflexia, and clonus with hepatic encephalopathy

WORKUP

- Liver function tests: Transaminase levels are often extremely elevated in acute viral or toxic injury to the liver. Less marked elevations (two to three times normal) with AST higher than ALT are suggestive of alcoholic liver injury. If alkaline phosphatase, conjugated bilirubin, or GGTP is significantly elevated (>two to three times normal) in the setting of only mildly elevated transaminases, biliary tract obstruction should be considered.
- Hepatitis serologies should be drawn. The presence of immunoglobulin M (IgM) against HAV is diagnostic for acute hepatitis A infection. Acute infection with hepatitis B shows HBsAg, anti-HBs IgM, and anti-hepatitis B core antigen (HBcAg) IgM. The presence of immunoglobulin G (IgG) against HAV or HBsAg (normally written as HBsAb) is representative of either past infection, prior immunization, or acute infection that has been present long enough for the production of IgG to occur. Antibody tests are also available against HCV and HDV.

COMMENTS AND TREATMENT CONSIDERATIONS

Treatment is largely supportive and directed at controlling symptoms. Avoid use of phenothiazines as antiemetics because they may produce cholestasis. Patients who are unable to tolerate oral fluids and those who have signs or symptoms suggestive of fulminant liver failure should be admitted.

In cases of possible exposure to hepatitis B, postexposure prophylaxis (PEP) should be given when indicated (Table 23–1).

TABLE 23–1
POSTEXPOSURE HEPATITIS B PROPHYLAXIS

VACCINATION AND ANTIBODY RESPONSE STATUS OF EXPOSED PERSON	TREATMENT		
	Source HBsAg Positive	Source HBsAg Negative	Source Unknown or Not Available for Testing
Unvaccinated			
	HBIG ×1 and initiate series	Initiate HB vaccine series	Initiate HB vaccine series
Previously Vaccinated			
Known responder (adequate levels of serum antibodies to HBsAg, i.e., ≥10 mIU/ml)	No treatment	No treatment	No treatment
Known nonresponder (inadequate levels of serum antibodies to HBsAg, i.e., <10 mIU/ml)	HBIG ×1 and initiate revaccination (unless has already completed two 3-dose vaccine series) or HBIG ×2 (if has already completed two 3-dose vaccine series)	No treatment	If known high-risk source, treat as if source were HBsAg positive
Antibody response unknown	Test exposed person for anti-HBs If adequate, no treatment is necessary If inadequate, administer HBIG ×1 and vaccine booster	No treatment	Test exposed person for anti-HBs If adequate, no treatment is necessary If inadequate, administer vaccine booster recheck titer in 1-2 months

Adapted from Updated Public Health Service guidelines for the management of occupational exposures to hepatitis B, hepatitis C, and HIV and recommendations for postexposure prophylaxis, *MMWR Recomm Rep* 55(RR-11):1, 2001.
Persons who have previously been infected with HBV are immune to reinfection and do not require postexposure prophylaxis.
The dose of HBIG is 0.06 ml/kg intramuscularly.

For PEP in persons exposed to hepatitis A, a dose of 0.02 ml/kg of immune globulin can be given IM within 2 weeks of the exposure. The effectiveness of this, however, is controversial. Immune globulin and antiviral agents are not recommended for PEP after exposure to HCV-positive blood.

REFERENCES

Craig AS, Schaffner W: Prevention of hepatitis A with the hepatitis A vaccine, *N Engl J Med* 350:476, 2004.

Guss DA: Liver and biliary tract. In Marx JA, Hockberger RS, Walls RM, et al (eds): *Rosen's emergency medicine—concepts and clinical practice*, ed 5. St Louis, 2002, Mosby.

PHLS Hepatitis Subcommittee: Hepatitis C virus: guidance on the risks and current management of occupational exposure, *Commun Dis Rep CDR Rev* 3:R135, 1993.

Taliani G, Gaeta GB: Hepatitis A: post-exposure prophylaxis, *Vaccine* 21:2234, 2003.

Tran TT, Martin P: Hepatitis B: epidemiology and natural history, *Clin Liver Dis* 8:255, 2004.

Updated Public Health Service guidelines for the management of occupational exposures to hepatitis B, hepatitis C, and HIV and recommendations for postexposure prophylaxis, *MMWR Recomm Rep* 55(RR-11):1, 2001.

CHOLECYSTITIS, CHOLANGITIS, AND COMMON BILE DUCT OBSTRUCTION

See Chapter 1, Abdominal Pain.

HEMOLYSIS

Patients who present to the ED with jaundice caused by hemolysis often have known disorders such as sickle cell disease (SCD), glucose-6-phosphate dehydrogenase (G6PD) deficiency, or other hemoglobinopathies. In patients with these disorders, hemolysis can be induced by oxidative stress such as hypoxia, infection, acidosis, or oxidative drug usage. Hemolysis can also be due to mechanical or infectious causes such as microangiopathic hemolytic anemia (MAHA), repetitive extremity trauma, heart valve irregularities or prosthetic valves, hypersplenism, burns, malaria, or mycoplasma or parvovirus infection. Autoimmune hemolysis is also common.

SYMPTOMS

- Fatigue, weakness, lightheadedness
- Syncope or near-syncope especially if concomitant vascular disease

- Dyspnea or exertion or palpitations
- Bleeding if associated with DIC
- Nausea/vomiting and right upper quadrant pain if hemolysis is due to HELLP syndrome
- Hemoglobinuria on voiding after sleep if due to paroxysmal nocturnal hemoglobinuria

SIGNS
- Pallor
- Jaundice
- Splenomegaly (absent in adults with SCD)
- Shock, tachypnea, tachycardia, congestive heart failure, and mental status changes if the drop in hematocrit is severe and acute.

WORKUP
- Hematocrit
- Haptoglobin (haptoglobin bound to iron released from hemolyzed red blood cells is removed by the reticuloendothelial system, so haptoglobin is decreased in hemolysis)
- Reticulocyte count (if not elevated, may indicate aplastic crisis in SCD; one third of cases of autoimmune hemolysis have reticulocytopenia)
- LFTs and bilirubin (bilirubin: indirect > direct in hemolysis, LFTs typically normal)
- Peripheral blood smear—to look for signs of hemolysis
- LDH (increased in hemolysis)
- For diagnosis of immune or autoimmune hemolysis, direct Coombs test may be ordered.

CHAPTER 23

COMMENTS AND TREATMENT CONSIDERATIONS
Transfusion may be necessary if anemia is severe and there is no evidence of reticulocytosis. Febrile patients with SCD should have workup to identify the source of infection and be treated with antibiotics if indicated.

Women in the third trimester of pregnancy who present with jaundice may be suffering from acute fatty liver of pregnancy or from preeclampsia/eclampsia that has progressed to the HELLP syndrome (hemolysis, elevated liver enzymes, and low platelets). Patients with HELLP syndrome suffer from nausea, vomiting, and right upper quadrant pain and are at risk for bleeding and the rare complication of spontaneous liver rupture. Patients with acute fatty liver of pregnancy can present with jaundice, encephalopathy, and coagulopathy. Both syndromes require emergent delivery and ICU care.

REFERENCES

Claster S, Vichinsky EP: Managing sickle cell disease, *BMJ* 327:1151, 2003.

Clenney TL, Viera AJ: Corticosteroids for HELLP (haemolysis, elevated liver enzymes, low platelets) syndrome, *BMJ* 329:270, 2004.

Dhaliwal G, Cornett PA, Tierney LM Jr: Hemolytic anemia, *Am Fam Physician* 69:2599, 2004.

Heilpern, KL, Quest TE: Jaundice. In Marx JA, Hockberger RS, Walls RM et al (eds): *Rosen's emergency medicine—concepts and clinical practice*, ed 5. St Louis, 2002, Mosby.

 ACETAMINOPHEN OVERDOSE

See Chapter 37, Toxic Exposure, Approach to.

Joint Pain
Samuel Ong

Nontraumatic joint pain may be monoarticular, polyarticular, or migratory. Although most patients presenting to the emergency department with nontraumatic joint pain are experiencing an acute exacerbation of a chronic arthritis, a small proportion of these patients have septic arthritis, a true medical emergency. Joint swelling and pain characterize septic arthritis. Nongonococcal septic arthritis is generally, although not always, monoarticular and most commonly involves the knee but may involve any joint, including the hip. Gonococcal arthritis is the most common cause of bacterial arthritis in sexually active adults and is generally migratory and asymmetric. It often has an associated typical rash.

Distinguishing septic arthritis from other generally monoarticular "inflammatory arthritides" (e.g., crystal induced) can be exceedingly difficult on clinical grounds alone. A history of gout or pseudogout and typical location of swelling (e.g., first metatarsophalangeal joint in foot in gout) can be helpful. In most cases, however, arthrocentesis is *required* to rule out a septic cause of swelling because of the serious implications of a missed infection. Both septic and crystal-induced arthritis generally lead to an increase in synovial fluid WBC >20,000. Visualization of crystals under polarized light establishes the diagnosis of crystal disease, although rarely an infection coexists. Gram staining that shows organisms is relatively insensitive but specific (i.e., if present, establishes the diagnosis; if absent, does not rule out septic joint). Full recovery can be expected if treatment is initiated within the first few days of symptoms. It is also important to remember that osteomyelitis accompanies septic arthritis in about half of the cases seen in neonates and young infants because of vessels that cross the physis before formation of the epiphyseal plate (at 6 months to 1 year). Occasionally, spirochetal infections (e.g., Lyme disease, syphilis) and rarely systemic diseases can also cause monoarticular arthritis. A detailed history, physical examination, and history of possible tick exposure direct the investigation of these conditions.

Polyarticular arthritis can be caused by a number of systemic illnesses, including rheumatoid arthritis, rheumatic fever, Reiter syndrome (nongonococcal urethritis, asymmetric polyarthritis, and conjunctivitis), Lyme disease, serum sickness, SLE, and viral arthritis. Nonarticular signs and symptoms are the key to suspecting these diagnoses in most cases.

Other conditions such as slipped capital femoral epiphysis, Legg-Calvé-Perthes disease, or osteomyelitis may mimic arthritis and should be considered when appropriate.

 SEPTIC ARTHRITIS OF THE HIP

See Chapter 25, Limping Child/Child Won't Walk.

 SEPTIC ARTHRITIS (NONGONOCOCCAL)

The knee is by far the most commonly affected joint (>50%) followed in order by the hip, ankle, wrist, elbow, and shoulder. The small joints of the hand and foot are infrequently affected in the absence of trauma. The majority of adults have some underlying joint abnormality, most commonly rheumatoid arthritis or osteoarthritis. Children frequently have no underlying disease. A history of trauma, intravenous drug use, or diseases that affect the immune system such as malignancy, diabetes, sickle cell disease, and chronic liver or kidney failure are risk factors.

SYMPTOMS
- Swelling
- Joint pain
- Decreased mobility
- Fever ++

SIGNS
- Erythema, warmth, and joint effusion are usually present but are neither sensitive nor specific for septic arthritis.
- Fever ++
- Monoarticular ++++
- Polyarticular ++
- Most specific sign is limitation of active and passive movement of the joint, but its absence cannot be used reliably to exclude septic arthritis, particularly in very mobile joints such as the shoulder.

WORKUP

- Arthrocentesis is required.
- Joint fluid aspirate WBC >20,000 ++++
- Joint fluid aspirate PMNs >75% ++++
- Most aspirates with WBC >50,000 and PMNs >85% are septic.
- Inoculate blood culture bottles because recent studies have found fastidious organisms.
- A low glucose and elevated protein in the synovial fluid are neither sensitive nor specific, but if glucose is markedly reduced (<2.8 mmol), increased specificity for septic cause.
- Gram stain and culture of joint fluid +++
- Polarizing microscopy to look for crystals
- Blood cultures +++ may be warranted because they may be positive when synovial fluid cultures are not. Some data also suggest that blood cultures have prognostic value; when positive, the outcome is worse.
- Elevated blood WBC and ESR are poorly discriminatory.
- Consider Lyme serology
- Plain radiographs are useful for diagnosing bone disease (e.g., slipped femoral capital epiphysis, Legg-Calvé-Perthes disease, or osteomyelitis) but are not useful for diagnosing septic effusion.
- Ultrasound of the hip is sensitive for effusions and, if negative, essentially excludes the diagnosis of septic arthritis for that joint. Hip effusions should be aspirated under ultrasound guidance by a physician skilled in the procedure.

COMMENTS AND TREATMENT CONSIDERATIONS

Treatment of septic arthritis consists of intravenous antibiotics, ED orthopedic consultation, and hospital admission. When the history, physical examination, and joint fluid analysis suggest the diagnosis, the patient should be admitted to the hospital and treated presumptively for septic arthritis pending the results of cultures. Choice of antibiotics depends on age, comorbidities, and presence of articular foreign body. Antibiotics should cover *Staphylococcus aureus* and *Streptococcus* spp in addition to other organisms as indicated. A short course of dexamethasone may reduce residual joint dysfunction in children.

REFERENCES

Del Beccaro MA, Champoux AN, Bockers T, Mendelman PM: Septic arthritis versus transient synovitis of the hip: the value of screening laboratory tests, *Ann Emerg Med* 21:1418, 1992.

Kaandorp CJ, Krijnen P, Bernelot Moens HJ, et al: The outcome of bacterial arthritis: a prospective, community-based study, *Arthritis Rheum* 40:884, 1997.

CHAPTER 24

Li SF, Henderson J, Dickman E, Darzynkiewicz R: Laboratory Tests in Adults with Monoarticular Arthritis: Can They Rule Out a Septic Joint?, *Acad Emerg Med.* 11:276, 2004.

Odio CM, Ramirez T, Arias G, Abdelnour A, et al: Double blind, randomized, placebo-controlled study of dexamethasone therapy for hematogenous septic arthritis in children. *Pediatr Infect Dis J.* 10:883, 2003.

Shmerling RH, Delbanco TL, Tosteson ANA, Trentham DE: Synovial fluid tests: what should be ordered? *JAMA* 264:1009, 1990.

 DISSEMINATED GONOCOCCAL INFECTION

Disseminated gonococcal infection is commonly manifested by arthritis, tenosynovitis, and a characteristic rash (arthritis-dermatitis syndrome). Other, less common complications of gonococcal infection include abscesses, pyomyositis, osteomyelitis, pericarditis, and perihepatitis (Fitz-Hugh–Curtis syndrome). Gonococcal arthritis, unlike other causes of bacterial arthritis, has a very good prognosis; full recovery of the joint is the norm. The groups at highest risk include women who are pregnant, postpartum, or near menstruation (1 week) and promiscuous homosexual men.

SYMPTOMS
- Polyarthralgia +++, which is frequently migratory and occasionally progresses to septic arthritis. The wrist, ankle, or knee is commonly involved.
- Periarticular pain ++++ is slightly more common than monoarthritis.
- Rash ++++
- Fever and chills +++

SIGNS
- Rash ++++; painful red papules on digits and distal extremities. May have gray necrotic center +++. The lesions are usually few in number ("countable" and often <10). More than 100 suggests the possibility of infection with *Neisseria meningitidis*.
- Tenosynovitis is most commonly seen in the wrist and fingers, whereas arthritis is usually found in the knee, ankle, hip, or elbow.

WORKUP
- Arthrocentesis
- Synovial fluid WBC usually >20,000 (i.e., inflammatory) ++++
- Gram stain and culture have limited sensitivity +++.
- Small studies have shown gonococcal polymerase chain reaction to be positive in all culture-proven gonococcal infections as well as some that were culture negative.

- Genitourinary tract cultures are highest yield ++++.
- Pharynx and rectum cultures are occasionally diagnostic. Cultures are frequently positive in the absence of localizing symptoms.
- Blood cultures +++

COMMENTS AND TREATMENT CONSIDERATIONS

Hospitalization for intravenous antibiotics (e.g., ceftriaxone) is generally required, although outpatient parenteral therapy with close supervision may be appropriate in some cases.

REFERENCES

Bardin T: Gonococcal arthritis, *Best Pract Res Clin Rheumatol* 17:201, 2003.

Garcia-De La Torre I: Advances in the management of septic arthritis, *Rheum Dis Clin North Am* 29:61, 2003.

Wise CM, Morris CR, Wailaukas BL, Salzer WL: Gonococcal arthritis in an era of increasing penicillin resistance: presentations and outcomes in 41 recent cases (1985-1991), *Arch Intern Med* 154:2690, 1994.

CHAPTER 24

Limping Child/Child Won't Walk
Alisa McQueen and Beverly Bauman

Determining the cause of acute limping in a child can be a diagnostic challenge, particularly in the very young child who is unable to describe and localize symptoms. Whereas many of the possible causes are benign, the differential diagnosis includes conditions that can lead to major morbidity or death if not detected early. The history, presentation, and frequency of these disorders change with age.

REFERENCES
Joffe MD, Loiselle JM: Orthopedic emergencies. In Fleisher GR, Ludwig S (eds): *Textbook of pediatric emergency medicine*, ed 5. Philadelphia, 2006, Lippincott Williams & Wilkins, pp 1689-1708.
Kost S: Limp. In Fleisher GR, Ludwig S (eds): *Textbook of pediatric emergency medicine*, ed 5. Philadelphia, 2006, Lippincott Williams & Wilkins, pp 415-420.

 SEPTIC ARTHRITIS

Bacterial infection in a joint is a medical emergency because delay in its diagnosis and treatment can lead to destruction of the joint cartilage and permanent disability. Although septic arthritis can occur in any joint, the most commonly affected joints in the pediatric age group are the hip (38%) and knee (32%). The bacterial etiology and clinical presentation change with age. Toxic or transient synovitis is an inflammatory disease that may cause hip or knee pain and low-grade fever. Aspiration of the hip may be required to distinguish this entity, which is treated on an outpatient basis with nonsteroidal anti-inflammatory agents, from a septic joint, which requires aggressive management. Specific information relevant to pediatrics is noted here; see Septic Joints in Chapter 24, Joint Pain, for more information.

SYMPTOMS
- Refusal to bear weight or use the affected joint
- "Pseudoparalysis" or prevention of joint movement in infants

SIGNS
- The infected joint is held in a position that helps to decrease intracapsular pressure and subsequent pain. A septic hip is held in flexion, external rotation, and abduction. The knee is held in mild flexion. The ankle is held in mild plantar flexion.
- Active or passive movement of the infected joint causes severe pain.
- Warmth of the skin overlying the joint
- Erythema of the skin overlying the joint
- Joint swelling with or without a palpable effusion
- Fever >38° C has limited sensitivity +++.

WORKUP
See Chapter 24, Joint Pain.
- Elevated erythrocyte sedimentation rate and leukocytosis may be seen but are frequently absent. An elevation in either value should prompt careful consideration of septic arthritis.
- Blood cultures ++ may guide later therapy.
- Ultrasound of the hip; if positive, joint should be aspirated by a physician skilled in the procedure.
- X-rays may demonstrate subtle changes of increased joint space widening from an effusion, soft tissue swelling, or obliteration of normal fat lines around the joint. Osteomyelitis can occur in association with septic joints, particularly in infants and young children, who have blood vessels that cross the growth plate. The sensitivity of plain radiographs is poor for both evidence of septic arthritis and osteomyelitis. Their greatest use is to rule out fracture.
- Urethral, pelvic, or pharyngeal cultures for *Neisseria gonorrhoeae* should be obtained if sexually transmitted diseases could be present at those sites.

COMMENTS AND TREATMENT CONSIDERATIONS
Treatment consists of prompt joint drainage and antibiotic administration. Hematogenous spread is the most common mode of joint infection in children. A thorough physical examination to investigate other sites of infection is mandatory. *Staphylococcus aureus* is the most common organism. In neonates, *S. aureus* and group A and group B streptococci predominate. *Neisseria gonorrhoeae* should be suspected in sexually active adolescents. Adolescent intravenous drug abusers are at risk for gram-negative organisms. The incidence of *Haemophilus influenzae* septic arthritis has fallen

CHAPTER **25**

dramatically with the routine administration of HIB vaccine. History of immunization compliance is important to ascertain.

Differentiation between septic arthritis and transient synovitis is paramount. In one study, the presence of three or more of the following variables was highly predictive of septic arthritis: refusal to bear weight, history of fever, ESR >40 mm/hr, and leukocytosis >12,000. Orthopedic consultation is indicated for all highly suspected and confirmed cases of septic arthritis.

REFERENCES

Kocher MS, Mandiga R, Zurackowski D, et al: Validation of a clinical prediction rule for the differentiation between septic arthritis and transient synovitis of the hip in children, *J Bone Joint Surg Am* 86:1629, 2004.

Shah SS: Abnormal gait in a child with fever: diagnosing septic arthritis of the hip, *Pediatr Emerg Care* 21:336, 2005.

 SLIPPED CAPITAL FEMORAL EPIPHYSIS

Slipped capital femoral epiphysis (SCFE) is a displacement of the normal relationship between the femoral head and femoral neck through the growth plate. It is the most common hip disorder in adolescents, occurring during the peak of the growth spurt. It is more common in overweight boys and is occasionally associated with hypothyroidism and other endocrine disorders. SCFE is preceded by trauma in only 25% of cases. A substantial minority of children with this diagnosis present with knee pain only, often leading to delay in diagnosis and an increased risk of complications.

SYMPTOMS

- Pain (hip, knee, thigh, or groin pain) often exacerbated by movement of the hip or ambulation. Hip pain is frequently referred to the medial knee.
- Altered gait
- Pain and limp can be acute or chronic. Small amounts of slippage can occur over a period of months, and an acute slip may be superimposed on chronic slippage after relatively minor trauma (the so-called acute-on-chronic slip).

SIGNS

- The hip is held in relative flexion and external rotation.
- External rotation upon passive hip flexion.
- Internal rotation and abduction may be limited.
- Atrophy of the thigh and a "toe-out" gait if symptoms have been long-standing

- Shortening of the affected lower extremity depends on the degree of slippage.

WORKUP

X-ray (anteroposterior view of the pelvis and frog-leg lateral views of both hips) may show subtle findings or gross displacement of the femoral epiphysis on the proximal femoral metaphysis, depending on the degree of slippage. Early slips may just show slight irregularity and widening of the epiphysis. On the AP view, a line is drawn from the lateral edge of the femoral neck cephalad toward the joint on the same side. The portion of the epiphysis lateral to this line should be symmetric on both hips. If it is not, SCFE should be suspected. On the frog-leg view, more advanced slips look like a scoop of ice cream slipping off the cone. The slip may be bilateral (++), and careful examination and radiographic evaluation of the contralateral hip, even if asymptomatic, are indicated.

COMMENTS AND TREATMENT CONSIDERATIONS

Hospital admission and strict bed rest with no weight bearing prevent further slippage of the femoral epiphysis. An orthopedic surgeon should be consulted because the condition usually requires surgical pinning. Delay in diagnosis is particularly common among children presenting with knee pain. Up to 50% of missed SCFE diagnoses occurred in patients who had only knee complaints. If unrecognized prior to growth plate closure, untreated SCFE leads to significant deformity and dysfunction.

REFERENCES

Loder R, Aronsson D, Doobs M, et al: Slipped capital femoral epiphysis, *J Bone Joint Surg Am* 82:1170, 2000.

Perron A, Miller M, Brady W: Orthopedic pitfalls in the ED: slipped capital femoral epiphysis, *Am J Emerg Med* 20:484, 2002.

 OSTEOMYELITIS

Osteomyelitis should be considered in all patients with bone pain or tenderness, particularly in the setting of fever (although fever is frequently absent), or if the evaluation does not provide another diagnosis. A history of trauma is often given and may represent a precipitating event or simply be a coincidence of normal childhood.

See Chapter 4, Back Pain, Lower.

SYMPTOMS

- Bone pain
- Fever (frequently absent)

289

- Smaller children and infants may have vague symptoms of irritability and poor feeding or may appear toxic or septic.

SIGNS
- Bone tenderness +++ in toddlers and young children. The older the patient, the easier it is to detect the exact site of tenderness on examination.
- Limp or refusal to walk +++
- Fever +++. The absence of fever does not exclude the diagnosis, particularly among patients who have been taking pain medication with antipyretic effects.
- Overlying erythema
- Joint motion can be limited from the local muscle spasm caused by inflammation.

WORKUP
- Bone scan ++++; the method of choice for detecting early pediatric osteomyelitis, particularly when the precise location of the infection is unclear
- MRI of the affected area demonstrates presence of abscesses and abnormal marrow signal.
- C-reactive protein is highly sensitive even in early osteomyelitis.
- Erythrocyte sedimentation rate ++++ peaks in 3 to 5 days but may be normal in early osteomyelitis.
- Blood cultures may help direct therapy +++ but are positive in only 30% of cases.
- WBC has low sensitivity ++.
- X-rays are negative early in the disease process but may detect another cause for a limp (e.g., fracture or neoplasm). Before bone changes of osteomyelitis are evident, an x-ray may reveal soft tissue swelling and blurring of the adjacent fat planes. The characteristic finding of periosteal elevation may be seen within 7 to 10 days.
- Joint aspiration is indicated if septic arthritis is suspected because this may coexist with osteomyelitis. Infants and young children are at high risk for coexisting septic arthritis because of blood vessels that cross the growth plate in this age group.
- Aspiration of fluid beneath the periosteum for culture may be considered by a consulting orthopedist.

COMMENTS AND TREATMENT CONSIDERATIONS
Over half of pediatric osteomyelitis cases involve bones of the lower extremity. Overall, the most common cause of osteomyelitis is *Staphylococcus aureus*. In neonates, group B *Streptococcus* and enteric gram-negative organisms are also found. In infants and toddlers who have not been adequately immunized, *H. influenzae*

should be considered. *Salmonella* is a common cause of osteomyelitis in patients with sickle cell anemia. *Pseudomonas aeruginosa* is often associated with puncture wounds of the foot, especially those sustained while wearing tennis shoes. Community-acquired *methicillin-resistant Staphylococcus aureus* has become an increasingly common pathogen and should be considered in areas where this organism is prevalent.

The most common source of osteomyelitis is hematogenous spread from another site of infection, and the bone metaphysis is the most common site of seeding. Extension from a local skin or muscle infection can also occur. Consider tuberculosis or a fungal cause in appropriate patients.

REFERENCES

Darville T, Jacobs R: Management of acute hematogenous osteomyelitis in children, *Pediatr Infect Dis J* 23:255, 2004.

Ferguson L, Beattie T: Lesson of the week: osteomyelitis in the well looking afebrile child, *BMJ* 324:1380, 2002.

McCarthy JJ, Dormans JP, Kozin SH, et al: Musculoskeletal infections in children: basic treatment principles and recent advancements, *J Bone Joint Surg Am* 86:850, 2004.

 SPINAL EPIDURAL ABSCESS

See Epidural Abscess in Chapter 4, Back Pain, Lower.

REFERENCES

Auletta J, John C. Spinal epidural abscesses in children: a 15-year experience and review of the literature, *Clin Infect Dis* 32:9, 2001.

 MALIGNANCIES

Malignant bone and soft tissue tumors are uncommon causes of limping in children. However, early diagnosis is critical and can be lifesaving. Leukemia is the most frequent childhood malignancy. The skeleton is often the first body system to display overt manifestations of the acute form of the disease. Osteogenic sarcoma, Ewing sarcoma, leukemia, spinal cord tumors, soft tissue sarcomas, and metastatic tumors of the extremities may cause limb pain or limping.

SYMPTOMS

- Knee pain is a common complaint in adolescents, but the two most common sites for bone tumors are the distal femur and proximal tibia. Knee pain that occurs at rest or at night should be a cause for concern.

- Musculoskeletal pain +++ in cases of acute leukemia is often intermittent, sharp, and migratory in nature.
- Fatigue or lethargy
- Fever

SIGNS
- Focal tenderness at the site of a bone tumor may be elicited by direct palpation.
- Thorough general physical examination may show hepatosplenomegaly, lymphadenopathy, pallor, purpura, or bleeding, which can be signs of leukemia or of other malignancies.
- Palpation of the muscles in the lower extremity may reveal a soft tissue mass as evidence of a rhabdomyosarcoma or other soft tissue tumor.
- Hyperreflexia or weakness of the lower extremities can point to a tumor in the spinal area.

WORKUP
- Plain films of the site of localized pain. Referred pain should be kept in mind and further distal radiographic studies considered if initial ones are negative.
- CBC including leukocyte differential and platelet count

COMMENTS AND TREATMENT CONSIDERATIONS
A history of trauma is often present, which may be coincidental or may indicate a weakened bone predisposed to a pathologic fracture. Appropriate consultation after diagnosis or for further evaluation is required.

REFERENCES
Arndt CA, Crist WM: Common musculoskeletal tumors of childhood and adolescence, *N Engl J Med* 341:342, 1999.

Ortiz EJ, Isler MH, Navia JE, et al: Pathologic fractures in children, *Clin Orthop Relat Res* 432:116, 2005.

Trueworthy RC, Templeton KJ: Malignant bone tumors presenting as musculoskeletal pain, *Pediatr Ann* 31:355, 2002.

 LEGG-CALVÉ-PERTHES DISEASE

Legg-Calvé-Perthes disease is avascular necrosis of the femoral head that occurs most commonly in boys between 5 and 9 years of age and is generally insidious in onset. Hip pain and limp are noted. X-rays may initially be negative; bone scan and MRI are more sensitive. Orthopedic consultation is required because prompt diagnosis and successful treatment decrease the risk of developing osteoarthritis in the affected hip.

REFERENCES
Lecuire F: The long-term outcome of primary osteochondritis of the hip (Legg-Calve-Perthes' disease), *J Bone Joint Surg Br* 84:636, 2002.

Wall E: Legg-Calvé-Perthes disease, *Curr Opin Pediatr* 11:76-80, 1999.

 ## PSOAS ABSCESS AND APPENDICITIS

Occult retroperitoneal, abdominal, or pelvic infections may cause limping in a young child.

See Chapter 1, Abdominal Pain.

SYMPTOMS
- Patients with psoas abscess may present with hip, groin, abdomen, lower back, buttock, or upper thigh pain associated with fever and limping.

SIGNS
- Hip held in flexion, abduction, and external rotation (like septic arthritis of the hip). Psoas abscess may be differentiated from the septic hip by increased pain with extension related to stretching of the iliopsoas muscle. Gentle internal and external rotation is less painful with a psoas abscess than with a septic hip.
- Rectal examination may occasionally reveal a mass and tenderness on the affected side.
- Scoliosis to the side of the abscess
- Gait disturbance manifested by a cautious, slow gait and flexion of the trunk may be observed with appendicitis.

WORKUP
- CT scan is sensitive for psoas abscess and appendicitis.
- Abdominal ultrasound may reveal evidence of appendicitis or other pathologic conditions of the pelvis but frequently misses a psoas abscess because of the presence of abdominal gas. The value of ultrasound in evaluating for appendicitis is operator dependent.

COMMENTS AND TREATMENT CONSIDERATIONS
Appendicitis is the most common surgical emergency of childhood. CT imaging is now commonly used to establish the diagnosis, particularly in cases with an equivocal history, physical examination,

CHAPTER 25

and laboratory findings. Admission to the hospital for observation and repeated abdominal examinations remains a reasonable alternative. Surgical consultation is needed when appendicitis and psoas abscess are suspected because the treatment is surgical.

REFERENCES

Mormino MA, Esposito PW, Raynor SC: Peripelvic abscesses: a diagnostic dilemma, *J Pediatr Orthop* 19:161,1999.

Song J, Letts M, Monson R: Differentiation of psoas muscle abscess from septic arthritis of the hip in children, *Clin Orthop Relat Res* 391:258, 2001.

 CHILD ABUSE

See Chapter 22, The Irritable Child.

Mass Casualty Exposure
Rick G. Kulkarni, Gregory J. Moran, and Scott R. Votey

Mass casualty exposures may occur by accident or arise from an intentional attack. Although evaluation and treatment of victims of an intentional attack share common features with those of other exposures, the agent may be unknown, altered from familiar agents, or include a mix of agents and methods designed to create maximal death and disability. In addition, attacks are often phased so that first responders and others fall victim to a second wave of attack. It is critical that medical and law enforcement personnel work closely together at the scene of a mass casualty event.

There are five categories of exposures, which are often abbreviated as CBRNE: *c*hemical, *b*iological, *r*adiological *n*uclear explosions, and conventional *e*xplosives. An understanding of these agents and their health effects is essential to provide effective care to victims and minimize risk to caregivers.

AN APPROACH TO THE UNKNOWN THREAT

If there is a chemical, biological, or radiological exposure, care providers are not likely to know which agent was used. This is particularly true in the early stages of an event, when people first begin to become ill. Because many agents are likely to be used covertly, it may not even be known that an attack has occurred until many people have fallen ill.

The Unknown Threat Algorithm (Fig. 26–1) is meant to guide care following a mass casualty chemical or biological attack involving an unknown agent. The goal of this approach is to allow identification of the causative agent of an "outbreak" of illness sufficiently to (1) provide appropriate treatment to limit morbidity and mortality and (2) take measures to contain the outbreak within a larger population that might develop illness either because of the initial exposure or from secondary spread. The algorithm does not include

295

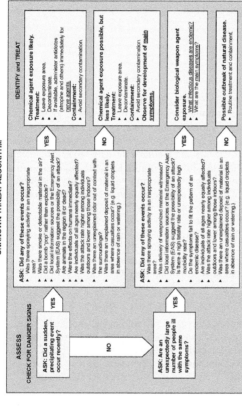

UNKNOWN THREAT ALGORITHM

ASSESS
CHECK FOR DANGER SIGNS

ASK: Did a sudden, precipitating event occur recently? — YES →

ASK: Did any of these events occur?
- Was there spraying activity in an inappropriate area?
- Was there smoke or detectable material in the air?
- Did a bomb "pop" rather than explode?
- Did local information sources or the Emergency Alert System (EAS) suggest the possibility of an attack?
- Were the effects on humans immediate?
- Are animals in the region ill or dead?
- Were individuals of all ages nearly equally affected?
- Was the attack rate higher among individuals outdoors and lower among those indoors?
- Was there an unexplained odor or out of context with the surroundings?
- Was there an unplanned deposit of material in an area where casualties occur? (e.g. liquid droplets in absence of rain or watering.)

YES →

IDENTIFY and TREAT

Chemical agent exposure likely.
Treatment:
- Leave exposure area.
- Decontaminate.
- If available, administer antidotes (atropine and others) immediately for nerve agents.
Containment:
- Avoid secondary contamination.

NO →

Chemical agent exposure possible, but less likely.
Treatment:
- Leave exposure area.
- Decontaminate.
Containment:
- Avoid secondary contamination.
- Observe for development of <u>main symptoms.</u>

ASK: Are an unexpectedly large number of people ill with the same symptoms? — YES →

ASK: Did any of these events occur?
- Was there spraying activity in an inappropriate area?
- Was delivery of weaponized material witnessed?
- Did local information sources or the Emergency Alert System (EAS) suggest the possibility of an attack?
- Is there an high fatality rate or unexpectedly high morbidity rate?
- Do the symptoms fail to fit the pattern of an endemic disease?
- Are individuals of all ages nearly equally affected?
- Was the attack rate higher among individuals outdoors and lower among those indoors?
- Was there an unplanned deposit of material in an area where casualties occur? (e.g. liquid droplets in absence of rain or watering.)

YES →

Consider biological weapon agent exposure.
- What infectious diseases are endemic?
- What are the <u>main symptoms?</u>

NO →

Possible outbreak of natural disease.
- Routine treatment and containment.

THEN ASK ABOUT MAIN SYMPTOMS
- Seizures or focal neurological abnormalities?
- Cough or trouble breathing?
- Diarrhea and/or vomiting?
- Rash or other skin signs?

Continued

Fig. 26–1 Unknown Threat Algorithm.

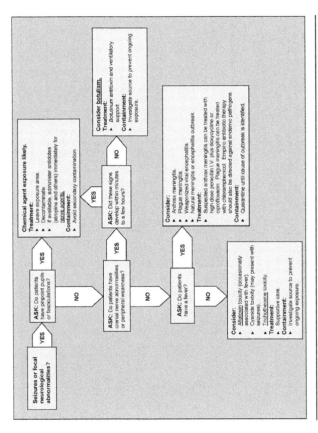

Fig. 26–1 cont'd

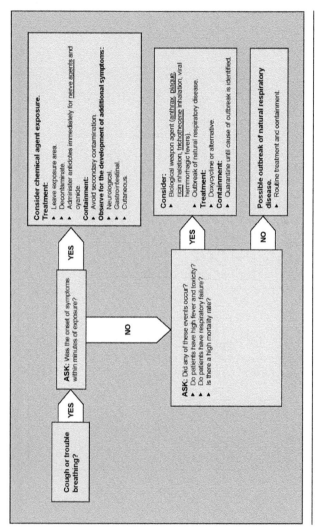

Cough or trouble breathing?

YES →

ASK: Was the onset of symptoms within minutes of exposure?

YES → **Consider chemical agent exposure.**
Treatment:
- Leave exposure area.
- Decontaminate.
- Administer antidotes immediately for nerve agents and cyanide.

Containment:
- Avoid secondary contamination.

Observe for the development of additional symptoms:
- Neurological.
- Gastrointestinal.
- Cutaneous.

NO →

ASK: Did any of these events occur?
- Do patients have high fever and toxicity?
- Do patients have respiratory failure?
- Is there a high mortality rate?

YES → **Consider:**
- Biological weapon agent (anthrax, plague, ricin inhalation, trichothecene inhalation, viral hemorrhagic fevers).
- Outbreak of natural respiratory disease.

Treatment:
- Doxycycline or alternative.

Containment:
- Quarantine until cause of outbreak is identified.

NO → **Possible outbreak of natural respiratory disease.**
- Routine treatment and containment.

Fig. 26–1 cont'd

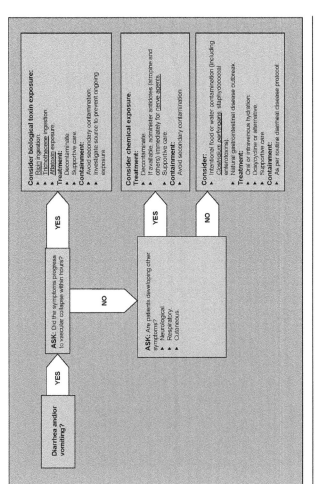

Diarrhea and/or vomiting? — YES →

ASK: Did the symptoms progress to vascular collapse within 1 hours? — YES →

Consider biological toxin exposure:
- Ricin ingestion.
- Trichothecene ingestion
- Aflatoxin exposure.

Treatment:
- Decontaminate
- Supportive care.

Containment:
- Avoid secondary contamination.
- Investigate source to prevent ongoing exposure.

NO ↓

ASK: Are patients developing other symptoms?
- Neurological.
- Respiratory.
- Cutaneous.

YES →

Consider chemical exposure.

Treatment:
- Decontaminate
- If available, administer antidotes (atropine and others) immediately for nerve agents.
- Supportive care.

Containment:
- Avoid secondary contamination

NO →

Consider:
- Intentional food or water contamination (including *Clostridium perfringens* staphylococcal enterotoxins).
- Natural gastrointestinal disease outbreak.

Treatment:
- Oral or intravenous hydration.
- Doxycycline or alternative.
- Supportive care

Containment:
- As per routine diarrheal disease protocol

Fig. 26-1   cont'd

CHAPTER **26**

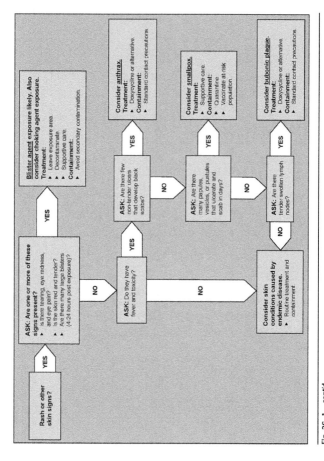

Fig. 26–1 cont'd

SELECT INFECTIONS REPORTED IN THE UNITED STATES

Bacterial Infections:
- Anthrax (Vaccine, limited availability)
- Brucellosis
- Cholera (Vaccine not generally recommended)
- *Clostridia botulinum* (Botulism)
- *Clostridia perfringens*
- Cryptosporidiosis
- Coccidiomycosis
- Diptheria (Vaccine)
- Enterotoxigenic Escherichia coli
- Gonorrhea
- *Haemophilus influenzae*
- Legionellosis
- Listeriosis
- Lyme Disease
- Meningococcal meningitis (Vaccine)
- Pertussis (Vaccine)
- Plague (No effective vaccine for inhalational exposure)
- Pneumococcus
- Psittacosis
- Relapsing fever (*Borrelia recurrentis*, tick- and louse-borne)
- Salmonellosis
- Shigellosis
- Streptococcal Disease, Invasive (Group A)
- Syphilis
- Tetanus (Vaccine)
- Tuberculosis
- Tularemia
- Trachoma
- Typhoid fever (Vaccine)

Viral Infections:
- Dengue
- Hepatitis A (Vaccine)
- Hepatitis B (Vaccine)
- Hepatitis C
- HIV/AIDS
- Influenza (Vaccine)
- Measles (Vaccine)
- Polio (no cases reported in 2002) (Vaccine)
- Rabies (Vaccine)
- Rocky Mountain Spotted Fever
- Rotavirus
- Varicella (Vaccine available in some countries)
- West Nile Fever

Rickettsial Infections:
- Q fever (*Coxiella burnetii*) (Vaccine, limited availability)
- Typhus (*Rickettsia typhi*, flea-borne)
- Typhus (*Rickettsia prowazekii*, louse-borne)

Fungal Infections:
- Histoplasmosis

Protozoal Infections:
- Amebiasis (*Entamoeba histolytica*)
- Giardiasis
- Leishmaniasis (cutaneous and visceral)
- Malaria

SELECT BIOLOGICAL WEAPON AGENTS NOT ENDEMIC TO THE UNITED STATES

- Smallpox
- Viral hemorrhagic fevers (e.g. Ebola, Marburg, Lassa)
- Russian spring/summer encephalitis
- Venezuelan equine encephalitis

Fig. 26-1 cont'd

CHAPTER **26**

every possible agent, only those believed to be credible risks (Table 26–1). The algorithm is based entirely on a brief history and visual inspection of the patient. Laboratory tests or radiographs are not necessary. In addition, in light of the potential risks to caregivers, who may be caught unprepared, its use does not require touching patients who could be contaminated by a chemical or ill with a contagious disease. Patients can be assessed and treatment begun within minutes. Although the algorithm will not usually identify the precise causative agent, identification is sufficiently specific to guide treatment and determine containment strategies. As additional information or resources become available, care providers should use this information to enhance or supplant the basic algorithmic approach.

Many chemical agent exposures result in symptoms immediately, creating awareness of the exposure and often allowing identification of the class of agent used. In contrast, most biological agent exposures do not result in immediate symptoms, so that exposures are unlikely to be identified until people become ill later. Once symptoms have developed, agents may often be identified on the basis of their predominant symptoms and signs. The algorithm cannot be used to identify a radiation exposure. In the absence of a nuclear weapon attack, intentional radiation exposure would probably be from the detonation of a dirty bomb (i.e., a radioactive material dispersion device). If a bomb were to be used for dispersion, the explosion would be apparent. The release of radioactive materials, however, would not be discernible without the use of detection devices.

Treatment recommendations are intended to be feasible and the medications used broadly available and preferably inexpensive. Containment recommendations are based on the safest practice for care for providers and populations at risk. If medical personnel cannot distinguish between agents with different transmission risks, we recommend implementing a higher level of containment measures to minimize spread.

CHEMICAL WEAPONS

Chemical weapons are devices that use hazardous chemicals to incapacitate, injure, or kill intended victims. For weapon use, the chemicals are generally in a gas or liquid form and are dispersed through the air. Some chemical weapon agents have local effects on the eyes, skin, or airways (e.g., chlorine); others have only systemic effects (e.g., hydrogen cyanide); and some have both (e.g., nerve agents). With few exceptions (e.g., sulfur mustard), their effects are typically immediate and dramatic. Although not classified as chemical weapon agents, many industrial chemicals

TABLE 26–1
CHEMICAL AND BIOLOGICAL WEAPON AGENTS

	AGENTS	NEUROLOGIC	RESPIRATORY	GASTROINTESTINAL	SKIN	ONSET AFTER EXPOSURE	PROGRESSION	DEATH (POSTEXPOSURE)
Chemical Weapon Agents	Nerve agents (sarin, tabun, VX)	X	X	X		Minutes–hours	Minutes–hours	Minutes–hours
	Blister agents (sulfur mustard)		X		X	Hours	Hours	Uncommon
	Choking agents (chlorine, phosgene)		X		X	Minutes–hour	Hours	Days
	Blood agents (hydrogen cyanide)	X	X			Seconds–minutes	Minutes	Minutes
	Incapacitating agents (BZ, LSD)	X				Minutes	Minutes	Rare
	Riot control agents (tear gases)		X			Seconds–minutes	Minutes	Rare

Continued

CHAPTER **26**

TABLE 26-1
CHEMICAL AND BIOLOGICAL WEAPON AGENTS—CONT'D

	AGENTS	NEUROLOGIC	RESPIRATORY	GASTROINTESTINAL	SKIN	ONSET AFTER EXPOSURE	PROGRESSION	DEATH (POSTEXPOSURE)
	Anthrax (*Bacillus anthracis*)							
	Skin				X	Days	Days	Uncommon
	Gastrointestinal			X		Days	Days	Days
	Inhalational		X			Days	Hours–days	Hours–days
	Botulism (*Clostridium botulinum* toxin)							
	Inhaled	X				Hours–days	Days	Days
	Ingested	X				Hours–days	Days	Days
	Plague (*Yersinia pestis*)							
	Pneumonic	X	X			Days	Days	Days
	Bubonic	X	(X)	(X)	(X)	Days	Days	Days
	Smallpox (*variola* virus)				X	2 weeks	Days	Weeks
	Viral hemorrhagic fevers (e.g., Ebola, Marburg)	X	(X)	X	X	Days–weeks	Days	Days–weeks
	Tularemia (*Francisella tularensis*), inhaled	(X)	X		(X)	Days–weeks	Days	Days

Biological Weapon Agents · CDC Category A

	Brucellosis (Brucella species)	X		Days-weeks	Days-weeks	Weeks
	Clostridium perfringens (organism or toxins) Ingested			Hours	Hours	Rare
	Injected		X	Hours-days	Hours-days	Hours-days
	Food- and waterborne pathogens		X	Hours-days	Hours-days	Hours-days
B	Glanders (Burkholderia mallei)		X	Days	Weeks	Weeks
	Melioidosis (Burkholderia pseudomallei)		X	Days-years	Days-years	Days-weeks
	Psittacosis (Chlamydia psittaci)	X	X	Weeks	Weeks	Weeks-months
	Q fever (Coxiella burnetii)	(X)	X	Weeks	Weeks-months	Uncommon

CHAPTER 26

Continued

TABLE 26-1
CHEMICAL AND BIOLOGICAL WEAPON AGENTS—CONT'D

	AGENTS	NEUROLOGIC	RESPIRATORY	GASTROINTESTINAL	SKIN	ONSET AFTER EXPOSURE	PROGRESSION	DEATH (POSTEXPOSURE)
B	Ricin (a biotoxin)							
	Inhaled		X			Hours	Hours	Hours–days
	Ingested			X		Hours	Hours	Days
	Staphylococcal enterotoxin B							
	Inhaled		X	X		Hours	Hours–days	Rare
	Ingested			X		Hours	Hours–days	Rare
	Typhus *(Rickettsia prowazekii)*				X	Days	Days	Days
	Viral encephalitis (e.g., Venezuelan equine encephalitis)	X				Days	Days	Days
Other	Aflatoxin, ingested	X		X		Hours	Days	Days–years

	Minutes–hours Hours	Minutes–hours Hours	Minutes–days Days–weeks
Trichothecene mycotoxins Inhaled or skin	X	X	X
Ingested		X	

X = Major symptoms

(X) = Less prominent or variably present symptoms

Notes:

1. Fever, chills, headache, and generalized aches (i.e., "flu-like" symptoms) may be seen with any biological agent (but toxins less likely).
2. Anything delivered by aerosol can have a respiratory presentation.
3. Food– and waterborne pathogens include *Salmonella* species, *Shigella dysenteriae*, *Escherichia coli* O157:H7, *Vibrio cholerae*, and *Cryptosporidium parvum*.

CDC category A agents: Highest priority designation because of the following attributes:

- Can be easily disseminated from person to person
- Result in high mortality rates and have the potential for major public health impact
- Might cause public panic and social disruption
- Require special action for public preparedness

CDC category B agents: Second highest priority designation because of the following attributes:

- Moderately easy to disseminate
- Result in moderate morbidity rates and low mortality rates
- Require specific enhancements of CDC's diagnostic capacity and enhanced disease surveillance

CHAPTER **26**

307

can be hazardous if deliberately or accidentally released into the environment.

Chemical weapon agents are classified by their clinical effects: nerve agents, blister agents (also called vesicants), blood agents, choking agents, and incapacitating agents. Unlike the other agents that are intended to cause serious injury or death, the incapacitating agents are intended to disable victims only temporarily.

 NERVE AGENTS

Nerve agents are chemically similar to organophosphate pesticides. They act by binding and irreversibly inactivating acetylcholinesterase (AChE) receptors. Excessive acetylcholine leads to overstimulation of nicotinic and muscarinic receptors. Death results from respiratory failure caused by respiratory muscle paralysis or severe bronchoconstriction. Physicians practicing in agricultural areas occasionally encounter workers suffering the effects of accidental exposure to organophosphate pesticides.

Nerve agents include tabun (GA), sarin (GB), soman (GD), GF, and VX. All are highly lethal. Nerve agents exist in a liquid form with variable volatility (tendency to form a gas or vapor): VX and tabun have a low degree of volatility, whereas sarin is highly volatile. Agents with low volatility can persist in the environment for several days. High-volatility agents are a greater inhalation hazard but disperse more rapidly.

SYMPTOMS
Specific symptoms and signs and the rate of progression vary depending on route and quantity of exposure (Fig. 26–2).

SIGNS
- Muscarinic receptor activation leads to excessive salivation, lacrimation, vomiting, bronchoconstriction, diarrhea, and urinary and fecal incontinence.
- Nicotinic receptor activation leads to excessive sweating, muscle flaccidity, seizures, coma, and respiratory depression.
- Exposure to high concentrations can lead to rapid loss of consciousness, paralysis, and respiratory failure.

WORKUP
- Treatment cannot wait for laboratory confirmation of exposure and must be based on clinical findings.
- Measure percent reduction in erythrocyte cholinesterase.
- ABG to assess the level of respiratory impairment
- ECG may demonstrate muscarinic receptor–mediated bradydysrhythmias or conduction defects.

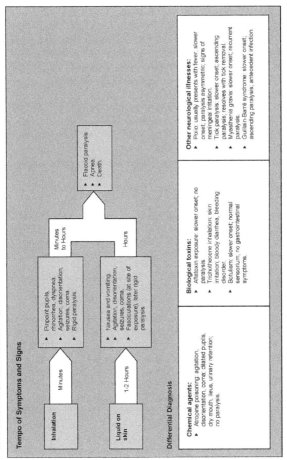

NERVE AGENTS (Sarin, Tabun, VX, etc.)

Tempo of Symptoms and Signs

Inhalation — Minutes →
- Pinpoint pupils, rhinorrhea, dyspnea.
- Agitation, disorientation, seizures, coma.
- Rigid paralysis.

Minutes to Hours →
- Flaccid paralysis.
- Apnea.
- Death.

Liquid on skin — 1-2 Hours →
- Nausea and vomiting.
- Agitation, disorientation, seizures, coma.
- Fasciculations (at site of exposure), later rigid paralysis.

Hours →

Differential Diagnosis

Chemical agents:
- Atropine poisoning: agitation, disorientation, coma; dilated pupils, dry mouth, ileus, urinary retention; no paralysis.

Biological toxins:
- Aflatoxin exposure: slower onset; no paralysis.
- Trichothecene inhalation: skin irritation, bloody diarrhea, bleeding disorder.
- Botulism: slower onset, normal sensorium, no gastrointestinal symptoms.

Other neurological illnesses:
- Polio: usually presents with fever, slower onset, paralysis asymmetric; signs of meningeal irritation.
- Tick paralysis: slower onset, ascending paralysis; resolves with tick removal.
- Myasthenia gravis: slower onset; recurrent paralysis.
- Guillain-Barré syndrome: slower onset; ascending paralysis, antecedent infection.

Fig. 26-2 Nerve agents.

CHAPTER 26

COMMENTS AND TREATMENT CONSIDERATIONS

All patients with suspicion of nerve agent exposure should be immediately decontaminated thoroughly by removing all clothing, rinsing copiously with water, and washing the skin with a solution of soap and water. Rescue and medical personnel can become victims from secondary exposure and should wear personal protective equipment (PPE) while treating victims. Early endotracheal intubation and ventilatory support are essential in severely affected patients. Immediate and aggressive treatment with atropine in 2-mg increments should be administered IV until respiratory secretions have dried. Pralidoxime chloride (2-PAM) prevents the permanent inactivation of AChE and should be administered as soon as possible.

See Table 37–2, Poisons and Their Antidotes, in Chapter 37, Toxic Exposure, Approach to.

REFERENCES

Arnold J: CBRNE—nerve agents, G-series: tabun, sarin, soman, eMedicine.com, Inc, 2004.

Benitez F: CBRNE—nerve agents, V-series: VE, VG, VM, VX, eMedicine.com, Inc, 2004.

Holstege CP, Kirk M, Sidell FR: Chemical warfare: nerve agent poisoning, *Crit Care Clin* 13:923, 1997.

Sidell FR, Borak J: Chemical warfare agents: II. nerve agents, *Ann Emerg Med* 21:865, 1992.

 BLISTER AGENTS (VESICANTS)

Blister agents, also known as vesicants, include mustard agents, lewisite, and phosgene oxime. Named for their ability to cause vesicular lesions of the skin or blistering, they are damaging to any tissue with which they come in contact, including the eyes and lungs. In sufficient concentrations, they can be fatal. Sulfur mustard is the only blister agent that has been used in battle, first in World War I and more recently in the 1980–1988 war between Iran and Iraq.

Blister agents exist as an oily liquid with variable volatility. All easily penetrate clothing and skin. Because these liquids generally have relatively low volatility, they may persist for more than a week, depending on environmental conditions. They may have a characteristic odor (e.g., mustard-like) or be odorless.

SYMPTOMS

Most of the blister agents (e.g., mustards) have similar effects and onset (Fig. 26–3), with the exception of lewisite, which causes more immediate-onset symptoms. Severity of symptoms

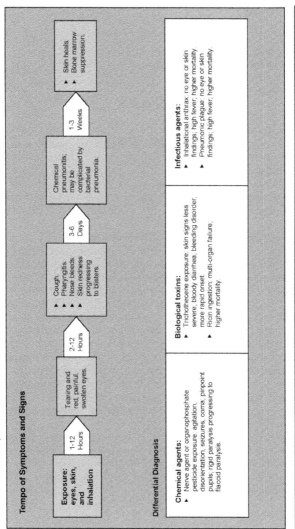

BLISTER AGENTS (Sulfur Mustard and Others)

Tempo of Symptoms and Signs

| Exposure: eyes, skin, and inhalation | 1-12 Hours → | Tearing and red, painful, swollen eyes. | 2-12 Hours → | Cough. Pharyngitis. Nose bleeds. Skin redness progressing to blisters. ▲▲▲▲ | 3-6 Days → | Chemical pneumonitis; may be complicated by bacterial pneumonia. | 1-3 Weeks → | Skin heals. Bone marrow suppression. ▲▲ |

Differential Diagnosis

Chemical agents:
- Nerve agent or organophosphate pesticide exposure: agitation, disorientation, seizures, coma, pinpoint pupils, rigid paralysis progressing to flaccid paralysis.

Biological toxins:
- Trichothecene exposure: skin signs less severe; bloody diarrhea, bleeding disorder, more rapid onset
- Ricin ingestion: multi-organ failure, higher mortality.

Infectious agents:
- Inhalational anthrax: no eye or skin findings; high fever, higher mortality.
- Pneumonic plague: no eye or skin findings; high fever, higher mortality.

Fig. 26-3   Blister agents.

CHAPTER 26

varies depending on the exposure dose. Additional symptoms may include:
- Nausea
- Hoarseness

SIGNS
- Conjunctivitis and hemorrhagic keratitis
- Pseudomembranous pharyngitis
- Vesiculobullous rash
- Respiratory distress
- Hypovolemic shock with hypotension

WORKUP
- No specific laboratory test exists to identify or quantify exposure.
- Chest radiography may demonstrate findings consistent with a chemical pneumonitis.
- Baseline laboratory investigations including a CBC, metabolic panel, and coagulation profile are appropriate for patients with significant exposure.

COMMENTS AND TREATMENT CONSIDERATIONS
Decontamination of exposed victims with plain soap and water must be carried out within minutes of exposure to prevent tissue damage. The eyes must also be thoroughly irrigated. If a shower is not available, victims may be decontaminated using 0.5% sodium hypochlorite solution (prepared by diluting one part household bleach with nine parts water), the military decontamination kit, or an absorbent powder such as flour, talcum, or Fuller's earth. Delayed decontamination does not prevent injury but remains important to prevent ongoing exposure and secondary contamination of others. Following decontamination measures, patients need supportive care (e.g., wound care, pain control, hydration, and nutrition). Attention must be given to infection control measures and to treating any ensuing skin infection. Inhaled beta-agonists may help victims with respiratory distress.

There are no specific antidotes for the mustard agents or phosgene oxime. Lewisite exposure can be treated with intramuscular injections of dimercaprol or British Anti-Lewisite (BAL).

See Table 37–2, Poisons and Their Antidotes, in Chapter 37, Toxic Exposure, Approach to.

REFERENCES
Borak J, Sidell FR: Agents of chemical warfare: sulfur mustard, *Ann Emerg Med* 21:303, 1992.

Dire D: CBRNE—vesicants, mustard: Hd, Hn1-3, H, eMedicine.com, Inc, 2004.

Fitzgerald G: CBRNE—vesicants, organic arsenicals: L, ED, MD, PD, HL, eMedicine.com, Inc, 2004.

Pons P, Dart RC: Chemical incidents in the emergency department: if and when, *Ann Emerg Med* 34:223, 1999.

BLOOD AGENTS (CYANIDES)

Blood agents cause illness by disrupting the enzyme complex responsible for the intracellular utilization of oxygen. These agents are highly lethal, and there is a very narrow margin between levels sufficient to cause symptoms and levels that cause death. The agents most likely to be weaponized are cyanogen chloride and hydrogen cyanide, two colorless gasses with pungent odors. Cyanogen chloride differs from hydrogen cyanide in that it irritates the eyes, airways, and lungs, similar to choking agents. All blood agents are highly volatile, and they tend to dissipate rapidly upon release into the air.

SYMPTOMS
Specific symptoms vary depending on the exposure dose.
- Anxiety
- Dizziness
- Lacrimation
- Nausea
- Respiratory distress

SIGNS
- Bronchorrhea
- Seizures
- Apnea
- Cyanosis
- Cardiac arrest

WORKUP
- Arterial and venous blood gas demonstrate a normal PaO_2 and an abnormally high PvO_2 because of impaired cellular oxygen utilization. Severe acidemia may be present.
- High erythrocyte cyanide levels are confirmatory in the post-mortem examination.

COMMENTS AND TREATMENT CONSIDERATIONS
If extrication of the victim is possible in a safe and timely manner, prompt administration of the cyanide antidote kit is potentially lifesaving. (See Cyanide in Chapter 37, Toxic Exposure, Approach to.)

CHAPTER 26

REFERENCES

Baud FJ, Barriot P, Toffis V, et al: Elevated blood cyanide concentrations in victims of smoke inhalation, *N Engl J Med* 325:1761, 1991.

Murphy-Lavoie H: CBRNE—cyanides, cyanogen chloride, eMedicine.com, Inc, 2004.

 CHOKING AGENTS

Choking agents (phosgene, phosphine, ammonia, chlorine, hydrogen chloride, and nitrogen oxides) are chemicals that irritate and damage the throat, airway, and lungs, leading to the sensation of choking and shortness of breath. Concentrated or prolonged exposure results in chemical pneumonitis and acute respiratory distress syndrome (ARDS). There have been many instances of accidental industrial releases of choking agents. Most of the deaths in the 1984 Bhopal, India, industrial accident resulted from the lung irritant effects caused by the release of methyl isocyanate gas. Chlorine and the more potent phosgene were used in World War I. Phosgene gas accounted for a majority of gas-related deaths during the war.

SYMPTOMS

Onset may be immediate (e.g., chlorine) or delayed (e.g., phosgene). Symptoms vary with the agent but generally include:

- Irritation of the eyes, nose, mouth, and throat
- Stridor or wheezing
- Coughing
- Chest tightness
- Shortness of breath
- Nausea
- Dermal irritation may also occur if exposed in high concentrations.
- Dizziness

SIGNS

- Bronchorrhea
- Tachypnea
- Tachycardia
- Apnea
- Cyanosis
- Vomiting
- Ventilatory failure
- Cardiovascular collapse

WORKUP

- Pulse oximetry or blood gas analysis demonstrates hypoxemia.
- Chest x-ray: chemical pneumonitis or the diffuse infiltrates of ARDS.

COMMENTS AND TREATMENT CONSIDERATIONS

There are no antidotes for choking agents. Management involves minimizing exposure, decontamination, and supportive care. Death that results from choking agent exposure is generally the result of hypoxemia and eventual ventilatory muscle fatigue. Oxygen, bronchodilators, and, if necessary, ventilatory assistance are the standard treatments for severe cases. Corticosteroids have been recommended for patients with chemical pneumonitis, but their value has not been established. Prophylactic antibiotics are not recommended and diuretics are contraindicated. Survivors of severe inhalation injury may suffer residual chronic lung disease.

 INCAPACITATING AGENTS

Incapacitating agents are designed to incapacitate temporarily rather than kill their intended victims. Their effects are transient, and supportive care typically results in full recovery. Groups of agents that have these effects include hallucinogens (e.g., BZ and LSD), vomiting agents (e.g., adamsite), and tearing agents (e.g., tear gas [CS] and Mace 7 [CN]). Some experts refer to all three groups of agents as incapacitating agents, whereas others refer to tearing agents as riot control agents.

SYMPTOMS AND SIGNS

- Hallucinogenic agents: confusion, sleepiness, inability to concentrate, hallucinations, and delirium. Effects can last for hours to days.
- Vomiting agents: irritation of the eyes and throat with coughing and sneezing followed within minutes by headache, nausea, vomiting, diarrhea, and abdominal cramps. Symptoms typically persist for an hour of more after exposure.
- Tearing agents: immediate severe burning of the eyes, nose, and throat with copious tearing. The agents can also cause cough, shortness of breathing, and vomiting. Symptoms begin to improve in minutes and resolve within several hours.

COMMENTS AND TREATMENT CONSIDERATIONS

- Hallucinogenic agents: there are no antidotes. The principal concern is to prevent the patient from inadvertent injury. Sedation with a benzodiazepine may be helpful.
- Vomiting agents: in most cases the effects resolve spontaneously within an hour of exposure and no treatment is necessary.

- Tearing agents: remove victim from the source of exposure and thoroughly irrigate the eyes. Inhaled beta-agonists may help victims with respiratory distress.

BIOLOGICAL WEAPONS
Classification of Biological Weapons

The United States Centers for Disease Control and Prevention (CDC) has created a list of "Bioterrorism Agents of Concern." The list classifies the agents in terms of the severity of health risk that they pose. The list also takes into consideration the ease of use of each agent in deployment as a biological weapon. Category A agents are viewed as being most likely to be weaponized and to pose the highest potential health risk to the greatest numbers of people. Category B agents are less easy to disseminate and are likely to cause only moderate morbidity and low mortality. Category C agents include emerging pathogens that have the potential for mass dissemination. Although the CDC list is extensive, not all potential biological weapon agents are included (see Table 26–1).

 ANTHRAX

Anthrax is the illness caused by the bacterium *Bacillus anthracis*, a large spore-forming gram-positive rod endemic in many parts of the world. Disease is contracted through contact with the spores, which are very durable, remaining capable of causing infection for many years. Anthrax is principally an infection of animals, but it can be transmitted to humans. Naturally acquired human anthrax occurs through exposure to infected animals or contaminated animal products. There are three different forms of illness caused by *B. anthracis* depending on the route of exposure: cutaneous contracted through direct contact with the skin, inhalational contracted through inhalation of the bacterial spores, and gastrointestinal contracted through ingesting contaminated meat or soil. Worldwide, there are approximately 100,000 cases each year, predominantly in developing countries. The cutaneous form is most common (~95%), with the remainder inhalational (5%) and gastrointestinal (1%). Anthrax is rare in the United States. Although most cases occur naturally following an identifiable contact with infected animal materials, any case of human anthrax should prompt investigation for intentional exposure as a biological terrorism agent. In 2001, 22 cases disseminated through the United States Postal Service were identified. Time from exposure to onset of symptoms is widely variable, typically 1 to 14 days, but may be as long as 60 days.

SYMPTOMS

Specific symptoms and signs vary depending on infection route (Fig. 26–4). Intentional exposure would be most likely to cause inhalation anthrax.

SIGNS

- Cutaneous anthrax begins as an erythematous, papulovesicular lesion with surrounding edema. The lesion is described as a "malignant pustule" for its necrotic appearance and progresses over several days to form a characteristic black eschar. Up to 20% of untreated cases disseminate systemically.
- Inhalational anthrax typically begins as a nonspecific febrile flu-like illness. It progresses into a severe sepsis with ARDS and hypoxia, cyanosis, and hypotension. Stridor resulting from tracheal compression from enlarged mediastinal lymphadenopathy can develop. A decreased level of consciousness and meningismus from meningeal involvement occur in up to 50% of cases.
- Gastrointestinal anthrax begins with vomiting and fever, followed by severe abdominal pain and bloody diarrhea. Massive mesenteric lymphadenopathy may cause bowel obstruction. Peroration can occur, and lower gastrointestinal bleeding can result in shock.

WORKUP

- Blood culture is a sensitive test to identify *B. anthracis*. The bacterium is occasionally visible on Gram stain of blood but usually not until later in the course of illness.
- Biochemical tests can differentiate *B. anthracis* from other members of the genus. The laboratory should be informed if anthrax is suspected so that gram-positive rods are not discarded as "contaminants" without characterization.
- An enzyme-linked immunosorbent assay (ELISA) is 98% sensitive for the IgG antibody to *B. anthracis*, but this test cannot be used for the early identification of disease.
- With inhalational anthrax, chest x-ray often demonstrates a prominent mediastinum and hilum caused by massive lymphadenopathy. Pleural effusions are also common.
- Computed tomography of the chest may show hemorrhagic mediastinal and hilar lymphadenopathy and pleural effusions.
- Skin lesions can be biopsied for culture and Gram stain.
- Meningitis is present in approximately half of inhalational and disseminated cutaneous cases, and the organism can be identified on Gram stain of CSF.

CHAPTER **26**

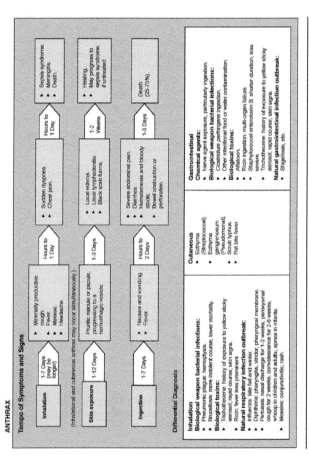

Fig. 26-4 Anthrax.

COMMENTS AND TREATMENT CONSIDERATIONS

Anthrax is not communicable between humans, but patients who have recently been exposed may still be contaminated with spores. All patients with suspicion of recent exposure to spores should be decontaminated in the field or upon presentation. A shower and disposal of clothing are adequate. Anthrax is a reportable disease.

Both ciprofloxacin and doxycycline are effective for postexposure prophylaxis and treatment of most naturally occurring cutaneous anthrax. Patients with inhalational anthrax, cutaneous anthrax of the head and neck, or cutaneous anthrax with systemic signs need hospitalization and intravenous treatment with ciprofloxacin and an additional agent such as clindamycin, an aminoglycoside, or rifampin.

Anthrax vaccine adsorbed (AVA) is available for individuals with high risk of exposure and use in postexposure prophylaxis. The anthrax Vaccine Immunization Program in the U.S. Army Surgeon General's Office can be reached at 1-877-GETVACC (1-877-438-8222), http://www.anthrax.osd.mil. Persons exposed to anthrax should be immunized if possible and treated with at least a 30-day course of ciprofloxacin or doxycycline. If the anthrax vaccine is unavailable, postexposure prophylaxis entails antibiotic treatment for a period of 60 days.

CHAPTER 26

REFERENCES

Bell DM, Kozarsky PE, Stephens DS: Clinical issues in the prophylaxis, diagnosis, and treatment of anthrax, *Emerg Infect Dis* 8:222, 2002.

Cranmer H: CBRNE—anthrax infection, eMedicine.com, Inc, 2004.

Dixon TC, Meselson M, Guillemin J, Hanna PC: Anthrax, *N Engl J Med* 341:815, 1999.

Inglesby TV, Henderson DA, Bartlett JG, et al: Anthrax as a biological weapon: medical and public health management, *JAMA* 281:1735, 1999.

Moran GJ: Update on emerging infections from the Centers for Disease Control and Prevention. Bioterrorism alleging use of anthrax and interim guidelines for management—United States, 1998, *Ann Emerg Med* 34:229, 1999.

Pile JC, Malone JD, Eitzen EM, Friedlander AM: Anthrax as a potential biological warfare agent, *Arch Intern Med* 158:429, 1998.

 BOTULISM

Botulism is a paralytic disease caused by neurotoxins of spore-forming anaerobic bacteria of the *Clostridium* genus. The most common bacterium is *C. botulinum*. The neurotoxins permanently bind to the presynaptic membrane of neurons at peripheral cholinergic synapses, preventing release of acetylcholine, thereby blocking neurotransmission and effectively paralyzing muscle cells. Botulism is characterized by an acute, symmetric, descending, flaccid paralysis with prominent facial muscle weakness in an alert patient. The toxins can cause ventilatory failure and death by paralyzing respiratory muscles. Severity of illness varies depending on the degree of toxin exposure, ranging from minimal weakness to full paralysis.

The toxins may enter the body in several ways, resulting in different forms of botulism. For use as a biological weapon, botulinum toxins could be used to contaminate food or delivered as an aerosol for inhalation. Inhalational botulism does not occur naturally but has been reported in laboratory workers.

See also Botulism in Chapter 44, Weakness and Fatigue for a discussion of naturally occurring botulism.

SYMPTOMS
- Diplopia
- Dysphagia and dysarthria
- Dry mouth
- Muscle weakness

SIGNS
Symmetric descending motor paralysis begins with cranial nerve involvement and progresses to the muscles of respiration, the upper extremities, and finally to the lower extremities (Fig. 26–5).
- Eyes: impaired extraocular movements, ptosis, nystagmus, nonreactive pupils
- Dysarthria
- Ataxia
- Motor weakness
- Respiratory distress
- Urinary retention
- Constipation

WORKUP
- The diagnosis of botulism is usually made clinically. Routine laboratory studies are not helpful in confirming the clinical suspicion of botulism.
- Toxin bioassay on serum sample is confirmatory in 40% of cases. This test is not widely available and takes several days for results.
- Standard culture on fecal or gastric sample is confirmatory in 50% of cases of intestinal or infant botulism but would not be positive with intentional toxin exposure.

BOTULISM

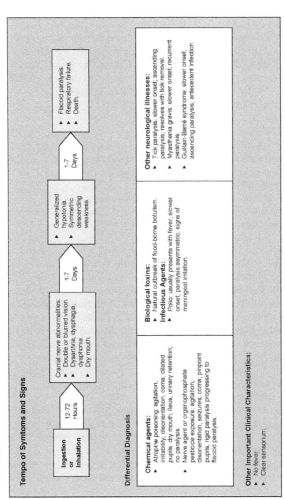

Tempo of Symtoms and Signs

Ingestion or Inhalation → 12-72 Hours → Cranial nerve abnormalities:
▲ Double or blurred vision.
▲ Dysarthria, dysphagia, dysphonia.
▲ Dry mouth.

→ 1-7 Days → Generalized hypotonia. Symmetric descending weakness.
▲
▲

→ 1-7 Days → Flaccid paralysis. Respiratory failure. Death.
▲
▲
▲

Differential Diagnosis

Chemical agents:
▲ Atropine poisoning: agitation, irritability, disorientation, coma, dilated pupils, dry mouth, ileus, urinary retention; no paralysis.
▲ Nerve agent or organophosphate pesticide exposure: agitation, disorientation, seizures, coma, pinpoint pupils, rigid paralysis progressing to flaccid paralysis.

Biological toxins:
▲ Natural outbreak of food-borne botulism.
Infectious Agents:
▲ Polio: usually presents with fever; slower onset, paralysis asymmetric, signs of meningeal irritation.

Other neurological illnesses:
▲ Tick paralysis: slower onset, ascending paralysis; resolves with tick removal.
▲ Myasthenia gravis: slower onset, recurrent paralysis.
▲ Guillain-Barré syndrome: slower onset; ascending paralysis, antecedent infection.

Other Important Clinical Characteristics:
▲ No fever.
▲ Clear sensorium.

Fig. 26–5   Botulism.

CHAPTER 26

COMMENTS AND TREATMENT CONSIDERATIONS

Botulism is not communicable between humans, but patients who have recently been exposed may still be contaminated with the toxin. All patients with suspicion of recent exposure to botulinum toxin should be decontaminated in the field. Enemas, cathartics, and emetics may assist in decreasing the toxin load, but their value has not been established. Treatment is therefore generally supportive, with ventilatory support the key to survival. A trivalent equine derived antitoxin is available in limited supply from state health departments and the CDC. It has been shown to decrease fatality, presumably by neutralizing unbound toxin. Botulism is a reportable disease.

REFERENCES

Arnon SS, Schechter R, Inglesby TV, et al: Botulinum toxin as a biological weapon, *JAMA* 285:1059, 2001.

Hatheway CL: Botulism: the present status of the disease, *Curr Top Microbiol Immunol* 195:55, 1995.

Kim J: CBRNE—botulism, eMedicine.com, Inc, 2004.

Schmidt RD, Schmidt TW: Infant botulism: a case series and review of the literature, *J Emerg Med* 10:713, 1992.

PLAGUE

Plague is the illness caused by *Yersinia pestis*, a facultative anaerobic, intracellular, gram-negative bacillus. Hundreds of millions of people have succumbed to plague over the history of humankind. Although the incidence of plague has declined with improvement of hygiene, the World Health Organization reports 1000 to 3000 cases of naturally occurring plague worldwide every year. Modern medical care has reduced the mortality rate, but plague remains a serious illness. Approximately 14% of plague cases in the United States are fatal.

Plague is a disease of rodents (rats, squirrels, etc.). Naturally occurring human infection is usually transmitted from a rodent through the bite of an insect vector (e.g., flea, tick, or human louse), although inhalational acquisition is also possible. As with anthrax, the route of exposure influences the characteristics of the resulting illness, giving rise to two common forms of plague—bubonic and pneumonic—either of which can be complicated by septicemia.

Bubonic plague accounts for 80% to 90% of cases in the United States. The word bubo is derived from the Latin for owls' eyes; bubonic plague gets its name from the large, tender lymph nodes resembling owls' eyes that develop in infected patients. Onset is usually 2 to 6 days after exposure. Initial manifestations include fever, headache, and general malaise, followed by the development of painful, swollen regional lymph nodes. Occasionally, buboes cannot be detected for a day or so after the onset of the initial symptoms. The disease progresses rapidly and, in up to a quarter of patients, the bacteria invade the bloodstream to produce secondary pneumonic plague or septicemic plague. Septicemic plague is characterized by hypotension, disseminated intravascular coagulopathy (DIC), and multiorgan failure. Often there is necrosis of the skin, which produces a black discoloration—hence the term Black Death. Without treatment, the fatality rate is high (50%).

Inhalation of the plague bacterium results in a severe pneumonia referred to as pneumonic plague. Naturally occurring pneumonic plague is uncommon. If the plague bacterium were to be used as a weapon, it would most likely be spread as an aerosol to result in pneumonic plague. The incubation period for pneumonic plague is usually 1 to 3 days. As with inhalational anthrax and bubonic plague, the initial manifestations of pneumonic plague are nonspecific with fatigue, fever, headache, and sore throat. Patients then rapidly develop a severe pneumonia with high fever, chills, cough, bloody sputum, and shortness of breath. Untreated, patients often rapidly progress to respiratory failure, sepsis, and death (50%). In contrast to inhalational anthrax, pneumonic plague can be transmitted from person to person through respiratory secretions.

SYMPTOMS
Specific symptoms and signs vary depending on infection route (Fig. 26–6).

SIGNS
- Fever ++++ in all forms of plague
- Bubonic: characteristic large tender lymph nodes
- Pneumonic: cough with blood-tinged sputum, hypoxia
- Septicemic: hypotension, purpura, necrosis of the distal extremities

WORKUP
- *Yersinia pestis* can be identified from culture and Gram stain of lymph node aspirate, sputum, or blood. The organism has a characteristic bipolar gram-negative appearance. A direct fluorescent antibody stain is also available.
- Chest x-ray may reveal a consolidating pneumonia.

COMMENTS AND TREATMENT CONSIDERATIONS
Pneumonic plague is highly contagious, and all patients suspected of having plague should be placed in respiratory droplet isolation. Management of patients with plague begins with general supportive and resuscitation measures. Ciprofloxacin, doxycycline, and

CHAPTER 26

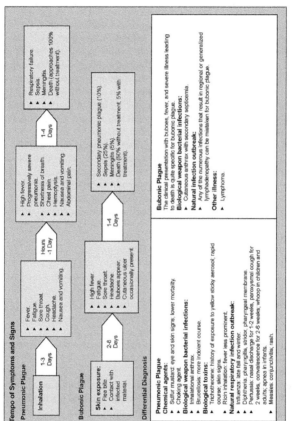

Fig. 26-6   Plague.

gentamicin are considered first-line antibiotics. A two-drug regimen (e.g., ciprofloxacin and gentamicin) is suggested for severe cases. The treatment duration should be 10 days. Antibiotic postexposure prophylaxis for 7 days should be considered for those with a high probability of exposure. Plague is a reportable disease.

REFERENCES

Inglesby TV, Dennis DT, Henderson DA, et al: Plague as a biological weapon, *JAMA* 283:2281, 2000.

Perry RD, Fetherston JD: *Yersinia pestis*—etiologic agent of plague, *Clin Microbiol Rev* 10:35, 1997.

Rotz LD, Khan AS, Lillibridge SR, et al: Public health assessment of potential biological terrorism agents, *Emerg Infect Dis* 8:225, 2002.

Velendzas D: CBRNE—plague, eMedicine.com, Inc, 2004.

SMALLPOX

Smallpox is caused by the variola virus, a member of the *Orthopoxvirus* genus. Smallpox was declared eradicated by the World Health Organization in 1977. It represents a potentially devastating biologic weapon if reintroduced, with an expected mortality rate of approximately 30% in unvaccinated individuals. Used as a biological weapon, the virus could lead to a major outbreak given the lack of immunity of the general population in the United States and around the world. The virus is acquired through inhalation of as little as 10 to 100 particles but can also be transmitted through contact with infected surfaces for up to 1 week. Only two laboratories are known to keep the smallpox virus, CDC in Atlanta, Georgia and the Russian State Research Center of Virology and Biotechnology in Koltsovo, but the potential for other stores of virus remains a concern.

SYMPTOMS

There is an incubation asymptomatic period of 7 to 17 days, followed by a febrile prodrome before the characteristic rash develops (Fig. 26–7). Prodromal symptoms include:
- Fever +++++ and rigors
- Headache
- Myalgias
- Malaise and exhaustion
- Vomiting

SIGNS

- Oropharyngeal ulcers are the earliest characteristic sign.
- An initial macular rash progresses to papules, then to vesicles, and finally to firm umbilicated pustules deep in the dermis.

325

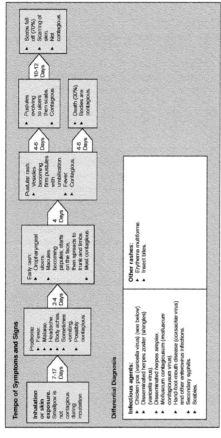

SMALLPOX

Tempo of Symptoms and Signs

| Inhalation or skin exposure. Smallpox is not contagious during incubation | 7-17 Days | Prodrome: ▲ Fever. ▲ Malaise. ▲ Headache. ▲ Body aches. ▲ Sometimes vomiting. ▲ Possibly contagious. | 2-4 Days | Early rash: ▲ Oropharyngeal ulcers. ▲ Macules becoming papules; starts on the face, then spreads to trunk and limbs. ▲ Most contagious. | 4 Days | Pustular rash: ▲ Vesicles becoming firm pustules with umbilication. ▲ Fever. ▲ Contagious. | 4-6 Days | Pustules evolving to ulcers then scabs. ▲ Contagious. | 10-12 Days | Scabs fall off (70%). ▲ Scarring of skin. ▲ Not contagious. |

Death (30%). Bodies are contagious. (4-6 Days)

Differential Diagnosis

Infectious agents:
▲ Chicken pox (varicella virus) (see below)
▲ Disseminated herpes zoster (shingles) (varicella virus).
▲ Disseminated herpes simplex.
▲ Molluscum contagiousum (molluscum contagiosum virus).
▲ Hand-foot-mouth disease (coxsackie virus) and other enterovirus infections.
▲ Secondary syphilis.
▲ Scabies.

Other rashes:
▲ Erythema multiforme
▲ Insect bites.

Comparison of Smallpox and Chicken Pox

Feature	Smallpox	Chicken pox
Prodrome	Fever, headache, malaise, vomiting	None
Character of lesions.	Uniform in stage; umbilicated.	Variable in stage.
Depth of lesions.	Deep in dermis.	Superficial in dermis.
Pattern of lesions.	Starts on the face, then spreads to the extremities proximally to distal.	Starts on the torso, then spreads to the extremities and the face.

Fig. 26-7 Smallpox.

The rash of smallpox is synchronous (all lesions at the same stage at any one time) with monomorphic lesions (all lesions appear similar to one another). Lesions mostly favor ventral surfaces with a concentration on the face and dorsal surfaces of the hands and feet. They spare the axillae, palms, and soles.

WORKUP
- A viral swab of pharynx or freshly opened pustule should be obtained. Suspected samples should be sent to a Biosafety Level 4 (BSL-4) laboratory. In the United States, the CDC in Atlanta and the U.S. Army Medical Research Institute of Infectious Disease in Ft. Detrick, Maryland have BSL-4 capability.
- Standard viral culture, polymerase chain reaction, and ELISA techniques are available for isolation and identification of the variola virus.
- Fluorescent antibody testing or PCR of fresh lesion material can be used to rule out varicella.

COMMENTS AND TREATMENT CONSIDERATIONS
All patients with suspicion of potential exposure to smallpox should have strict respiratory and contact precautions instituted immediately. All exposed health care personnel and patient contacts from up to 17 days prior to illness should be quarantined in isolation until a definitive diagnosis is established. Illness can be prevented or attenuated if the vaccine is administered within 4 days after smallpox exposure. Smallpox is a reportable disease.

CHAPTER **26**

REFERENCES
Franz DR, Jahrling PB, Friedlander AM, et al: Clinical recognition and management of patients exposed to biological warfare agents, *JAMA* 278:399, 1997.

Gordon SM: The threat of bioterrorism: a reason to learn more about anthrax and smallpox, *Cleve Clin J Med* 66:592, 1999.

Henderson DA, Inglesby TV, Bartlett JG, et al: Smallpox as a biological weapon: medical and public health management. Working Group on Civilian Biodefense, *JAMA* 281:2127, 1999.

Hogan C: CBRNE—smallpox, eMedicine.com, Inc, 2004.

 TULAREMIA

Tularemia is caused by *Francisella tularensis*, a gram-negative bacillus endemic to the continental United States and the Northern Hemisphere except for the United Kingdom. Like plague, tularemia is a disease of animals that may be transmitted to humans, hence its common names of "rabbit fever" and "deer tick fever." Many small mammals, including mice, squirrels, rabbits, and hares, are natural reservoirs of infection. Natural human infection occurs through bites by infected ticks, fleas, or mosquitos; handling infectious animal tissues; ingestion of contaminated food or water; or inhalation of infective aerosols. Humans can develop severe and sometimes fatal illness but do not transmit the disease to others. The disease is characterized as an acute, febrile, granulomatous illness with specific manifestations and mortality primarily determined by the mode of transmission. The organism is very infectious; a small number (10 to 50 or so organisms) can cause disease. If *F. tularensis* were used as a biological weapon, the bacteria would probably be aerosolized for inhalational exposure.

SYMPTOMS

There is an asymptomatic incubation period of 3 to 5 days. Specific symptoms vary depending on the route of exposure.

- Dermal or tickborne exposure leads to ulceroglandular tularemia: painful skin ulcer and tender lymphadenopathy.
- Ingestion leads to oropharyngeal tularemia: sore throat, abdominal pain, nausea, and diarrhea.
- Inhalation exposure leads to pneumonic tularemia: dry cough, dyspnea, and pleuritic chest pain.
- Any exposure route can be associated with a nonspecific febrile illness known as typhoidal tularemia: fever, malaise, myalgias, and headache.

SIGNS

- Painful regional lymphadenopathy
- Ulcerated skin lesions
- Purulent conjunctivitis
- Exudative pharyngotonsillitis
- Pulmonary rales
- Erythema nodosum

WORKUP

- Routine laboratory testing is generally not helpful.
- Elevated creatine phosphokinase indicates associated rhabdomyolysis.
- The bacillus is not isolated in routine cultures. Laboratory should be notified if tularemia is suspected; with proper media it can be isolated from blood, wounds, sputum, or other sources.
- Tularemia tube agglutination serology is presumptive at titers above 1:160 but is usually not positive until after 2 weeks of illness.
- Biopsy of lymph nodes is definitive.

COMMENTS AND TREATMENT CONSIDERATIONS

Tularemia can be effectively treated with antibiotics. Streptomycin or an aminoglycoside are the drugs of choice. Doxycycline or ciprofloxacin are preferred in the postexposure prophylaxis or mass casualty setting. Isolation is not recommended for tularemia patients because person-to-person transmission is unlikely. However, laboratory personnel should be notified when tularemia is a concern because culture specimens may pose a risk.

REFERENCES

Chang M, Glynn MK, Groseclose SL: Endemic, notifiable bioterrorism-related diseases, United States, 1992-1999, *Emerg Infect Dis* 9:556, 2003.

Cleveland KO: CBRNE—tularemia, eMedicine.com, Inc, 2004.

Dennis DT, Inglesby TV, Henderson DA, et al: Tularemia as a biological weapon: medical and public health management, *JAMA* 285:2763, 2001.

 VIRAL HEMORRHAGIC FEVERS

Viral hemorrhagic fevers (VHFs) are a group of highly lethal febrile syndromes characterized by increased vascular permeability that are caused by a variety of infectious RNA viruses. The four viral families known to cause VHF are Arenaviridae (Lassa, Junin), Bunyaviridae (Rift Valley, Crimean-Congo, hantavirus pulmonary syndrome), Filoviridae (Marburg, Ebola), and Flaviviridae (yellow, dengue). The transmission vector is usually a rodent or mosquito but in some cases is unknown. Internationally, these viruses affect millions of individuals in endemic regions and have mortality rates ranging from less than 10% to over 90% in the case of Ebola-Zaire. They are typically spread by close contact with body fluids but can potentially be spread by fine particle aerosol and are considered a possible biological weapon.

SYMPTOMS

There is an asymptomatic incubation period of 2 to 21 days, followed by:
- High fever
- Headache
- Myalgias
- Fatigue
- Abdominal pain
- Prostration

SIGNS
- Hematemesis
- Generalized mucous membrane hemorrhage
- Altered mental status
- Hypotension
- Nondependent edema
- Petechial or ecchymotic rash

WORKUP
Because of risks associated with handling infectious material, minimal laboratory testing is indicated.
- Complete blood count demonstrates leukopenia and thrombocytopenia.
- Elevated creatine phosphokinase indicates associated rhabdomyolysis.
- Disseminated intravascular coagulation profile and elevations in prothrombin time, partial thromboplastin time, and the international normalized ratio are present.
- Specific tests using ELISA and PCR are available for most viruses. These tests are conducted in only a limited number of BSL-4 laboratories.

COMMENTS AND TREATMENT CONSIDERATIONS
All patients with suspicion of a VHF should be kept under strict contact precautions unless respiratory symptoms are present, in which case respiratory isolation is indicated. Administer blood products as clinically indicated and implement general resuscitation and supportive measures. Prevent nonessential staff from coming into contact with affected individuals and avoid antiplatelet agents as well as invasive procedures. No specific antiviral therapy is available, although ribavirin may have efficacy for some VHF agents such as Lassa, Congo-Crimean, or Rift Valley fever. Vaccines are readily available for some agents (e.g., yellow fever), and others are under development.

REFERENCES
Borio L, Inglesby T, Peters CJ, et al: Hemorrhagic fever viruses as biological weapons: medical and public health management, *JAMA* 287:2391, 2002.

Pigott DC: CBRNE—viral hemorrhagic fevers, eMedicine.com, Inc, 2004.

 RICIN

Ricin is a potent toxin derived from the beans of the castor plant (*Ricinus communis*). Castor beans are commonly used in the production of castor oil and automotive fluids. The toxin inhibits protein synthesis and leads to cellular death. Routes of exposure include dermal, inhalational, gastrointestinal, and parenteral. Used as a biological weapon, the agent would probably be used to contaminate food or water supplies, leading to the disabling of large populations. Since 1991, there have been three cases involving the use of ricin in the United States. In February 2004, three Senate offices were closed after ricin was found in an adjoining mailroom.

SYMPTOMS AND SIGNS
Symptoms and signs vary depending on whether the toxin is inhaled or ingested (Fig. 26–8).
- Inhalational exposure results in rapid deterioration with cyanosis, hypoxia, respiratory distress, tachycardia, and eventual respiratory failure.
- Gastrointestinal exposure leads to vomiting and diarrhea with secondary hypovolemia; this may be followed by hematemesis and hematochezia or melena.
- Parenteral exposure results in pain, induration, and erythema at the site of exposure prior to the onset of systemic findings.

WORKUP
- Disseminated intravascular coagulation profile in severe cases.
- An ELISA is under development.
- Chest radiograph demonstrates ARDS in inhalational exposure.

COMMENTS AND TREATMENT CONSIDERATIONS
Ricin illness is not communicable, but patients with recent exposure may have residual contamination. Therefore, all patients with suspicion of recent exposure to ricin should be decontaminated in the field. Management of patients with exposure to ricin consists of general supportive and resuscitation measures. Activated charcoal should be administered to patients whose exposure is by ingestion to reduce toxin absorption. Ricin-related illness should be reported to local public health authorities.

REFERENCES
Balint GA: Ricin: the toxic protein of castor oil seeds, *Toxicology* 2:77, 1974.

Kortepeter MG, Parker GW: Potential biological weapons threats, *Emerg Infect Dis* 5:523, 1999.

Mirarchi F: CBRNE—ricin, eMedicine.com, Inc, 2004.

Moran GJ: Threats in bioterrorism: CDC category B and C agents, *Emerg Med Clin North Am* 20:311, 2002.

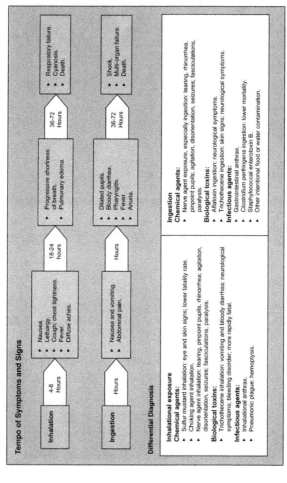

RICIN

Tempo of Symptoms and Signs

Inhalation → 4-8 Hours → Nausea. Lethargy. Cough; chest tightness. Fever. Diffuse aches. → 18-24 hours → Progressive shortness of breath. Pulmonary edema. → 36-72 Hours → Respiratory failure. Cyanosis. Death.

Ingestion → Hours → Nausea and vomiting. Abdominal pain. → Hours → Dilated pupils. Bloody diarrhea. Pharyngitis. Fever. Anuria. → 36-72 Hours → Shock. Multi-organ failure. Death.

Differential Diagnosis

Inhalational exposure
Chemical agents:
- Sulfur mustard inhalation: eye and skin signs; lower fatality rate.
- Choking agent inhalation.
- Nerve agent inhalation: tearing, pinpoint pupils, rhinorrhea; agitation, disorientation, seizures; fasciculations, paralysis.

Biological toxins:
- Trichothecene inhalation: vomiting and bloody diarrhea; neurological symptoms; bleeding disorder; more rapidly fatal.

Infectious agents:
- Inhalational anthrax.
- Pneumonic plague: hemoptysis.

Ingestion
Chemical agents:
- Nerve agent exposure, especially ingestion: tearing, rhinorrhea, pinpoint pupils; agitation, disorientation, seizures; fasciculations, paralysis.

Biological toxins:
- Aflatoxin ingestion: neurological symptoms.
- Trichothecene ingestion: skin signs; neurological symptoms.

Infectious agents:
- Gastrointestinal anthrax.
- *Clostridium perfringens* ingestion: lower mortality.
- Staphylococcal enterotoxin B.
- Other intentional food or water contamination.

Fig. 26-8 Ricin.

RADIOLOGICAL MATERIALS

 DIRTY BOMB

A dirty bomb is a radioactive material dispersion device consisting of a conventional explosive, such as dynamite, attached to radioactive material. The detonation of a dirty bomb results in immediate damage from the explosion itself and the dispersion of radioactive materials into the surrounding environment. Although contamination can be spread over several square kilometers, there is very little chance of radiation injury outside the immediate blast area. Even within the blast area, ionizing radiation from a dirty bomb is unlikely to be sufficient to cause immediate or rapid death. In addition to the damage caused by the explosion, a dirty bomb could cause widespread panic and environmental contamination. Resulting health effects can be minimized by removing radioactive particles from people and the environment. This decontamination process is likely to be labor intensive and expensive.

CHAPTER 26

SYMPTOMS
- Immediate symptoms of victims within the blast area are likely to be due to blunt and penetrating injury from the explosion.
- High levels of radiation cause acute radiation syndrome. Symptoms can include nausea, weakness, abdominal cramping, confusion, and headache.

SIGNS
- There are not likely to be any immediate signs attributable to the radiation exposure; all initial signs would be due to the effects of the explosion.

WORKUP
- Complete blood cell count and differential count. The degree of absolute lymphocyte count drop is prognostic.
- Save bodily secretions for analysis of dosage received.

COMMENTS AND TREATMENT CONSIDERATIONS
Each facility should have a radiation safety plan with provisions for decontamination areas, personal protective equipment, and radiation detection equipment (e.g., a Geiger counter) available to evaluate for contamination. Stabilizing life-threatening conventional injuries from the blast takes priority, but precautions must be taken for radioactive contamination. After stabilization, all patients with radiation exposure from a dirty bomb should be thoroughly decontaminated. Removal of all clothing, washing with soap and water, and rinsing the eyes and mouth effectively remove the preponderance of external contamination. Patients should be instructed not to

eat, drink, or smoke to reduce internal contamination until after they have left the area of exposure, completed decontamination, and been evaluated for residual radioactive contamination. Wounds must be irrigated and radioactive shrapnel removed. Definitive care of injuries should follow decontamination. Chelating or blocking agents, such as potassium iodide for exposure to radioactive iodide, should be considered in consultation with experts.

REFERENCES

Forrow L, Blair BG, Helfand I, et al: Accidental nuclear war—a post-cold war assessment, *N Engl J Med* 338:1326, 1998.

Leonard RB, Ricks RC: Emergency department radiation accident protocol, *Ann Emerg Med* 9:462, 1980.

Murphy-Lavoie H: CBRNE—cyanides, cyanogen chloride, eMedicine.com, Inc, 2004.

 ## THERMONUCLEAR DEVICE

Nuclear weapon explosions have devastating effects. Nuclear energy is derived from the processes of fission and fusion of atomic nuclei. Tremendous amounts of energy are released as a result of these processes. The immediate health effects of nuclear weapon detonation include blast injuries and burn injuries in the area of detonation. The exact extent of the burn and blast injury zone depends on the strength of the nuclear weapon, measured in kilotons (KT). Radiation injury causes a greater proportion of deaths with lower energy nuclear weapons. In contrast, blast and burn injuries account for most deaths with sophisticated nuclear weapons. Large amounts of nuclear radiation (e.g., gamma rays) are immediately released with detonation. Concurrently, radioactive materials (e.g., neutrons, alpha particles, and beta particles) are dispersed into the air and radio-active fallout is created. Many victims exposed to a nuclear weapon explosion will sustain high-level radiation exposure and develop acute radiation syndrome (ARS). The severity and rapidity of onset of acute radiation syndrome depend on several factors including exposure dose, age of the victim, preexisting comorbidities, and portion of the body exposed.

SYMPTOMS

- Immediate symptoms of victims within the blast area are likely to be due to blunt and penetrating injury and burns from the explosion.
- Early ARS symptoms occur only following severe radiation exposure but can include a burning sensation of the skin, nausea, weakness, abdominal cramping, confusion, and headache.

SIGNS
- There are not likely to be any immediate signs attributable to the radiation exposure; all initial signs would be due to the effects of the explosion.
- There are no early signs of ARS except in cases of extreme, lethal radiation exposure, in which case there may be fever, vomiting, seizures, coma, and hemodynamic collapse.

WORKUP
- Baseline complete blood cell count and differential count. The degree of absolute lymphocyte count drop is prognostic.
- Save bodily secretions for analysis of dosage received.

COMMENTS AND TREATMENT CONSIDERATIONS
Initial management of patients surviving a nuclear weapon explosion to present at a functioning medical facility is the same as for a dirty bomb explosion victim. Development and progression of ARS is far more likely.

REFERENCES
Forrow L, Blair BG, Helfand I, et al: Accidental nuclear war—a post-cold war assessment, *N Engl J Med* 338:1326, 1998.

Leonard RB, Ricks RC: Emergency department radiation accident protocol, *Ann Emerg Med* 9:462, 1980.

Pemberton L: CBRNE—nuclear radiation exposure, eMedicine.com, Inc, 2004.

CONVENTIONAL EXPLOSIVES
Conventional explosives can result in thermal and blast injury. Blast injury is categorized by mechanism (Table 26–2).

Explosions in enclosed spaces tend to result in a high incidence of morbidity and mortality. Lung injuries, including pulmonary contusion, pneumothorax, hemothorax, or air embolism, are common. Injury to the abdomen is more commonly noted in the gas-containing organs, such as small and large intestine, than solid organs, such as liver, spleen, and kidney. Limited injuries to the bowel can progress in time resulting in perforations in the bowel. Perforation of the tympanic membrane is the most common ear injury seen after an explosion. More significant blasts can damage the inner ear. Injury to the eye purely from a blast wave is rare but often results from debris propelled into the eye by the blast.

SYMPTOMS
- Respiratory distress
- Decreased hearing

TABLE 26–2
MECHANISM OF INJURY BY TYPE OF BLAST

TYPE OF BLAST INJURY	MECHANISM OF INJURY
Primary	Injury caused by the effect of the blast wave on the body. Primary blast injury occurs principally in the gas-filled organs and results from extreme pressure differentials developed at body surfaces. Organs most susceptible include the middle ear, lung, and bowel.
Secondary	Injury caused by flying debris and fragments, propelled mostly by the blast winds generated by an explosion. Most commonly produces penetrating injury to the body. At very close distance to the explosion, may cause limb amputation or total body disruption.
Tertiary	Injury results from victim being displaced through space by the blast wind and striking a stationary object.
Quaternary	Injury suffered as a result of all other effects of bomb blasts, including crush injury from a collapsed structure, inhalation of toxic gasses and debris, thermal burns, exposure to radiation, and exacerbation of prior medical illnesses.

- Extremity pain
- Abdominal pain

SIGNS
- Hypoxia
- Hypotension
- Blunt trauma
- Penetrating trauma
- Asphyxiation
- Crush injury

WORKUP
- Carboxyhemoglobin level measurement if explosion associated with smoke or fire exposure to rule out carbon monoxide poisoning
- Laboratory investigations such as urinalysis, serial complete blood count, coagulation profile, and a creatinine phosphokinase should be considered.
- Chest radiography in victims with respiratory symptoms or those exposed to high-pressure injury (especially if associated tympanic membrane rupture).
- Abdominal computed tomography in patients with abdominal symptoms and potential or known mechanism for penetrating or blunt abdominal injury

COMMENTS AND TREATMENT CONSIDERATIONS

All patients involved in an explosion should have a thorough evaluation including liberal use of radiographic imaging. Blast injury often results in serious internal injury without external signs of trauma, and even serious penetrating injury may be easily overlooked. Small metal objects such as nails and ball bearings are frequently used in bombs, resulting in inapparent or trivial-appearing wounds but serious internal injury. The possibility of associated ionizing radiation, biological agent, or chemical agent exposure must also be investigated.

See Chapter 39, Trauma, Approach to and Chapter 40, Trauma, Burns.

REFERENCES

Lavonas E: Blast injuries, eMedicine.com, Inc, 2004.

Stein M, Hirshberg A: Medical consequences of terrorism: the conventional weapon threat, *Surg Clin North Am* 79:1537, 1999.

Wightman JM, Gladish SL: Explosions and blast injuries, *Ann Emerg Med* 37:664, 2001.

CHAPTER 26

CHAPTER 27

Mental Status Change and Coma
Julian G. Lis

Altered mental status (AMS) represents a spectrum of disability, from mild confusion to deep coma. It is a common occurrence, with approximately 1% of patients arriving at emergency departments comatose and many more (up to 5%) arriving with an altered sensorium. The differential diagnosis is large (Table 27–1) and includes numerous life-threatening conditions. An organized approach begins with a rapid initial standard evaluation and stabilization plan that is applicable to most patients. The aim of the initial evaluation is to identify and treat potential immediate threats to life, such as ventilatory failure or hypoxia, cardiac dysrhythmia, and

TABLE 27–1
DIFFERENTIAL DIAGNOSIS OF ALTERED MENTAL STATUS

(See specific diagnoses throughout text)

RESPIRATORY	VASCULAR	INFECTION	NEUROLOGIC
Hypercarbia	Hypotension	Sepsis	Head trauma
Hypoxia	Stroke	Meningitis	Intracranial hemorrhages
	Hypertensive	Encephalitis	Intracranial tumors
	Encephalopathy	Other intracranial	Hydrocephalus
	Thrombotic	infections (abscess,	Cerebral edema
	thrombocytopenic	subdural empyema)	Seizures, including
	purpura (TTP)	Other non-CNS	nonconvulsive
	CNS vasculitis	infections	status epilepticus,
			temporal lobe
			epilepsy, and
			postictal state

hypotension, as well as conditions that are easily treated, such as hypoglycemia.

As the patient is stabilized, possible causes for the change in mental status are considered. Potential general causes include primary CNS processes (e.g., infection, bleeding, seizure, and infarction), conditions that reduce CNS perfusion (e.g., hypotension from any cause), decreased oxygen content in the blood (hypoxia or alteration in hemoglobin binding to oxygen), ventilatory failure (hypercapnia), sepsis, toxic or metabolic abnormalities, and other rare conditions. In the setting of possible bacterial meningitis or sepsis, antibiotics should not be unreasonably delayed for any test (including CT or LP). In general, blood and urine cultures should be obtained and antibiotics administered early in the ED evaluation. Only after an exhaustive medical evaluation, which is rarely possible to complete in the ED, can an abnormal mental status be ascribed to psychiatric disease.

INITIAL EVALUATION AND STABILIZATION

A systematic approach is necessary to diagnose and appropriately manage the gamut of causes of AMS. As with all true emergency patients, *evaluation and treatment begin with the ABCs* before a complete history and physical examination are performed. The initial approach is essentially the same for all AMS patients, with physical assessment, diagnostic studies, treatment, and consideration of the differential diagnosis occurring simultaneously.

TABLE 27-1
DIFFERENTIAL DIAGNOSIS OF ALTERED MENTAL STATUS—CONT'D

TOXINS	ENVIRONMENTAL	ENDOCRINE AND METABOLIC	PSYCHIATRIC
See Chapter 37, Toxic Exposure, Approach to	Heat Stroke Hypothermia	Adrenal insufficiency Hypoglycemia DKA HHNK Thyroid storm Myxedema coma Hypercalcemia Hyponatremia Hypernatremia Hepatic encephalopathy Uremia Wernicke-Korsakoff syndrome	Psychosis Mania Catatonia Hysteria Malingering

27

CHAPTER

1. Assess and stabilize the ABCs.
2. Establish intravenous access.
3. Check pulse oximetry.
4. Initiate cardiac monitoring.
5. Perform rapid bedside capillary glucose.
    a. *Hypoglycemia*: In the context of AMS, administer glucose for a measured glucose <60.
    b. *Hyperglycemia*: Consider DKA and hyperosmolar hyperglycemic syndrome (HHS) (note: BS should generally be >600 to be considered the cause of AMS).
6. Check vital signs.
    a. Blood pressure
        (1) Hypotension (usually <90 mm Hg systolic to cause AMS): see Chapter 21, Hypotension.
        (2) Blood pressure: >180/120, consider sympathomimetic abuse, thyroid storm, hypertensive encephalopathy, or primary CNS vascular event (stroke).
        (3) Heart rate: if >150 or <45 and signs of poor perfusion are present, the arrhythmia may be the primary cause of the AMS.
    b. Temperature
        (1) If elevated or depressed, consider sepsis. Temperature may also be normal in patients with sepsis.
        (2) >104° F: consider thyroid storm, neuroleptic malignant syndrome (NMS), malignant hyperthermia, heat stroke, and infection.
        (3) <95.0° F: consider myxedema coma, hypothermia.
    c. Respiratory rate
        (1) Tachypnea: consider hypoxia, altered hemoglobin oxygen binding, acidosis, sepsis.
        (2) Bradypnea: consider opiate abuse; beware of agonal respirations with impending respiratory collapse.
7. Assess level of consciousness. If comatose, does the patient need immediate intubation for airway protection? (If the patient lacks a gag reflex or the Glasgow Coma Scale score <8, generally "Yes.")
8. Administer thiamine 100 mg IV. Thiamine is given to alcoholics and others at risk for vitamin deficiency to prevent possible precipitation of Wernicke's encephalopathy by glucose-containing intravenous fluids. (This is probably not a truly emergent action but is generally done before glucose administration.)
9. Check pupils. Pinpoint pupils and bradypnea or apnea strongly suggest overdose of opiate (rarely other causes, such as pontine hemorrhage) and often dramatically respond to naloxone. A unilateral, dilated, nonreactive pupil indicates probable brain stem herniation from increased intracranial

pressure. Emergent management includes intubation, mild hyperventilation, immediate neurosurgical consultation, and mannitol administration as a bridge to surgery. An emergent cranial CT scan is indicated.

10. Consider occult trauma. Examine the head and neck. Consider cervical spine immobilization and x-rays.

11. Perform a brief, focused neurologic examination. Emergent cranial CT scanning is a top priority if trauma is evident or focal neurologic deficits are present.

After the immediate life-threatening conditions have been addressed, a more complete history and physical examination can be performed. The circumstances surrounding the onset of the AMS, as well as the patient's past medical history (including medications and any psychiatric history), are often the most helpful factors in determining the cause of AMS. Obtaining a history often entails using all potential sources of information regarding the patient (e.g., calling the nursing home from which the patient was transferred, speaking directly to the paramedics who were on scene, reviewing the patient's empty pill bottles, calling the patient's primary care physician or family members.).

Common drug overdose toxidromes should be considered when examining patients with AMS (see Chapter 37, Toxic Exposure, Approach to).

Specific populations of patients require additional considerations. For children, consider Reye's syndrome and intussusception. For the elderly, consider polypharmacy and drug interactions, sepsis and other non-CNS infections, dementia, and fluid and electrolyte disorders. For pregnant women, consider HELLP syndrome and eclampsia. For immunocompromised patients, consider opportunistic intracranial infections, intracranial tumors, and hypercalcemia in certain cancer patients. Agitation with AMS suggests a number of possible conditions (e.g., delirium tremens, thyroid storm, adrenergic drug overdose, serotonin syndrome, anticholinergic overdose, NMS, and heat stroke).

DIAGNOSTIC TESTING

Diagnostic studies can be divided into tests reasonably performed routinely whenever the etiology of AMS is uncertain and those performed only as the specifics of the patient's presentation indicate.

ROUTINE STUDIES
- Urinalysis: especially in the elderly, in whom urosepsis is a frequent cause of AMS
- ECG (and possibly biomarkers of cardiac injury): in cognitively marginal elderly individuals, an acute myocardial infarction may

manifest as AMS. ECG may also be useful in suspected overdoses of cyclic antidepressants (see Chapter 32, Seizure, Adult), type Ia antiarrhythmics (QT prolongation), and digoxin (arrhythmias and heart block).

- Chest x-rays: pneumonia may cause AMS in the frail elderly, who may present without cough, fever, hypoxia, or definitive physical findings. Concomitant sepsis or meningitis must be considered.
- Calcium: hypercalcemia, especially in known malignancy and in the elderly.
- Electrolytes, BUN, creatinine, and glucose: hyponatremia, hypernatremia, hyperkalemia (in adrenal insufficiency), anion gap, BUN and creatinine for renal failure, serum glucose to confirm the rapid bedside glucose.
- CBC: although of questionable utility, the WBC is commonly used to detect occult infection, especially in the afebrile elderly. Hemolytic anemia with decreased platelets and AMS suggests thrombotic thrombocytopenic purpura (TTP).

SPECIFIC STUDIES
- Lumbar puncture (LP): emergent for patients with AMS and evidence of either meningitis or fever without source. Whenever bacterial meningitis is a concern and the LP will be delayed, antibiotics should be given before LP.
- Head CT: all AMS patients should have a cranial CT scan to exclude structural lesions unless a definitive cause for AMS has already been established by the initial evaluation.
- Blood cultures: when considering sepsis. Most useful in the elderly, children <36 months, immunocompromised patients, and when fever accompanies AMS.
- ABG: With AMS and COPD, to detect hypercarbia. When acidosis is suspected (i.e., increased respiratory rate without hypoxia), such as with DKA or toxic ingestions that cause an increased anion gap acidosis, a venous blood gas may be substituted.
- Certain laboratory tests are useful when specific toxic ingestions are under consideration, including serum osmolality (e.g., for methanol or ethylene glycol), cooximetry (e.g., for CO or methemoglobinemia), and possibly qualitative or quantitative toxin screens (see Chapter 37, Toxic Exposure, Approach to).
- Ethanol level: although ethanol is a common cause of AMS in every ED, obtaining an alcohol level is not necessary for every AMS patient. While supporting a diagnosis of ethanol intoxication, a high level does not preclude an occult subdural hematoma or other coexistent pathologic condition. A level of "0" in a patient who was presumed drunk should encourage a more aggressive pursuit of alternative causes for the AMS. Alcohol level can also

be used to calculate the osmolal gap (see Chapter 37, Toxic Exposure, Approach to).

- Liver function tests (AST, ALT, total/direct bilirubin, ammonia level, PT): in children to rule out Reye's syndrome and in patients of any age with suggestive symptoms or physical findings to confirm previously undiagnosed liver disease. Hepatic encephalopathy, however, especially in known chronic liver disease, is largely a clinical diagnosis, and test results rarely change management.
- TSH and free T_4: results often not available in the ED, but supports diagnosis of thyrotoxicosis or myxedema coma.
- Serum cortisol: results often not available in the ED, but supports diagnosis of adrenal crisis.

There are a number of causes of AMS for which no rapidly available specific test exists and which can be diagnosed only on clinical grounds in the ED (see the accompanying box). Many of these conditions have specific treatments and carry high mortality if untreated.

Occasionally, the cause of AMS remains unknown despite a thorough evaluation. In these cases the patient should generally have cultures and be given antibiotics, hospitalized (usually to a monitored bed), and observed. Further diagnostic evaluation and treatment should be individualized.

CHAPTER 27

REFERENCES

American College of Emergency Physicians: Clinical policy for the initial approach to patients presenting with altered mental status, *Ann Emerg Med* 33:251, 1999.

Kanich W, Brady WJ, Huff JS, et al: Altered mental status: evaluation and etiology in the ED, *Am J Emerg Med* 20:613, 2002.

Mick N, Brown DF, Nadel ES: Pediatric altered mental status, *J Emerg Med* 25:193, 2003.

CAUSES OF ALTERED MENTAL STATUS THAT MUST BE DIAGNOSED ON CLINICAL GROUNDS

- Adrenal crisis
- Delirium tremens
- Heat stroke
- Hypertensive encephalopathy
- Myxedema coma
- Postictal state
- Psychogenic (always a diagnosis of exclusion)
- Sepsis
- Thyroid storm
- Toxicologic causes (e.g., anticholinergic toxicity, cholinergic crisis, and serotonin syndrome)
- Wernicke's encephalopathy

HYPOGLYCEMIA

Hypoglycemia is most often encountered in diabetic patients who fail to balance caloric intake, caloric expenditure, and the amount of insulin or hypoglycemic agent taken. Less commonly, hypoglycemia occurs in fasting alcoholics (owing to the inhibition of gluconeogenesis by alcohol), patients with hepatic dysfunction, and otherwise healthy elderly adults after a prolonged fast. Hypoglycemia also occurs in infants with poor caloric intake (inadequate glycogen stores) and children who ingest alcohol (owing to inhibition of gluconeogenesis and poor glycogen stores).

Many other medications stimulate insulin secretion or inhibit gluconeogenesis (e.g., pentamidine, propranolol, quinine, and salicylates, among others) and can cause hypoglycemia in overdose. Rarely, an insulinoma is the cause of hypoglycemia.

SYMPTOMS

Signs and symptoms can be categorized into hyperadrenergic (owing to release of counterregulatory hormones, such as epinephrine, secreted in response to a falling serum glucose) and neuroglucopenic (cerebral dysfunction because of insufficient glucose). Hyperadrenergic manifestations may be absent in (1) patients with long-standing diabetes because of diabetic autonomic neuropathy and (2) patients who have had recent severe episodes of hypoglycemia that results in down-regulation of the autonomic response.

- *Neuroglucopenic*: progress from subtly diminished ability to concentrate to impaired judgment and memory, confusion, drowsiness, and disorientation
- *Hyperadrenergic*: sweating, tremor, sensation of warmth, generalized weakness, hunger, palpitations, and dizziness

SIGNS

- AMS: confusion ++++, bizarre behavior suggestive of a psychiatric disturbance ++, stupor ++, coma ++
- Seizures ++
- Focal neurologic deficit +; focal neurologic deficit occurs most commonly in patients who have had a previous stroke but who had recovered function. The hypoglycemia-related deficits often mimic the prior stroke, manifesting in the same manner. Hypoglycemia-related focal neurologic deficits resolve after the hypoglycemia is treated.

WORKUP

- In the setting of appropriate symptoms, a rapid finger-stick glucose <55 mg/dl establishes the diagnosis. If the diagnosis remains in doubt, dextrose should be given and the low glucose concentration confirmed by the laboratory.

- Renal function (BUN and creatinine) should be checked in diabetics if the cause of the episode is unclear because worsening renal function may cause insulin or hypoglycemics to accumulate.
- Liver function tests should be considered if hepatic gluconeogenic function is a concern.

COMMENTS AND TREATMENT CONSIDERATIONS

Symptoms and glucose concentrations correlate imperfectly. Some patients are symptomatic with glucose >60, whereas others appear asymptomatic with glucose <40.

Treatment in adults consists of an immediate intravenous bolus of 50 ml (one ampule) of dextrose 50% (D50). In children, 2 to 4 ml/kg of D25 is given intravenously. Neonates should receive D10 intravenously. Glucagon (1 mg subcutaneously or intramuscularly for adults; 0.02 to 0.03 mg/kg for children, to maximum of 1 mg) may be given if venous access is delayed. Glucose determination should be repeated in 30 minutes, and additional dextrose may be administered as necessary. Patients should be fed as soon as they are able to eat safely. One ampule of D50 has only 25 g of carbohydrate, the equivalent of one glass of orange juice.

A period of ED observation with rechecks of serum glucose after feeding is necessary for all patients with an episode of hypoglycemia. Recurrent hypoglycemia is common with long-acting insulins and oral hypoglycemics. Hospital admission for observation should be considered if a patient has recurrent or intractable hypoglycemic episodes.

In approximately two thirds of episodes the cause of hypoglycemia can be found, with inadequate caloric intake being the most common cause in diabetics. Increased activity or delayed meals are also frequent causes.

Prevention of subsequent episodes is crucial; this may require decreasing the insulin dose.

REFERENCES

Banarer S, Cryer PE: Hypoglycemia in type 2 diabetes, *Med Clin North Am* 88:1107, 2004.

Cryer PE: Diverse causes of hypoglycemia-associated autonomic failure in diabetes, *N Engl J Med* 350:2272, 2004.

Lee PH, Bank DE, Flomenbaum N: Hypoglycemia and the ABC'S (sugar), *Ann Emerg Med* 36:278, 2000.

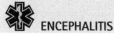 **ENCEPHALITIS**

Encephalitis is an inflammatory disorder of the brain. Common etiologies in immune competent individuals include herpes simplex virus (HSV), arboviruses (including West Nile virus), and a postviral syndrome mediated by the autoimmune system (30%). In immunocompromised patients, cytomegalovirus (CMV), toxoplasmosis, and fungal infections can cause encephalitis.

There are currently approximately 20,000 cases of encephalitis in the United States per year. Since its introduction into the United States in 1999, West Nile virus (WNV) has spread to 46 states and in 2004 caused 900 reported cases of encephalitis and 88 deaths. However, despite its media attention, WNV in neither as prevalent nor as deadly as the other forms of encephalitis, such as toxoplasmosis, CMV, and HSV encephalitis. In addition, HSV has a specific treatment (acyclovir) that greatly affects mortality, making detection of HSV encephalitis a priority for the clinician dealing with an immunocompetent patient. HSV causes 2000 cases of encephalitis annually in the United States, with no specific age-related, geographic, or seasonal preference. Mortality is 70% in untreated individuals, and patients with advanced disease almost always become permanently disabled. Herpes encephalitis can cause bizarre behavior that may be misdiagnosed as a psychiatric disorder.

Although the signs and symptoms discussed here pertain specifically to HSV encephalitis, most features are shared by the encephalitides caused by other entities.

SYMPTOMS
- AMS +++++: personality changes ++++, drowsiness ++++
- Onset may be insidious or abrupt.
- Headache +++
- History of an antecedent prodromal influenza-like illness +++
- Seizures +++: focal (85%), generalized (15%)

SIGNS
- AMS +++++
- Fever ++++
- Focal neurologic signs +++++, hemiparesis +++
- Of those conscious, difficulty speaking or complete aphasia +++
- Meningismus +++
- Evidence of increased intracranial pressure (papilledema or elevated opening pressure on LP) +++

WORKUP
- CT scan +++; approximately 80% specific for temporal lobe lesions typical of HSV at the time of presentation, increases to ++++ and approximately 90% specific after 6 days of symptoms.
- MRI provides earlier detection and better visualization of lesions than CT.
- CSF analysis initially can be normal and becomes progressively abnormal as illness progresses.

- WBC: range 0 to 545 WBC/mm³ (but usually >5 WBC/hpf)
- RBC: elevated +++, range 12 to 4000 RBC/mm³ (hemorrhagic CSF that does not clear is a sensitive and specific feature of HSV encephalitis)
- Protein: elevated in ++++; range, 0.34 to 2.8 g/L
- Glucose: normal ++++
- Pressure is usually elevated.
- PCR analysis of cerebrospinal fluid (CSF-PCR) for herpes simplex virus DNA ++++; approaches 100% specificity
- EEG ++++, but only 33% specific. Diffuse slowing or unilateral (or bilateral) periodic discharges in the temporal lobes. Slow-wave complexes at regular intervals of two or three per second are classic findings.

COMMENTS AND TREATMENT CONSIDERATIONS

Acyclovir (10 mg/kg IV q8h) has decreased 6-month mortality from 70% to 19% and should be administered. Early diagnosis is essential, and in most cases presumptive treatment with acyclovir until CSF-PCR results return is indicated whenever the diagnosis is entertained. Think of HSV encephalitis in the febrile patient with AMS whose CSF shows "meningitis" but is also hemorrhagic. When in doubt, give acyclovir along with antibiotics for meningitis until an HSV-PCR is determined to be negative.

REFERENCES:

Gendelman HE, Persidsky Y: Infections of the nervous system, *Lancet Neurol* 4:12, 2005.

Schneider JI: Rapid infectious killers, *Emerg Med Clin North Am* 22:1099, 2004.

Tyler KL: Herpes simplex virus infections of the central nervous system: encephalitis and meningitis, including Mollaret's, *Herpes* 11(Suppl 2):57A, 2004.

 DIABETIC KETOACIDOSIS

Diabetic ketoacidosis (DKA) is a syndrome defined by a constellation of clinical findings and laboratory abnormalities (typically blood glucose >250, pH <7.30, serum HCO_3^- <15 to 20 mmol/L, and ketonemia >1:4 dilution). Between 60% and 80% of DKA occurs in known diabetics; the remaining 20% to 40% occurs with the onset of diabetes. Relative or absolute insulin deficiency is the cause of DKA.

As a result of insulin deficiency, peripheral glucose uptake is impaired and hepatic gluconeogenesis increases, resulting in hyperglycemia. As the glucose concentration rises, the renal threshold for glucose is exceeded; glucosuria ensues, creating an

Chapter 27

347

osmotic diuresis, which in turn leads to volume depletion. A serum glucose greater than 400 in a patient with normal renal function implies a significant total body water deficit. Increasing serum osmolarity causes progressive obtundation. Fat cells, without the action of insulin, release fatty acids into the blood, which are converted by the liver into ketoacids. Acidosis accounts for the symptoms of tachypnea, Kussmaul respirations, nausea, vomiting, and abdominal pain.

SYMPTOMS
Symptoms vary with severity of the DKA episode.
- Polydipsia and polyuria
- Weight loss
- Fatigue ++++
- Muscle cramps +++
- Abdominal pain, nausea, and vomiting +++
- AMS ++: confusion and lethargy to coma ++

SIGNS
- Vital signs: tachypnea ++++, tachycardia ++++, hypotension ++, hypothermia
- Evidence of volume depletion: dry oral mucosa, dry skin ++++
- AMS (50% to 60%): drowsiness to coma
- Kussmaul respirations ++++
- Odor of acetone on breath +++
- Abdominal tenderness without rebound +++ or less commonly with rebound and guarding +

WORKUP
- Serum glucose to confirm bedside glucose
- Electrolytes: HCO_3^- to determine the severity of the acidosis. The potassium concentration is critically important. Rehydration and insulin therapy, with correction of the acidosis, acutely decrease the serum potassium concentration, which must be monitored closely. The measured serum sodium may be low initially owing to the dilutional effect of the movement of water from the intracellular to the extracellular space because of the osmotic effect of serum hyperglycemia, a condition referred to as "pseudo-hyponatremia"; the "corrected" sodium concentration can be calculated by adding 1.6 mEq/L for every 100 mg/dl elevation of glucose over the normal value of 100 mg/dl.
- BUN, creatinine: to assess renal function
- Serum ketones
- ECG: for evidence of hyperkalemia (peaked T waves), hypokalemia (U waves), presence of acute myocardial infarction
- Consider CBC, blood and urine cultures, and chest x-rays as appropriate.

- ABG: if the patient appears severely ill, to assess the severity of the acidosis (may not be needed if quick electrolytes are rapidly available) and ventilatory status

COMMENTS AND TREATMENT CONSIDERATIONS

The most important treatment in the ED management of DKA is volume replacement (generally at least 2 L of normal saline in adults who are not at risk for CHF). Fluid management of DKA in children is more controversial because of the rare (incidence approximately 0.8%) but life-threatening complication of cerebral edema that may develop during treatment. Although the volume of fluid administered has not been demonstrated to be causative, the American Diabetes Association recommends no more than 50 ml/kg over the first 4 hours. Unless the ECG shows evidence of hyperkalemia, insulin therapy is not needed immediately and should generally be held until the potassium level is known, as insulin can cause life-threatening hypokalemia.

In addition to intravenous fluids, insulin therapy is required in order to stop ketogenesis and subsequent acidosis. Bicarbonate is generally not indicated. Regular insulin (0.1 units/kg/hr in adults and children) may be given by intravenous infusion with or without a bolus dose (0.1 units/kg of regular insulin). The blood sugar may drop before ketogenesis is reversed (generally monitored by normalization of the anion gap). Therefore, glucose should be added to intravenous fluids when the blood sugar begins to approach "normal" levels (usually glucose is added to IVF when level is 200 to 250 mg/dl). Intravenous potassium replacement is also necessary even when initial serum K is "normal" because total body potassium is decreased and insulin therapy further decreases extracellular levels. Glucose and potassium levels should be monitored closely (approximately every hour) during initial treatment. Potassium (20 to 40 mEq/L) is usually added to the IV fluids when serum K drops to 4.0 to 4.5 mEq/L provided the patient is not in oliguric renal failure.

A search for the precipitating cause of the episode of DKA is necessary. Common precipitating factors include insufficient insulin (including noncompliance and new onset), infection +++, alcohol or drug abuse ++, pancreatitis or other abdominal disorders +, and acute myocardial infarction + (age older than 50 ++).

REFERENCES
Dunger DB, Sperling MA, Acerini CL, et al: ESPE/LWPES consensus statement on diabetic ketoacidosis in children and adolescents, *Arch Dis Child* 89:188, 2004.

Glaser N, Kuppermann N: Diabetic ketoacidosis, *Pediatr Emerg Care* 21:76, 2005.

CHAPTER 27

Hardern RD, Quinn ND: Emergency management of diabetic ketoacidosis in adults, *Emerg Med J* 20:210, 2003.

Kitabchi AE, Umpierrez GE, Murphy MB, et al: Hyperglycemic crises in diabetes, *Diabetes Care* 27(Suppl 1):S94, 2004.

HYPEROSMOLAR HYPERGLYCEMIC SYNDROME

HHS is a condition that usually occurs in older type 2 diabetics in whom severely elevated serum glucose results in an osmotic diuresis, electrolyte abnormalities, profound dehydration, and frequently AMS. HHS is defined as a serum glucose >600 mg/dl, serum osmolarity >320 to 330 mOsm/L, arterial pH >7.30, and negative or trace serum ketones. HHS has an incidence roughly equivalent to that of DKA, and the two syndromes have significant overlap. HHS differs from DKA in the more severely elevated glucose levels reached and the absence of ketoacidosis. Approximately half of patients with HHS do not have a history of known diabetes. Many patients have precipitant medical or surgical conditions such as infection, AMI, or stroke.

SYMPTOMS
- Weakness ++++
- Polyuria ++++
- Polydipsia +++
- Anorexia +++
- Nausea and vomiting +++
- Dizziness ++
- Confusion

SIGNS
- Volume depletion +++++: dry oral mucosa, dry skin with poor turgor, orthostatic hypotension, and tachycardia (moderate to severe +++; mild ++)
- AMS: alert ++, lethargic +++, comatose +++. Mental status correlates with serum osmolarity; coma is rare with an osmolarity <350 mOsm/L.
- Seizures ++
- Altered mental status

WORKUP
- Glucose: 800 to 1000 mg/dl
- Electrolytes, BUN, creatinine, and serum osmolarity. Severe hyperglycemia results in a pseudo-hyponatremia; the corrected sodium concentration should be calculated by adding 1.6 mEq/L for every 100 mg/dl elevation of glucose over the normal value of 100 mg/dl.

- Serum ketones to differentiate from DKA
- Search for a precipitating cause: chest x-rays, urinalysis and urine culture, and blood cultures for infection
- ECG (and possibly biomarkers of cardiac injury) to investigate acute MI
- Head CT or MRI to look for a concomitant stroke

COMMENTS AND TREATMENT CONSIDERATIONS

Hydration, initially with intravenous normal saline, is the cornerstone of therapy. Insulin is routinely administered but is less crucial than with DKA and lower doses are required. Otherwise treatment is similar to that for DKA, that is, fluids, insulin, replacement of electrolytes, and specific treatments for precipitant illnesses. Hyperglycemia and hyperosmolarity should be corrected gradually to prevent hypokalemia and cerebral edema caused by rapid shifting of fluid into the intracellular space.

Mortality has ranged from 10% to 17% in recent series and is predominantly related to the severity of the precipitating illness. A higher serum osmolarity and higher serum sodium also correlate with a poor outcome.

REFERENCES

Gaglia JL, Wyckoff J, Abrahamson MJ: Acute hyperglycemic crisis in the elderly, *Med Clin North Am* 88:1063, 2004.

Kitabchi AE, Umpierrez GE, Murphy MB, et al: Hyperglycemic crises in diabetes, *Diabetes Care* 27(Suppl 1):S94, 2004.

Pinies JA, Cairo G, Gaztambide S, Vazquez JA: Course and prognosis of 132 patients with diabetic nonketotic hyperosmolar state, *Diabete Metab* 20:43, 1994.

Yared Z, Chiasson JL: Ketoacidosis and the hyperosmolar hyperglycemic state in adult diabetic patients. Diagnosis and treatment, *Minerva Med* 94:409, 2003.

CHAPTER **27**

 HYPERCALCEMIA

Malignancy is the most common cause of severe hypercalcemia resulting in AMS. Malignancies most likely to cause hypercalcemia are breast cancer (30% to 40%), multiple myeloma (20% to 40%), squamous cell carcinomas of the lung (12% to 35%), the head, neck, or esophagus (19%), non-Hodgkin's lymphoma (3% to 13%), leukemias (2% to 11%), renal cell carcinoma (8%), cervical carcinoma (7%), and colon cancer (5%). Of these, the only malignancies that commonly present *initially* with signs of hypercalcemia are adult T-cell lymphoma (45%) and multiple myeloma. Although hyperparathyroidism is a more common cause of hypercalcemia, most patients with that disorder have less severe hypercalcemia and are asymptomatic. Hypercalcemic crisis is usually defined as a serum calcium concentration >14 mg/dl with acute signs and symptoms.

SYMPTOMS

Although symptoms are determined by both the absolute serum calcium concentration and the rate of rise, certain generalizations apply (Table 27–2).

- Polyuria and polydipsia ++++ related to inhibition of ADH
- Nausea and vomiting

SIGNS

- Evidence of extreme dehydration: dry mucous membranes, tachycardia, and orthostasis
- Increased vascular tone may lead to normal blood pressures despite severe dehydration.
- Coma, if present, usually occurs at concentrations >15 mg/dl.

WORKUP

- Total or ionized serum calcium concentrations. Total serum calcium must be corrected for low-albumin states (such as cancer) because ionized levels may be normal.

Total serum calcium corrected for albumin level =
[(normal albumin – patient's albumin) × 0.8] + patient's measured total calcium

These corrections can be avoided by measuring ionized serum calcium directly (normal range, 4.2 to 4.8 mg/dl).

- Check electrolytes for evidence of hypokalemia, hypomagnesemia, and hypernatremia.
- ECG: shortening of the QT interval; bradyarrhythmias, heart block, and asystole can occur.

COMMENTS AND TREATMENT CONSIDERATIONS

Initial treatment consists of hydration with normal saline because correction of volume depletion increases calcium excretion.

TABLE 27–2

CORRELATION OF CALCIUM CONCENTRATION WITH SYMPTOMS OF HYPERCALCEMIA

CALCIUM CONCENTRATION	SYMPTOMS
<12 mg/dl	Often asymptomatic; polyuria and polydipsia may be present
12-14 mg/dl	Moderate weakness and fatigue
14-16 mg/dl	Extreme weakness, lethargy, and confusion

Furosemide may also be used. Other pharmacologic therapy is not usually begun in the ED.

Serum phosphate is low but should not be replaced because of the danger of precipitating calcium phosphate crystals in the blood and tissues.

REFERENCES

Ariyan CE, Sosa JA: Assessment and management of patients with abnormal calcium, *Crit Care Med* 32(4 Suppl):S146, 2004.

Body JJ: Hypercalcemia of malignancy, *Semin Nephrol* 24:48, 2004.

Edelson GW, Kleerekoper M: Hypercalcemic crisis, *Med Clin North Am* 79:79, 1995.

Ziegler R: Hypercalcemic crisis, *J Am Soc Nephrol* 12(Suppl 17):S3, 2001.

 DELIRIUM TREMENS AND ALCOHOL WITHDRAWAL

CHAPTER 27

Delirium tremens (DTs) occurs in chronic alcoholics who are withdrawing from alcohol. Alcohol withdrawal causes a spectrum of clinical manifestations from mild tremulousness to seizures, hallucinations (may be auditory or visual and are often dramatic, e.g., bugs crawling on patient, or persecutory), and delirium. Aggressive treatment with benzodiazepines is required when early symptoms and signs are present to prevent progression of alcohol withdrawal syndrome. DTs can lead to death.

SYMPTOMS
Depend on stage of withdrawal
- Early: Shaking, anxious, nausea, vomiting
- Late: Seizures, altered mental status

SIGNS
Depend on stage of withdrawal
- Early: tremor, increasing levels of autonomic activity as condition progresses (tachycardia, hypertension, hyperreflexia)
- Late: diaphoresis, seizures, hallucinations, delirium

WORKUP
- Clinical diagnosis
- Rule out other conditions such as infection or CNS trauma that frequently coexist (e.g., urinalysis, chest x-rays, CT, LP as indicated).
- Electrolytes, glucose, magnesium (frequently low)
- CBC

COMMENTS AND TREATMENT CONSIDERATIONS
The mainstay of treatment is benzodiazepine administration. Large doses of IV benzodiazepines are often required. Thiamine 100 mg IV

should also probably be given because of the possibility of inducing Wernicke's encephalopathy with delivery of glucose-containing solutions. Patients are generally given magnesium because they are frequently hypomagnesemic. Patients with DTs require hospital admission, often to the ICU. Patients with mild withdrawal controlled with benzodiazepine administration in the ED may be discharged. Caution needs to be exercised in prescribing benzodiazepines for outpatient alcoholic patients because the combination of alcohol and benzodiazepines can lead to lethal respiratory depression.

REFERENCES

Bayard M, McIntyre J, Hill KR, et al: Alcohol withdrawal syndrome, *Am Fam Physician* 69:1443, 2004.

Chang PH, Steinberg MB: Alcohol withdrawal, *Med Clin North Am* 85:1191, 2001.

Kosten TR, O'Connor PG: Management of drug and alcohol withdrawal, *N Engl J Med* 348:1786, 2003.

 HYPERNATREMIA

Hypernatremia is defined as a serum sodium concentration >145 mmol/L. Hypernatremia is unlikely to be the cause of AMS until the sodium concentration is >155 mEq/L.

Hypernatremia generally occurs in infants, the debilitated, and the elderly, that is, generally in those who do not control their own dietary intake. Even a slight increase in serum sodium levels (3 mEq/L) above baseline triggers an intense thirst response in patients with normal physical abilities, mentation, and an intact thirst mechanism. This triggers water intake and a correction of the serum sodium before significant hypernatremia ensues.

Hypernatremia is usually precipitated by an illness that increases water loss or, less commonly, by excessive sodium intake. Diarrhea accounts for the majority of cases in young children (40% to 90%). Other precipitants in pediatric patients include pneumonia (10%), urinary tract infections, various CNS diseases, and inadequately diluted infant formulas. Complications include intracranial hemorrhages and arterial thrombosis. Permanent brain damage affects 10% to 15% of survivors.

Half of elderly patients with hypernatremia live in nursing homes. Hypernatremia is frequently precipitated by infection (pneumonia, 39%; urinary tract infections or urosepsis, 28%; bacteremia, 17%). In adults, comorbidities contribute to a higher mortality (40% to 60%) and incidence of permanent neurologic sequelae (38%).

Undiagnosed diabetes insipidus (DI) is a rare cause of hypernatremia in the ED but should be considered in patients who have recently undergone intracranial surgery. Persistently high urine output with concomitant volume depletion is a clue to this diagnosis.

SYMPTOMS
- AMS +++++, with severe hypernatremia causing lethargy to coma. Infants may be irritable and have a high-pitched cry.
- Infants are more likely to have seizures +++ to ++++, depending on severity of hypernatremia and rapidity of rise, than adults ++.
- Anorexia (infants: decreased feeding), nausea, and vomiting
- Oliguria ++++
- Symptoms stemming from the precipitating illness may predominate; diarrhea (90%) in infants, infection in any age group.

SIGNS
- AMS: lethargy to coma
- The features of volume depletion (weak pulses, and poor capillary perfusion) may be absent until late in the course.
- A doughy consistency of the skin is common.

WORKUP
- A workup for sepsis (chest x-rays, blood and urine cultures, and often an LP) is indicated.
- Electrolytes, BUN, creatinine, and glucose: the serum sodium concentration establishes the diagnosis of hypernatremia.
  The serum sodium concentration must be corrected if severe hyperglycemia is present (see Hyperosmolar Hyperglycemic Syndrome).
- A cranial CT scan may be indicated to rule out an intracranial hemorrhage, especially in children.
- Urine specific gravity is inappropriately low with DI.

CHAPTER 27

COMMENTS AND TREATMENT CONSIDERATIONS
Initial treatment of hypernatremia caused by dehydration is saline 0.9% IV until the intravascular volume is restored as indicated by normalization of pulse, BP, and urine output. Correction can then continue with 0.45% saline. Correction of serum Na^+ should be gradual to prevent cerebral edema.

REFERENCES
Adrogue HJ, Madias NE: Hypernatremia, *N Engl J Med* 342:1493, 2000.

Moritz ML, Ayus JC: Disorders of water metabolism in children: hyponatremia and hypernatremia, *Pediatr Rev* 23:371, 2002.

Weiss-Guillet EM, Takala J, Jakob SM: Diagnosis and management of electrolyte emergencies, *Best Pract Res Clin Endocrinol Metab* 17:623, 2003.

HEPATIC ENCEPHALOPATHY

Hepatic encephalopathy results from severe hepatic dysfunction. Patients' mental status varies from mildly depressed to coma in severe cases. Asterixis and sequelae of chronic liver disease may be found during physical examination, and plasma ammonia levels may be increased. Other conditions associated with liver failure, such as GI bleeding, must be considered. Treatments include lactulose and neomycin. Most patients are hospitalized while an evaluation for the precipitating cause is initiated.

REFERENCES

Als-Nielsen B, Gluud LL, Gluud C: Non-absorbable disaccharides for hepatic encephalopathy: systematic review of randomised trials, *BMJ* 328:1046, 2004.

Lizardi-Cervera J, Almeda P, Guevara L, et al: Hepatic encephalopathy: a review, *Ann Hepatol* 2:122, 2003.

Vaquero J, Chung C, Cahill ME, et al: Pathogenesis of hepatic encephalopathy in acute liver failure, *Semin Liver Dis* 23:259, 2003.

 MYXEDEMA COMA

Myxedema coma is the most severe expression of decompensated hypothyroidism. The true incidence is unknown; however, only 200 cases were reported between 1953 and 1986. It is more common in elderly (70% >60 years of age) women (80%), who almost invariably present during winter months (95%). Only approximately a third of patients have a history of hypothyroidism. The diagnosis is often delayed because of the coexistence of a precipitating factor (infection, stroke, hypothermia, sedative-hypnotic use, recent surgery, trauma, or other severe illness), which is presumed to be the cause of the patient's AMS. The diagnosis is then entertained only when initial management fails. Previous mortality was 80%; it is now 15% to 20%, principally because of the availability of intravenous levothyroxine.

SYMPTOMS

- AMS: lethargy, confusion, or psychosis; often a gradual deterioration over weeks
- Symptoms of hypothyroidism: fatigue, weakness, cold intolerance, muscle cramps, constipation, weight gain

SIGNS

- Coma +++
- Seizures: ++ in patients with coma

- Hypothermia (T < 35.5° C) ++++ in comatose patients
- Vital signs reflect the state of overall decreased metabolism: bradycardia ++++, SBP <100 +++, hypoventilation (with hypoxemia and hypercarbia).
- Signs of long-standing hypothyroidism: periorbital edema, macroglossia, hoarse voice, dry and cool skin, nonpitting edema of the lower extremities, fine hair texture with diminished eyebrows, and delayed relaxation of deep tendon reflexes
- Many of the signs of myxedema are indicative of a lowered basal metabolic rate and a lack of stimulation of beta-adrenergic receptors.
- Abdominal distention is common from either ileus or constipation; megacolon and fecal impaction can occur.
- Heart sounds are frequently distant because of pericardial effusion +++. Congestive heart failure is also frequent.
- Fever may develop and heart rate can be "normal" if sepsis is also present.

WORKUP
- Diagnosis is clinical in the ED setting.
- Serum TSH and free T_4 index are sent to the laboratory to confirm the clinical diagnosis. If available, a free T_3 and free T_4 by dialysis may be more clinically useful.
- A serum cortisol level is useful to exclude coexisting adrenal insufficiency.
- Other tests may assist in ruling out other conditions. Results are inconsistent in myxedema.
- Electrolytes: hyponatremia +++, hypochloremia +++, hypoglycemia +
- CK levels: frequently mildly elevated to 500 to 1000 U/L (MM fraction)
- CBC: macrocytic anemia; WBC rarely exceeds 10,000/mm^3 even with infection, although bandemia may be present.
- ECG: low voltage, sinus bradycardia, prolonged PR and QT intervals, and inverted or flattened T waves without ST segment changes
- LP: increased opening pressure and increased protein
- Chest x-rays: cardiomegaly
- Abdominal x-rays: constipation, ileus, or megacolon
- ABG: hypoxia ($Po_2 < 75$ mm Hg), hypercarbia, and respiratory acidosis

COMMENTS AND TREATMENT CONSIDERATIONS
Treatment must be initiated on the basis of clinical suspicion. Debate is ongoing concerning the optimal formulation and dose of thyroid hormone replacement in myxedema coma. Most experts recommend treatment with intravenous levothyroxine (T_4).

CHAPTER 27

357

Possible coexisting adrenal insufficiency should be treated empirically with hydrocortisone (100 mg IV q8h). Alternatively, dexamethasone phosphate (4 mg IV q6-8h) allows an ACTH stimulation test after initial cortisol measurement, although this may not be necessary in all patients.

REFERENCES

Fliers E, Wiersinga WM: Myxedema coma, *Rev Endocr Metab Disord* 4:137, 2003.

Ringel MD: Management of hypothyroidism and hyperthyroidism in the intensive care unit, *Crit Care Clin* 17:59, 2001.

Rodriguez I, Fluiters E, Perez-Mendez LF, et al: Factors associated with mortality of patients with myxoedema coma: prospective study in 11 cases treated in a single institution, *J Endocrinol* 180:347, 2004.

 NONCONVULSIVE STATUS EPILEPTICUS

Patients who have AMS, even to the point of being comatose, may occasionally be in nonconvulsive status epilepticus (NCSE). Nonconvulsive seizures occur in nonmotor areas of the brain (usually the temporal, frontal, or parietal regions) and can be simple or complex (relating to whether consciousness is affected) and focal (partial) or generalized. NCSE is defined as continuous or intermittent seizure activity for more than 30 minutes as evidenced by impaired mental status, without motor convulsions.

SYMPTOMS

Patients in NCSE are often unaware of their seizures and do not voice any complaint. Family members who become concerned about the patient's behavior typically bring him or her to medical attention.

SIGNS

- Automatisms, such as repetitive lip smacking, picking at clothes, smiling, head nodding, laughing inappropriately, and verbal perseveration are common.
- Level of consciousness often fluctuates. Patients may appear awake but withdrawn and confused. Alternatively, they may be drowsy and slow to respond or even comatose.
- NCSE may progress to convulsive seizure activity, resulting in focal signs such as clonic jerking of the eyelids or an extremity or tonic deviation of the head.

WORKUP

An EEG is ultimately needed to diagnose the seizure activity.

COMMENTS AND TREATMENT CONSIDERATIONS

NCSE is frequently misdiagnosed as psychiatric illness (40%), a metabolic encephalopathy, or a prolonged postictal phase. The diagnosis of NCSE should be considered in patients who (1) have AMS and fail to awaken after a seizure and all other medical workup is negative; (2) have AMS and exhibit automatisms or minor myoclonic jerking of the arms or facial region; or (3) have a new-onset "psychiatric" illness, especially if consciousness, symptoms wax and wane, or the patient has a history of seizure disorder.

Patients in NCSE often respond dramatically to diazepam, with improvement of their mental status within 4 to 5 minutes in many cases.

REFERENCES

Benson PJ, Klein EJ: New-onset absence status epilepsy presenting as altered mental status in a pediatric patient, *Ann Emerg Med* 37:402, 2001.

Fernandez-Torre JL, Diaz-Castroverde AG: Non-convulsive status epilepticus in elderly individuals: report of four representative cases, *Age Ageing* 33:78, 2004.

Scholtes FB, Renier WO: Non-convulsive status epilepticus: causes, treatment, and outcome in 65 patients, *J Neurol Neurosurg Psychiatry* 61:93, 1996.

Shneker BF, Fountain NB: Assessment of acute morbidity and mortality in nonconvulsive status epilepticus, *Neurology* 61:1066, 2003.

REYE SYNDROME

Reye syndrome is an acute, noninflammatory encephalopathy that usually occurs in children and is associated with fatty degeneration of the liver. Case fatality rates range from 26% to 42%, and any delay in recognition, aggressive management, or disposition is strongly associated with a poor outcome.

SYMPTOMS

- History of a prodromal illness in 75% to 95%, either influenza B or varicella infection ++++; followed by severe, repetitive vomiting 3 to 6 days later during apparent convalescence ++++ then altered behavior, usually irritability and lethargy
- History of therapeutic dosages of salicylate during the antecedent infection ++++; 75% to 95% sensitivity, limited specificity
- Approximately 75% of cases occur in winter months.
- Between 75% to 80% of cases occur in children 5 to 15 years old, the rest in children younger than 5. These cases may be more

difficult to detect because the differential diagnosis for vomiting and lethargy is large; adult cases are rare but can occur, following the same history, clinical course, and laboratory values as pediatric cases.
- Afebrile by the time of presentation

SIGNS
- Disease progresses in stages; 70% to 80% present in precomatose stages (I-II).
- Stage I—lethargy only
- Stage II—combative or stuporous; inappropriate verbalizing; sluggish pupillary reaction; conjugate deviation on doll's eyes maneuver; may have nonpurposeful response to pain; seizures
- Stage III—same as stage II except comatose with decorticate posture and response to pain
- Stage IV—same as stage III except decerebrate posture and response to pain, inconsistent or absent oculocephalic reflex
- Stage V—same as stage IV except flaccid with no response to pain, no pupillary response, no oculocephalic reflex
- Tachypnea ++++
- Lack of jaundice or nuchal rigidity ++++
- Hepatomegaly +++
- Dehydration ++
- Arrhythmias and myocarditis can occur rarely in advanced stages.

WORKUP
- Hypoglycemia occurs in 40% of all children and more commonly affects younger children; adults are rarely hypoglycemic.
- ALT and AST levels are 3 to 30 times normal but significantly lower than in fulminant hepatitis.
- PT abnormal in 90% ++++; low specificity
- CSF cell counts and bilirubin levels are normal ++++.
- Ammonia levels initially may be normal ++; levels greater than 300 µg% are associated with increased mortality; comatose patients have levels 3 to 20 times normal ++++.
- Salicylate levels help differentiate liver failure from toxicity; Reye syndrome occurs in the absence of toxicity.
- CT of the head should be done before LP in patients with neurologic symptoms; absence of papilledema does not reliably rule out increased intracranial pressure in children.

COMMENTS AND TREATMENT CONSIDERATIONS
All patients with Reye syndrome must be admitted to the hospital. Those with stage II or higher disease require admission to an ICU with ICP monitoring capability; stage III or higher generally require intubation.

REFERENCES

Casteels-Van Daele M, Van Geet C, Wouters C, Eggermont E: Reye syndrome revisited: a descriptive term covering a group of heterogeneous disorders, *Eur J Pediatr* 159:641, 2000.

Dezateux CA, Dinwiddie R, Helms P, Matthew DJ: Recognition and early management of Reye's syndrome, *Arch Dis Child* 61:647, 1986.

Glasgow JF, Middleton B: Reye syndrome—insights on causation and prognosis, *Arch Dis Child* 85:351, 2001.

METHEMOGLOBINEMIA

Many drugs and substances, including nitrates, benzocaine, and dapsone, can induce methemoglobinemia. Because of an alteration in the properties of hemoglobin and its subsequent ability to bind oxygen, the oxygen-carrying capacity of the blood is reduced. It is similar in mechanism to CO poisoning; patients have central cyanosis but "normal" blood gasses because dissolved oxygen (not bound to hemoglobin) in the blood (PaO_2) is unaffected by the process. Direct measurements of oxygen saturation of hemoglobin by cooximetry and methemoglobin levels confirm the diagnosis. Treatment is with methylene blue. See Chapter 37, Toxic Exposure, Approach to.

REFERENCES

Bradberry SM: Occupational methaemoglobinaemia. Mechanisms of production, features, diagnosis and management including the use of methylene blue, *Toxicol Rev* 22:13, 2003.

Rehman HU: Methemoglobinemia, *West J Med* 175:193, 2001.

HYPOMAGNESEMIA

Those at high risk for hypomagnesemia include chronic alcoholics, patients with cirrhosis or who are taking diuretics, malnourished patients, patients requiring tube feeding or total parenteral nutrition, and patients with renal failure. The clinical syndrome of hypomagnesemia is similar to hypocalcemia.

SYMPTOMS

- Anorexia
- Nausea and vomiting
- Fatigue
- Irritability
- Generalized weakness

SIGNS
- Tremor
- Muscular twitching and tetany
- Chvostek's sign
- Trousseau's sign
- Hyporeflexia
- Altered mentation: delirium, hallucinations
- Hypotension and hypothermia (occasional)
- Seizures (usually generalized)

WORKUP
- If a patient has signs or symptoms of hypomagnesemia or is in a high-risk group, serum magnesium, calcium, and electrolytes should be measured. However, serum magnesium levels do not reflect the total body tissue depletion of magnesium. Severe symptoms, such as seizures, are associated with serum magnesium levels below 1.5.
- ECG: a prolonged PR interval, prolonged QT interval, ST segment depression, and T wave abnormalities are characteristic of hypomagnesemia. Arrhythmias may be seen.

COMMENTS AND TREATMENT CONSIDERATIONS
Magnesium depletion is almost always associated with hypocalcemia and hypokalemia. Acid-base abnormalities are also common. In clinical practice, patients who are at high risk for hypomagnesemia typically also have many other risk factors for seizures (e.g., alcohol abuse or withdrawal, other electrolyte abnormalities). Seizures associated with hypomagnesemia are probably multifactorial. Experimentally induced hypomagnesemia in humans has failed to induce seizures.

REFERENCES
Shils ME: Experimental human magnesium depletion, *Medicine (Baltimore)* 48:61, 1969.

Suter C, Klingman WO: Neurologic manifestations of magnesium depletion states, *Neurology* 5:691, 1955.

Turnball TL, Vanden Hoek TL, Howes DS, Eisner RF: Utility of laboratory studies in the emergency department patient with a new-onset seizure, *Ann Emerg Med* 19:373, 1990.

Neck Pain and Stiffness
Thomas P. Graham

Patients with neck pain as a result of trauma should be considered to have a cervical spine fracture or ligamentous injury until proved otherwise. In the absence of trauma, meningitis and encephalitis must be excluded because bacterial meningitis can progress from an initially mild-appearing illness to death within hours. Subarachnoid hemorrhage, also potentially life threatening, may cause neck pain as a result of blood in the cerebral spinal fluid irritating the meninges. Carotid artery dissection can arise as neck pain associated with stroke symptoms and may be preceded by exertion or trauma.

Focal cervical spine tenderness without trauma should raise suspicion for potentially devastating processes such as epidural abscess, discitis, and vertebral osteomyelitis. These illnesses may arise with fever and usually but not invariably occur in immunocompromised patients, IV drug abusers, or elderly persons. Severe cervical disc herniation may occur with or without preceding trauma and often arises as neck pain with radicular pain radiating into an upper extremity. Neck pain in association with a sore throat and fever should prompt evaluation for epiglottitis/supraglottitis, retropharyngeal abscess, peritonsillar abscess, or other deep tissue infection. Other structures in the neck, such as the thyroid gland, can also cause neck pain.

Dystonic reactions are common after short- or long-term neuroleptic use and often manifest as neck stiffness. Patients with dystonia are often very uncomfortable, and urgent treatment is required. Tetanus causes neck and back stiffness in association with trismus and dysphagia, most commonly in unimmunized individuals and particularly the elderly. Although rare in countries where immunization is widespread, tetanus can be fatal.

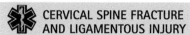

CERVICAL SPINE FRACTURE AND LIGAMENTOUS INJURY

Patients with significant head or cervical spine trauma, in particular those with neck pain, cervical spine tenderness, alteration in mentation, or distracting injuries, must be immobilized with a hard cervical collar until a fracture is excluded. Those who can not or will not maintain a neutral position of the spine with a collar alone should also be placed on a backboard with their head, neck, and trunk immobilized. Patients who are able to turn their head or move their body off the board have not been adequately immobilized. Immobilized patients must be monitored to prevent aspiration and asphyxiation.

SYMPTOMS
- Neck pain occurring at rest or during range of motion ++++. Patients may not complain of neck pain if they have an altered level of alertness (related to intoxication, head trauma, or other causes) or have distracting injuries (e.g., other fractures, intra-abdominal bleeding, or extensive lacerations). Neck pain is present in nearly 100% of patients with fractures in the absence of these factors.
- Weakness, numbness, paresthesias, or pain in a radicular pattern suggests possible concurrent spinal cord injury.
- Dysesthesias, paresthesias, or weakness of the upper extremities out of proportion to the lower extremities may indicate a central spinal cord injury (central cord syndrome) and may occur in the absence of significant neck pain or abnormal neurologic findings in the lower extremities.

SIGNS
- Midline neck tenderness ++++
- Neck pain with active range of motion (patients who are not fully alert, are intoxicated, or have distracting injuries should not be put through range of motion).
- Soft tissue swelling is usually not appreciated.
- Weakness, paresthesias, or sensory deficit ++ may occur with spinal cord involvement.

WORKUP
Rule out bone injury.
- Three-view x-ray series of the cervical spine (Figs. 28–1 to 28–3). A cervical spine series must contain (1) a lateral film showing C1 through and including the entire upper border of T1, (2) an anteroposterior (AP) view, and (3) an open-mouth odontoid view demonstrating the dens and the lateral masses of C1.

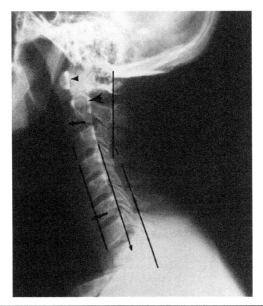

Fig. 28–1 Lateral view of normal cervical spine. Predental space *(arrowhead)*. Harris' ring *(barbed arrow)*. Prevertebral soft tissues *(arrows)*. Posterior cervical line, anterior and posterior body lines, spinolaminar lines *(long arrows)*. (Courtesy of Michael Zucker, MD, Los Angeles.)

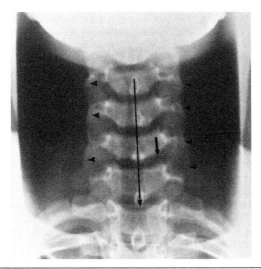

Fig. 28–2 Anteroposterior view of normal cervical spine. Lateral masses *(arrowheads)*. Spinous processes are aligned *(line)*. (Courtesy of Michael Zucker, MD, Los Angeles.)

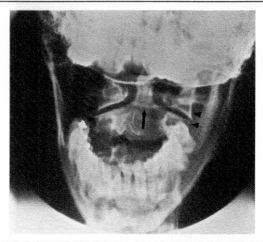

Fig. 28-3 Open-mouth odontoid view of normal cervical spine. Lateral masses C1-2 are aligned *(arrowheads)*. Dens is unremarkable *(arrow)*. (Courtesy of Michael Zucker, MD, Los Angeles.)

These films must be of adequate quality to view clearly the prevertebral soft tissue as well as the cervical vertebrae and their alignment. It may be necessary to apply gentle downward traction to both arms during the lateral x-ray in order to visualize the lower cervical spine in obese or muscular patients. Traction should not be applied if neurologic deficits are present, however. (Examples of cervical spine fractures are shown in Figs. 28–4 to 28–7.)

- When one fracture is seen, other less obvious fractures are often present.
- Transaxillary ("swimmer's") view. This view may be useful to evaluate the lower cervical spine if the initial three-view series cannot visualize all the way down to the level of T1.
- Oblique views, in combination with the AP view, may assist in diagnosing facet dislocations (Figs. 28–8 and 28–9).
- CT scan of the cervical spine is indicated to evaluate a fracture or suspicious finding noted on x-ray. CT is also indicated when plain films are normal but clinical suspicion for fracture is high (e.g., in the presence of neurologic signs/symptoms or persistent neck pain). Current practice at many trauma centers is to perform helical CT scan instead of cervical spine plain films in trauma patients with moderate to high risk for cervical spine fracture. In these instances, a single lateral x-ray may be utilized to screen for obvious fractures pending CT evaluation.

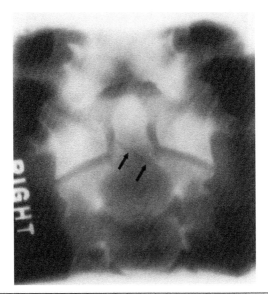

Fig. 28–4 Anteroposterior tomogram of dens fracture, type II. Oblique fracture at base of dens *(arrows)*. (Courtesy of Michael Zucker, MD, Los Angeles.)

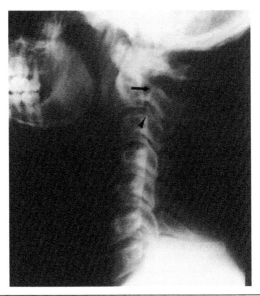

Fig. 28–5 Lateral view of pars fracture of C2 (hangman's fracture) *(arrow)*. Mild subluxation *(arrowhead)*. (Courtesy of Michael Zucker, MD, Los Angeles.)

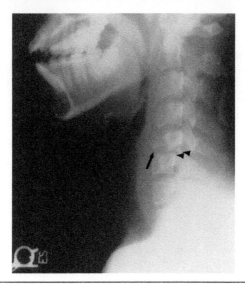

Fig. 28–6 Lateral view of hyperflexion teardrop fracture–dislocation of C5 *(arrow)*. Posterior subluxation of C5 and C6 *(arrowheads)*. (Courtesy of Michael Zucker, MD, Los Angeles.)

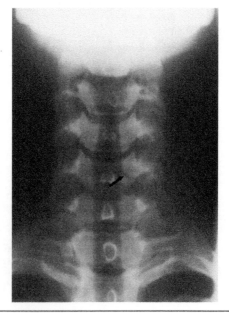

Fig. 28–7 Anteroposterior view of burst fracture of C6. Oblique fracture line *(arrow)*. (Courtesy of Michael Zucker, MD, Los Angeles.)

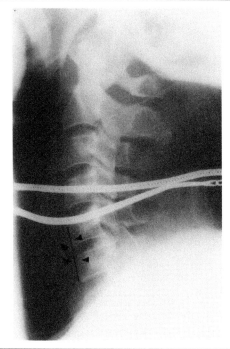

Fig. 28–8   Lateral view of unilateral interfacetal dislocation of C5-6. Subtle anterior subluxation of C5 on C6 *(arrowheads* and *line).* (Courtesy of Michael Zucker, MD, Los Angeles.)

Rule out ligamentous injury.

- Flexion-extension views of the cervical spine were previously widely used to evaluate ligamentous stability in patients with persistent neck pain and a normal three-view cervical spine series. Flexion-extension x-rays, however, are not adequately sensitive or specific to be useful in the acute setting.
- MRI is superior to flexion-extension views or CT in demonstrating ligamentous injury, spinal cord injury, and intervertebral disc herniation. CT scan is preferred when evaluating for fractures.

COMMENTS AND TREATMENT CONSIDERATIONS

Cervical spine precautions must be observed until a fracture or ligamentous injury has been reliably excluded. Large prospective studies have investigated whether cervical spine fractures can be ruled out by clinical examination. The National Emergency X-Radiography Utilization Study (NEXUS) reported five criteria that, when all are present, approach 100% sensitivity for detecting

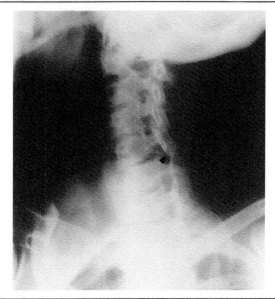

Fig. 28–9 Oblique view of unilateral interfacetal dislocation of C5-6. Facets are reversed *(arrowhead)*. (Courtesy of Michael Zucker, MD, Los Angeles.)

patients at extremely low risk for cervical spine injury after blunt trauma (Table 28–1). These criteria are commonly used in emergency departments to identify patients who do not require imaging studies.

If significant midline neck pain persists after negative cervical spine x-rays, ligamentous injury may be present. MRI should be considered in these cases if available. Alternatively, patients with possible ligamentous injury but without any neurologic signs or symptoms may be discharged with a hard collar (e.g., Aspen collar, Philadelphia collar, or Miami collar) in place. These patients require orthopedic or neurosurgical follow-up.

TABLE 28–1

NEXUS CRITERIA FOR SELECTING PATIENTS AT EXTREMELY LOW RISK FOR CERVICAL SPINE INJURY AFTER BLUNT TRAUMA

All five criteria must be present:
1. The absence of midline cervical tenderness
2. The absence of neurologic deficit
3. Normal alertness
4. The absence of intoxication
5. The absence of painful, distracting injury

Adapted from Hoffman JR, Mower WR, Wolfson AB, et al: Validity of a set of clinical criteria to rule out injury to the cervical spine in patients with blunt trauma, *N Engl J Med* 343:94, 2000.

Cervical spine fractures in children are uncommon. However, because of the higher incidence of subluxation and spinal cord injury without radiographic abnormality (SCIWORA) in children, careful neurologic assessment and imaging should be performed for all pediatric trauma patients who have a mechanism for or clinical evidence of neck injury. CT to rule out fracture and/or MRI to rule out ligamentous injury should be performed if plain x-rays are normal but suspicion for serious injury remains.

The majority of cervical spine fractures occur at level C2 and C5-6. In the elderly, odontoid fractures predominate. Any spinal column fracture, whether cervical or thoracolumbar, should heighten suspicion for other (often noncontiguous) spinal column fractures.

REFERENCES

Grogan EL, Morris JA Jr, Dittus RS, et al: Cervical spine evaluation in urban trauma centers: lowering institutional costs and complications through helical CT scan, *J Am Coll Surg* 200:160, 2005.

Hoffman JR, Mower WR, Wolfson AB, et al: Validity of a set of clinical criteria to rule out injury to the cervical spine in patients with blunt trauma, *N Engl J Med* 343:94, 2000.

Mower WR, Hoffman JR, Pollack CV Jr, et al: Use of plain radiography to screen for cervical spine injuries, *Ann Emerg Med* 38:1, 2001.

Widder S, Doig C, Burrowes P, et al: Prospective evaluation of computed tomographic scanning for the spinal clearance of obtunded trauma patients: preliminary results, *J Trauma* 56:1179, 2004.

 MENINGITIS

Neck pain and stiffness may be due to inflammation of the meninges. Meningismus in association with a headache should be considered a medical emergency until proved otherwise.

See Chapter 18, Headache.

 SUBARACHNOID HEMORRHAGE

Neck pain and stiffness may be due to inflammation of the meninges. Meningismus in association with a headache should be considered a medical emergency until proved otherwise.

See Chapter 18, Headache.

 CAROTID ARTERY DISSECTION

Carotid artery dissection may occur in any age group and accounts for a significant percentage of strokes in young people.

Trauma is sometimes but not invariably present. When trauma is reported, symptom onset is often delayed. A high degree of suspicion should exist for this condition when patients present with neck pain in association with transient ischemic attack (TIA) or stroke findings or Horner's syndrome. Abuse of cocaine or amphetamines may cause dissections in previously healthy patients.

SYMPTOMS
- Neck pain, sometimes but not always related to a traumatic event or neck manipulation
- Headache
- Amaurosis fugax
- Symptoms of TIA or stroke
- Syncope

SIGNS
- Horner's syndrome (ptosis, miosis, and anhidrosis)
- Cranial nerve dysfunction
- Signs of TIA or stroke may be present.
- Carotid bruit may be present but is not specific.

WORKUP
- Laboratory studies are not diagnostic but may be useful to exclude coagulopathy or other concurrent disease processes.
- Carotid artery duplex is noninvasive and usually diagnostic.
- MRI/MRA is usually diagnostic if available and if the patient is stable.
- CT angiogram may show a dissection but appears to lack the sensitivity of MRI/MRA.
- Contrast arteriography is invasive but may be required to confirm the diagnosis.

COMMENTS AND TREATMENT CONSIDERATIONS
The diagnosis is often difficult because of the nonspecific nature of presenting symptoms. If the diagnosis is confirmed, emergent consultation with a vascular surgeon is required. Anticoagulation may be indicated if there are no contraindications. Surgical intervention may also be indicated.

REFERENCES
Chaves C, Estol C, Esnaola MM, et al: Spontaneous intracranial internal carotid artery dissection: report of 10 patients, *Arch Neurol* 59:977, 2002.

Chen YC, Lee TH, Chen CJ, et al: Spontaneous common carotid artery dissection: a case report and review of the literature, *Eur Neurol* 50:58, 2003.

Scovell SD, Masaryk T: Carotid artery dissection, *Semin Vasc Surg* 15:137, 2002.

 CERVICAL SPINE DISC HERNIATION

SYMPTOMS
- Neck pain that may radiate to the scalp, shoulder, or down an extremity in a radicular pattern
- Vibration (e.g., driving) or certain position may exacerbate symptoms.
- Numbness of the distal upper extremities

SIGNS
- Weakness or sensory deficit of the upper extremities
- Fasciculations
- Loss of deep tendon reflexes
- Atrophy of muscles in the affected nerve distribution may be present in chronic cases.

WORKUP
- MRI is the study of choice to evaluate for disc herniation and spinal cord compression.
- Cervical spine x-rays are usually negative in the setting of disc herniation but are helpful in ruling out other causes of neck pain. Oblique views may indicate bone impingement of cervical nerve roots causing similar symptoms.
- CT-myelography can be useful to diagnose severe cases if MRI is unavailable.

COMMENTS AND TREATMENT CONSIDERATIONS
Acute motor weakness or significant sensory deficit may indicate spinal cord compression. MRI (if available) and urgent neurosurgical consultation should be obtained for these cases. Chronic disc disease may arise as a slow progression of symptoms. Disc levels most commonly involved are C5-6 and C6-7. Conservative treatment with analgesics is usually indicated. Neurologic or neurosurgical consultation should be obtained for significant neurologic symptoms or signs.

REFERENCES
Connell MD: Natural history and pathogenesis of cervical disk disease, *Orthop Clin North Am* 23:369, 1992.
Kuroki T, Kumano K, Hirabayashi S: Usefulness of MRI in the preoperative diagnosis of cervical disk herniation, *Arch Orthop Trauma Surg* 112:180, 1993.

28

CHAPTER

Schimandle JH, Heller JG: Nonoperative treatment of degenerative cervical disk disease, *J South Orthop Assoc* 5:207, 1996.

 CERVICAL SPINE EPIDURAL ABSCESS, OSTEOMYELITIS, DISCITIS, AND TUMOR

Neck pain and midline cervical spine tenderness not associated with trauma may indicate one of these serious pathologic conditions.

See Chapter 4, Back Pain, Lower.

 EPIGLOTTITIS/SUPRAGLOTTITIS AND PERITONSILLAR/RETROPHARYNGEAL ABSCESSES

Neck pain associated with a sore throat, especially in a febrile patient, suggests a potential serious soft tissue infection. Such infections have the potential to cause airway compromise.

See Chapter 35, Sore Throat.

 THYROIDITIS

See Chapter 29, Palpitations and Tachycardia.

 DYSTONIC REACTION

Neuroleptic agents, antiemetics (e.g., prochlorperazine [Compazine] or metoclopramide [Reglan]), and occasionally other agents can cause extrapyramidal side effects, including dystonia, akathisia, and akinesis. These reactions are generally responsive to treatment; tardive dyskinesia occurs after longer term neuroleptic therapy and is usually not reversible. Patients with dystonia are most likely to seek treatment in the ED because symptoms are acute in onset and severe. Dystonia may develop hours or days after drug exposure.

The diagnosis of dystonia should be entertained in patients currently taking a suspected medication (including those who have recently taken a single dose) and reporting the characteristic muscle spasms of the neck or face. The presentation is often dramatic but, if recognized, is easily treated. Cocaine use may predispose patients to dystonic reactions.

SYMPTOMS
- Severe neck discomfort and stiffness
- Difficulty with speech

SIGNS
- Acute torticollis
- Neck muscle spasm and/or trismus

- Elevation of the shoulder
- Upward deviation of the eyes (oculogyric crisis)
- Protrusion of tongue
- Arching of back (opisthotonos)

WORKUP
- Diagnosis is established by the physical examination in the setting of an appropriate medication history.
- Laboratory tests are of no value for diagnosing dystonic reactions.

COMMENTS AND TREATMENT CONSIDERATIONS
Treatment with an anticholinergic agent such as diphenhydramine (an antihistamine with anticholinergic effects; adults: 50 mg IV/IM; children: 1 to 2 mg/kg IV/IM) or benztropine mesylate (adults: 1 to 2 mg IM; children (over 3 years only): 0.02 to 0.05 mg/kg IM) is therapeutic. Rapid relief of symptoms should occur; if not, other disease processes should be considered. If discharged, patients should be instructed to continue oral diphenhydramine or benztropine therapy for 3 or 4 days.

REFERENCES
Corre KA, Niemann JT, Bessen HA: Extended therapy for acute dystonic reactions, *Ann Emerg Med* 13:194, 1984.

McCormick MA, Manoguerra AS: Dystonic reactions. In Harwood-Nuss A, Linden CH, Luten RC, et al (eds): *The clinical practice of emergency medicine*, ed 2. Philadelphia, 1996, JB Lippincott.

Peiris RS, Peckler BF: Cimetidine-induced dystonic reaction, *J Emerg Med* 21:27, 2001.

 TETANUS

Tetanus is an acute illness characterized by severe generalized muscle rigidity and spasms. It is caused by the toxin tetanospasmin, which is secreted by the anaerobic gram-positive rod bacterium *Clostridium tetani*. The highly resistant spores of *C. tetani* are ubiquitous in soil and feces worldwide. Tetanospasmin, a potent neurotoxin, diffuses into the nervous system, where it causes disinhibition of the autonomic and motor nervous systems. Although the incubation period can be as short as 1 day or as long as 1 month, symptom onset is usually 1 to 2 weeks after the initial injury. A shorter incubation period portends a more severe course. Although rare in the United States, tetanus causes an estimated 200,000 deaths per year worldwide, principally as a result of neonatal tetanus.

Tetanus should be strongly considered in individuals with neck stiffness or trismus and a history of inadequate tetanus immunization. Of particular concern are older or immunocompromised patients, intravenous drug users, and those with recent wounds (contaminated, operative, or burns). In some cases, no history of skin break is noted.

SYMPTOMS
- Jaw pain or tightness
- Neck or back pain or stiffness
- Dysphagia
- Extremity pain, especially in the wounded extremity
- Cranial nerve palsies +

SIGNS
- Trismus
- Tetanic spasms, especially in the face (risus sardonicus) and back muscles (opisthotonus)
- Hypersympathetic autonomic disturbances: tachycardia, labile blood pressure, hyperpyrexia, dysrhythmias

WORKUP
A reliable history of active immunization within the past 10 years makes the diagnosis very unlikely. Unfortunately, immunization status reported by patients is frequently inaccurate.
- No diagnostic studies exist for tetanus. In anticipation of intensive supportive care, routine studies such as a chest x-ray, EKG, CBC, electrolytes, calcium, BUN, creatinine, creatine kinase, and urinalysis are usually performed.
- An ABG and vital capacity are indicated if ventilatory failure is a concern.
- The site of infection should be sought.

COMMENTS AND TREATMENT CONSIDERATIONS
Unless treated, symptoms progress from pain and stiffness to rigidity and violent convulsive spasms. The early stages of tetanus may mimic dystonia or hypocalcemic tetany, whereas a more severe episode must be differentiated from strychnine poisoning. Unlike tetanus, dystonic reactions respond to anticholinergic medications. Strychnine poisoning, in contrast to tetanus, usually spares the jaw muscles, and muscle rigidity is absent between spasms.

Treatment of tetanus consists of five components:
1. Aggressive supportive care including, in severe cases, intubation and paralysis to ensure adequate ventilation
2. Human tetanus immune globulin (TIG) to neutralize circulating and wound tetanospasmin
3. Treatment of muscle spasm with benzodiazepines in milder cases and with paralysis in severe cases

4. Antibiotics (penicillin 4 million U IV q6h or metronidazole 500 mg IV q6h)
5. Wound débridement

All patients with suspected tetanus should be admitted to an ICU. The typical duration of illness is 4 to 6 weeks. Patients who have recovered from tetanus require active immunization because the disease does not confer immunity.

REFERENCES

Cook TM, Protheroe RT, Handel JM: Tetanus: a review of the literature, *Br J Anaesth* 87:477, 2001.

Groleau G: Tetanus, *Emerg Med Clin North Am* 10:351, 1992.

Thwaites CL, Farrar JJ: Preventing and treating tetanus, *BMJ* 326:117, 2003.

CHAPTER 28

Palpitations and Tachycardia
Mel E. Herbert and Mary L. Lanctot-Herbert

Palpitations are a common and frequently perplexing presenting complaint in emergency medicine. Patients ultimately may have a life-threatening disease, a benign rhythm disturbance, or simply "anxiety." Definitive diagnosis on initial presentation to the ED is uncommon. The ED physician must distinguish high-risk patients needing treatment or hospitalization from low-risk patients who can be evaluated in an outpatient setting. The sensation of a beating heart is normal in many situations. The normal contraction and movement of the heart are generally not felt at rest. A normal sinus tachycardia may be noted during exercise, high-stress situations, or after drug ingestion.

CAUSES
1. Arrhythmias (ultimately diagnosed in 45% of unselected patients): Almost any arrhythmia can cause palpitations; however, most arrhythmias are clinically silent. Sinus pause or extrasystole may be felt as a pounding in the chest. Paradoxically, patients with serious heart disease frequently have the most arrhythmias and the least sensation of palpitation.
2. High-output states: Patients with anemia, fever, or thyrotoxicosis may feel the compensatory sinus tachycardia associated with the underlying condition.
3. Caffeine: Coffee, various teas, and even sodas high in caffeine
4. Illicit drugs: Stimulants including cocaine, amphetamines
5. Prescribed drugs: Inhaled beta-agonists (albuterol and others), aminophylline, and thyroid replacement medications
6. Anxiety (ultimately diagnosed in 30% of unselected cases): A common cause of palpitations, but this diagnosis should be made only after serious diseases have been excluded.

SYMPTOMS

Although it remains good practice to determine the onset, timing, rate, and rhythm of the palpitations, the usefulness of many of these features is in doubt (Table 29–1).

1. Palpitations associated with the following suggest potentially serious cardiac disease and generally require hospital admission:
   a. Syncope or near-syncope suggests hypoperfusion caused by an arrhythmia and is usually an indication for admission and monitoring; unfortunately, the results of inpatient evaluation frequently fail to diagnose the cause of the syncope.
   b. History of underlying ischemic heart disease. A history of prior myocardial infarction (MI) or congestive heart failure (CHF) is a major risk factor for ventricular arrhythmias. Patients with this history and with palpitations should generally be admitted to the hospital to rule out a malignant arrhythmia such as ventricular tachycardia.
   c. Chest pain. A history of ischemic-sounding chest pain in association with palpitations is cause for concern. Tachycardia stresses the heart in a manner analogous to an exercise stress test. Symptoms of cardiac ischemia accompanying rapid palpitations suggest the patient has significant coronary artery disease.
   d. Shortness of breath. Although many patients with rapid palpitations experience some shortness of breath, more prolonged or severe shortness of breath may indicate the pulmonary congestion of heart failure. Patients with palpitations in the setting of CHF are more likely to have a serious arrhythmia such as ventricular tachycardia.

CHAPTER 29

TABLE 29–1	
PATIENT HISTORY AND POSSIBLE ARRHYTHMIC EVENTS	
HISTORICAL FEATURE	CONSIDER
Isolated skips or jumps	Dropped beats or extrasystole
Paroxysms of rapid *irregular* palpitations	Atrial fibrillation, atrial flutter with variable block, MAT
Paroxysms of rapid *regular* palpitations	SVT or VT
On standing or change in posture	Postural hypotension
In women, associated with sweating and flushing	Menopause

2. Palpitations associated with the following suggest a potentially serious cardiac condition but may not require hospital admission:
   a. Sustained palpitations. Patients who have palpitations that last more than 5 minutes frequently have a cardiac cause of their symptoms.
   b. Irregular palpitations. Palpitations clearly described as irregular are strongly predictive of an underlying cardiac cause. Rapid irregular palpitations are usually episodes of atrial fibrillation.

SIGNS

- The physical examination is rarely helpful in patients with palpitations, as they have generally resolved. If palpitations occur during the examination, a rhythm strip should be obtained. A normal physical examination does not rule out a serious cause for the palpitation.
- Underlying signs of cardiac disease should be sought (e.g., cardiomegaly, signs of heart failure, and murmurs).
- Conditions that could cause a high-output state should be investigated (e.g., goiter from thyroid disease, anemia from GI bleed, and so forth).

WORKUP

1. ECG in patients currently *symptomatic* allows a diagnosis to be made in most cases. If present, an arrhythmia should be treated appropriately. If no arrhythmia is noted, this information can be used to reassure the patient or as evidence for an alternative, frequently psychiatric, diagnosis. Patients should be questioned about stress and suicidal or homicidal thoughts.
2. ECG in patients currently *asymptomatic* yields limited information. A completely normal, one-time ECG is consistent with a cardiac cause. However, ECG may show the following:
   a. *Evidence of old myocardial infarction (pathologic Q waves).* Patients with ECG evidence of an old MI are at higher risk of ventricular arrhythmias.
   b. *Evidence of preexcitation.* The most common form of preexcitation is Wolff-Parkinson-White syndrome (WPW). The usual manifestations are a short PR interval and a delta wave. WPW is associated with a number of arrhythmias that can present as palpitations (Fig. 29–1).
   c. *Long QT interval.* Prolongation of the QT interval is associated with ventricular arrhythmia and sudden death. Long QT syndrome may be congenital or the result of drug or electrolyte abnormalities. Many ECGs provide the QTc, or it may be calculated as QTc = QT/square root of the R-R interval. A simplified approach to determining whether the QT interval is long

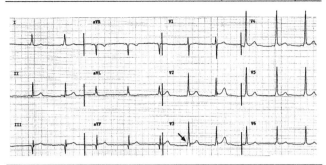

Fig. 29-1 Wolff-Parkinson-White syndrome. Note delta wave.

CHAPTER **29**

is to divide the R-R interval in half. If the T wave lies past the midpoint of the R-R interval, a long QT interval is present.

d. *Conduction blocks.* Although conduction blocks are common in patients without symptoms, their presence should suggest the possibility of an intermittent high-grade block that may cause palpitations.

e. *Brugada syndrome.* An inherited disease manifested by an electrocardiographic pattern of ST segment elevation in leads V1 to V3 and incomplete or complete right bundle branch block. It is associated with sudden death and is an indication for an AICD.

3. Event and Holter monitoring: Most ED patients require an event or Holter monitor because generally an ECG cannot be obtained during symptoms. These tests are performed in the outpatient setting in low-risk patients. Event monitors are by far the more useful and cost-effective test. Approximately 30% of patients initially given a psychiatric diagnosis for their palpitations have arrhythmias noted on subsequent investigation.

COMMENTS AND TREATMENT CONSIDERATIONS

Traditionally, all patients with syncope, near-syncope, pulmonary edema, or ischemic-sounding chest pain in association with palpitations have been admitted to the hospital. For many of these patients, unfortunately, the yield of inpatient evaluation is low. Nonetheless, the inability to distinguish between patients with serious and benign causes of palpitations warrants the admission of high-risk patients.

Many discharged patients should have event monitoring performed to rule out cardiac arrhythmia as the cause of palpitations.

THYROTOXICOSIS AND THYROID STORM

Thyrotoxicosis and the more severe form—thyroid storm—are uncommon but important causes of palpitations. Symptoms and signs of mild thyrotoxicosis are those expected from catecholamine excess. Patients with mild symptoms require no immediate treatment or only symptomatic therapy in the ED. Undiagnosed or undertreated Graves' disease is the most common cause of thyrotoxicosis.

Thyroid storm is a medical emergency that may mimic or complicate other conditions such as sepsis, sympathomimetic intoxication, or drug withdrawal. Findings defining thyroid storm include the following:

- Elevated temperature +++++ (T >38.7° C, but may be as high as 41° C)
- CNS dysfunction ++++ (anxiety, emotional lability, delirium)
- Cardiovascular dysfunction
- Gastrointestinal dysfunction (nausea, vomiting, hyperdefecation or diarrhea, crampy abdominal pain)

SYMPTOMS
- Anxiety
- Tremor
- Weakness
- Heat intolerance
- Weight loss
- Hyperdefecation
- Sweating
- Angina and CHF may be present even in the absence of prior known heart disease. Angina tends to indicate the unmasking of a previously existing coronary artery disease, whereas severe hyperthyroidism may precipitate heart failure in an otherwise healthy heart.

SIGNS
- Sinus tachycardia is almost always present in thyrotoxicosis and serves as a marker of the severity of catecholamine excess.
- PACs and PVCs may be present.
- Atrial fibrillation ++
- Enlarged thyroid gland may be palpable or have bruit on physical examination.
- Proptosis and other eye findings indicative of Graves' disease
- Brisk reflexes

WORKUP
- Primarily a clinical diagnosis in the ED because the results of thyroid function tests (TFTs) are generally not immediately available.

The differentiation between hyperthyroidism and thyroid storm is based on clinical judgment. Laboratory values for hyperthyroidism without storm and true storm overlap.

- TFTs are used to confirm the clinical diagnosis. In general, an elevated free T_4 and a suppressed (unmeasurably low) TSH establish the diagnosis.
- Glucose (may be elevated)
- ECG

COMMENTS AND TREATMENT CONSIDERATIONS

In most cases of mild thyrotoxicosis, patients can be referred for outpatient evaluation and treatment without ED therapy. In patients who are symptomatic but not acutely ill, beta-adrenergic blockade (e.g., with propranolol 1 mg slow IV bolus, may repeat) alone is generally adequate with a discharge prescription for ongoing beta-blockade until follow-up is obtained. Angina should be treated with a beta-blocker. The treatment of CHF with thyroid storm is controversial. Because the underlying precipitant is beta-agonist excess, cautious beta-adrenergic blockade with propranolol or esmolol is the best approach. Patients in thyroid storm require admission to a monitored setting.

Only the sickest patients (i.e., those with thyroid storm) need more specific treatment in the ED. Treatment of *thyroid storm* consists of five components:

1. Supportive care including cooling measures
2. Inhibition of thyroid hormone synthesis: propylthiouracil (PTU) 100 to 200 mg po tid
3. Inhibition of thyroid hormone release: iodine (e.g., SSKI gtt 4 po tid); wait at least 1 hour after PTU administration.
4. Inhibition of peripheral conversion of T_4 to T_3: dexamethasone 2 mg IV or po q6h. PTU and propranolol have minor effects.
5. Blockade of peripheral thyroid hormone effects: beta-adrenergic blockade with propranolol. As an alternative, an esmolol drip (an intravenous beta-blocker with a short half life) can be considered.

It is also imperative to consider other processes as precipitants of thyroid storm or as the primary cause of the symptoms. These include infection, surgery, trauma, contrast studies, DKA/HHS, and emotional stress. Patients in thyroid storm require ICU admission and consultation with an endocrinologist.

CHAPTER **29**

 ATRIAL FIBRILLATION

Atrial fibrillation is a common cause of palpitations. Patients are most commonly elderly but may be in their 30s or 40s. Atrial fibrillation is one of the more benign causes of palpitations. In general, palpitations with a ventricular origin are far more serious. The search for the cause of the atrial fibrillation is generally more important than the disease itself as it may occasionally be caused by a serious medical condition (e.g., MI, hypertension, pulmonary embolism, hyperthyroidism, alcohol withdrawal or use, hypertension, or valvular disease).

SYMPTOMS
- Palpitations, irregular beating
- Chest pain, shortness of breath, if decompensated from the arrhythmia
- Syncope (rarely)
- Symptoms of the cause of the atrial fibrillation (see earlier)

SIGNS
- Generally rapid (but the rate may be normal or slow) irregular heartbeat
- Peripheral pulse, heart beat dissociation (i.e., more heartbeats heard than felt at the radial pulse)
- Signs of CHF, if decompensated
- Slow irregular heartbeat can occur if concomitant AV node disease.
- No signs (between episodes)
- Signs of the underlying cause

WORKUP
- ECG is diagnostic and assists in evaluating for ischemia.
- Chest x-ray is used to evaluate for heart failure or evidence of valvular disease (calcified valve or atrial hypertrophy).
- Outpatient event monitoring is appropriate for patients in normal sinus rhythm who are otherwise medically stable for discharge but for whom there is a concern of paroxysmal atrial fibrillation or other arrhythmia.

COMMENTS AND TREATMENT CONSIDERATIONS
The goal of therapy for ED patients with rapid atrial fibrillation is rate control. In patients without evidence of end-organ compromise (e.g., no CHF or chest pain and stable blood pressure), rate control can be achieved with a number of agents including diltiazem (dose 5 mg IVP administered q5min to a heart rate of approximately 80 and SBP >100; initial rate control is generally achieved with a maximum dose of 20 to 30 mg; diltiazem infusion can follow at 5 to 15 mg/hr) or a beta-blocker. Most patients should be anticoagulated (and/or evaluated for thrombus) before cardioversion because of the risk of embolization after return to a normal rhythm. This includes patients who give a history of recent onset of palpitations because patients' symptoms may not correlate with the time of

onset of atrial fibrillation and because of rare instances of clot pre-existent to the current episode of atrial fibrillation. Conversion to sinus rhythm is a secondary goal, usually best performed as an inpatient procedure if at all.

Emergent ED cardioversion at 200 J (increase as needed) should be reserved for unstable patients and is considered a form of rate control. It is frequently unsuccessful in patients with chronic atrial fibrillation or underlying heart disease.

REFERENCES

Abbott AV: Diagnostic approach to palpitations, *Am Fam Physician* 71:743, 2005.

Barsky AJ: Palpitations, arrhythmias, and awareness of cardiac activity, *Ann Intern Med* 134:832, 2001.

Brugada P, Gursoy S, Brugada J, et al: Investigation of palpitations, *Lancet* 341:1254, 1993.

Kinlay S, Leitch JW, Neil A, et al: Cardiac event recorders yield more diagnoses and are more cost-effective than 48-hour Holter monitoring in patients with palpitations: a controlled clinical trial, *Ann Intern Med* 124:16, 1996.

Lochen ML, Snaprud T, Zhang W, et al: Arrhythmias in subjects with and without a history of palpitations: the Tromso study, *Eur Heart J* 15:345, 1994.

Mattu A: The Brugada syndrome. *Am J Emerg Med* 21:146, 2003.

Zimetbaum P, Josephson M: Current concepts: evaluation of patients with palpitations, *N Engl J Med* 19:338, 1998.

CHAPTER **29**

CHAPTER 30

Rash
Pamela L. Dyne and Carin Van Zyl

The evaluation and treatment of a patient with a chief complaint
of rash can be very intimidating because, to the uninitiated,
all rashes look alike. However, only four principal categories
of rashes exist: (1) erythematous and maculopapular,
(2) petechial and purpuric, (3) vesiculobullous, and (4) urticarial.
From an emergency physician's perspective, a rash is generally
only one component of a constellation of signs and symptoms
that can be brought together to establish a definitive diagnosis.
Although most illnesses with an associated rash are not life
threatening, a few emergent conditions must be understood and
recognized readily.

TERMINOLOGY
Macule: flat, nonpalpable discoloration <1 cm
Patch: flat, nonpalpable discoloration >1 cm
Papule: solid, raised, palpable lesion <1 cm
Nodule: rounded, raised, palpable lesion >1 cm
Plaque: flat-topped, raised, palpable lesion <1.5 cm
Maculopapular: flat or raised red, pink, or tan discoloration of
     varying sizes and textures
Vesicle: well-circumscribed, fluid-filled, raised lesion <1 cm
Bullae: well-circumscribed, fluid-filled, raised lesion >1 cm
Pustule: well-circumscribed, pus-filled, raised lesion
Wheal: pink, raised, usually pruritic, transient lesion
Purpura: blue to purple lesion, secondary to hemorrhage into the
     skin, usually nonblanching
Petechia: round, pinpoint, flat purplish spot caused by intradermal
     or subdermal hemorrhage
Excoriation: linear erosion, usually from scratching

ERYTHEMATOUS AND MACULOPAPULAR RASHES

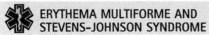

ERYTHEMA MULTIFORME AND STEVENS-JOHNSON SYNDROME

Erythema multiforme (EM) and Stevens-Johnson (SJ) syndrome constitute two ends of a spectrum of the same disease. EM is the mild form; SJ is the more severe, potentially fatal form. In patients who have SJ syndrome, the skin eruption generally involves the mucous membranes. Patients appear clinically ill and may suffer from multisystem dysfunction. EM/SJ is usually the result of a hypersensitivity (allergic) reaction either to a medication or to infection (*Mycoplasma pneumoniae* and herpes simplex most frequently), although a cause is not identified in half of the cases.

SYMPTOMS
- SJ usually begins with a prodrome: upper respiratory tract infection, fever, headache, malaise.
- Rash

SIGNS
- *EM*: rash usually begins as erythematous macules and papules, found symmetrically on the hands and feet. The rash spreads and evolves into the classic target-appearing lesions (dark center with a lighter outside ring) (Fig. 30–1).
- *SJ*: erythematous blisters are also seen on the mucous membranes of the eyes, mouth, and genitalia. The lesions may progress to bullae and then slough. The patient's lips may have a characteristic thick hemorrhagic crust.

WORKUP
The diagnosis is made clinically.

COMMENTS AND TREATMENT CONSIDERATIONS
In EM, topical corticosteroids can be used but should not be applied to eroded areas. The use of systemic steroids is controversial. A 3- to 5-day course probably provides some benefit with a limited risk of complications. Analgesics and antipruritics or antihistamines should be provided and follow-up with a dermatologist arranged.

Patients with SJ should generally be admitted to the hospital because their condition can rapidly deteriorate. Nutrition, analgesia, and other supportive care should be provided and fluid and electrolyte balance maintained. An ophthalmologist should be consulted for eye care. Sitz bath and whirlpool are used for wound care. Patients with severe symptoms may be best served in a burn center. Topical and systemic antibiotics are used for specific infections only.

CHAPTER 30

387

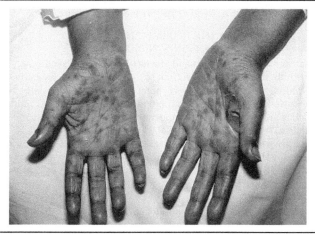

Fig. 30–1 Erythema multiforme. "Target" lesions on the palms. (Courtesy of Anthony J. Mancini, MD, Chicago.)

 TOXIC EPIDERMAL NECROLYSIS

Toxic epidermal necrolysis (TEN) is a rare, life-threatening syndrome characterized by erythema and exfoliation of the skin. TEN is usually the result of a drug hypersensitivity reaction, although it may rarely be seen as a manifestation of graft-versus-host disease in a transplant recipient.

SYMPTOMS
- 24- to 48-hour prodrome of high fever, headache, intense malaise, myalgias, arthralgias, diarrhea, vomiting, conjunctival irritation, and skin tenderness

SIGNS
- Lesions are usually a morbilliform ("sandpaper") eruption or diffuse macular erythema. The skin is often tender. The lesions can progress to form vesicles, which then coalesce and slough, leaving large denuded areas (Fig. 30–2).
- Mucous membranes are often involved, with erosions and sloughing occurring as well.
- Fingernails and toenails may slough or develop Beau's lines.

WORKUP
- Diagnosis is generally made clinically.

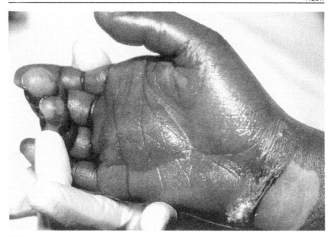

Fig. 30–2 Toxic epidermal necrolysis. Blisters and epidermal sloughing. (Courtesy of Anthony J. Mancini, MD, Chicago.)

- Skin biopsy shows necrosis of the epidermis with detachment from the dermis.

COMMENTS AND TREATMENT CONSIDERATIONS

Treatment is similar to that for severe burns. Patients are admitted to an ICU or burn unit and are provided with aggressive intravenous hydration, nutritional support, infection control, and measures to stop the effects of the offending drug. The use of systemic corticosteroids is controversial. Antibiotic coverage for *Staphylococcus aureus* should be considered because the differential diagnosis includes staphylococcal scalded skin syndrome (see later).

Researchers disagree on whether TEN is related to EM and SJ.

 NECROTIZING FASCIITIS

Necrotizing fasciitis ("flesh-eating" bacteria) is an invasive soft tissue bacterial infection of the skin, often developing in patients who have had minor skin trauma (50% to 85%). The disease is also seen in immunocompromised and postoperative patients. If the area of infection involves the perineum, the disease is called Fournier's gangrene.

SYMPTOMS

- Patients usually have severe pain in a localized area. This is the earliest and most consistent symptom.

SIGNS

- May be very minimal initially (i.e., pain is out of proportion to physical findings).
- Erythema and swelling without demarcated margins initially.
- Rapidly evolves to include the development of reddish purple patches and then bullae.
- Area becomes necrotic, edematous, and possibly crepitant.
- Surrounding surface becomes involved as the infection spreads along the subcutaneous tissue and fascia. Pain may then be remote from visibly affected tissue.
- Fever is common as disease progresses.

WORKUP

- X-rays of the area involved may demonstrate subcutaneous gas, although they may be negative.
- Blood cultures
- Electrolytes may reveal hyponatremia.
- Wound culture is required to determine bacterial etiology (*Streptococcus*, *Clostridium*, or polymicrobial).
- During surgical exploration, the surgical instrument easily passes through planes of fascia.

COMMENTS AND TREATMENT CONSIDERATIONS

This is a disease for which a high index of suspicion can be life- or limb-saving. Patients present along the continuum of disease, with those in the early stages showing only minimal local symptoms. This aggressive infection rapidly advances to involve contiguous areas, eventually causing generalized sepsis. Early diagnosis is made by a high level of concern for patients complaining of intense pain without significant physical findings.

Regardless of the severity of illness at presentation, this is a surgical emergency. The patient needs immediate, wide surgical débridement along with antibiotic treatment. The antibiotics chosen should cover gram-negative and gram-positive organisms and anaerobes. Clindamycin 900 mg IV q8h plus penicillin G 24 million units/day IV divided q4-6h and an aminoglycoside is reasonable first-line therapy. A penicillinase-resistant penicillin is added if a skin source is suspected. Patients in shock need aggressive supportive care in an ICU setting after surgical débridement.

REFERENCE

Brenner BE, Vitullo M, Simon RR: Necrotizing fasciitis, *Ann Emerg Med* 11:384, 1982.

Kotrappa KS, Bansal RS, Amin NM: Necrotizing fasciitis, *Am Fam Physician* 53:1691, 1996.

 TOXIC SHOCK SYNDROME

Toxic shock syndrome (TSS) is a multisystem illness caused by an exotoxin usually produced by certain strains of *Staphylococcus aureus*. The site of the S. *aureus* infection is often a tampon (85%), catheter, nasal packing, or other foreign body but may be a skin infection including an abscess or infected wound. A very similar illness can also be caused by a toxin-producing streptococcal infection. The diagnostic criteria include any group A streptococcus infection associated with shock and organ failure and may or may not include a maculopapular rash.

SYMPTOMS
- Fever +++++
- Chills and rigors ++
- Diarrhea ++++
- Dizziness
- Headache ++++
- Myalgias ++++
- Sore throat +++
- Red, nonpruritic rash that includes the palms and soles

SIGNS
- Diffuse, nonpruritic, blanching macular (or maculopapular or petechial) erythematous rash.
- Patient may appear clinically ill with hypotension and other clinical signs of shock.
- Desquamation of skin (usually hands or feet) may occur by the second to fifth day.

WORKUP
- Culture: blood, urine, sites of potential foreign bodies (vagina, nares, etc.), abscesses, and wounds
- Laboratory evaluation for possible multiorgan dysfunction: CBC, platelet count, PT/PTT, electrolytes, liver function tests, urinalysis.

COMMENTS AND TREATMENT CONSIDERATIONS
The offending foreign body, if any, needs to be sought and subsequently removed. Patients should be admitted to the hospital

CHAPTER 30

and the infection treated with beta-lactamase–resistant antistaphylococcal antibiotics. Aggressive supportive care is essential for patients in shock.

REFERENCE
Strausbaugh LJ: Toxic shock syndrome: are you recognizing its changing presentations? *Postgrad Med* 94:107, 1993.

 ## STAPHYLOCOCCAL SCALDED SKIN SYNDROME

Staphylococcal scalded skin syndrome (SSSS) is an illness caused by an exfoliative exotoxin produced by certain strains of *S. aureus.* The primary infection (of the nose, conjunctiva, or umbilicus) is often clinically inapparent. SSSS usually occurs in children.

SYMPTOMS
- Rash
- Fever
- Malaise
- Irritability

SIGNS
- Diffuse, tender, red rash, sometimes with a sandpaper texture initially.
- Bullae and vesicles may appear over the course of a few days.
- Exfoliation of large sheets of epidermis with a positive Nikolsky sign (the skin sloughs easily if the examiner applies lateral pressure to the area) may follow (Fig. 30–3).

WORKUP
Definitive diagnosis is usually made by skin biopsy.

COMMENTS AND TREATMENT CONSIDERATIONS
Large volume losses may occur in these patients secondary to insensible losses without intact skin. Fluid resuscitation is initiated and electrolyte abnormalities are corrected. Attempts should be made to identify the source of the staphylococcal infection. SSSS is treated with beta-lactamase–resistant antistaphylococcal antibiotics (e.g., nafcillin 100 mg/kg/day divided q4-6h).

 ## KAWASAKI'S DISEASE (MUCOCUTANEOUS LYMPH NODE SYNDROME)

Kawasaki's disease is an idiopathic disease of children younger than 5 years. It is characterized by a systemic illness and usually has mucosal and cutaneous manifestations.

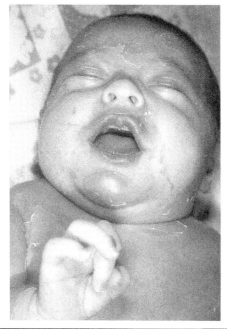

Fig. 30–3 Staphylococcal scalded skin syndrome. Epidermolysis in a 3-week-old infant. (Courtesy of Anthony J. Mancini, MD, Chicago.)

SYMPTOMS

- Sore throat
- Headache
- Malaise
- Nausea, vomiting, diarrhea
- Rash

SIGNS

DIAGNOSTIC FEATURES

- Fever prolonged more than 5 days ++++
- Acute cervical lymphadenopathy; usually unilateral and >1.5 cm ++++
- Oral mucosal findings ++++: dry, fissured lips (Fig. 30–4), strawberry tongue, or pharyngitis.
- Extremity findings: peripheral edema +++; erythema of palms and soles +++; desquamation of the fingertips ++++ is a late finding occurring at 1 to 2 weeks.

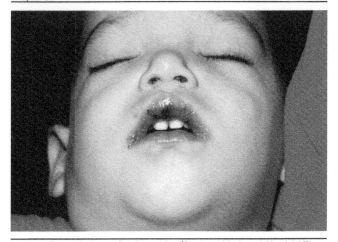

Fig. 30-4 Kawasaki's disease. Dry, fissured lips. (Courtesy of Anthony J. Mancini, MD, Chicago.)

- Bilateral, painless, nonpurulent bulbar conjunctivitis that spares the limbic portions ++++
- Polymorphic rash: may be any nonvesicular rash, although usually is maculopapular; commonly involves the perineum ++++

OTHER MANIFESTATIONS
- Polyarthralgia
- Urethritis with sterile pyuria ++++
- Abdominal pain and diarrhea ++
- Aseptic meningitis ++
- Cardiac disease ++: pericardial effusion, congestive heart failure, arrhythmias.
- Obstructive jaundice with acute gallbladder hydrops

WORKUP
The diagnosis is made clinically based on the presence of the preceding signs and symptoms. However, these children need to be evaluated for the complications of this disease, namely cardiac abnormalities, which occur in 20% of cases. They require cardiac echocardiography at the time of diagnosis to evaluate for coronary artery aneurysm or pericardial effusions. Consultation with a pediatric cardiologist or a pediatric infectious disease specialist is recommended.

COMMENTS AND TREATMENT CONSIDERATIONS

Many patients need to be admitted for further evaluation and treatment. Intravenous immunoglobulin and oral salicylates, in addition to supportive measures, are suggested by most pediatric cardiologists because they may decrease cardiac complications.

 LYME DISEASE

Lyme disease is a multisystem infection caused by the bite of a tick infected with the spirochete *Borrelia burgdorferi*. Systemic dissemination can occur within days to weeks. The symptoms tend to occur in stages, somewhat arbitrarily divided into early localized, early disseminated, and late. Prompt diagnosis is crucial because early treatment is highly effective, whereas late disease is more difficult to eradicate. In addition to the symptoms and signs, the history of *possible* exposure to ticks is extremely important, as there is a history of tick bite in less than 30% of cases. In patients with later manifestations of Lyme disease, there may be a history of earlier manifestations (e.g., in a patient presenting with seventh nerve palsy, history of prior rash should be solicited).

CHAPTER 30

SYMPTOMS
EARLY LOCALIZED DISEASE
- Rash: solitary erythema migrans (EM, see the following), which may be pruritic, painful, or neither ++++
- Flu-like symptoms: fatigue, headache, fever, stiff neck

EARLY DISSEMINATED DISEASE (MAY OCCUR IN VARIOUS COMBINATIONS)
- Rash: multiple EM
- Flu-like illness with fevers, chills, fatigue
- Neurologic: facial weakness or paralysis, headache and stiff neck, painful or weak limb, dysesthesias.
- Cardiac (more common in males): palpitation, dyspnea, syncope, chest pain.
- Musculoskeletal: arthralgias, pain over muscles, tendons, and bursae.
- Ocular (resulting from conjunctivitis, iritis, or keratitis): red eye, eye pain, blurred vision.

SIGNS (MAY OCCUR IN VARIOUS COMBINATIONS)
EARLY LOCALIZED DISEASE
- EM: large (median size, 15 cm), red, usually flat, round, or oval eruption at the site of tick bite. Rash morphology can be variable. It is typically located at skin creases or thorax and appears 1 to 33 days after exposure, typically between 7 and 10 days (Fig. 30–5).

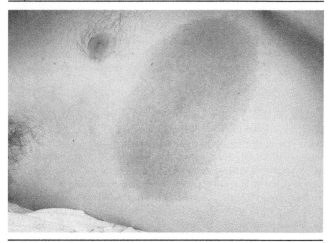

Fig. 30–5 Lyme disease, erythema migrans.

EARLY DISSEMINATED DISEASE
- Fever with or without rash
- Cutaneous: multiple EM (secondary lesions are usually smaller and lack the central punctum).
- Neurologic: most commonly facial nerve palsy, which can be bilateral.
- Cardiac: irregular pulse, cardiac rub or gallop.
- Ocular: conjunctival injection, corneal fluorescein uptake from keratitis, cells in the anterior chamber; rarely, disc edema and retinal changes from vasculitis or inflammation.
- Musculoskeletal: frank synovitis occasionally found in this stage.
- GI: rarely, hepatomegaly or splenomegaly.

WORKUP
- In patients with typical EM, diagnosis is clinical. No testing (including serologic testing) is indicated.
- In patients with symptoms of early disseminated and late disease, Lyme serology is usually positive.
- In patients with isolated facial palsy, some practitioners recommend examining the cerebrospinal fluid for a pleocytosis, which, if present, argues for parenteral rather than oral therapy. Definitive data are lacking.
- ECG: in patients with cardiac symptoms or disseminated disease
- Hepatic transaminases: in an atypical case, this may support the diagnosis (at least one LFT is elevated in +++ of cases of Lyme disease) and can also be a clue to ehrlichiosis.

COMMENTS AND TREATMENT CONSIDERATIONS

In patients with prominent flu-like illness or atypical manifestations, coinfection with *Babesia microti* and human *Ehrlichia* pathogens should be considered. Treatment is as follows:

- Early localized disease: 21 days of oral doxycycline (100 mg bid), amoxicillin (500 mg tid), or cefuroxime axetil (500 mg bid). Doxycycline cannot be used in children younger than 9 years or in pregnant or lactating women; in others, it has the advantage of covering coinfected ehrlichiosis.
- Early disseminated disease: Without CSF pleocytosis or second- or third-degree heart block, treatment is same as for solitary EM. If either of these is present, treat with ceftriaxone, 2 g/day IV for 2 to 4 weeks, depending on clinical variables and response to treatment (in children, ceftriaxone 75 mg/kg/day IV).
- Early antibiotic prophylaxis after a tick bite is controversial but may be appropriate for individuals with prolonged tick attachment (>48 hours) in highly endemic areas. A single 200-mg dose of doxycycline within 72 hours of tick removal appears to be effective.

Follow-up by a primary care physician is important to confirm success of the treatment. Late disease, mainly arthritis (most commonly of the knee) and neurologic syndromes (most commonly encephalopathy and peripheral neuropathy), requires prompt referral for diagnosis and treatment.

CHAPTER 30

REFERENCES

Abramowicz A (ed): Treatment of Lyme disease, *Med Lett Drugs Ther* 47:41, 2005.

Edlow JA: The multiple faces of Lyme disease and other common tickborne conditions, *Emerg Med Rep* 18:103, 1997.

Feder HM Jr, Whitaker DL: Misdiagnosis of erythema migrans, *Am J Med* 99:412, 1995.

Magnarelli LA: Current status of laboratory testing for Lyme disease, *Am J Med* 98:10, 1995.

Nadelman RB, Wormser GP: Erythema migrans and early Lyme disease, *Am J Med* 98:15, 1995.

Steere AC: Lyme disease, *N Engl J Med* 345:115, 2001.

 SYPHILIS

A sexually transmitted disease previously in decline, syphilis is now on the rise especially in immigrant and HIV-infected populations. It is transmitted by the spirochete *Treponema pallidum* through direct contact with intact mucous membranes or abraded skin. There are three stages of infection, separated by latency. The primary stage presents with a genital chancre that is painless and spontaneously resolves. The secondary stage presents with characteristic rash and systemic symptoms. The tertiary stage, presenting many years later, has neurologic, cardiovascular, and musculoskeletal findings and is rarely seen. Diagnosis and treatment are important to prevent spread of disease and prevent significant morbidity and mortality.

SYMPTOMS
- Constitutional symptoms: malaise, headache, anorexia, myalgia, fever.
- Rash begins to appear 2 to 10 weeks after infection and is most apparent 3 to 4 months later.
- History of painless genital ulcers

SIGNS
- Symmetric pale red or pink macules 5 to 10 mm in diameter over trunk and proximal extremities, later more papular, on flexor surfaces, palms and soles.
- Painless lymphadenopathy
- Silver gray mucous membrane erosions with red areola.
- Patchy alopecia

WORKUP
- VDRL, RPR, or new ICE serologies, confirmed with darkfield microscopy, direct antitreponemal fluorescent antibody testing (FTA-Abs), or microhemagglutination tests.
- Punch biopsy of lesion if needed

TREATMENT CONSIDERATIONS
Penicillin remains the antibiotic of choice; penicillin G benzathine 2.4 million units IM is given IM once for disease of less than a year's duration and once a week for 3 weeks in disease longer than a year. Penicillin-allergic patients should be skin tested and desensitized. There is no demonstrated penicillin resistance. Alternatively, doxycycline 100 mg po bid for 2 weeks is recommended.
The disease is also reportable—notify local health authorities.
Consider ancillary sexually transmitted disease and HIV testing.

REFERENCES
Baugh RE, Musher DM: Secondary syphilitic lesions, *Clin Microbiol Rev* 18:206, 2005.

 PEDIATRIC RASHES

Rash is a common pediatric complaint. Certain rashes are seen predominantly in children. Each of these rashes has a characteristic appearance and associated symptoms and signs that facilitate diagnosis. See Table 30–1.

REFERENCES

Bialecki C, Feder HM Jr, Grant-Kels JM: The six classic childhood exanthems: a review and update, *J Am Acad Dermatol* 5:891, 1989.

Braun DK, Dominguez G, Pellett PE: Human herpesvirus 6, *Clin Microbiol Rev* 10:521, 1997.

Jacobs PH: Seborrheic dermatitis: its causes and management, *Cutis* 41:192, 1988.

Keeler MC: Human parvovirus B19: not just a pediatric problem, *J Emerg Med* 10:39, 1992.

Thomas I, Kannigan CK: Hand, foot, and mouth disease, *Cutis* 52:265, 1993.

PETECHIAL AND PURPURIC RASHES

 MENINGOCOCCEMIA

Meningococcemia is a disease caused by the gram-negative diplococcal bacteria *Neisseria meningitidis* and is usually seen in people younger than 20 years. This infection can cause pharyngitis, meningitis, sepsis, or a combination of CNS and systemic infection. Infection usually begins 3 to 4 days after exposure and can progress from very mild symptoms to death in a few hours.

SYMPTOMS
- Rash
- Headache
- Fever
- Nausea
- Sore throat
- Vomiting
- Myalgias
- Arthralgias
- Stiff neck
- Confusion

SIGNS
- Rash classically begins as petechiae (extremities, trunk, palms, soles, head, and mucous membranes).
- Petechiae develop into palpable purpura with gray necrotic centers (Fig. 30–6).
- Rash can also manifest as urticaria, hemorrhagic vesicles, macules, and maculopapules.

CHAPTER 30

TABLE 30-1
PEDIATRIC RASHES

DISEASE AND AGENT	RASH APPEARANCE	ASSOCIATED FEATURES	PEAK AGES	TREATMENT	COMPLICATIONS
Hand, foot, and mouth disease (Coxsackie A16, echovirus, enteroviruses)	Maculopapular rash evolving to vesicles then ulcers (in mouth) with a red halo. Distributed over palms, soles, mouth, around nails, more on the hands than the feet. May include an MP rash on the buttocks.	Low-grade fever, URI symptoms, oral pain.	Usually younger than 10 yr	Supportive. Lidocaine or diphenhydramine rinses. Acyclovir shown to help severe cases, especially in the immunocompromised in small trials.	Superinfection of skin lesions, dehydration in patients with severe oral pain. Very contagious by contact with saliva.
Measles (measles virus)	Red maculopapular rash becoming confluent on the face, then spreading to trunk, palms, soles. Desquamation after a week. *Modified measles* after vaccination, has longer viral prodrome and more mild symptoms. *Atypical measles* is due to incomplete immunity, has no viral prodrome, and the rash spreads peripheral to central and may be polymorphic.	Fever, cough, coryza, conjunctivitis with limbal sparing Koplik's spots on buccal mucosa, just prior to rash.	Younger than 12 mo, second peak at school age.	Supportive. Vitamin A supplementation. Ribavirin on an experimental basis only. Reportable disease.	Encephalitis, giant cell pneumonia in the immunocompromised. Subacute sclerosing panencephalitis.

Seborrheic dermatitis (*Malassezia furfur*, *Candida* spp, abnormal immune responses)	Greasy, scaly crusting with reddened skin, on scalp, trunk, hairline, sebum-rich areas. Nasolabial sparing	Increased with stress, weather changes, sweating, heat	Onset mostly in puberty. In infants, called cradle cap.	Ketoconazole, coal tar, salicylate shampoos. Tacrolimus or pimecrolimus creams.	Steroids cause rebound phenomenon. Super-infection from excoriation.
Rubella (rubella virus)	Pink maculopapular rash spreading from face to trunk	Malaise, fever, conjunctivitis, posterior auricular and posterior chain lymph nodes, soft palate petechiae	Most cases between 15 and 45 yr	Supportive.	Congenital rubella syndrome. Arthritides lasting up to a year.
Roseola (human herpes virus 6)	Faint pink maculopapular rash spreading from trunk to extremities, blanching, nonpruritic	High fever that resolves prior to rash. Some-times seen with periorbital edema prior to rash	Younger than 2 yr	Supportive.	Febrile seizures Diarrhea Hepatitis Mononucleosis-like syndrome Encephalitis

Continued

TABLE 30-1
PEDIATRIC RASHES—cont'd

DISEASE AND AGENT	RASH APPEARANCE	ASSOCIATED FEATURES	PEAK AGES	TREATMENT	COMPLICATIONS
Erythema infectiosum (parvovirus B19)	"Slapped cheek" rash with nasolabial fold and perioral sparing. Lacy rash on trunk and extremities that may wax and wane for weeks.	Prodrome of arthralgias, fever, URI symptoms	5-15 yr	Supportive. IV IgG in immunocompromised, or aplastic crisis	Aplastic crisis Fetal hydrops Polyarthropathies, mostly in fingers.
Candida (C. albicans, other sp)	Angry, beefy rash in skin folds, diaper area, often with smaller satellite lesions. In the mouth, white patches that bleed when scraped.	Often seen after antibiotics, in diabetics, other immunocompromised	First year	Nystatin mouth washes Nystatin cream, miconazole cream. Fluconazole	Keep skin clean and dry, with barrier ointments.

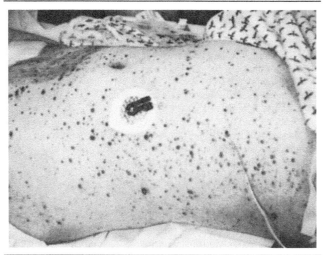

Fig. 30-6 Meningococcemia. Purpura and petechiae. (Courtesy of Javier Gonzalez del Rey, MD.)

- Occasionally presentation as fulminant meningococcal disease characterized by shock, with petechial and ecchymotic areas ++. Purpura fulminans, a severe form of disseminated intravascular coagulation, may develop in these patients. Some affected ecchymotic areas become necrotic and gangrenous and must be amputated.

WORKUP
- Antibiotics must not be delayed for tests, including lumbar puncture.
- Diagnosis is often made clinically: an ill patient with rapidly progressive symptoms, a petechial rash, fever, headache, and altered mental status.
- Blood cultures
- Lumbar puncture
- Gram stain of the skin lesions

COMMENTS AND TREATMENT CONSIDERATIONS
Immediate treatment with a third-generation cephalosporin (e.g., ceftriaxone, adult: 2 g IV; child: 40 mg/kg IV) after rapidly obtaining blood cultures, if possible. Supportive care and hemodynamic stabilization are provided as needed in an intensive care unit with

isolation from other patients. Once the diagnosis is confirmed, penicillin is the drug of choice.

Patients should be placed in respiratory isolation. Because this is a very contagious and severe illness, individuals who have been in close proximity to the patient's oral secretions or have had prolonged exposure to the patient's respiratory secretions should be treated with antibiotics to help prevent subsequent contraction of the illness. The current CDC recommendation for prophylaxis for those exposed to *N. meningitides* is a single dose of ciprofloxacin 500 mg po (avoid in pregnant women and children). Rifampin is recommended in children (10 mg/kg po q12h for 2 days) and ceftriaxone in pregnant women (250 mg in a single IM dose).

See Chapter 18, Headache.

 ROCKY MOUNTAIN SPOTTED FEVER

Rocky Mountain spotted fever (RMSF) is a multisystem disease caused by the parasite *Rickettsia rickettsii*. The parasite is usually transmitted through the bite of an infected wood or dog tick. However, 40% of patients do not recall being exposed to a tick at the time of diagnosis. RMSF must be suspected in a patient with possible tick exposure. A clinical triad of fever, headache, and myalgias is commonly present. There is a regional distribution of this disease to the central and southern Atlantic seaboard states, and it is most common in children.

SYMPTOMS
- Common triad, usually presenting 1 week after tick bite: fever +++++, headache ++++, myalgias ++++
- Rash begins approximately 4 days after these symptoms begin ++++.
- Rash: palms and soles ++++
- Nausea and vomiting +++
- Abdominal pain +++
- Confusion ++
- Diarrhea ++
- Meningismus ++

SIGNS
- Rash commonly begins on the wrists and ankles and then spreads more centrally to the palms and soles, proximal extremities, trunk, and face.
- Rash consists of blanching macules or maculopapules, which evolve into diffuse petechiae over 2 to 4 days.
- Systemic signs develop if multiorgan (e.g., cardiovascular, renal) involvement.

WORKUP
- Diagnosis is usually clinical.
- Diagnosis can be confirmed with a rise in antibody titer after 10 days to 2 weeks or by immunofluorescent staining of skin biopsy.

COMMENTS AND TREATMENT CONSIDERATIONS
Doxycycline (100 mg po bid for 7 days or for 2 days after normal temperature; do not use in children and pregnant women) or chloramphenicol (50 mg/kg/day) should be used to treat RMSF. Remove any ticks and provide supportive care as needed. Without appropriate antibiotic treatment, there is a high rate of mortality related to complications, some of which include shock, congestive heart failure, renal insufficiency, meningitis, DIC, and hepatic dysfunction.

REFERENCES
Brady WJ, DeBehnke D, Crosby DL: Dermatological emergencies, *Am J Emerg Med* 12:217, 1994.
Rosenstein N, Perkins B, Stephens D, et al: Meningococcal disease, *N Engl J Med* 344:1378, 2001.
Silber JL: Rocky Mountain spotted fever, *Clin Dermatol* 14:245, 1996.

 HENOCH-SCHÖNLEIN PURPURA

Henoch-Schönlein purpura (HSP) is an immune-mediated anaphylactoid reaction to bacterial or viral infection (especially beta-hemolytic streptococcus), drugs (penicillin, sulfonamides, and sedatives), and chemical toxins. It is idiopathic and causes vasculitis of the small vessels. It most commonly affects school-aged children.

SYMPTOMS
- Migratory joint pain and swelling
- Colicky abdominal pain
- Rash on the lower extremities or dependent regions

SIGNS
- Physical findings of this illness are the result of showers of immune complexes throughout the body with resultant microhemorrhages at sites of deposition. The skin, joints, gut, and kidney are affected.
- Rash is purpuric with isolated petechiae at the ankles, lower extremity, and buttocks, along with edematous plaques, vesicles, and central necrosis (Fig. 30–7).

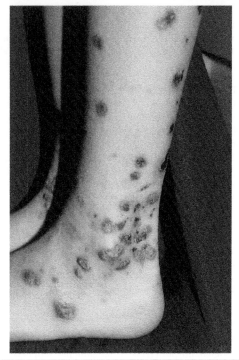

Fig. 30-7 Henoch-Schönlein purpura. Raised, palpable hemorrhagic lesions on a child's leg. (Courtesy of Anthony J. Mancini, MD, Chicago.)

WORKUP
- Diagnosis is made clinically.
- Evaluation of the patient's renal function, urine, and CBC to evaluate for hematuria and proteinuria is indicated.

COMMENTS AND TREATMENT CONSIDERATIONS
Treatment is generally supportive only, with NSAIDs given as needed for arthralgias. Steroids may be indicated in some cases. Renal insufficiency, hypertension, and GI bleeding are complications.

REFERENCES
Brady WJ, DeBehnke D, Crosby DL: Dermatological emergencies, *Am J Emerg Med* 12:217, 1994.

VESICULOBULLOUS RASHES

PEMPHIGUS VULGARIS

Pemphigus vulgaris (PV) is a blistering disease caused by the development of autoantibodies against epidermal intercellular material. PV usually affects the middle-aged and elderly. A genetic link may be associated with this disease, but other etiologic factors include drug associations or other autoimmune diseases.

SIGNS AND SYMPTOMS
- Blisters on erythematous skin (Fig. 30–8) and on mucous membranes with positive Nikolsky's sign (lateral stress to the skin causes exfoliation).
- Tremendous epidermal disruption is possible, resulting in large fluid and electrolyte disturbances, causing potentially serious illness.

WORKUP
- Skin biopsy: immunofluorescent and histopathologic studies

COMMENTS AND TREATMENT CONSIDERATIONS
Treatment initially consists of intravenous corticosteroids and aggressive supportive care. Adjunct immunosuppressive therapy may be added (cyclophosphamide [Cytoxan], azathioprine [Imuran], and similar drugs); antibiotics to cover skin flora may be

CHAPTER 30

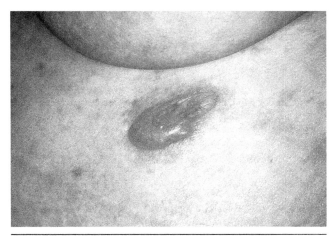

Fig. 30–8 Pemphigus vulgaris. Vesicle. (Courtesy of Anthony J. Mancini, MD, Chicago.)

considered. With current therapies and early diagnosis, the mortality rate is low.

REFERENCES

Becker BA, Gaspari AA: Pemphigus vulgaris and vegetans, *Dermatol Clin* 11:429, 1993.

 CHICKEN POX

Varicella-zoster virus causes both chicken pox and herpes zoster (shingles). Chicken pox presents as a generalized viral infection with a typical skin eruption. The rash is initially maculopapular and becomes vesicular after several days. Chicken pox in adults, especially those who are pregnant or immunocompromised, can cause life-threatening pneumonitis or encephalitis. Live attenuated varicella vaccines are approximately 90% effective in preventing disease in the immunocompetent; conversely, this means that up to 10% of previously vaccinated individuals develop disease if exposed. Rash, sometimes resembling varicella, is common following vaccination and is due to infection with the vaccine strain of the virus. Intravenous acyclovir and varicella-zoster immunoglobulin (VZIG) have been shown to decrease mortality in immunocompromised patients. Routine use of oral acyclovir for treatment of children with chicken pox is controversial.

REFERENCES

Fitzpatric TB, Johnson RA, Polano MK, et al: *Color atlas and synopsis of clinical dermatology*, ed 2. New York, 1994, McGraw-Hill.

Polis MA: Viral infections in emergency medicine. In Rosen P, Barkin RM, Hockberger RS (eds): *Emergency medicine: concepts and clinical practice*, ed 4. St Louis, 1998, Mosby.

URTICARIAL RASHES

There are many causes of urticarial rashes. Most of these rashes are the result of mild allergic reactions to skin or GI contacts. They are self-limited or respond to oral antihistamines (e.g., diphenhydramine 25 to 50 mg po q6h). More serious eruptions may require topical or oral steroid treatment. Patients who do not respond to this treatment and who are otherwise clinically well should be referred to a dermatologist for further evaluation.

Occasionally, allergic reactions are more serious and cause life-threatening respiratory or hemodynamic compromise. These patients require intravenous antihistamine, steroids, epinephrine, and possibly advanced airway management.

See Chapter 34, Shortness of Breath.

Scrotal Pain
Brian Robert Miura

A patient who has acute scrotal pain must be evaluated promptly because testicular torsion, one of the key diagnostic considerations, has a time-dependent testicular salvage rate (90% salvageable if detorsion occurs within 6 hours of pain onset; 20% salvageable if greater than 12 hours). Other diagnoses not to miss include strangulated inguinal hernia, Fournier's gangrene, abdominal aortic aneurysm, and appendicitis.

All patients with scrotal pain warrant an abdominal examination, and all male patients with lower abdominal pain require a scrotal examination because pain can often be referred and poorly localized. Testicular torsion, frequently misdiagnosed as epididymo-orchitis, should be the key diagnosis to entertain in any patient with unilateral testicular pain or tenderness. In patients with scrotal pain but a normal scrotal examination, referred causes of scrotal pain such as appendicitis and abdominal aortic aneurysm must be considered. Ureterolithiasis can also cause scrotal pain but is diagnosed only after determining that an emergent condition is not present.

 TESTICULAR TORSION VERSUS EPIDIDYMO–ORCHITIS
(Table 31–1)

Patients with any of the following clinical features should be considered to have testicular torsion:

1. Age <18
2. Recent history of similar painful episodes resolving spontaneously
3. Sudden onset of testicular pain
4. Absent or diminished ipsilateral cremasteric reflex
5. Horizontal testicular lie of ipsilateral or contralateral testis
6. High-riding ipsilateral testicle
7. Absence of pyuria

TABLE 31-1
SIGNS AND SYMPTOMS OF TESTICULAR TORSION AND EPIDIDYMO-ORCHITIS

SIGNS AND SYMPTOMS	TESTICULAR TORSION	EPIDIDYMO-ORCHITIS
Age	Newborn to 20 years (80%)	Adolescent to adult
Risk factors	Prior orchiopexy	Sexually active, genitourinary anomalies, recent genitourinary instrumentation
Onset of pain	Sudden (90%)	Gradual
History of similar painful episodes	30%	Rare
History of trauma	Possible	Possible
Nausea or vomiting	30%	Rare
Dysuria	Rare	Common
Fever >101° F	Rare	30%
Tenderness, swelling	Testicle/global	Epididymis/global
Cremasteric reflex present	Substantial minority	Many
Testicle position (standing)	Usually high-riding and horizontal lie (50%)	Normal position and vertical lie
Contralateral testicle	Horizontal lie (if "bell clapper deformity")	Normal vertical lie
Pyuria (>10 WBC/hpf)	<10%	50%

In some patients it may not be possible to distinguish by history and physical examination between testicular torsion and epididymo-orchitis.

WORKUP
Immediate urologic evaluation is required when testicular torsion is suspected. A delay in urologic evaluation and definitive operative treatment repair while performing ancillary tests can lead to "castration by neglect."

Color Doppler ultrasonography ++++ should be performed in patients with an equivocal presentation and in pediatric patients who are suspected of having epididymo-orchitis. If color Doppler ultrasonography is not available, nuclear scintigraphy can be performed.

A Doppler ultrasound stethoscope +++ can be a quick bedside test (listen for arterial flow at the inferior pole of the testicle). Although insensitive, a diminished or absent testicular pulse compared with the contralateral testicle strongly supports the diagnosis.

COMMENTS AND TREATMENT CONSIDERATIONS
No single clinical feature or diagnostic test can absolutely exclude testicular torsion, and surgical exploration is required when an alternative diagnosis is not clear. The diagnosis of epididymo-orchitis should be made hesitantly in the pediatric patient.

 ## INCARCERATED OR STRANGULATED INGUINAL HERNIA

Incarcerated or strangulated inguinal hernias are typically noted as firm, tender masses in the inguinal canal or superior scrotum. The ipsilateral testicle and scrotum are normal. Nausea, vomiting, and other signs of bowel obstruction may develop. Tachycardia, low-grade fever, and toxic appearance are also common.

See Chapter 1, Abdominal Pain.

 ## FOURNIER'S GANGRENE

Fournier's gangrene, a rapidly progressive scrotal infection from mixed bacterial flora, occurs most commonly in diabetic or other immunocompromised patients between 50 and 70 years of age. Fever, toxic appearance, scrotal edema and erythema, focal necrotic areas, crepitus, and foul odor and discharge are some of the common features. This is a medical-surgical emergency and requires aggressive treatment.

See Chapter 30, Rash.

 ## ABDOMINAL AORTIC ANEURYSM

Expanding or leaking abdominal aortic aneurysms should be considered in older men with scrotal pain but with unimpressive findings on genital examination. Pain is usually severe and constant and may persist for weeks.

See Chapter 1, Abdominal Pain.

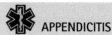

APPENDICITIS

Appendicitis is an uncommon cause of referred pain to the scrotum but should be considered in a patient who has a normal genital examination and no other explanation for the pain. Patients may have fever, vomiting, anorexia, right lower abdominal tenderness, a positive iliopsoas or obturator sign, and hypoactive bowel sounds. Mild pyuria can be noted secondary to ureteral irritation from an adjacent retrocecal inflamed appendix.

See Chapter 1, Abdominal Pain.

REFERENCES

Baker L, Sigman D, Mathews R, et al: An analysis of clinical outcomes using color doppler testicular ultrasound for testicular torsion, *Pediatrics* 105:604, 2000.

Burgher SW: Acute scrotal pain, *Emerg Med Clin North Am* 16:781, 1998.

Hawtrey C: Assessment of acute scrotal symptoms and findings. A clinician's dilemma, *Urol Clin North Am* 25:715, 1998.

Karmazyn B, Steinberg R, Kornreich L, et al: Clinical and sonographic criteria of acute scrotum in children: a retrospective study of 172 boys, *Pediatr Radiol* 35:302, 2005.

Marcozzi D, Suner S: The nontraumatic acute scrotum, *Emerg Med Clin North Am* 19:547, 2001.

Nelson C, Williams J, Bloom D: The cremasteric reflex: a useful but imperfect sign in testicular torsion, *J Pediatr Surg* 38:1248, 2003.

Stehr M, Boehm R: Critical validation of colour Doppler ultrasound in diagnostics of acute scrotum in children, *Eur J Pediatr Surg* 13:386, 2003.

Seizure, Adult
Michelle Kalinski

With a lifetime incidence of 2% to 5%, seizure is a common complaint among patients seeking ED care, accounting for at least 1% of ED visits. Seizures can present in a variety of ways including single isolated events, recurrent seizures, and status epilepticus. Status epilepticus has been defined in a number of ways. The broadest definition uses 30 minutes of sustained seizure activity or repeated seizures without returning to a normal baseline mental state. Some authors, however, recommend shortening the time criterion to 5 minutes. The incidence of status epilepticus increases at the extremes of age, and about 50 persons per 100,000 suffer this condition. Up to 25% of status epilepticus cases present with altered mental status and no convulsions in what is termed "nonconvulsive status epilepticus." EEG monitoring is required to establish this diagnosis. Mortality rates for status epilepticus are as high as 20% to 25%.

Patients with chronic recurrent seizures are generally easily managed within the ED. If a thorough history and physical examination exclude any exacerbating illness leading to a lower seizure threshold or a significant change in the chronic seizure pattern, then most patients with recurrent seizures require nothing more than (1) observation until the postictal state resolves and the patient's neurologic baseline is reached and (2) measurement of serum concentration (if available) of any anticonvulsants that the patient is known to be taking to help assess whether dose adjustment is indicated.

The evaluation of a new-onset seizure is of greater concern because many disease processes can cause seizures, with significant morbidity or mortality if not promptly diagnosed. Even in recurrent seizures it is important to realize that new medical conditions can precipitate increased seizure activity. A directed search for an underlying cause is appropriate in patients with an increase in seizure activity or with clinical suspicion of another process (as suggested by fever, persistent or new focal neurologic findings, shortness of breath, and so forth), as well as in patients whose mental status and neurologic function fail to normalize within the first hour of their evaluation.

Initial evaluation must include an assessment of airway, breathing, and circulation followed by a careful history and physical examination. If airway control is required, do not use long-acting paralytics without continuous EEG monitoring. Patients who are seizing on arrival to the ED should have an immediate check of a glucose level and administration of intravenous dextrose if hypoglycemia is present (consider concomitant treatment with thiamine 100 mg IV in appropriate patients). If intravenous access is unavailable and the patient is hypoglycemic, glucagon 1 mg subcutaneously or intramuscularly may be administered. Diagnostic tests and subsequent treatment should be directed toward an identifiable cause of seizure that can be specifically treated. Whenever meningitis is a serious consideration, dexamethasone 10 mg IV and appropriate antibiotics should be given (after quickly obtaining blood cultures and before LP if a delay in obtaining CSF is anticipated). Emergent CT neuroimaging is warranted for patients who are at risk for a structural intracranial lesion. Many drugs and toxins can cause seizures, and administration of charcoal and specific antidotes should be considered.

Most nonhypoglycemic seizures cease spontaneously or respond to the administration of a benzodiazepine. Options include:

1. Lorazepam (Ativan)—0.05 to 0.1 mg/kg administer at 1 to 2 mg/min, maximum of 10 mg IV/IM. The anticonvulsant duration is several hours.
2. Diazepam (Valium)—0.1 to 0.2 mg/kg at 5 mg/min IV. Diazepam may also be given IM in 5-mg increments or rectally at 0.3 to 0.5 mg/kg using the standard IV formulation or a gel form (Diastat). The anticonvulsant duration is 20 minutes.
3. Midazolam (Versed)— 0.05 to 0.1 mg/kg IV or IM at 1 to 2 mg/min; midazolam can also be administered intranasally.

In cases of status epilepticus, additional treatment is required. Phenytoin (Dilantin) may be given only intravenously (adults: 20 mg/kg at <50 mg/min). Fosphenytoin (Cerebyx) dosing (15 to 20 mg phenytoin equivalents per kilogram) is similar to that of phenytoin. It may be given intravenously at a rate of 100 to 150 phenytoin sodium equivalents/min or intramuscularly. If the seizures do not abate with this treatment, the patient is said to be in refractory status epilepticus. Treatment options include:

1. High-dose phenytoin (mean dose 24 mg/kg IV). One study showed a 38% reduction in the need for third-agent therapy.

The Epilepsy Foundation of America's working group recommends that up to 30 mg /kg of phenytoin be given with hemodynamic monitoring before dosing another drug.

2. Phenobarbital (20 mg/kg IV at 60 to 100 mg/min) may be administered. The VA Cooperative Study showed it to be equally efficacious to phenytoin and benzodiazepines alone or in combination at terminating status epilepticus. Phenobarbital IV at this dose and rate results in profound respiratory depression, and the ability to manage the airway is imperative.

3. Continuous barbiturate infusion (with pentobarbital and others) has also been effective at suppressing electrical discharges.

4. Valproate (average dose 10 to 15 mg/kg IV, maximum load 20 mg/kg at an infusion rate of 20 mg/min) has been shown to be effective in small studies in Europe. It has not yet been approved for this use in the United States, and its use is contraindicated in the setting of hepatic dysfunction.

5. Propofol (1 to 2 mg/kg IV followed by 2 to 10 mg/kg/hr infusion) has been shown in small studies to be effective about 60% of the time in refractory status epilepticus.

6. Continuous benzodiazepine infusion resulted in seizure suppression up to 80% of the time.

CHAPTER 32

REFERENCES

Bradford JC, Kyriakedes CG: Evaluation of the patient with seizures: an evidence based approach, *Emerg Med Clin North Am* 17:203,1999.

Claassen J, Hirsch LJ, Emerson RG, et al: Treatment of refractory status epilepticus with pentobarbital, propofol, or midazolam: a systematic review, *Epilepsia* 43:146, 2002.

Clinical Policy: Critical issues in the evaluation and management of adult patients presenting to the emergency department with seizures, *Ann Emerg Med* 43:605, 2004.

De Gans J, Van De Beek D: Dexamethasone in adults with bacterial meningitis, *N Engl J Med* 347:1549, 2002.

Eisner RF, Turnbull TL, Howes DS, et al: Efficacy of a "standard" seizure workup in the emergency department, *Ann Emerg Med* 15:33, 1986.

Henneman PL, De Roos F, Lewis RJ: Determining the need for admission in patients with new-onset seizures, *Ann Emerg Med* 24:1108, 1994.

Jagoda A, Colucciello S: Seizures: accurate diagnosis and effective treatment, *Emerg Med Pract* 2:1, 2000.

Mower WR, Biros MH, Talan DA, et al: Selective tomographic imaging of patients with new-onset seizure disorders, *Acad Emerg Med* 9:43, 2002.

Neufeld MY, Chistik V, Vishne TH, et al: The diagnostic aid of routine EEG findings in patients presenting with a presumed first-ever unprovoked seizure, *Epilepsy Res* 42:197, 2000.

Pellegrino TR: An emergency department approach to first time seizures, *Emerg Med Clin North Am* 12:925, 1994.

Roth HL, Drislane FW: Seizures, *Neurol Clin* 16:257, 1998.

Turnbull TL, Vanden Hoek TL, Howes DS, Eisner RF: Utility of laboratory studies in the emergency department patient with a new-onset seizure, *Ann Emerg Med* 19:373, 1990.

 HYPOXIA

Adequacy of ventilation and oxygen saturation should be checked for all patients who are seizing. Hypoxia may be a cause of seizure or be caused by ventilatory insufficiency as a result of the seizure. Initial airway and ventilatory stabilization must take priority over ancillary testing. Paralytic agents used for airway management prevent the motor activity seen with many seizures without suppressing the underlying seizure activity in the brain. In the absence of motor activity, caregivers may fail to recognize ongoing seizure activity. Continuous EEG monitoring should be used for patients at risk for ongoing seizure activity whenever long-acting paralytic agents are administered.

See Chapter 34, Shortness of Breath.

 HYPONATREMIA

Hyponatremia may be the cause of new-onset seizures in up to 5% of patients with an identifiable cause. The severity of the clinical manifestations of hyponatremia depends on the absolute reduction in serum sodium and the rapidity with which this reduction has occurred. Hyponatremia can be life threatening and requires laboratory testing for diagnosis. Hyponatremia is unlikely to be the cause of seizures until the sodium concentration is less than 120 mEq/L. Ultraendurance athletes represent a group of healthy young adults who may have acute hyponatremia as the cause of their seizure in the setting of a prolonged athletic event.

SYMPTOMS
- Lethargy
- Confusion or agitation
- Headaches
- Nausea and vomiting
- Muscle cramps or generalized weakness
- Seizures

SIGNS
- Altered mentation: agitation, lethargy, and coma
- Seizures are usually generalized and may be refractory or recurrent.

WORKUP
- Serum sodium level confirms the diagnosis of hyponatremia.
- CT scan may be indicated to rule out a CNS process.

COMMENTS AND TREATMENT CONSIDERATIONS
If hyponatremia is present, a thorough investigation is necessary to identify its cause. Causes of hyponatremia include retention of water (SIADH, CHF, cirrhosis, etc.) and sodium losses (GI tract, skin, renal). Severe hyperglycemia and, depending on the assay used, hypertriglyceridemia and hyperproteinemia cause a "pseudohyponatremia" (measured sodium concentrations are low without actual hyponatremia), which does not cause seizures. Hyponatremic seizures are frequently refractory to standard anticonvulsant therapy and require serum sodium supplementation for seizure abatement. Controlled delivery of hypertonic saline (3%) is the treatment of choice. Careful attention to the rate in the rise of serum sodium is crucial to prevent central pontine myelinolysis and other brain demyelination syndromes.

CHAPTER 32

REFERENCES
American College of Emergency Physicians: Clinical policy for the initial approach to patients presenting with a chief complaint of seizure who are not in status epilepticus, *Ann Emerg Med* 29:706, 1997.

Davis DP, Videen JS, Marino A, et al: Exercise-associated hyponatremia in marathon runners: a two-year experience, *J Emerg Med* 21:47, 2001.

Speedy DB, Rogers I, Safih S, et al: Hyponatremia and seizures in an ultra distance triathlete, *J Emerg Med* 18:41, 2000.

HYPERNATREMIA
Hypernatremia is a rare cause of new-onset seizures. Patients at risk for hypernatremia are generally debilitated individuals who do not control their own dietary intake. Patients with normal mentation and intact thirst mechanisms have an intense thirst response to even a slight increase in the serum sodium level (3 mEq/L) above baseline. This triggers water intake and a correction of the serum sodium. Seizures are usually generalized.

See Chapter 27, Mental Status Change and Coma.

HYPOCALCEMIA

Hypocalcemia is the cause of new-onset seizures in up to 4% of patients with an identifiable cause. Most of these individuals have other signs of or risk factors for hypocalcemia (pancreatitis, renal failure, and thyroid surgery with hypoparathyroidism). Alert patients without signs of or risk factors for hypocalcemia are very unlikely to have hypocalcemia as the cause of seizure.

SYMPTOMS
- Anorexia
- Nausea and vomiting
- Fatigue
- Paresthesias (especially perioral)
- Muscle twitching
- Generalized weakness

SIGNS
- Tremor
- Muscular twitching
- Chvostek's sign: tapping over the facial nerve causes twitching of the mouth
- Trousseau's sign: carpal spasm induced by inflating the blood pressure cuff between the systolic and diastolic pressures and leaving it inflated for 3 minutes
- Tetany and hyperreflexia
- Altered mentation: delirium and hallucinations
- Seizures are usually generalized and may be recurrent or refractory.

WORKUP
- Ionized calcium should be measured in patients with seizures who have signs and symptoms of or risk factors for hypocalcemia. Hypocalcemia is defined as ionized calcium <2.0 mEq/L. Serious effects, however, are not usually seen until the level falls below 1.6 mEq/L.
- Electrolytes, magnesium, phosphorus, and creatinine should be measured.
- ECG: a prolonged QT interval is characteristic of hypocalcemia.

COMMENTS AND TREATMENT CONSIDERATIONS
Patients with hypocalcemic seizures require parenteral calcium replacement with 10 ml of 10% calcium gluconate given slowly (over 5 to 10 minutes) and repeated until the hypocalcemia is

corrected and the seizures resolve. Patients should be on a cardiac monitor while calcium is infused.

REFERENCES

American College of Emergency Physicians: Clinical policy for the initial approach to patients presenting with a chief complaint of seizure who are not in status epilepticus, *Ann Emerg Med* 22:875, 1993.

Aminoff MJ, Simon RP: Status epilepticus: causes, clinical features, and consequences in 98 patients, *Am J Med* 69:657, 1980.

Eisner RF, Turnbull TL, Howes DS, Gold IW: Efficacy of a "standard" seizure workup in the emergency department, *Ann Emerg Med* 15:33, 1986.

Powers RD: Serum chemistry abnormalities in adult patients with seizures, *Ann Emerg Med* 14:416, 1985.

Wijdicks EFM, Sharbrough FW: New-onset seizures in critically ill patients, *Neurology* 43:1042, 1993.

Working Group on Status Epilepticus: Treatment of convulsive status epilepticus, *JAMA* 270:854, 1993.

HYPOMAGNESEMIA

Hypomagnesemia accounts for <1% of new-onset seizures and is usually seen in patients who have many other risk factors for seizures. It is likely that seizures associated with hypomagnesemia are multifactorial. Experimentally induced hypomagnesemia in humans has failed to induce seizures.

See Chapter 27, Mental Status Change and Coma.

UREMIA

Renal failure only rarely causes seizures. Seizures in renal failure patients are more commonly seen as part of the dialysis dysequilibrium syndrome (headache, nausea, muscle cramps, agitation, delirium, and convulsions), which typically occurs near the end of or just after a rapid dialysis or ultrafiltration procedure. Seizures generally respond well to conventional therapy. Many anticonvulsant drug dosages have to be adjusted in renal failure.

See Chapter 27, Mental Status Change and Coma.

REFERENCES

Wijdicks EFM, Sharbrough FW: New-onset seizures in critically ill patients, *Neurology* 43:1042, 1993.

CHAPTER **32**

HYPOGLYCEMIA

Hypoglycemic seizures generally occur in patients with a history of treatment for diabetes and do not resolve until the hypoglycemia is corrected. These patients present in status epilepticus until therapy is initiated. Patients with cirrhosis, alcoholism, sepsis, and malnutrition are also predisposed to hypoglycemia. In up to 10% of patients with hypoglycemia, a seizure is the principal manifestation of the hypoglycemia.

A finger-stick glucose is a rapid, safe, inexpensive screening test that should be performed for all patients with altered mental status or seizures. The treatment of hypoglycemic seizures consists of dextrose (consider concomitant thiamine 100 mg IV in appropriate patients), not standard anticonvulsants. If IV access is not available, glucagon 1 mg IM/SC may be given to increase serum glucose levels transiently. Careful serial examinations and a thorough search for the cause of the hypoglycemia are required.

See Chapter 27, Mental Status Change and Coma.

REFERENCES

American College of Emergency Physicians: Clinical policy for the initial approach to patients presenting with a chief complaint of seizure who are not in status epilepticus, *Ann Emerg Med* 29:706, 1997.

Aminoff MJ, Simon RP: Status epilepticus: causes, clinical features, and consequences in 98 patients, *Am J Med* 69:657, 1980.

Browning RG, Olson DW, Steven HA, Mateer JR: 50% dextrose: antidote or toxin? *Ann Emerg Med* 19:683, 1990.

Jones JL, Ray VG, Gough JE, et al: Determination of prehospital blood glucose: a prospective, controlled study, *J Emerg Med* 10:679, 1992.

Rosenthal RH, Heim ML, Waeckerle JF: First time major motor seizures in an emergency department, *Ann Emerg Med* 9:242, 1980.

Wijdicks EFM, Sharbrough FW: New-onset seizures in critically ill patients, *Neurology* 43:1042, 1993.

Working Group on Status Epilepticus: Treatment of convulsive status epilepticus, *JAMA* 270:854, 1993.

HYPERGLYCEMIA, DIABETIC KETOACIDOSIS, AND HYPEROSMOLAR HYPERGLYCEMIC SYNDROME (HHS)

Mild hyperglycemia (glucose < 200 mg/dl) may occur after generalized seizures. Seizures attributable to hyperglycemia, however, usually occur in the setting of severe hyperglycemia and multiple metabolic abnormalities. The mechanism is thought to involve hyperosmolality. Hyperglycemia accounts for up to 4% of new-onset seizures in patients with an identifiable cause. The majority of patients with seizures attributable to hyperglycemia have a history of diabetes; however, up to two thirds of patients with HHS do not have a history of diabetes.

Hyperglycemia associated seizures frequently do not respond to anticonvulsant therapy, and correction of the metabolic abnormalities including a reduction in serum glucose is often required to terminate them. The underlying cause (infection, myocardial infarction, stroke, noncompliance, etc.) of the complicated hyperglycemia must be thoroughly investigated.

See Chapter 27, Mental Status Change and Coma.

REFERENCES

American College of Emergency Physicians: Clinical policy for the initial approach to patients presenting with a chief complaint of seizure who are not in status epilepticus, *Ann Emerg Med* 22:875, 1993.

Aminoff MJ, Simon RP: Status epilepticus: causes, clinical features, and consequences in 98 patients, *Am J Med* 69:657, 1980.

Aquino A, Gabor AJ: Movement-induced seizures in non-ketotic hyperglycemia, *Neurology* 30:600, 1980.

Maccario M, Messis CP, Vastola EF: Focal seizures as a manifestation of hyperglycemia without ketoacidosis, *Neurology* 15:195, 1965.

Rosenthal RH, Heim ML, Waeckerle JF: First time major motor seizures in an emergency department, *Ann Emerg Med* 9:242, 1980.

Vastola EF, Maccario M, Homan R: Activation of epileptogenic foci by hyperosmolarity, *Neurology* 17:520, 1967.

Wijdicks EFM, Sharbrough FW: New-onset seizures in critically ill patients, *Neurology* 43:1042, 1993.

Working Group on Status Epilepticus: Treatment of convulsive status epilepticus, *JAMA* 270:854, 1993.

HYPOTHYROIDISM

Hypothyroidism is a rare cause of seizures in adults, and the seizures that have been reported occur in the presence of myxedema coma. Patients usually have a history of hypothyroidism and other manifestations of myxedema coma, although seizures may be the initial presentation in up to 25% of patients. The mortality from myxedema coma is greater than 50%.

See Chapter 27, Mental Status Change and Coma.

REFERENCES

Catz B, Russell S: Myxedema, shock, and coma: seven survival cases, *Arch Intern Med* 108:407, 1961.

 HYPERTHYROIDISM

Seizures attributable to hyperthyroidism are associated with thyrotoxicosis and are limited to case reports in the literature.

REFERENCES

Urbanic RC, Mazzaferri EL: Thyrotoxic crisis and myxedema coma, *Heart Lung* 7:435, 1978.

Waldstein SS, Slodki SJ, Kaganiec GI, et al: A clinical study of thyroid storm, *Ann Intern Med* 52:626, 1960.

 INTRACEREBRAL HEMORRHAGE, EPIDURAL AND SUBDURAL HEMATOMAS

Intracranial hemorrhages account for about 2% of new-onset seizures, and subdural hematomas are the most common type of hemorrhage associated with seizures. The seizures may be focal or generalized, and status epilepticus is not uncommon. Seizures occur in up to 15% of patients with lobar parenchymal brain hemorrhages (secondary to tumors, arteriovenous malformations, hypertension, angiomas, and so forth), and 70% of these patients have recurrent seizures. Patients with a significant head injury should receive prophylactic anticonvulsant therapy without delay because seizures may worsen the outcome of the head injury.

See Chapter 18, Headache.

REFERENCES

American College of Emergency Physicians: Clinical policy for the initial approach to patients presenting with a chief complaint of seizure who are not in status epilepticus, *Ann Emerg Med* 29:706, 1997.

American College of Emergency Physicians, American Academy of Neurology, American Association of Neurologic Surgeons, and the American Society of Neuroradiology: Practice parameter: neuroimaging in the emergency patient presenting with seizure (summary statement), *Ann Emerg Med* 27:114, 1996.

Aminoff MJ, Simon RP: Status epilepticus: causes, clinical features, and consequences in 98 patients, *Am J Med* 69:657, 1980.

Lobato RD, Rivas JJ, Gomez PA, et al: Head-injured patients who talk and deteriorate into coma, *J Neurosurg* 75:256, 1991.

Ramirez-Lassepas M, Cipolle RJ, Morillo LR, Gumnit RJ: Value of computed tomographic scan in the evaluation of adult patients after their first seizure, *Ann Neurol* 15:536, 1984.

Reinus WR, Wippold FJ, Erickson KK: Seizure patient selection for emergency computed tomography, *Ann Emerg Med* 22:1298, 1993.

Wijdicks EFM, Sharbrough FW: New-onset seizures in critically ill patients, *Neurology* 43:1042, 1993.

SUBARACHNOID HEMORRHAGE

Seizures occur in about 6% to 8% of patients at the onset of bleeding from a subarachnoid hemorrhage. Some studies have shown that seizures are a poor prognostic indicator in the setting of a subarachnoid hemorrhage. Nonconvulsive status epilepticus occurs in up to 8% of subarachnoid hemorrhage patients with an unexplained coma or neurologic deterioration.

See Chapter 18, Headache.

REFERENCES

Arboix A, Marti-Vilalta JL: Predictive clinical factors of very early in-hospital mortality in subarachnoid hemorrhage, *Clin Neurol Neurosurg* 101:100, 1999.

Butzkueven H, Evans AH, Pitman A, et al: Onset seizures independently predict poor outcome after subarachnoid hemorrhage, *Neurology* 55:1315, 2000.

Dennis LJ, Claassen J, Hirsch LJ, et al: Nonconvulsive status epilepticus after subarachnoid hemorrhage, *Neurosurgery* 51:1136,2002.

Fontanarosa PB: Recognition of subarachnoid hemorrhage, *Ann Emerg Med* 18:1199, 1989.

Mayberg MR, Batjer HH, Dacey R, et al: Guidelines for the management of aneurysmal subarachnoid hemorrhage, *Circulation* 90:2592, 1994.

Pinto AN, Canhao P, Ferro JM: Seizures at the onset of subarachnoid hemorrhage, *J Neurol* 243:161, 1996.

Rhoney DH, Tipps LB, Murry KR, et al: Anticonvulsant prophylaxis and timing of seizures after aneurysm subarachnoid hemorrhage, *Neurology* 55:258, 2000.

van der Wee N, Rinkel GJ, Hasan D, et al: Detection of subarachnoid hemorrhage on early CT: is lumbar puncture still needed after a negative CT scan? *J Neurol Neurosurg Psychiatry* 58:357, 1995.

CHAPTER 32

STROKE

Stroke is a common cause of a new-onset seizure in patients older than 50; up to 20% of new-onset seizures in older adults may be caused by stroke. Conversely, a seizure is the presenting symptom of a stroke in less than 7% of patients. Recurrent seizures occur in as many as one third of patients after a stroke.

See Chapter 44, Weakness and Fatigue.

REFERENCES

American College of Emergency Physicians: Clinical policy for the initial approach to patients presenting with a chief complaint of seizure who are not in status epilepticus, *Ann Emerg Med* 29:706, 1997.

American College of Emergency Physicians, American Academy of Neurology, American Association of Neurologic Surgeons, and the American Society of Neuroradiology: Practice parameter: neuroimaging in the emergency patient presenting with seizure (summary statement), *Ann Emerg Med* 27:114, 1996.

Aminoff MJ, Simon RP: Status epilepticus: causes, clinical features, and consequences in 98 patients, *Am J Med* 69:657, 1980.

Ettinger AB, Shinnar S: New-onset seizures in an elderly hospitalized population, *Neurology* 43:489, 1993.

Greenberg MK, Barsan WG, Starkman S: Neuroimaging in the emergency patient presenting with seizure, *Neurology* 47:26, 1996.

Gupta SR, Naheedy MH, Elias D, Rubino FA: Postinfarction seizures: a clinical study, *Stroke* 19:1477, 1988.

Reinus WR, Wippold FJ, Erickson KK: Seizure patient selection for emergency computed tomography, *Ann Emerg Med* 22:1298, 1993.

Wijdicks EFM, Sharbrough FW: New-onset seizures in critically ill patients, *Neurology* 43:1042, 1993.

Working Group on Status Epilepticus: Treatment of convulsive status epilepticus, *JAMA* 270:854, 1993.

MENINGITIS AND ENCEPHALITIS

Central nervous system infections account for up to 4% of new-onset seizures and up to 14% of cases of status epilepticus in patients with an identifiable cause. Many patients have a mild transient elevation in CSF white blood cell count following a generalized seizure. Nevertheless, patients with a mild CSF pleocytosis should be treated as if they have a CNS infection if there is any doubt.

See Chapter 18, Headache, and Chapter 27, Mental Status Change and Coma.

REFERENCES

American College of Emergency Physicians: Clinical policy for the initial approach to patients presenting with a chief complaint of seizure who are not in status epilepticus, *Ann Emerg Med* 29:706, 1997.

American College of Emergency Physicians, American Academy of Neurology, American Association of Neurologic Surgeons, and the American Society of Neuroradiology: Practice parameter: neuroimaging in the emergency patient presenting with seizure (summary statement), *Ann Emerg Med* 27:114, 1996.

Hauser WA: Status epilepticus: epidemiologic considerations. *Neurology* 40(Suppl 2):9, 1990.

Schmidley JW, Simon RP: Postictal pleocytosis, *Ann Neurol* 9:81, 1981.

Simon RP: Physiologic consequences of status epilepticus, *Epilepsia* 26(Suppl 1):58, 1985.

Wijdicks EFM, Sharbrough FW: New-onset seizures in critically ill patients, *Neurology* 43:1042, 1993.

Working Group on Status Epilepticus: Treatment of convulsive status epilepticus, *JAMA* 270:854, 1993.

 BACTERIAL BRAIN ABSCESSES

In most studies, bacterial brain abscesses account for less than 2% of new-onset seizures, although up to 50% of patients with brain abscesses have seizures during the course of their illness. Brain abscesses are frequently misdiagnosed on initial presentation because of an absence of physical signs.

See Chapter 18, Headache.

REFERENCES

American College of Emergency Physicians: Clinical policy for the initial approach to patients presenting with a chief complaint of seizure who are not in status epilepticus, *Ann Emerg Med* 29:706, 1997.

American College of Emergency Physicians, American Academy of Neurology, American Association of Neurologic Surgeons, and the American Society of Neuroradiology: Practice parameter: neuroimaging in the emergency patient presenting with seizure (summary statement), *Ann Emerg Med* 27:114-118, 1996.

Reinus WR, Wippold FJ, Erickson KK: Seizure patient selection for emergency computed tomography, *Ann Emerg Med* 22:1298, 1993.

Rosenblum ML, Mampalam TJ, Pons VG: Controversies in the management of brain abscesses, *Clin Neurosurg* 33:603, 1986.

 BRAIN TUMOR

See Chapter 18, Headache.

CYCLIC ANTIDEPRESSANT TOXICITY

Cyclic antidepressants (CAs) account for approximately 25% of drug-induced seizures, and 20% to 30% patients with significant CA overdose have seizures. Although CA-induced seizures can occur without cardiac toxicity, most CAs are major cardiotoxins, and patients with seizures frequently manifest serious cardiovascular toxicity as well. Risk of mortality is significant.

See Chapter 37, Toxic Exposure, Approach to.

REFERENCES

Glaser J: Tricyclic antidepressant poisoning, *Cleve Clin J Med* 67:717, 2000.

Olson KR, Kearney TE, Dyer JE, et al: Seizures associated with poisoning and drug overdose, *Am J Emerg Med* 11:565, 1993.

 ISONIAZID TOXICITY

The classic triad of acute isoniazid (INH) neurotoxicity is coma, metabolic acidosis, and refractory seizures. INH toxicity should be considered in any patient who has intractable seizures (typically associated with severe metabolic acidosis) unresponsive to standard anticonvulsants. This is particularly true in patients from high-risk groups who are likely to have ready access to INH (e.g., AIDS patients, recent immigrants, Native Americans, homeless patients, and patients who have tuberculosis or are living with someone who has tuberculosis). Empirical treatment with pyridoxine should be considered in such cases (see later).

SYMPTOMS
- Anorexia
- Nausea and vomiting
- Dizziness
- Elevated temperature
- Altered mentation
- Slurred speech
- Photophobia and blurred vision
- Symptoms usually occur within 2 hours of ingestion.

SIGNS
- Hyperpyrexia, hyperreflexia, tachypnea, tachycardia, hypotension, and altered mental status are common.
- Other manifestations include nystagmus, mydriasis, ataxia, and cyanosis.
- Seizures are usually generalized tonic-clonic seizures.

426

WORKUP

- INH toxicity can be difficult to diagnose and commonly is identified after the multidrug-resistant seizures are terminated with pyridoxine.
- Glycosuria, hyperglycemia, and an anion-gap metabolic acidosis (mean pH 7.05) are typical laboratory findings.
- Electrolytes, glucose, magnesium, and calcium should be checked to identify other causes of seizure unless it is clear from the history that INH is the etiologic agent.
- An ECG and acetaminophen and aspirin levels should be obtained to screen for coingestants if an intentional overdose is suspected.
- Liver enzymes should be measured to screen for INH hepatotoxicity.

COMMENTS AND TREATMENT CONSIDERATIONS

All patients should be admitted to a monitored critical care area. Ingestion of 80 to 150 mg/kg usually results in severe seizures and high mortality. Pyridoxine is the specific antidote for neurotoxicity after INH ingestion and can be dosed as 1 g of pyridoxine (vitamin B_6) per gram of INH ingested or a 5-g repeat dosing regimen if the amount ingested is unknown. Up to one third of hospitals did not have enough pyridoxine in stock to treat a single INH overdose.

Because most patients become symptomatic and rapidly decline within 2 hours of ingestion, treatment must be rapid and aggressive. Rapid administration of activated charcoal with or without initial decontamination (i.e., lavage) is required. Alkalinization has been used to correct profound acidosis. Hemodialysis removes INH but is usually unnecessary because pyridoxine is a safe and effective antidote for INH toxicity.

REFERENCES

Brent J, Vo N, Kulig K, Rumack BH: Reversal of prolonged isoniazid induced coma by pyridoxine, *Arch Intern Med* 150:1751, 1990.

Kunisaki T, Augenstein L: Drug and toxin induced seizures, *Emerg Med Clin North Am* 12:1027, 1994.

Olson KR, Kearney TE, Dyer JE, et al: Seizures associated with poisoning and drug overdose, *Am J Emerg Med* 11:565, 1993.

Santucci KA, Shah BR, Linakis JG: Acute isoniazid exposures and antidote availability, *Pediatr Emerg Care* 15:99, 1999.

 THEOPHYLLINE TOXICITY

Although theophylline use is decreasing as other therapies for asthma and emphysema are increasingly being recognized as more efficacious, it remains an important cause of drug-induced seizures. Because of a narrow toxic-therapeutic ratio and multiple drug interactions, theophylline toxicity is common. Among individuals taking theophylline, the incidence of toxicity has been reported to be as high as 20%. Theophylline toxicity can be acute, acute on chronic, or chronic. Seizures are more common with chronic toxicity. Seizures associated with theophylline can be prolonged and fatal. Mortality rates as high as 60% have been reported.

SYMPTOMS
- GI: anorexia, nausea, vomiting, and abdominal pain
- Tremor
- Anxiety or agitation
- Palpitations
- The symptoms of a serious chronic overdose are frequently subtle and nonspecific and may lead to a missed diagnosis.

SIGNS
- Agitation, confusion, and tremor are common and frequently precede seizures.
- Seizures may be focal or generalized, are frequently refractory, and portend a very high risk of morbidity and mortality. Seizures can occur without concomitant gastrointestinal or cardiac toxicity.
- Other common signs of toxicity include tachycardia, cardiac arrhythmias, hypotension, and hyperventilation.

WORKUP
- In acute ingestions, the severity of the toxicity tends to correlate with the peak serum level. Serum levels, however, are less predictive of toxicity in acute on chronic or chronic exposures.
- Seizures may occur with therapeutic serum theophylline levels.
- Because theophylline has multiple sustained-released formulas and drug interactions, serum levels are of limited use in guiding the initial treatment and therapy.
- Serial levels measured 2 hours apart show whether a peak level has been reached.
- Electrolytes, glucose, and an ABG should be checked because these patients are usually acidotic, hypokalemic, and hypoglycemic. All these abnormalities must be corrected because they worsen the signs of theophylline toxicity.
- Consider obtaining baseline calcium, PT/PTT, platelets, and a CBC in the event that extracorporeal drug removal is necessary.

COMMENTS AND TREATMENT CONSIDERATIONS
All patients with suspected theophylline toxicity must have intravenous access and critical care monitoring. Theophylline is

effectively eliminated with charcoal hemoperfusion (HP). Any seizure or cardiac event associated with theophylline toxicity should prompt the initiation of HP. Theophylline is eliminated somewhat less effectively with hemodialysis (HD), but HD is an acceptable alternative if HP is unavailable.

For less severe toxicity, multidose activated charcoal is the treatment of choice. The predictors of major toxicity vary depending on the type of overdose, with peak serum levels being the best predictor in acute overdose and age older than 60 being the main predictor in chronic overmedication. Benzodiazepines and phenobarbital are the drugs of choice for treating theophylline-induced seizures, which may be difficult to control.

REFERENCES

Chu NS: Caffeine- and aminophylline-induced seizures, *Epilepsia* 22:85, 1981.

Olson KR, Kearney TE, Dyer JE, et al: Seizures associated with poisoning and drug overdose, *Am J Emerg Med* 11:565, 1993.

Roberts JR: Drug-induced seizures: theophylline, *Emerg Med News* 19:4, 1997.

 STIMULANT-INDUCED SEIZURES

Stimulants (including cocaine, amphetamines, 3,4-methylenedioxymethamphetamine [MDMA, ecstasy], phencyclidine, and ephedrine) account for approximately 30% of drug-induced seizures. As illicit and prescription stimulants continue to become more widely used, seizures associated with these substances continue to increase in frequency. Stimulants are more likely than other drugs to produce brief, self-limited seizures. Cocaine is the most common stimulant that produces seizures. Amphetamine and other stimulant intoxications present in a similar manner to cocaine intoxication. Other forms of cocaine-induced neurotoxicity include subarachnoid hemorrhage, cerebral infarction, vasculitis, TIAs, and toxic delirium. Many of these can be complicated by seizures (e.g., subarachnoid hemorrhage), and therefore a complete investigation is required.

See Chapter 37, Toxic Exposure, Approach to.

REFERENCES

Choy-Kwong M, Lipton RB: Seizures in hospitalized cocaine users, *Neurology* 39:425, 1989.

Ernst AA, Sanders WM: Unexpected cocaine intoxication presenting as seizures in children, *Ann Emerg Med* 18:774, 1989.

Jerrard DA: "Designer drugs"—a current perspective, *J Emerg Med* 8:733, 1990.

Mody CK, Miller BL, McIntyre HB, et al: Neurologic complications of cocaine abuse, *Neurology* 38:1189, 1988.

Olson KR, Kearney TE, Dyer JE, et al: Seizures associated with poisoning and drug overdose, *Am J Emerg Med* 11:565, 1993.

Roberts JR: Cocaine-related seizures, *Emerg Med News* 19:8, 1997.

Steele MT, Westdorp EJ, Garza AG, et al: Screening for stimulant use in adult emergency department seizure patients, *J Toxicol Clin Toxicol* 38:609, 2000.

ALCOHOL AND SEIZURES

Alcohol abuse increases an individual's risk of having a seizure, and up to 10% of people with active withdrawal have seizures. Alcohol withdrawal seizures usually occur 6 to 48 hours after an individual stops drinking. Although seizures are typically associated with an overt withdrawal syndrome, some patients with withdrawal seizures have few other signs or symptoms of withdrawal. Alcohol abuse and withdrawal are frequently associated with concomitant trauma and other underlying medical issues. For this reason, a first-time withdrawal seizure warrants a complete and thorough investigation including neuroimaging.

See Chapter 27, Mental Status Change and Coma.

SYMPTOMS
- The most common CNS symptoms in alcoholic withdrawal are shaking, headache, altered mentation, hallucinations, and seizures.
- Nausea and vomiting are common.

SIGNS
- Patients with withdrawal seizures typically have other signs of alcohol withdrawal including tachycardia, altered mental status, and tremors.
- Many patients show signs of chronic liver disease.

WORKUP
- A complete workup for a first-time seizure in an alcoholic must be performed. This should include complete laboratory studies and neuroimaging because alcoholics have so many comorbid medical conditions.

COMMENTS AND TREATMENT CONSIDERATIONS
Seizures can usually be controlled with intravenous benzodiazepines. There is also good evidence to support the administration of

benzodiazepines (specifically lorazepam) in patients who are not actively seizing as it has been shown to reduce recurrent seizures related to alcohol use. Intravenous phenytoin is relatively ineffective in the treatment of alcohol-related seizures or withdrawal seizures.

REFERENCES

Chance J: Emergency department treatment of alcohol withdrawal seizures with phenytoin, *Ann Emerg Med* 20:520, 1991.

D'Onofrio G, Rathlev N, Ulrich A, et el: Lorazepam for the prevention of recurrent seizures related to alcohol, *N Engl J Med* 340:915, 1999.

Lynch RM, Greaves I: Regular attenders to the accident and emergency department, *J Accid Emerg Med* 17:351, 2000.

McMicken D, Freeland E: Alcohol-related seizures: pathophysiology, differential diagnosis, evaluation, and treatment, *Emerg Med Clin North Am* 12:1057, 1994.

Ng S, Hauser A, Brust J, et al: Alcohol consumption and withdrawal in new onset seizures, *N Engl J Med* 319:666, 1988.

Rathlev N, D'Onofrio G, Fish S, et al: The lack of efficacy of phenytoin in the prevention of recurrent alcohol-related seizures, *Ann Emerg Med* 23:513, 1994.

Rathlev N, Ulrich A, Fish S, et al: Clinical characteristics as predictors of recurrent alcohol related seizures, *Acad Emerg Med* 7:886, 2000.

CHAPTER 32

 AIDS

HIV must be considered as a diagnostic possibility in any patient with a new-onset seizure. CNS disease is seen in most AIDS patients during the course of their illness. In 10% to 20% of AIDS patients, CNS disease is the initial manifestation of AIDS. Up to 50% of AIDS patients with seizures have no specific CNS lesion identified, and the seizure is presumed to be caused by HIV infection. Secondary causes of seizures include toxoplasmosis, cryptococcal meningitis, herpes encephalitis, syphilis, lymphoma, and tuberculosis. Toxoplasmosis is the most common opportunistic infection that causes seizures in AIDS patients.

See Chapter 19, HIV/AIDS Patient, Approach to the.

SYMPTOMS
• The most common neurologic symptoms in HIV-positive patients are seizures, altered mentation, headache, and neuropathy.

SIGNS
• The examination can range from normal to very abnormal, but patients with AIDS-related seizures often have other signs of AIDS (thrush, wasting, Kaposi's lesions, and so forth).

- Many patients with a secondary CNS infection as the cause of seizure have focal neurologic deficits on examination.

WORKUP
- CT scans of the brain with and without contrast (or MRI if available)
- If the CT scans are normal, a lumbar puncture is required. Fluid should be sent for routine testing, as well as for the following: VDRL, AFB, India ink, cryptococcal antigen, herpes PCR, fungal cultures, and viral cultures. Opening and closing pressures are crucial because these may be the only abnormalities in early cryptococcal meningitis. Coccidioidomycosis titers and toxoplasmosis and cryptococcal antigens should also be obtained.

COMMENTS AND TREATMENT CONSIDERATIONS
Because infections frequently result in seizures, initial therapy is directed at correcting the underlying etiology. Seizures can usually be controlled with intravenous benzodiazepines. Intravenous phenytoin or barbiturates are useful for prolonged, refractory, or repeated seizures.

REFERENCES
Berger JR, Moskowitz L, Fischl M, et al: The neurologic complications of AIDS: frequently the initial manifestation, *Neurology* 34(Suppl 1):134, 1984.

Hollander H: Cerebrospinal fluid abnormalities and abnormalities in individuals infected with human immunodeficiency virus, *J Infect Dis* 158:855, 1988.

Holtzman DM, Kaku DA, So YT: New-onset seizures associated with human immunodeficiency virus infection: causation and clinical features in 100 cases, *Am J Med* 87:173, 1989.

McArthur JW: Neurologic manifestations of AIDS, *Medicine (Baltimore)* 66:407, 1987.

Pesola GR, Westfal RE: New-onset generalized seizures in patients with AIDS presenting to the emergency department, *Acad Emerg Med* 5:905, 1998.

Wong MC, Suite NDA, Labar DR: Seizures in human immunodeficiency virus infection, *Arch Neurol* 47:640, 1990.

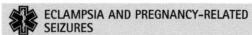 **ECLAMPSIA AND PREGNANCY-RELATED SEIZURES**

The most common cause of seizures in pregnancy is idiopathic epilepsy. Approximately 0.5% of women of childbearing age have epilepsy. Between 20% to 40% of women have an increase in seizure frequency when they become pregnant. Fewer than 15% of women with their first seizure in pregnancy have gestational seizures; the remainder have idiopathic epilepsy.

Although other conditions must be considered, eclampsia is the likely cause of seizures in pregnant patients who have a new onset of seizures in their third trimester or in the early postpartum period. Eclampsia is rare (<1% incidence) in the United States but is associated with a maternal mortality rate above 10%. The hallmark of preeclampsia, which is more common, is (relative) hypertension with proteinuria or edema. Risk factors for eclampsia include chronic hypertension, nulliparity, a family history of eclampsia, multiple gestations, molar pregnancies, diabetes, extremes of age, and fetal hydrops. Seizures before the third trimester or more than 48 hours postpartum are far less likely to be due to eclampsia. Seizures in pregnant women can also be caused by the same conditions found in nonpregnant patients.

COMMENTS AND TREATMENT CONSIDERATIONS

Eclampsia should be considered in any pregnant woman who has seizures and is past 20 weeks' gestation. Obstetric consultation should be obtained immediately because delivery of the fetus is the definitive therapy.

Aggressive seizure control with magnesium (4 g IV over 10 to 20 minutes followed by 2 g/hr) and standard measures such as benzodiazepine administration (if needed) are indicated. Monitoring of deep tendon reflexes (DTRs) is essential when magnesium is being administered, as a loss of reflexes generally precedes ventilatory arrest caused by hypermagnesemia. Antidote for hypermagnesemia is 10 to 20 ml of calcium gluconate 10% solution IV. Hypertension is often initially treated with hydralazine 5 to 10 mg IV (may repeat) or labetalol.

See Preeclampsia and Eclampsia in Chapter 20, Hypertension.

REFERENCES

Aminoff MJ, Simon RP: Status epilepticus: causes, clinical features, and consequences in 98 patients, *Am J Med* 69:657, 1980.

Chelsey C: History and epidemiology of preeclampsia-eclampsia, *Clin Obstet Gynecol* 27:801, 1984.

Clifford DB: Seizures in pregnancy, *Am Fam Physician* 29:271, 1984.

Hachinski V: Magnesium sulfate in the treatment of eclampsia, *Arch Neurol* 154:267, 1988.

Jagoda A, Riggio S: Emergency department approach to managing seizures in pregnancy, *Ann Emerg Med* 20:80, 1991.

Knight AH, Rhind EJ: Epilepsy and pregnancy: a study of 153 pregnancies in 59 patients, *Epilepsia* 16:99, 1976.

CHAPTER 32

Lucas M, Leveno K, Cunningham G: A comparison of magnesium sulfate with phenytoin for the prevention of eclampsia, *N Engl J Med* 333:201, 1995.

Schmidt D, Canger R, Avanzini G, et al: Changes of seizure frequency in pregnant epileptic women, *J Neurol Neurosurg Psychiatry* 46:751, 1983.

The Eclampsia Trial Collaborative Group: Which anticonvulsant for women with eclampsia? *Lancet* 345:1455, 1995.

Will A, Lewis K, Hinshaw D, et al: Cerebral constriction in toxemia, *Neurology* 37:1555, 1987.

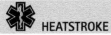 **HEATSTROKE**

See Chapter 15, Fever (Elevated Temperature).

Seizure, Pediatric
Richard Sonner

Up to 6% of children have a seizure by the age of 16 years.
Seizures in children are usually self-limited and have a good
prognosis, but they may represent a medical or surgical emergency with significant morbidity and mortality. In addition,
seizures resulting from trauma or toxic exposure may indicate
child abuse or neglect and have a poor prognosis if not correctly
identified. A careful history and physical examination are the
most important aspects of a seizure workup and should guide
the use of neuroimaging and laboratory tests. Neuroimaging for a
child with a generalized seizure and normal examination is very
unlikely to show clinically significant abnormalities in the
absence of "predisposing conditions" (sickle cell disease,
bleeding disorders, cerebral vascular disease, malignancy,
human immunodeficiency virus infection, hemihypertrophy,
hydrocephalus, and travel to an area endemic for cysticercosis)
or significant head injury. In many cases, well-appearing
children without risk factors may be discharged without
emergency scanning if follow-up is arranged. Similarly, lumbar
puncture and serum chemistries (including toxicologic studies)
are unlikely to show clinically significant abnormalities in the
absence of historical or physical findings that suggest the need
for such tests.

REFERENCES
Freeman JM: Commentary: less testing is needed in the emergency
room after a first afebrile seizure, *Pediatrics* 111:194, 2003.
Sharma S, Riviello JL, Harper MB, Baskin MN: The role of emergent
neuroimaging in children with new-onset afebrile seizures,
Pediatrics 111:1, 2003.

TRAUMA AND CHILD ABUSE

Homicide is the leading cause of injury-related death in infants (children <1 year of age) in the United States, with death most often caused by head injury. Child abuse accounts for 64% of head injuries and 95% of intracranial injuries in infants. Brain trauma represents 7% to 44% of injuries in abused children. Posttraumatic seizures are seen in 5% of minor head injuries and 35% of major head injuries in children. A history of trauma may be difficult to obtain from young children and may be misrepresented by caretakers. In children with a history of trauma, inquire about the exact mechanism of injury and associated symptoms.

See Chapter 22, The Irritable Child.

SYMPTOMS (INFANTS)
- Poor feeding
- Vomiting
- Lethargy
- Irritability.

SIGNS
- Signs of basilar skull fracture (Battle sign, hemotympanum, otorrhea) or focal neurologic abnormalities (focal motor deficit, pupillary asymmetry) predict >57% chance of abnormal head CT.
- Glasgow Coma Scale score <13 correlates with an abnormal head CT in >50% of children with head trauma.
- Infants with shaken baby syndrome may not suck or swallow well; may not follow movements, smile, or vocalize; and usually have retinal hemorrhages (75% to 90%).
- Respiratory difficulty or bradycardia may occur in children with severe brain injury.
- Cervicocephalic soft tissue injury confirms trauma; associated injuries may demonstrate abuse. Complete physical examination includes a search for bone and soft tissue injuries.

WORKUP
- Head CT is indicated in all children with posttraumatic seizures. Abnormal head CT occurs in 36% of older children and 14% of those younger than 2 years with posttraumatic seizures.
- Cervical spine radiographs are indicated if injury cannot be ruled out clinically.
- Skeletal survey of long bone, skull, spine, and rib radiographs may show past fractures in various stages of healing in an abused child.

COMMENTS AND TREATMENT CONSIDERATIONS

There is no "gold standard" for the detection of child abuse; thus, diagnosis may be difficult. Consider abuse in the presence of physical or radiographic findings inconsistent with history, injuries in various stages of healing, or intracranial injury in an infant. Retinal hemorrhages are never seen in trivial accidental head injury and have not been demonstrated in postseizure patients in several studies. Subdural hematomas often result from abuse; epidural hematomas rarely result from abuse. Xanthochromic CSF indicates past cerebral trauma, not a bloody spinal tap. Suspected child abuse must be reported to the appropriate legal authorities. Phenytoin prophylaxis does not reduce the incidence of early posttraumatic seizures in children and is not recommended for routine use.

REFERENCES

Hahn YS, Fuchs S, Flannery AM, et al: Factors influencing post-traumatic seizures in children, *Neurosurgery* 22:864, 1988.

Ramundo ML, KcKnight T, Kempf J, Satkowiak L: Clinical predictors of computed tomographic abnormalities following pediatric traumatic brain injury, *Pediatr Emerg Care* 11:1, 1995.

Young KD, Okada PJ, Sokolove PE, et al. A randomized, double-blind, placebo-controlled trial of phenytoin for the prevention of early posttraumatic seizures in children with moderate to severe blunt head injury, *Ann Emerg Med* 43:435, 2004.

 FEBRILE SEIZURES AND MENINGITIS

Seizure associated with fever usually represents a benign event but may be symptomatic of life-threatening central nervous system infection. Simple febrile seizures are generalized seizures associated with fever, occurring in children 6 months to 5 years of age, lasting less than 15 minutes, and not recurring within 24 hours. Febrile seizures occur in 2% to 5% of all children. Children rarely develop their first febrile seizure before 6 months of age or after 3 years of age. Of children presenting with seizures and a fever, 1.8% to 5.4% were reported to have meningitis prior to widespread vaccination against *H. influenzae* and *S. pneumoniae.* Several subsequent studies show much lower incidence of meningitis. Of children with meningitis, 13% to 16% present with seizure, although meningitis rarely, if ever, presents without complex seizure features (focal, prolonged, or recurrent) or other symptoms of meningitis after infancy.

See Meningitis and Encephalitis in Chapter 18, Headache, and Chapter 16, Fever in Children under 2 Years of Age.

SYMPTOMS OF MENINGITIS

- Altered level of consciousness: lethargy to coma. The postictal state is usually very short in simple febrile seizures so that a prolonged altered level of consciousness should increase suspicion for intracranial infection.
- Irritability or paradoxical irritability (infant becomes more irritable on being held or rocked)
- Vomiting
- Complex seizure features (focal, prolonged, or recurrent)
- Patients who have recently been treated with antibiotics may lack clinical signs of meningitis.

SIGNS OF MENINGITIS

- Fever
- Lethargy +++
- Irritability +++
- Vomiting +++
- Nuchal rigidity ++
- Bulging fontanel ++
- Kernig's sign ++
- Brudzinski's sign ++
- Petechiae ++
- "Toxic appearing" ++
- Headache ++
- Apnea +
- Coma +
- Patients with central nervous system infection may also present with focal neurologic signs, cyanosis, hypotension, grunting respirations, or rash.

WORKUP

- Lumbar puncture (LP) is used to diagnose or exclude meningitis. In patients presenting with a seizure and a fever, LP should be strongly considered for ages <12 months, considered for ages 12 to 18 months, and performed in the presence of clinical signs or symptoms of intracranial infection in ages >18 months. LP should also be performed in any child with a febrile seizure who was recently treated with antibiotics.
- Blood studies and neuroimaging are generally not useful in evaluation unless other clinical indications are present.
- A bedside glucose should be checked if the postictal state is prolonged.

COMMENTS AND TREATMENT CONSIDERATIONS

Signs and symptoms of meningitis may be minimal or absent in children <12 months and "subtle" in children 12 to 18 months of age. Consider herpes encephalitis and need for antiviral therapy for CSF pleocytosis with negative Gram stain, especially in children with focal neurologic findings or coma. Consider mycobacterial or fungal infection for very low CSF glucose without identified bacterial cause.

Children with simple febrile seizures are not at increased risk for serious bacterial illness. Their evaluation should focus on identifying the source of the fever based on clinical features other than the occurrence of the seizure.

REFERENCES

American Academy of Pediatrics: Practice parameter: the neuro-diagnostic evaluation of the child with a first simple febrile seizure, *Pediatrics* 97:769, 1996.

National Institute for Neurological Diseases, National Institutes of Health: www.ninds.nih.gov.

Rosenberg NM, Meert K, Marino D, De Baker K. Seizures associated with meningitis, *Pediatr Emerg Care* 8:67, 1992.

Trainor JL, Hampers LC, Krug SE, Listernick R: Children with first-time simple febrile seizures are at low risk of serious bacterial illness, *Acad Emerg Med* 8:781, 2001.

 ELECTROLYTE ABNORMALITY AND HYPOGLYCEMIA

Pediatric patients presenting with seizure rarely have clinically significant abnormalities in glucose, electrolytes, calcium, or magnesium. Neonates and children with status epilepticus are more likely to have serum chemistry abnormalities. In children <1 year of age with status epilepticus, the most common disorders are hyponatremia/hypernatremia (23%), hypoglycemia (5%), and hypocalcemia (2%). Increased risk of serum abnormalities occurs in children with vomiting, diarrhea, poor feeding, and inappropriate feeding practices (water intoxication caused by overdilution of formula or use of excessive free water in the treatment of dehydration.).

SYMPTOMS
- Vomiting
- Diarrhea
- Poor feeding

SIGNS
- Prolonged seizures
- Altered mental status
- Clinical evidence of dehydration or shock

- Hypothermia (rectal temperature < 36.5° C) ++++ in infants with hyponatremic seizures

WORKUP

- Medical history and physical findings should guide the use of laboratory studies. Serum electrolytes are indicated only for children at increased risk for a serum chemistry abnormality requiring treatment, specifically neonates or young infants, children with seizure activity in the emergency department, children with gastrointestinal symptoms, and children with symptoms or signs suggesting an electrolyte disturbance.
- Children with normal mental status and physical examination are at low risk and do not need laboratory testing.

COMMENTS AND TREATMENT CONSIDERATIONS

Seizures caused by metabolic abnormalities often respond better to correction of the metabolic defect than to anticonvulsant drug use. Retrospective studies have shown that when serum chemistry abnormalities are detected in clinically well children who have had seizures, test results rarely change management. A prolonged postictal state should prompt search for causes other than the seizure. Pyridoxine deficiency should be considered in neonates with status epilepticus.

REFERENCES

Lacroix J, Deal C, Gauthier M, et al: Admissions to a pediatric intensive care unit for status epilepticus: a 10-year experience, *Crit Care Med* 22:827, 1994.

Nypaver MM, Reynolds SL, Tanz RR, et al. Emergency department laboratory evaluation of children with seizures: dogma or dilemma? *Pediatr Emerg Care* 8:13, 1992.

Valencia I, Sklar E, Blanco F, et al: The role of routine serum laboratory tests in children presenting to the emergency department with unprovoked seizures, *Clin Pediatr* 42:511, 2003.

TOXIC INGESTIONS

Toxic causes of seizures in all age groups reported to a poison control center included antidepressants (29%), cocaine and other stimulants (29%), diphenhydramine and other antihistamines (7%), theophylline (5%), and isoniazid (5%). The diagnosis is primarily made on the basis of exposure history, associated symptoms, and physical examination (toxidrome). Consider the patient's current medications as well as possible exposure to other medications or toxins as potential causes of seizure. Teenagers are at risk for intentional overdose.

See Chapter 37, Toxic Exposure, Approach to, and Chapter 32, Seizure, Adult.

SIGNS
- Complications associated with drug-induced seizures in all age groups include respiratory compromise necessitating intubation ++, cardiac arrhythmias ++, hypotension ++, hyperthermia ++, rhabdomyolysis ++, and death ++.
- Seizures may occur in cyclic antidepressant overdose ++ and may be prolonged or multiple ++, leading to cardiovascular instability +++, intubation +++, or death ++.
- Neurologic abnormalities associated with cocaine exposure in children younger than 8 years include seizure ++++, obtundation ++, and ataxia ++; those in children older than 8 years include obtundation +++, delirium ++, drooling ++, and dizziness ++.
- Antihistamine overdose causes anticholinergic signs and seizures that are usually self-limited.
- Salicylate toxicity may cause fever, tachypnea, vomiting, agitation, and coma in addition to seizures.
- Carbon monoxide toxicity may cause dyspnea, tachycardia, lethargy, and coma, with seizures occurring in severe exposures.

WORKUP
- The diagnosis is primarily based on exposure history, associated symptoms, and physical examination.
- In some cases (e.g., acetaminophen, salicylates, digoxin, lithium, theophylline, anticonvulsants), serum drug levels may be useful in confirming the diagnosis or guiding therapy.
- In salicylate toxicity, arterial blood gas classically shows respiratory alkalosis with metabolic acidosis, but mixed acidosis is common in children.
- Arterial or venous carboxyhemoglobin levels evaluate for carbon monoxide poisoning.
- Cases involving isoniazid often present with severe metabolic acidosis.
- In cyclic antidepressant overdose, EKG may show QRS prolongation +++.

COMMENTS
Standard seizure treatment, including assessing airway, breathing, and circulation and anticonvulsant medication for persistent seizures, is often all that is necessary for toxin-induced seizures. Theophylline overdose may require hemodialysis or hemoperfusion. Isoniazid overdose requires treatment with high-dose pyridoxine.

CHAPTER 33

Cocaine-induced seizures tend to be self-limited, but child abuse or neglect must considered.

REFERENCES

Kunisaki TA, Augenstein WL: Drug- and toxin-induced seizures, *Emerg Med Clin North Am* 12:1027, 1994.

Mott SH, Packer RJ, Soldin SJ: Neurologic manifestations of cocaine exposure in childhood, *Pediatrics* 93:557, 1994.

Olson KR, Kearney TE, Dyer JE, et al: Seizures associated with poisoning and drug overdose, *Am J Emerg Med* 12:392, 1994.

Shortness of Breath
Luis M. Lovato

Few medical complaints require more prompt and efficient evaluation and management than acute shortness of breath. Adherence to the universal dictum of airway/breathing/circulation is important to optimize patients' outcome. Patients with acute severe shortness of breath often deteriorate rapidly if critical interventions are not initiated during the primary assessment.

Many causes of acute shortness of breath, or dyspnea, can be life threatening. A detailed history may not be possible because of severity of symptoms. For critical clinical signs related to dyspnea (Table 34–1), initiate interventions during or immediately

TABLE 34–1	
ACUTE DYSPNEA: CRITICAL SIGNS AND IMMEDIATE INTERVENTIONS	
CRITICAL SIGN	IMMEDIATE INTERVENTION
Hypoxia	Supplemental oxygen with reservoir mask, regular mask, nasal cannula depending on the severity
Wheezing	Beta-agonists
Stridor	Steroids, epinephrine, prepare for intubation or foreign body extraction
AMS/fatigue	Consider noninvasive positive-pressure ventilation (NiPPV), especially if suspected pulmonary edema or chronic obstructive pulmonary disease (COPD). Prepare for intubation.
Unilateral breath sounds	Immediate chest x-ray, thoracostomy if patient is unstable

after the ABCs. Once the patient is stabilized, deriving a differential diagnosis of acute dyspnea, based on a more detailed history, physical, and the response to initial interventions, becomes possible. This chapter focuses on common causes of acute dyspnea, categorized by etiology: pulmonary, cardiovascular, obstructive, systemic, environmental, neuromuscular, and psychiatric. Several important causes of dyspnea (acute coronary syndrome, pulmonary embolism, pneumonia) are discussed in other chapters.

PULMONARY

 ASTHMA

The diagnosis of asthma is based on (1) episodic symptoms of airflow obstruction, (2) partial reversibility, and (3) exclusion of alternative diagnoses. Prevalence of asthma is 5% of U.S. adults. Approximately 50% of asthma has an adult onset. Asthma results in approximately 5000 deaths per year in the United States. When evaluating the patient:

- Consider triggers: infectious, pharmacologic, allergic, exercise related, occupational, environmental, vagal, and emotional. The most common trigger is a viral infection, but in many asthmatics the trigger is multifactorial.
- Assess risk for fatal asthma: prior ICU admission, prior intubation, current oral steroid use, hospitalization >2/year, ED visits >3/year, ED visit within the last month, poor access to primary care, psychiatric illness, and illicit drug use.

SYMPTOMS
- Dyspnea; when severe precludes speaking
- Cough
- Chest tightness

SIGNS
- Tachypnea
- Tachycardia
- Wheezing or diminished breath sounds (no breath sounds if severe)
- Work of breathing: posture, accessory muscle use, nasal flaring
- Hypoxia with or without cyanosis (a late finding)
- Altered mental status (agitation, confusion, stupor) from hypercapnia or hypoxia

WORKUP

- The severity of the acute exacerbation is best determined by clinically assessing the patient's ability to ventilate and oxygenate satisfactorily (Table 34–2).
- Pulse oximetry: oxygenation is generally maintained until ventilatory status is severely compromised.
- Peak flow: quantifies severity of initial obstruction and response to therapy. However, normal peak flows often vary with type of meter, ethnicity, effort, and position. Best to compare ED peak flow with the patient's personal best. Many exacerbations require no further workup.
- ABG is useful only when the clinical diagnosis of ventilatory failure is uncertain or if there is a need to assess status by following acid-base and CO_2 status over a long period.
- ECG and cardiac monitor: consider in moderate and severe exacerbations with aggressive beta-agonist use, uncorrectable hypoxia, concurrent risk of ischemia, or in atypical exacerbations.
- Routine laboratory tests (WBC, potassium, etc.) are not useful in most exacerbations.
- Theophylline level: check whether patient is taking theophylline because the drug has a low toxic/therapeutic ratio, frequent serious side effects, and levels are frequently outside the therapeutic range.
- Chest x-ray is not routinely necessary. Consider for severe exacerbations, inadequate response to aggressive therapy, the diagnosis of asthma is new, or if pneumonia, pneumothorax, foreign body, or other comorbidities (HIV, cancer) are suspected.

COMMENTS AND TREATMENT CONSIDERATIONS

- Initiate beta-agonist therapy. Inhaled beta-2 selective agents (e.g., albuterol) are the mainstay of treatment and can be used aggressively and safely in nearly all patients including those with coronary artery disease. Reversing the underlying airway constriction with albuterol generally helps normalize vital signs including tachycardia. Evidence suggests that a metered-dose inhaler (MDI) with a chamber is equivalent to a hand-held nebulizer (HHN). Albuterol has minimal side effects and a high toxic/therapeutic ratio. More frequent administration is more effective. Use continuous therapy in more severe exacerbations. Continuous nebulizer treatments generally use a dose of 15 mg/hr.
- Glucocorticosteroids: early oral prednisone in the ED results in fewer admissions, and treating with oral steroids after discharge results in fewer relapses. Although there is no absolute agreement on dosing, 40 mg daily for 5 days without a taper is a reasonable course of treatment for a mild/moderate flare. There is no benefit

TABLE 34–2
GRADING THE ACUTE ASTHMA EXACERBATION

	MILD	MODERATE	SEVERE	PREARREST
Dyspnea	With walking	With talking	At rest	
Mental status	Normal	Anxious	Agitated	Lethargic, coma
Accessory muscle use	None	Common	Usual	Paradoxical
Speech	Sentences	Phrases	Words	Unintelligible or none
Breath sounds	Expiratory wheezing	Inspiratory and expiratory wheezing	Diminished, often no wheezing	Faint or none
Heart rate	< 100	100–120	>120	???
Room air pulse oximetry	>95%	91–95%	<91%	<<91%
Peak flow as % of normal	>80%	50–80%	<50%	Unable

Adapted from National Asthma Education and Prevention Program: Guidelines for the Diagnosis and Management of Asthma, Expert Panel Review NIH Publication No. 97–4051 (1997). Available on line at http://www.nhlbi.nih.gov/guidelines/asthma/asthgdln.htm.

of intravenous steroids over oral prednisone in the ED or hospitalized patients unless the patient is unable to take oral medications.

- Inhaled glucocorticosteroids are not currently recommended for use in the ED. Consider prescribing at discharge for patients with chronic persistent asthma (requiring use of albuterol more often than twice a week at baseline) in order to prevent recurrences.

- Inhaled anticholinergic agents: there appears to be minimal or no benefit to the addition of anticholinergic agents to adequate beta-agonist therapy. Use in the ED is controversial. These agents have no role in the chronic management of asthma.

- Admission guidelines: poor response to therapy, worsening symptoms, persistent hypoxia, continued dyspnea, peak flow <50% of patient's personal best, unreliable patient, and presence of risk factors for fatal asthma

- Discharge guidelines: subjective (dyspnea) and objective (peak flow, lung sounds) improvement, able to ambulate without recurrent symptoms or hypoxia

- Discharge patients with (1) albuterol MDI with chamber to and instructions on use, (2) fixed dose oral prednisone for 3 to 10 days, (3) inhaled steroids if history of persistent asthma, (4) a peak flow meter, and (5) scheduled follow-up.

ADDITIONAL THERAPIES FOR MODERATE TO SEVERE EXACERBATIONS

- Intravenous (IV) epinephrine can be lifesaving for patients in extremis but carries risks of arrhythmia, MI, and other serious complications. Administration is titrated to pulse, blood pressure, and clinical results. IV epinephrine must be given in dilute form, preferably in a 1:100,000 dilution or in a drip on an IV pump. Dose and administration: draw 1 ml of 1:10,000 (0.1 mg) in a 10-ml syringe, fill remainder of syringe with 9 ml of NS (achieving a concentration of 0.01 mg/ml or 10 μg/ml), administer in 2- to 5-ml aliquots over 1 to 10 minutes intravenously depending on acuity, repeat as needed. Consider following with a titrated epinephrine drip at 2 to 10 μg/min. Subcutaneous epinephrine (adult dose 0.3 mg [0.3 ml of 1:1,000 dilution]) is less effective than adequate doses of inhaled beta-agonists for the treatment of asthma and is no longer commonly used.

- Magnesium: safe and inexpensive, it may provide an incremental benefit in severe asthma when administered as an IV bolus followed by drip.

- Methylxanthines (theophylline, aminophylline) are not recommended because there is no evidence of benefit if adequate doses of beta-agonists are used. Methylxanthines have many drug interactions, low toxic/therapeutic ratios, and serious side effects including arrhythmias and seizure.

- The role of leukotriene modulators in acute asthma exacerbations is controversial, and they are not currently recommended.
- Heliox: a helium/oxygen mixture that theoretically improves laminar flow through small airways. Limited evidence supports a trial of heliox in severe asthma unresponsive to other interventions as a means to prevent need for intubation.
- Noninvasive positive-pressure ventilation (NiPPV): there is no evidence that NiPPV decreases the need for intubation of asthmatics experiencing severe exacerbations.
- Endotracheal intubation: avoid if possible. If unavoidable, consider use of ketamine as the induction agent because it is a bronchodilator. The ventilator strategy of permissive hypercapnia (allowing mild CO_2 retention by using low tidal volume [6 ml/kg]) significantly reduces barotrauma and ventilator-associated complications and improves morbidity and mortality. Adequate sedation is essential because the sense of suffocation is severe as CO_2 rises.

REFERENCES

Adams BK, Cydulka RK: Asthma evaluation and management, *Emerg Med Clin North Am* 21:315, 2003.

National Asthma Education and Prevention Program: Guidelines for the Diagnosis and Management of Asthma, NIH Publication No. 97-4051 (1997) and No. 02-5074 (2003). Available on line at http://www.nhlbi.nih.gov/guidelines/asthma/index.htm.

Rodrigo GJ, Rodrigo C, Hall JB: Acute asthma in adults: a review, *Chest* 125:1081, 2004.

 CHRONIC OBSTRUCTIVE PULMONARY DISEASE

Chronic obstructive pulmonary disease (COPD) is typically characterized by late adult onset, slowly progressive symptoms, and a history of significant smoking. The airflow limitation of COPD is not fully reversible, is usually progressive, and is associated with an abnormal inflammatory response to noxious particles or gases, particularly tobacco smoke. A COPD exacerbation can be defined as a change in baseline dyspnea, cough, and/or sputum beyond the usual day-to-day variability sufficient to warrant change in management. Chronic bronchitis is a form of COPD characterized by excessive sputum production for 3 months or more in 2 consecutive years with other diagnoses excluded. A flare of symptoms is referred to as an acute exacerbation of chronic bronchitis. Emergency management is the same as for a COPD exacerbation.

SYMPTOMS
- Dyspnea
- Cough
- Increased sputum purulence or volume
- Recent upper respiratory infection symptoms
- Chest tightness

SIGNS
- Tachypnea
- Cough, especially with increased sputum production
- Wheezing or diminished breath sounds (no breath sounds if severe)
- Cyanosis
- Clubbing (often seen with chronic hypoxemic lung disease)
- Altered mental status (agitation, confusion, stupor) caused by hypercapnia or hypoxia

WORKUP
- Pulse oximetry reveals hypoxia, which in this setting is generally chronic, except in a severe flare.
- Peak flow
- Chest x-ray is typically unnecessary in mild exacerbations. Consider for patients with advanced age, atypical presentations, requiring hospital admission, poor response to therapy, or to exclude alternative diagnoses (e.g., congestive heart failure, pneumonia).
- Cardiac monitoring and ECG: consider for moderate to severe exacerbations, older patients, concomitant ischemic heart disease risks, or atypical presentations.
- Arterial blood gas (ABG) or venous blood gas (VBG): consider in patients with severe exacerbations or altered mental status to assess degree of respiratory acidosis or response to NiPPV.

COMMENTS AND TREATMENT CONSIDERATIONS
- Beta-agonists and inhaled anticholinergics: although COPD is characterized by chronically irreversible airflow obstruction, inhaled albuterol and ipratropium bromide (Atrovent) may improve symptoms during an acute exacerbation.
- Oral glucocorticosteroids result in short-term improvement in pulmonary function and less treatment failure when given for acute exacerbations. A 10- to 14-day course of prednisone is typically given. Steroids may result in hyperglycemia, especially in patients with known diabetes.
- Oxygen: the goal for patients with chronic hypoxemia is to keep the oxygen saturation at approximately 90% to 92%.

CHAPTER 34

Administration of excessive oxygen to chronically hypoxic patients may worsen respiratory status by several mechanisms (decreased central drive, V/Q mismatch, decreased CO_2 carrying capacity of oxygenated hemoglobin), although the clinical consequence of this is not well established.

- Antibiotics: although evidence supports the use of antibiotics for COPD exacerbations, it remains controversial whether antibiotics should be used for all exacerbations, for severe exacerbations, or only when sputum volume or purulence increases. Emerging bacterial resistance complicates antibiotic selection. Consider using a graded approach to antibiotic therapy with no antibiotics or a less expensive antibiotic (e.g., doxycycline, trimethoprim-sulfamethoxazole) for very mild to moderate exacerbations and newer antibiotics (e.g., fluoroquinolones, cephalosporins) for patients with more severe exacerbations, multiple comorbidities, or required hospitalization.
- Methylxanthines: a Cochrane meta-analysis showed no established benefit from these agents in acute exacerbations of COPD. In addition, methylxanthines can cause serious adverse effects including seizures and arrhythmias.
- NiPPV: a Cochrane review concluded that NiPPV is beneficial in patients with acute exacerbations of COPD, improving many important outcomes such as hospital stay, need for intubation, and mortality. Treatment should be considered early, especially for patients with significant respiratory acidosis or altered mental status.

REFERENCES

American Thoracic Society/COPD: www.thoracic.org/copd.

CDC National Center for Health Statistics: www.cdc.gov/nchs/fastats/lcod.htm.

Celli BR, MacNee W: ATS/ERS Task Force: standards for the diagnosis and treatment of patients with COPD: a summary of the ATS/ERS position paper, *Eur Respir J* 23: 932, 2004.

Palm KH, Decker WW: Acute exacerbations of chronic obstructive pulmonary disease, *Emerg Med Clin North Am* 21:331, 2003.

Ram FSF, Picot J, Lightowler J, et al: Non-invasive positive pressure ventilation for treatment of respiratory failure due to exacerbations of chronic obstructive pulmonary disease, *Cochrane Database Syst Rev* (3), 2004.

Wood-Baker RR, Gibson PG, Hannay M, et al: Systemic corticosteroids for acute exacerbations of chronic obstructive pulmonary disease, *Cochrane Database Syst Rev* (1), 2005.

ACUTE LUNG INJURY AND ACUTE RESPIRATORY DISTRESS SYNDROME

Acute lung injury (ALI) and acute respiratory distress syndrome (ARDS) are both characterized by noncardiogenic pulmonary edema caused by lung injury. ALI and ARDS differ only in the degree of hypoxia, ARDS being more severe. A wide range of clinical conditions causing direct injury (e.g., aspiration, pulmonary infection, submersion, inhalation injury, pulmonary contusion) or indirect injury (e.g., sepsis, pancreatitis, high altitude exposure, multisystem trauma) to the lung can lead to ALI and ARDS.

Diagnostic criteria for ALI/ARDS are (1) chest x-ray with bilateral infiltrates; (2) no clinical evidence of left heart failure and, if measured, a pulmonary capillary wedge pressure <18 mm Hg, (3) severe hypoxemia on ABG manifested by high O_2 requirement (ALI: $po_2 < 300$ mm Hg on $Fio_2 = 100\%$, ARDS: $po_2 < 200$ mm Hg on $Fio_2 = 100\%$).

SYMPTOMS
- Dyspnea
- Fatigue
- Symptoms of causative underlying illness

SIGNS
- Tachypnea
- Hypoxia despite high oxygen delivery
- Wet crackles
- Altered mental status
- No S_3, hepatojugular reflux, or peripheral edema.
- Normal jugular venous pressure (JVP)
- Signs associated with the underlying illness, such as fever, hypotension, abdominal pain, multisystem organ failure.

WORKUP
- Chest x-ray: initial chest x-ray is often normal with subsequent rapid onset of bilateral infiltrates (required to make the diagnosis). Heart size is normal.
- ABG: Pao_2 must be measured for strict definition of ALI or ARDS.
- Pulmonary artery catheterization is used in some cases to measure capillary wedge pressure and guide therapy in the ICU.

COMMENTS AND TREATMENT CONSIDERATIONS
Both ALI and ARDS are associated with decreased lung compliance and pulmonary barotrauma. Low tidal volume ventilator management (6 ml/kg) rather than traditional tidal volumes (10 to 15 ml/kg.) along with low plateau pressures (<30 cm H_2O) significantly reduces days ventilated and mortality. Patients with ALI or ARDS

CHAPTER 34

may also benefit from other specialized ventilator strategies. Treatment of the causative condition is crucial, as is effective supportive care.

REFERENCES

Perina DG: Noncardiogenic pulmonary edema, *Emerg Med Clin North Am* 21:385, 2003.

The Acute Respiratory Distress Syndrome Network: Ventilation with lower tidal volumes as compared with traditional tidal volumes for acute lung injury and the acute respiratory distress syndrome, *N Engl J Med* 342:1301, 2000.

 PLEURAL EFFUSION

Dyspnea associated with pleural effusion may be caused by either the effusion itself or the associated medical condition (e.g., pneumonia, CHF). Based on diagnostic thoracentesis, effusions are classified as *transudative* or *exudative* to help identify the likely etiology. Transudative effusions are commonly associated with nonpulmonary, noninflammatory diseases, primarily CHF but also cirrhosis and nephrotic syndrome. Exudative effusions are associated with pleural-based disease and inflammatory conditions including pneumonia, other infections, malignancy, pancreatitis, collagen vascular disease, and uremia. Pulmonary embolism can present with either a transudative or exudative effusion.

SYMPTOMS
- Dyspnea
- Cough
- Pleuritic chest pain
- Symptoms of the underlying illness (e.g., chest pain, fever, abdominal pain, ascites, weight loss)

SIGNS
- Tachypnea
- Hypoxia
- Decreased breath sounds
- Dullness to percussion

WORKUP
- Chest x-ray: at least 200 ml of pleural fluid is necessary for an effusion to be clearly visible on an upright chest x-ray.
- Lateral decubitus chest x-ray or ultrasound: indication for thoracentesis is a free-flowing, nonloculated effusion greater than 10 mm wide when CHF is not suspected.

- Chest CT is often helpful in identifying the underlying cause of an effusion and can be used to guide chest tube placement with loculated effusions.
- Thoracentesis for primarily diagnostic purposes in stable patients is usually deferred to the primary physician, a pulmonologist, or other consultant. If performed in the ED, appropriate diagnostic studies should be ordered including serum and pleural fluid total protein and lactate dehydrogenase (LDH) levels. Consider checking pleural fluid and serum albumin. In the appropriate clinical settings, including larger effusions, larger volumes of fluid may be sent for cytology in search of malignancy. *Light's criteria* (Table 34–3) are used to classify the effusion type but may incorrectly classify some transudative effusions as exudative. If Light's criteria suggest an exudative process but a transudative effusion is highly suspected on clinical grounds, the serum albumin gradient is used to clarify further the effusion type. If exudative, further studies on pleural fluid include Gram stain, cell count, culture, glucose, and cytology. Do not delay infectious workup if pleural fluid protein and LDH results will be delayed because of laboratory resources.

COMMENTS AND TREATMENT CONSIDERATIONS

Characteristics of the effusion and the patient often provide clues to the cause and are helpful in guiding management.
- An effusion associated with CHF is usually bilateral, symmetrical, and usually resolves over 2 to 3 days with diuresis alone.
- A nonloculated parapneumonic (associated with pneumonia) effusion in an otherwise healthy patient may not require thoracentesis and may resolve with antibiotics alone.

TABLE 34–3
LIGHT'S CRITERIA TO DISTINGUISH EXUDATIVE FROM TRANSUDATIVE PLEURAL EFFUSION

	EXUDATIVE	TRANSUDATIVE
Pleural fluid/ serum protein	>0.5	<0.5
Pleural fluid/ serum LDH	>0.6	<0.6
Pleural fluid LDH	>2/3 of upper limits of normal for serum	<2/3 of upper limits of normal for serum
Serum–fluid	>1.2 g/dl (used only to reclassify an exudative effusion by Light's criteria to a transudative effusion)	<1.2 g/dl

- A loculated effusion with fever is presumed to be an empyema.

Emergent thoracentesis is reserved for patients with significant symptoms (shortness of breath at rest, hypoxia, pain) unresponsive to supportive care. An effusion associated with trauma is presumed to be blood (*hemothorax*) and requires tube thoracostomy. A grossly purulent effusion (*empyema*) upon thoracentesis also requires tube thoracostomy drainage.

REFERENCES
Light RW: Pleural effusion, *N Engl J Med* 346:1971, 2002.

 BRONCHIOLITIS

Bronchiolitis is an acute viral lower respiratory infection usually caused by the respiratory syncytial virus (RSV). RSV bronchiolitis is highly contagious, often occurring in epidemics during the winter months, usually in children younger than 2 years. In most patients, bronchiolitis is self-limited. It is characterized by profuse rhinorrhea, nasal congestion, and wheezing (especially when there is no asthma history). Mild cases are often unrecognized. In severe cases, RSV bronchiolitis can lead to progressive respiratory failure or unpredictable apnea, especially in younger children.

SYMPTOMS
- Dyspnea
- Rhinorrhea and nasal congestion
- Fever

SIGNS
- Tachypnea
- Nasal flaring and accessory muscle use
- Wheezing
- Wet crackles
- Fatigue
- Hypoxia with or without cyanosis

WORKUP
- Nasal swab for rapid RSV test
- Chest x-ray: may include atelectasis, hyperinflation, peribronchial cuffing, or diffuse interstitial infiltrates but is often normal. The chest x-ray is also useful to exclude other diagnoses such as pneumonia.
- Routine laboratory studies (CBC, chemistry, urinalysis, blood cultures) are not useful in the diagnosis of bronchiolitis but

may be performed depending on general appearance, height of fever, severity of disease, and likelihood of an alternative diagnosis.

COMMENTS AND TREATMENT CONSIDERATIONS

Management of bronchiolitis is supportive, centering on maintaining adequate oxygenation and hydration. Treatment with racemic epinephrine, inhaled beta-agonists, inhaled anticholinergics, or glucocorticosteroids can be considered, particularly in severe illness, but none of these therapies have been definitively shown to be beneficial in bronchiolitis. Admit children with persistent tachypnea or hypoxia or who appear toxic. Consider admission for all patients with risk factors for severe disease including prematurity, age younger than 3 months, chronic lung disease, congenital heart disease, or immunocompromise.

REFERENCES

Hartling L: Epinephrine for bronchiolitis, *Cochrane Database Syst Rev* (1), 2004.

Patel H, Platt R, Lozano JM, et al: Glucocorticoids for acute viral bronchiolitis in infants and young children, *Cochrane Database Syst Rev* (3), 2004.

Viswanathan M, King VJ, Bordley C: Management of bronchiolitis in infants and children, AHRQ Publication No. 03-E014, 2003. Available on line at www.ahrq.gov.

Wright RB, Pomerantz WJ, Luria JW: New approaches to respiratory infections in children: bronchiolitis and croup, *Emerg Med Clin North Am* 20:93, 2002.

 PNEUMONIA, PNEUMOTHORAX

See Chapter 7, Chest Pain.

CARDIOVASCULAR

 CONGESTIVE HEART FAILURE AND ACUTE PULMONARY EDEMA

Congestive heart failure (CHF) may be classified as systolic or diastolic. Chronic systolic heart failure is characterized by a decreased ejection fraction and is most commonly caused by previous myocardial infarction. Pump dysfunction worsens when exacerbated by volume overload. Decreased cardiac output leads to decreased blood pressure and compensatory vasoconstriction, which further worsens pump function. Diastolic heart failure is characterized by a normal ejection fraction but impaired myocardial relaxation. It is most commonly caused by chronic hypertension. Distinguishing between the two in the ED can be difficult. Fortunately, initial management is usually the same because volume overload is common to both systolic and diastolic dysfunction. Acute pulmonary edema (APE), the most acute and severe form of CHF, is often precipitated by an acute coronary syndrome.

SYMPTOMS
- Dyspnea, often worse with exertion ++++. Patients often present to the ED when their dyspnea has progressed to shortness of breath at rest ++++.
- Paroxysmal nocturnal dyspnea +++
- Orthopnea ++
- Fatigue and decreased exercise tolerance
- Cough, if APE may have pink frothy sputum
- Angina: an acute coronary syndrome is common in ED patients with CHF/APE, especially when symptoms are hyperacute.

SIGNS
- Vital signs: tachypnea and tachycardia
- Hypoxia
- S_3 gallop heard in systolic dysfunction ++ (>90% specific)
- S_4 gallop heard in diastolic dysfunction ++ (>90% specific)
- Jugular venous distention (>90% specific)
- Wet crackles, may have wheezing
- Peripheral edema ++ (80% specific)
- Murmur (often with valvular abnormalities)
- Hepatojugular reflux ++ (>90% specific)

WORKUP
- ECG: may show LVH with or without strain but is often normal. Look for evidence of acute ischemia.
- Chest x-ray: look for cardiomegaly, pulmonary vascular conges-tion, redistribution of pulmonary blood flow, bilateral pleural effusions, and Kerley B lines (short, horizontal lines in the lateral aspects of the lung).
- Electrolytes: often abnormal due to prerenal failure and diuretic/angiotensin-converting enzyme inhibitor (ACEI) use. It is important to obtain baseline levels because aggressive diuresis is usually part of therapy.
- Cardiac enzymes
- Echocardiogram: may help guide therapy if there is valve dysfunction or a new focal wall motion abnormality suggestive of ischemia.

- In most cases, the diagnosis of CHF is presumed on the basis of the clinical examination and confirmed by CXR. In some cases, B-type natriuretic peptide (BNP) may be helpful because it is elevated in patients with CHF and may be predictive of long-term morbidity and mortality. The utility of this assay in changing management of emergency department patients with acute dyspnea is still uncertain.

COMMENTS AND TREATMENT CONSIDERATIONS

The severity of the presentation guides the urgency of therapy. Immediate therapy is indicated for APE. Multiple therapeutic agents are often initiated simultaneously:

- Vasodilatory agents: the goal is to quickly reduce filling pressures and improve the overdistention of the ventricle. Sublingual nitroglycerin can be started immediately and acts within minutes. It can be followed by an intravenous infusion of nitroglycerin or nitroprusside. Care must be used in the setting of aortic stenosis because a rapid drop in preload can cause hypotension from which recovery is uncertain. Nesiritide, a natriuretic peptide analogue, requires further study before it can be recommended over nitroglycerin.
- Diuretics: loop diuretics (e.g., furosemide) are generally used. Choice of agent and dosing should include consideration of the patient's chronic regimen. Patients who are already receiving high-dose furosemide maintenance require higher doses than patients who are not taking a diuretic.
- Afterload reduction agents: decreasing afterload improves cardiac output acutely and improves long-term morbidity. Afterload reduction is best accomplished by use of an ACEI. Care must be taken not to drop blood pressure too precipitously. Initiate titrated doses of a short-acting ACEI as blood pressure allows.
- Morphine sulfate: has a historical role in managing pulmonary edema, but it has not been rigorously studied. Morphine may have a beneficial role in vasodilatation or may assist by decreasing the anxiety and discomfort associated with severe dyspnea. It is unlikely to be harmful in small doses.
- NiPPV: the benefit in preventing the need for intubation in patients with APE has been established, but the best mode of NiPPV in pulmonary edema patients remains controversial. Continuous positive airway pressure (CPAP) is clearly safe and effective. Bilevel positive airway pressure (BiPAP) may improve respiratory parameters better and faster than CPAP but has been weakly associated with increased myocardial infarction in pulmonary edema patients.
- Simultaneous management of acute coronary syndrome, including aspirin in all patients who do not have contraindications to

CHAPTER 34

457

aspirin therapy. Avoid beta-blockers in APE. For hypotensive patients consider pressor support, primary angioplasty, or an intra-aortic balloon pump.

REFERENCES

Jessup M, Brozena S: Heart failure, *N Engl J Med* 348:2007, 2003.

Maisel AS, Krishnaswamy P, Nowak RM: Rapid measurement of b-type natriuretic peptide in the emergency diagnosis of heart failure, *N Engl J Med* 347:161, 2002.

Nava S, Carbone G, DiBattista N, et al: Noninvasive ventilation in cardiogenic pulmonary edema, *Am J Respir Crit Care Med* 168:1432, 2003.

CARDIAC TAMPONADE, MYOCARDIAL INFARCTION, AND PULMONARY EMBOLISM

See Chapter 7, Chest Pain.

OBSTRUCTIVE

ANAPHYLAXIS

Allergic reactions are caused by release of intracellular mediators from mast cells and basophils. Symptoms can range from a mild pruritic rash to rapid airway obstruction and death. Although definitions vary, anaphylaxis can be considered an allergic reaction with systemic symptoms. Anaphylaxis is immune (IgE mediated), but anaphylactoid reactions are not. Anaphylaxis and anaphylactoid reactions are clinically similar, are managed in the same way, and are discussed here as a single entity. Shortness of breath from anaphylaxis is caused by either upper airway involvement (facial, tongue, or laryngeal edema) or lower airway involvement (bronchospasm and bronchorrhea). Common triggers include medications such as aspirin, NSAIDS, penicillins, Hymenoptera envenomation, and radiocontrast material. Often the trigger is never identified. Reactions can be delayed hours to days, but the most severe reactions usually occur within the first few minutes following exposure.

SYMPTOMS

- Pruritus
- Rash or swelling, flushing ++++
- Change in voice, hoarseness, sensation of throat tightness
- Dyspnea, sensation of chest tightness
- Lightheadedness
- Stridor

- Facial, oral, and generalized cutaneous edema
- Nausea, vomiting, and diarrhea may occur.

SIGNS
- Tachypnea
- Tachycardia
- Hypotension
- Blanching erythema or urticaria ++++
- Hoarseness
- Stridor or wheezing
- Syncope
- Nonpitting edema, commonly to lips, tongue, uvula, face, hands

WORKUP
- Pulse oximetry
- ECG monitoring

COMMENTS AND TREATMENT CONSIDERATIONS
Patients with hypotension or respiratory symptoms can deteriorate rapidly. Consider immediate endotracheal intubation for severe reactions. If swelling progresses, delay may make the airway inaccessible by direct laryngoscopy, and cricothyrotomy may be required.

Epinephrine is first-line therapy in moderate to severe anaphylaxis and should be given immediately. The risks of epinephrine (including hypertension, arrhythmias, and myocardial ischemia) are outweighed by its rapid and often lifesaving therapeutic benefits. In treating anaphylaxis, epinephrine can be given IM or IV.
- IM: most useful for patients with moderate anaphylaxis or patients with severe anaphylaxis while starting an IV. Dose: 0.3 to 0.5 ml of 1:1000 (0.3 to 0.5 mg); administer in the anterolateral thigh or deltoid. May repeat every 5 minutes as needed.
- IV: for patients unresponsive to IM epinephrine or in extremis. Dose and administration: draw 1 ml of 1:10,000 (0.1 mg) in a 10-ml syringe, fill remainder of syringe with 9 ml of NS (achieving a concentration of 0.01 mg/ml or 10 µg/ml), administer in 2- to 5-ml aliquots over 1 to 10 minutes intravenously depending on acuity, repeat as needed, consider following with a titrated epinephrine drip at 2 to 10 µg/min.
  Other agents that are useful in anaphylaxis include:
- Antihistamines: H1 blocking agents (e.g., diphenhydramine): 50 mg IM or IV depending on severity of symptoms. Consider H2 blocking agents (e.g. cimetidine or ranitidine) for additive effect.

459

CHAPTER 34

- Albuterol by nebulizer for bronchospasm
- Oral prednisone or intravenous methylprednisolone for serious reactions

Symptoms can be biphasic, recurring several hours after initial improvement. Patients who have had severe episodes of anaphylaxis should be admitted. Patients who have experienced mild to moderate episodes of anaphylaxis should be observed for at least several hours prior to discharge, particularly if they required epinephrine treatment. Patients who are stable for discharge should be prescribed H1 and H2 antihistamines, a short course of prednisone, and a means to self-inject epinephrine (EpiPen) if needed. Precautions regarding likely causative agent and potential need to carry epinephrine should be given.

REFERENCES

Anchor J, Settipane RA: Appropriate use of epinephrine in anaphylaxis, *Am J Emerg Med* 22:488, 2004.

Kemp SF, Lockey RF: Anaphylaxis: a review of causes and mechanisms, *J Allergy Clin Immunol* 110:341, 2002.

 ANGIOEDEMA

Angioedema is a focal, dermal, inflammatory reaction often involving the face and upper airways that can be either allergic or nonallergic. Nonallergic angioedema includes hereditary, acquired, and drug-related (especially ACEI) forms. Nonallergic angioedema can present with limited systemic signs until the airway is nearly completely obstructed.

SYMPTOMS

- Swelling often of the face, lips, tongue, or uvula
- Dyspnea

SIGNS

- Nonpitting edema with ill-defined margins
- Dyspnea
- Tachypnea
- Stridor
- Urticaria (if an allergic cause of angioedema)

WORKUP

- Often none is required in the ED, but if symptoms are severe consider appropriate workup on other affected systems, especially cardiac.

COMMENTS AND TREATMENT CONSIDERATIONS

All interventions for anaphylaxis (see previous section) may be used with allergic angioedema but are often ineffective for nonallergic angioedema. Because the cause is often uncertain and the risks of no treatment are high, treating all cases as allergic is often warranted. Avoid all likely causative agents, most notably ACEIs.

Consider the diagnosis of a hereditary form of angioedema associated with C_1-esterase inhibitor (C_1-INH) deficiency in patients with angioedema without urticaria, a preponderance of GI symptoms, frequent recurrences, and no identifiable cause. If a nonallergic cause is suspected and a patient is critically ill, fresh frozen plasma (FFP) can be administered as a substitute for C_1-INH concentrate, a therapy not available in the United States.

REFERENCES

Agostoni A, Aygoren-Pursen E, Binkley KE, et al: Hereditary and acquired angioedema: problems and progress: proceedings of the third C1 esterase inhibitor deficiency workshop and beyond, *J Allergy Clin Immunol* 114(3 Suppl):S51, 2004.

Sondhi D, Lippmann M, Murali G: Airway compromise due to angiotensin-converting enzyme inhibitor-induced angioedema, *Chest* 126:400, 2004.

CHAPTER 34

 FOREIGN BODY ASPIRATION

Foreign body (FB) aspiration occurs in all ages. In children, most FB aspirations occur between 1 and 3 years of age. In a child unable to crawl or walk, consider ingestion of an object provided by a sibling. Common foreign bodies include small toys and solid food (peanuts, hot dogs). If the diagnosis is missed, children may present with infectious complications such as pneumonia. Have a high index of suspicion in toddlers, especially when shortness of breath is hyperacute. In adults who are poor historians, consider risk factors such as poor dentition, intoxication, altered mental status, maxillofacial trauma, impaired reflexes or swallowing mechanism, mental retardation, or dementia.

SYMPTOMS

- Sudden onset choking ++++
- Cough: especially following a choking episode ++++, may be intractable.
- Dyspnea
- Throat or neck pain or a foreign body sensation
- Patients are occasionally asymptomatic

461

SIGNS
- Cough
- Stridor
- Wheezing (especially unilateral)
- Tachypnea
- Hypoxia
- Unilaterally decreased breath sounds
- Fever (if presentation delayed)
- Recurrent lobar pneumonia (especially in children)
- Cardiac arrest in a child

WORKUP
- Chest x-ray: many foreign bodies (especially food particles) are radiolucent and the initial x-ray may be normal. Findings may include atelectasis; pneumonia; signs of barotrauma such as pneumothorax, pneumomediastinum, and subcutaneous air; and air trapping (especially in children) manifesting as unilateral hyperinflation on expiratory film or on lateral decubitus with the affected side down. In children, FBs are usually in the upper airways and when found in the lower airways are equally common on both sides. In adults, FBs are more often in the lower airways and more often on the right.
- Chest CT
- Bronchoscopy may be both diagnostic and therapeutic.

COMMENTS AND TREATMENT CONSIDERATIONS
Direct laryngoscopy to attempt extraction of any FB visualized above the larynx is immediately indicated for the unconscious patient with a suggestive history and who is unresponsive to bag-valve-mask ventilation. If an FB is not visible, the patient should be intubated. If the FB is below the vocal cords and cannot be removed, in some cases the endotracheal tube may be used to push the FB deeper into the airway allowing at least partial ventilation. For the conscious but unstable patient consider the basic life support algorithms for FB aspiration including the Heimlich maneuver, abdominal thrusts, and back blows in children. For the stable patient with minimal symptoms, provide supportive care and initiate diagnostic workup.

Bronchoscopy is the "gold standard" for the diagnosis and management of aspirated FB. It is more commonly positive when signs and imaging are suggestive of FB aspiration, but it is often indicated on the basis of history alone.

REFERENCES
Baharloo F, Veyckemans F, Francis C, et al: Tracheobronchial foreign bodies: presentation and management in children and adults, *Chest* 115:1357, 1999.

Ciftci AO, Bingol-Kologlu M, Senocak ME, et al: Bronchoscopy for evaluation of foreign body aspiration in children, *J Pediatr Surg* 38:1170, 2003.

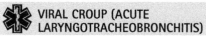

VIRAL CROUP (ACUTE LARYNGOTRACHEOBRONCHITIS)

Croup is the most common cause of stridor in the febrile child. Viruses of the parainfluenza group are most commonly implicated. Croup usually affects children younger than 6 years. The illness is typically benign and self-limited, resolving within 5 to 7 days. In severe cases, especially in younger children, it can cause respiratory failure from obstructive sublaryngeal edema.

SYMPTOMS
- High-pitched cough, often worse at night
- Dyspnea
- Fever

SIGNS
- Characteristic barking cough
- Stridor, especially with cough and agitation, more concerning when it occurs at rest
- Tachypnea
- Nasal flaring, intercostal retractions
- Hypoxia
- Fever

WORKUP
- Often no workup is necessary.
- Consider chest x-ray or lateral neck x-ray if considering FB aspiration, abscess, or epiglottitis. Chest x-ray may show characteristic sublaryngeal narrowing of the air column (*steeple sign*).

COMMENTS AND TREATMENT CONSIDERATIONS
- Cool mist is a common intervention in croup that has no evidence to support its use. A recent study showed no benefit from cool mist in patients treated with steroids. Low cost and likely safety argue for its continued use as long as treatments proven effective are not inappropriately withheld.
- Inhaled epinephrine, although not extensively studied, has been shown to improve symptoms temporarily. Inhaled L-epinephrine (the type used in ACLS) is as safe and effective as racemic (mixed D- and L-epinephrine) and is often more readily available. Because of the concern for transient improvement with subsequent

CHAPTER 34

463

deterioration, it is generally recommended that children receiving epinephrine should be observed for 2 to 3 hours before discharge.

- Systemic glucocorticosteroids have been shown to improve symptoms, result in shorter ED visits, reduce return visits, and shorten hospitalizations. Oral dexamethasone 0.6 mg/kg has been shown to be as effective as IM dexamethasone and is well tolerated when dexamethasone tablets are crushed and mixed with flavored syrup.
- Inhaled glucocorticosteroids may be beneficial, but additional studies are needed to determine their role, if any.

REFERENCES

Rittichier KK, Ledwith CA: Outpatient treatment of moderate croup with dexamethasone: intramuscular versus oral dosing, *Pediatrics* 106:1344, 2000.

Russell K, Wiebe N, Saenz A, et al: Glucocorticoids for croup, *Cochrane Database Syst Rev* (1), 2004.

 EPIGLOTTITIS

Epiglottitis is an acute infection of the epiglottis and upper airway. It was previously more common in children, but routine childhood vaccination against *Haemophilus influenzae* type b (Hib) and pneumococcus has almost entirely eliminated the disease in children. Now principally seen in adults, epiglottitis may be due to bacterial (Hib, *Streptococcus* species, and *Haemophilus parainfluenzae*) or other infections, but most often no etiology is identified.

SYMPTOMS

- Sore throat +++++
- Odynophagia ++++
- Fever ++++
- Dyspnea ++++
- Dysphagia ++++
- Change in voice

SIGNS

- Tachypnea
- Tripod position: uncomfortable seated posture with the body supported anteriorly by the extended arms, with a slightly extended neck and often a protruding tongue
- Drooling

- Stridor
- Anterior neck erythema or pain ++
- Hoarseness or muffled voice ++
- Cervical lymphadenopathy ++

WORKUP

- A lateral soft tissue neck x-ray is useful in stable patients as a screen but is often not definitive. Findings may include the "thumb sign," in which the epiglottis loses its normal elongated shape and resembles an adult thumb; and the "vallecula sign," in which the vallecula is abnormally narrowed, angled, or obliterated (the normal vallecula is a deep radiolucent air column between the tongue and epiglottis, parallel to the pharyngotracheal air column).

COMMENTS AND TREATMENT CONSIDERATIONS

Patients with epiglottitis can deteriorate rapidly and unexpectedly. Advanced airway equipment including a cricothyrotomy tray and rapid sequence intubation (RSI) medications should be ready at the bedside. Management strategies differ for children and adults because of the greater propensity for children with epiglottitis to develop airway obstruction. It is important to avoid stimulation of the child with epiglottitis with unnecessary manipulations, including pharyngeal examination, or attempting to place a close-fitting oxygen mask on the face. Fiberoptic laryngoscopy should generally be performed by a multidisciplinary team (surgery, ENT, anesthesia, pediatrics) in the operating room in the event that an emergent surgical airway is necessary. Oral intubation to secure the airway is indicated for severely ill and deteriorating adults in the ED. For all other adults, fiberoptic laryngoscopy is the procedure of choice to confirm the diagnosis and to secure the airway if obstruction is pending at visualization. Begin empirical treatment with broad-spectrum antibiotics (consider an extended spectrum penicillin or a second- or third-generation cephalosporin) until Gram stain or culture further guides therapy. All cases should be admitted to an ICU.

CHAPTER 34

REFERENCES

Carey MJ: Epiglottitis in adults, *Am J Emerg Med* 14:421, 1996.

Ducic Y, Hebert PC, MacLachlan L, et al: Description and evaluation of the vallecula sign: a new radiologic sign in the diagnosis of adult epiglottitis, *Ann Emerg Med* 30:1, 1997.

Miller K, Chang A: Acute inhalational injury, *Emerg Med Clin North Am* 21:533, 2003.

SYSTEMIC

METABOLIC ACIDOSIS

Increased minute ventilation is a compensatory response to metabolic acidosis driven by the decreased pH of the serum and CSF. Carbon dioxide excretion is increased through the lungs (compensatory respiratory alkalosis) in an attempt to maintain the pH in the normal range. If the metabolic acidosis is acute and severe, as occurs with many etiologies of anion gap acidosis, the patient often feels dyspneic. Four principal causes of anion gap metabolic acidosis are ketoacidosis, lactic acidosis, toxic ingestion, and renal failure. Clinical clues often lead the physician to the correct etiology of metabolic acidosis long before confirmatory test results.

ENVIRONMENTAL

See Inhalational Injuries in Chapter 40, Trauma, Burns.

NEUROMUSCULAR

Patients with a neuromuscular etiology of respiratory failure often have more prominent neurologic symptoms such as weakness as their chief complaint (See Chapter 44, Weakness and Fatigue). Prominent respiratory symptoms and signs such as tachypnea and hypoxia are often not present even when respiratory failure is imminent. Historical features that may suggest an etiology include a recent infection, ill contacts (botulism, heavy metal intoxication), recent travel (tick paralysis, poliomyelitis, diphtheria), history of similar episodes (myasthenia gravis, acute intermittent porphyria), or an incomplete vaccination history (poliomyelitis, diphtheria). Signs of impending neuromuscular respiratory failure include tachypnea, hypoxia, hypercapnia, or difficulty handling secretions. Patients with neuromuscular respiratory insufficiency should be placed in a monitored setting (often in the ICU) with serial bedside spirometry and close observation and treated supportively until the underlying problem resolves.

Guillain-Barré syndrome (GBS) is the most common etiology of emergent neuromuscular respiratory failure. In patients with GBS, a spirometric vital capacity (VC) of less than 20 ml/kg, a decrease in serial VC greater than 30%, and bulbar symptoms are all strongly associated with the need for mechanical ventilation.

REFERENCES

Lawn ND, Fletcher DD, Henderson RD, et al: Anticipating mechanical ventilation in Guillain-Barré syndrome, *Arch Neurol* 58:893, 2001.

PSYCHIATRIC

Shortness of breath is a common somatic complaint associated with anxiety. Nevertheless, clinicians must be cautious in attributing dyspnea to a psychiatric cause, especially if the patient is presenting for the first episode. Clinical clues suggestive of psychogenic dyspnea include having an anxiety or mood disorder, a stressor preceding the dyspnea, circumoral paresthesia, carpopedal paresthesia with or without spasm, or an erratic staccato breathing pattern. Consider a psychiatric cause only after an appropriate history and physical, observing the response to interventions (if any are given), and a reasonable workup depending on the likelihood of another etiology. A young dyspneic patient with prior similar episodes, a previously diagnosed anxiety disorder, a normal examination, and a response to benzodiazepines may not require any further workup. However, an anxious elderly patient with comorbid disease may require extensive testing and admission to rule out a causative medical disease before attributing acute dyspnea to a psychiatric cause.

REFERENCES

Merritt TC: Recognition and acute management of patients with panic attacks in the emergency department, *Emerg Med Clin North Am* 18:289, 2000.

CHAPTER 34

Sore Throat

Sukhjit S. Takhar and Richelle J. Cooper

Sore throat is a common presenting symptom in the emergency room and primary care setting. A variety of diagnoses and etiologic agents are associated with the symptom of a sore throat. The majority of these illnesses are benign and self-limited. However, a handful of diseases can be life threatening, and it is imperative for the ED physician to identify and treat these conditions in a timely fashion. Sore throat may be the presenting symptom of a disease process that can lead to rapid airway compromise or a deep space infection that can extend into the neck or mediastinal spaces and produce overwhelming sepsis. A sore throat in a toxic-appearing patient is a medical emergency.

PHARYNGITIS

Pharyngitis (and tonsillitis, or pharyngotonsillitis) is the most common cause of sore throat. It is the inflammation or irritation of the pharynx and tonsils and can be either noninfectious or infectious. The noninfectious causes of pharyngitis include gastroesophageal reflux, allergy, trauma, and caustic ingestions. Infectious etiologies, usually viral, are the most common cause of acute pharyngitis. We describe the common signs and symptoms of infectious pharyngitis and discuss group A beta-hemolytic streptococcal (GABHS) pharyngitis, the entity that, because of its potential sequelae, is the principal concern in emergency care. Several other viral and bacterial etiologies that have specific symptoms, signs, and diagnostic or treatment considerations are also discussed.

 INFECTIOUS (VIRAL AND BACTERIAL) PHARYNGITIS

SYMPTOMS
- Sore throat
- Fever

- Dysphagia
- Rhinorrhea
- Cough
- Malaise
- Rash

SIGNS
- Posterior oropharyngeal and palatal erythema, petechiae, or enanthem
- Symmetric oropharynx
- Fever
- Lymphadenopathy
- Tonsillar exudates may be present.
- Rhinorrhea

WORKUP
It is not possible to identify reliably the causative organism in infectious pharyngitis on the basis of history and physical examination. For example, the presence or absence of exudates is neither sensitive nor specific in differentiating bacterial from viral etiologies. Nevertheless, an adequate history and physical remain the most useful tools in evaluating the patient with a sore throat. History and physical identify the patients who need additional diagnostic testing or specific treatment, and in many cases no testing is required. In selected cases the following adjuncts may help establish a specific diagnosis:

- Rapid antigen screen for GABHS
- Throat culture
- Monospot (for suspected infectious mononucleosis)

COMMENTS AND TREATMENT CONSIDERATIONS
Most cases of pharyngitis, whether viral or bacterial, are self-limited and require no specific therapy. Despite this, more than 75% of adults and children with pharyngitis are treated with antibiotics. The true number of patients who should be treated is less than 20%; thus, in most instances antibiotics are inappropriately prescribed, contributing to antibiotic resistance. Taking time to explain why antibiotics are not needed, providing symptomatic relief, and identifying the minority of cases that require antibiotics or have more serious illnesses is the goal of the ED evaluation. Patients may be treated symptomatically with antipyretics. Analgesia, including the use of acetaminophen, ibuprofen, narcotic analgesia, and possibly topical anesthetics, is appropriate for patients with significant pain. Adjunctive use of steroids has been shown to hasten symptom relief, but probably only in the subgroup of patients with GABHS and only in those treated early

CHAPTER 35

in the course of illness (within the first 72 hours of symptom onset). There are two important caveats when considering the diagnosis of pharyngitis: (1) an asymmetric oropharynx is always abnormal; it may represent a peritonsillar abscess (see later) or another process and should be investigated further; and (2) patients who have severe symptoms and a relatively normal oropharyngeal examination may have a more serious disease process.

REFERENCES
Bisno AL: Acute pharyngitis, *N Engl J Med* 344:205, 2001.

Huovinen P, Lahtonen R, Ziegler T, et al: Pharyngitis in adults: the presence and coexistence of viruses and bacterial organisms, *Ann Intern Med* 110:612, 1989.

Little P, Williamson I: Sore throat management in general practice, *Fam Pract* 13:317, 1996.

 GROUP A BETA-HEMOLYTIC STREPTOCOCCAL PHARYNGITIS

GABHS is predominantly a disease of children aged 5 to 15 years, with a prevalence of about 30% in pediatric pharyngitis but only 5% to 15% in adult pharyngitis. The rate of carriage is also high in the pediatric population (15%), complicating the interpretation of diagnostic tests.

SIGNS
- Rapid-onset sore throat
- Odynophagia and dysphagia
- Fever
- Headache (predominantly in children [40%])
- Abdominal pain (predominantly in children)
- Nausea and vomiting (predominantly in children)
- No cough and/or rhinorrhea
- History of streptococcal exposure
- Highest incidence in winter months

SYMPTOMS
- Posterior oropharynx and tonsillar erythema (overall 95%, adults 90%)
- Tonsillopharyngeal exudates (70% to 75%)
- Petechiae on soft palate (children up to 40%, adults 9%)
- Uvular erythema
- Tender anterior cervical lymphadenopathy (70%)
- Fever (adults 30%)
- Scarlatiniform rash (predominantly in young children)

WORKUP

- The Centor clinical scoring system can be used in adults to determine which patients should be treated with antibiotics. The four Centor criteria for streptococcal pharyngitis (+++) are fever, anterior cervical lymphadenopathy, tonsillar exudates, and absence of cough. Adults meeting three or four of the Centor criteria have a high enough probability of a GABHS infection to warrant empirical therapy. Adults meeting at least two Centor criteria should undergo rapid antigen testing for GABHS. In children, a clinical scoring system alone is not sufficiently sensitive or specific to guide therapy but can be used to help select those who should be screened further with a rapid antigen test.
- ASO titers are not useful in guiding acute care.
- Use of throat culture is controversial because of problems with sensitivity and specificity and the difference between surface and core bacteria. Cultures take 2 to 3 days to return, and there are both false positives and false negatives.
- Rapid antigen screens, particularly the optical immunoassay, are generally considered sufficiently sensitive and specific to guide treatment decisions. Some experts, however, recommend a culture in children with a negative rapid antigen test.

COMMENTS AND TREATMENT CONSIDERATIONS

In the immunocompetent patient, without a past history of rheumatic fever or valvular heart disease, strategies that treat symptomatically and minimize the use of antibiotics are prudent. A case can be made for not treating any adult with antibiotics because the incidence of complications is much lower in adults. The most compelling reason to treat is to decrease the rate of acute rheumatic fever, a rare complication associated with specific strains of GABHS. Antibiotics may also slightly decrease the incidence of peritonsillar abscess (PTA), but in most studies patients with PTA present with the abscess on their first visit to the physician or have already been treated with antistreptococcal antibiotics. Antibiotics have no effect on the incidence of poststreptococcal glomerulonephritis.

Antibiotics are commonly administered with the goal of decreasing the duration of illness and infectivity. Antibiotics are only marginally effective in this capacity, hastening relief of symptoms by 12 to 24 hours if instituted within the first 48 to 72 hours of illness. In most patients, GABHS pharyngitis is a self-limited (~7 day) illness. Treatment of GABHS pharyngitis should be with a narrow-spectrum antibiotic, such as a 10-day course of oral penicillin V. Cephalexin is a reasonable alternative, and erythromycin is appropriate for penicillin-allergic patients. A single dose of intramuscular penicillin G benzathine or penicillin G benzathine combined with penicillin G procaine is an acceptable alternative in patients who may have trouble completing a full oral course.

REFERENCES

Centor RM, Witherspoon JM, Dalton HP, et al: The diagnosis of strep throat in adults in the emergency room, *Med Decis Making* 1:239, 1981.

Cooper RJ, Hoffman JR, Bartlett JG, et al: Principles of appropriate antibiotic use for acute pharyngitis in adults: background, *Ann Intern Med* 134:509, 2001.

Del Mar CB, Glasziou PP, Spinks AB: Antibiotics for sore throat, *Cochrane Database Syst Rev* 2004, issue 2, Art. No. CD000023. DOI: 10.1002/14651858.CD000023.pub2.

 PERITONSILLAR ABSCESS

Peritonsillar abscess is the most common deep space infection of the head and neck. It is a collection of pus between the tonsillar capsule, superior constrictor muscles, and the palatopharyngeal muscle. It is rare in young children (<6 years of age) and in the elderly. Infections are usually polymicrobial or anaerobic.

SYMPTOMS
- Progressive worsening of sore throat ++++
- Trismus +++
- Odynophagia ++++
- Dysphagia ++
- Dehydration ++
- Drooling ++++
- Voice change ++++

SIGNS
- Contralateral uvular deviation and inferomedial displacement of the tonsil ++++
- Unilateral fluctuance and peritonsillar edema ++++
- Exudative pharyngitis +++
- Cervical lymphadenopathy +++
- Fever +++
- Muffled voice +++
- Trismus ++++

WORKUP
The diagnosis of peritonsillar abscess is suspected from an asymmetric oropharynx examination and is confirmed with needle aspiration of pus. Intraoral ultrasound and CT scans of the neck can confirm

abscess, but imaging studies are generally not necessary because the diagnosis can usually be made clinically. Laboratory tests (WBC and blood cultures) do not influence management.

COMMENTS AND TREATMENT CONSIDERATIONS
Needle aspiration of the abscess is both diagnostic and therapeutic and has been shown to be as effective as incision and drainage. Drainage and oral antibiotics are effective in >80% of cases. If there is minimal fluctuance or no pus is aspirated, peritonsillar cellulitis is likely, and the patient can be treated with antibiotics alone. Penicillin has long been the drug of choice, but clindamycin or a cephalosporin may be superior. Complications of peritonsillar abscess include airway obstruction and extension into other deep spaces of the neck leading to sepsis. Consider imaging to exclude lateral extension into the parapharyngeal space if symptoms do not improve after drainage.

REFERENCES
Kieff DA, Bhattacharyya N, Siegel NS, Salman SD: Selection of antibiotics after incision and drainage of peritonsillar abscesses, *Otolaryngol Head Neck Surg* 120:57, 1999.

Spires JR, Owens JJ, Woodson GE, Miller RH: Treatment of peritonsillar abscess. A prospective study of aspiration versus incision and drainage, *Arch Otolaryngol Head Neck Surg* 113:984, 1987.

CHAPTER 35

SPECIFIC VIRAL INFECTIONS

HAND, FOOT, AND MOUTH DISEASE

This viral infection occurs most commonly in young children and is characterized by intraoral, hand, and foot lesions. Many patients have only oral lesions. Additional skin lesions on the buttock are common. In addition to the rash, common signs and symptoms include fever, sore throat, mild generalized lymphadenopathy, and malaise. Disease in adults and household outbreaks are not uncommon. The disease is more prevalent in the summer months. Following an incubation period, patients typically develop fever, followed in 2 or 3 days by oral lesions and other symptoms. The enanthem and rash typically appear over 1 to 2 days. The enanthem is characterized by small vesicles, usually on the posterior oropharynx and tongue, that become ulcerative. The lips and gingiva are usually spared. Hand and foot lesions occur on both the dorsal surfaces and the palms and soles. Initially erythematous, they progress into grayish papules and then vesicles. Buttock lesions are typically maculopapular. Lesions may be tender.

473

Coxsackievirus (types A and B) is the major cause of this syndrome, but cases due to *Enterovirus* also occur. The diagnosis is based on history and physical. This is a benign, self-limited illness. There is no specific therapy, but antipyretics and analgesics are often indicated for symptomatic relief

 ## HERPES SIMPLEX VIRUS 1 (STOMATITIS, GINGIVITIS, AND PHARYNGITIS)

Herpes simplex virus type 1 can infect multiple body sites, but the infection is most commonly oral and perioral. Primary infection may be asymptomatic or in children can present as herpes gingivostomatitis. Clinical appearance includes the rapid onset of multiple vesicular lesions on erythematous bases, usually on the gingiva and lips. Lesions are multiple and the gums may appear swollen. The symptomatic infections with multiple lesions may produce dehydration because of pain-related decrease in oral intake. Treating the pain and encouraging continued oral intake are important. Oral acyclovir started within the first 72 hours decreases the duration of symptoms by approximately 50%.

 ## ACUTE HUMAN IMMUNODEFICIENCY VIRUS TYPE 1 SEROCONVERSION

Up to 50% of patients with acute HIV infection develop a mononucleosis-like illness. Sore throat is often a prominent feature, along with fever, lymphadenopathy, rash, and myalgias. Elicit HIV risk factors and refer patients at risk for follow-up.

See Chapter 19, HIV/AIDS Patient, Approach to the.

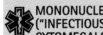 ## MONONUCLEOSIS–EPSTEIN BARR VIRUS ("INFECTIOUS MONONUCLEOSIS") AND CYTOMEGALOVIRUS

Mononucleosis is seen most commonly in the 15- to 30-year-old age group and is characterized by sore throat, lymphadenopathy (particularly posterior cervical), fever, malaise, and tonsillar exudates. Hepatosplenomegaly may occur. Therapy is supportive. Contact sports should be avoided for up to 2 months because of the possibility of splenic rupture following minimal trauma.

SPECIFIC BACTERIAL INFECTIONS

 ### *NEISSERIA GONORRHOEAE*

Gonococcal pharyngitis is a sexually transmitted disease that can occur in the absence of genital symptoms. It is more common in

adolescents and young adults. The presentation and severity of illness can vary. Patients complain of sore throat, and exudates are present in 20% of cases and fever and lymphadenopathy in about 10% of cases. Although an infrequent cause of pharyngitis, it should be considered in patients with potential exposure. The most common risk factor is oral sexual contact. Diagnosis can be made with throat swab, but the culture requires a chocolate agar medium. It is important to identify gonococcal pharyngitis because it can lead to gonococcemia. In uncomplicated cases a single dose of ceftriaxone IM is adequate therapy. A single dose of azithromycin or 1-week course of doxycycline should be considered to treat chlamydial infection, which is frequently coexistent.

 ### *CHLAMYDIA PNEUMONIAE* AND *MYCOPLASMA PNEUMONIAE*

Although sore throat may be a common symptom with these bacterial infections, there is no evidence that therapy for isolated pharyngitis (i.e., in the absence of lower respiratory tract disease) is of any benefit.

 ### *CORYNEBACTERIUM DIPHTHERIAE*

Because of immunization, diphtheria pharyngitis is a rare cause of illness in the United States and industrialized countries. Most cases occur in nonimmunized and underimmunized individuals, more commonly among lower socioeconomic classes. *C. diphtheriae* may cause cutaneous infections, but the pharyngeal infections, which can lead to airway compromise, are most concerning. Symptoms include fever, sore throat, dysphagia, and cough as well as cardiac and neurologic symptoms related to the exotoxin. Classic signs are gray to black exudates referred to as a pseudomembrane on the posterior oropharynx, tonsils, and palate and neurologic deficits including bulbar findings. Throat culture is diagnostic but requires a special medium (tellurite selective medium or Loeffler's medium). Therapy with antitoxin administration and erythromycin should be instituted before culture results are known if diphtheria is suspected. Because of the risk of airway compromise, patients in whom diphtheria is suspected should be admitted for observation.

OTHERS CAUSES

 ### KAWASAKI DISEASE

See Chapter 30, Rash.

GASTROESOPHAGEAL REFLUX DISEASE

Gastroesophageal reflux disease (GERD) is a common cause of sore throat, particularly chronic or recurrent sore throat and hoarse voice in adults in the absence of signs of infection. Upper airway and pulmonary symptoms are common, and up to 25% of patients have only head and neck symptoms without typical "heartburn" symptoms.

SYMPTOMS
- Sore throat or burning
- "Lump in the throat" sensation
- Hoarseness
- Odynophagia
- Dysphagia
- Chronic cough
- Symptoms may be worse in the morning or awaken the patient at night.
- Acid taste in mouth and substernal to epigastric burning pain (heartburn)
- In young children and infants, vomiting, apnea, and failure to thrive

SIGNS (PERTINENT TO THE OROPHARYNX)
- Posterior oropharynx erythema
- Posterior oropharynx "cobblestoning"
- Laryngeal mucosal erythema and edema

WORKUP
The history and physical examination are usually sufficient to make a tentative diagnosis of GERD. Often patients with sore throat related to GERD have a relatively benign-appearing oropharynx and hypopharynx. Direct visualization of the larynx can help make the diagnosis. The "gold standard" in diagnostic testing is a 24-hour pH probe.

COMMENTS AND TREATMENT CONSIDERATIONS
Therapy for GERD includes medication and lifestyle changes. Antacids, H2 blockers, and proton pump inhibitors provide symptomatic relief. Lifestyle modification including decreased use of caffeine, alcohol, and tobacco; avoiding meals 2 hours before sleeping; and sleeping more upright (using a wedge pillow or multiple pillows) can help decrease symptoms.

ALLERGIC PHARYNGITIS

Rhinosinusitis, allergic rhinitis, and associated postnasal drip can be a source of chronic sore throat. The history and physical examination, including the classic cobblestone appearance of the throat, should be sufficient to make the diagnosis and begin appropriate antiallergy therapy. Follow-up to assess resolution of symptoms is important in all patients with chronic sore throat to ensure that cancer is not the cause of symptoms.

 EPIGLOTTITIS

Epiglottitis is a rapidly progressive cellulitis of the epiglottis and the surrounding tissues, which can rapidly lead to airway obstruction and death. Historically, this was a disease caused by *Haemophilus influenzae* type b that primarily affected children. Over the past 15 years, widespread administration of the *H. influenzae* serotype b (Hib) vaccine has dramatically changed the microbiology of this disease and decreased the number of cases in children. Most cases now occur in adults, especially in patients with AIDS. Nonetheless, there are vaccination failures and underimmunized children still at risk. The presentation of this illness in adults is different from that in young children because of the relatively larger, more rigid trachea and less lymphoid tissue. Epiglottis has also been described from scalds and chemical ingestions.

CHAPTER 35

SYMPTOMS
INFANTS AND TODDLERS
- Dyspnea ++++
- Fever +++++
- Cough +++
- Dysphagia ++
- Sore throat +++
- Change in voice ++

ADULTS AND OLDER CHILDREN
- Dyspnea ++
- Fever ++
- Cough ++
- Change in voice +++
- Sore throat ++++
- Dysphagia and odynophagia ++++

SIGNS

INFANTS AND TODDLERS

- Fever +++++
- Stridor ++++
- Cervical lymphadenopathy +++
- Drooling +++
- Muffled voice ++++
- Neck tenderness +++
- Irritable +++
- Sitting with neck hyperextended or tripod position
- Barky or croupy cough

ADULTS AND OLDER CHILDREN

- Fever +++
- Stridor +++
- Respiratory distress +++
- Cervical lymphadenopathy +++
- Muffled voice ++++
- Tenderness of anterior neck ++++
- Sitting erect ++
- Drooling ++

WORKUP

INFANTS AND TODDLERS

- Patients with a classic presentation for epiglottis should be transferred to the operating room to undergo laryngoscopy and intubation. Epiglottitis is a rapidly progressive disease and airway protection is of paramount importance. Protocols for the rapid management of epiglottitis in the operating room have significantly decreased mortality. Intravenous catheter placement and other interventions that may agitate the child should be avoided.
- Patients presenting less severely ill, especially those in whom other diagnoses are a strong possibility, can be safely examined in the ED.
- Lateral neck radiograph ++++ may show "thumb sign." However, if the diagnosis is suspected clinically, one should not delay definitive visualization in the operating room for radiographs, and one should not exclude the diagnosis if clinically suspected if the radiograph appears normal.
- Indirect and direct laryngoscopy ++++ showing a cherry red epiglottis confirms the diagnosis.
- After the airway is secure, blood cultures and epiglottis cultures should be obtained.

ADULTS AND OLDER CHILDREN

- Workup is based on the severity of illness. Adults and older children typically have a less fulminant course than toddlers.

- Unstable patients need to have their airway secured; usually this is accomplished by direct laryngoscopy and intubation, with cricothyroidotomy as a backup.
- Lateral neck radiographs +++ are less sensitive in the adult.
- Indirect and direct laryngoscopy ++++ can confirm the diagnosis.

COMMENTS AND TREATMENT CONSIDERATIONS

Consider epiglottitis in all patients with sudden-onset severe sore throat, particularly if the oropharyngeal examination does not explain the severity of symptoms. The majority of patients who decompensate do so within the first 12 hours of presentation. Many case reports have described adverse events while patients were in radiology or in transport. If airway compromise is a possibility, it is of utmost importance to secure the airway first.

Currently, a variety of pathogens are implicated in acute infectious epiglottis including group A beta-hemolytic streptococcus, *Staphylococcus aureus*, and *Streptococcus pneumoniae*. These bacteria are generally less virulent than *Haemophilus influenza* type b, and as a result the disease severity has diminished when compared with the pre-Hib vaccine era. Appropriate empirical antibiotic therapy is a third-generation cephalosporin, with the addition of vancomycin in areas that have a high rate of methicillin-resistant *Staphylococcus aureus* (MRSA).

CHAPTER 35

REFERENCES

Frantz TD, Rasgon BM, Quesenberry CP Jr: Acute epiglottitis in adults. Analysis of 129 cases, *JAMA* 272:1358, 1994.

Gorelick MH, Baker MD: Epiglottitis in children, 1979-1992: effects of *Haemophilus influenzae* type b immunization, *Arch Pediatr Adolesc Med* 148:47, 1994.

Mayo-Smith MF, Spinale JW, Donskey CJ, et al: Acute epiglottitis. An 18-year experience in Rhode Island, *Chest* 108:1640, 1995.

Shah RK, Roberson DW, Jones DT: Epiglottitis in the *Haemophilus influenzae* type B vaccine era: changing trends, *Laryngoscope* 114:557, 2004.

 RETROPHARYNGEAL ABSCESS AND CELLULITIS

Most retropharyngeal abscesses occur in children ages 6 months to 6 years, probably as a result of the rupture of a suppurative retropharyngeal lymph node. This predilection for young children is probably related to the abundance of lymph tissue that atrophies as children age. In older patients, the infection usually starts with a direct inoculum from trauma or contiguous spread from local infections. Retropharyngeal abscesses are very serious infections because of their ability to spread rapidly to the mediastinum. Retropharyngeal abscess should be considered in any patient with a sore throat, fever, and limited neck mobility. Symptoms disproportionate to the physical examination findings should also raise the suspicion of a deep space infection. A recent upper respiratory tract infection is usually seen in infants, whereas oropharyngeal trauma or poor dentition is more common in older patients. Infants often present with poor feeding; older patients report pain.

SYMPTOMS
INFANTS AND TODDLERS
- Fever ++++
- Neck posturing or stiffness +++
- Sore throat +++
- Decreased oral intake +++
- Neck swelling +++
- Drooling

OLDER CHILDREN AND ADULTS
- Fever ++++
- Sore throat ++++
- Difficulty swallowing (odynophagia and dysphagia) +++
- Neck pain +++

SIGNS
INFANTS AND TODDLERS
- Neck mass +++
- Cervical lymphadenopathy +++
- Limited neck mobility +++
- Stridor +++
- Drooling ++
- Irritability ++
- Asymmetric bulge in the posterior pharynx ++
- Torticollis ++

ADULTS AND OLDER CHILDREN
- Neck mass +++
- Cervical lymphadenopathy +++
- Limited neck mobility +++
- Stridor +
- Asymmetric bulge in posterior pharynx ++

WORKUP

A constellation of symptoms suggests the diagnosis of a retropharyngeal abscess. Imaging is required for confirmation.

- Soft tissue lateral radiograph of neck ++++ (note prevertebral soft tissues; abnormal width >7 mm at C2 in all patients, >14 mm at C6 in children, and >22 mm at C6 in adults)
- CT scan of neck with IV contrast ++++ (this may differentiate an abscess from cellulitis)
- MRI with gadolinium ++++
- Ultrasound may be useful to differentiate abscess from cellulitis.
- Chest radiograph to evaluate for mediastinal involvement
- Blood cultures and cultures from abscess
- Palpation of pharynx is not recommended.

COMMENTS AND TREATMENT CONSIDERATIONS

Patients in respiratory distress must be promptly intubated. Empirical antibiotic therapy covering the typical causative organisms (*Streptococcus*, *Staphylococcus*, anaerobes, and gram negatives) such as ampicillin/sulbactam, clindamycin, or a third-generation cephalosporin with metronidazole must be initiated promptly. Older diabetic patients are susceptible to *Klebsiella* infections. Head and neck surgery needs to be consulted early for operative drainage of the abscess. Patients with mediastinal involvement also need thoracic surgery consultation. Patients with cellulitis or phlegmon without discrete abscess may be treated with intravenous antibiotics and in-hospital observation.

REFERENCES

Brook I: Microbiology and management of peritonsillar, retropharyngeal, and parapharyngeal abscesses, *J Oral Maxillofac Surg* 62:1545, 2004.

Gaglani MJ, Edwards MS: Clinical indicators of childhood retropharyngeal abscess, *Am J Emerg Med* 13:333, 1995.

Lee SS, Schwartz RH, Bahadori RS: Retropharyngeal abscess: Epiglottitis of the new millennium, *J Pediatr* 138:435, 2001.

Tannebaum RD: Adult retropharyngeal abscess: a case report and review of the literature, *J Emerg Med* 14:147, 1996.

 PARAPHARYNGEAL ABSCESS

The parapharyngeal space is located in the lateral aspect of the upper neck. Parapharyngeal abscesses are rare serious infections that arise from odontogenic infections, peritonsillar abscess, or various other infections in the neck. Parapharyngeal space infections can spread rapidly into the surrounding structures of the neck and the retropharyngeal space and can lead to airway obstruction, mediastinitis, and overwhelming sepsis.

SYMPTOMS
- Fever +++
- Pain and swelling of the neck ++++
- Sore throat +++
- Torticollis ++
- Odynophagia

SIGNS
- Palpable mass below angle of mandible ++++
- Trismus ++
- Medial displacement of tonsil ++
- Medial bulging of pharyngeal wall ++
- Swelling of upper neck +++

WORKUP
The diagnosis of a parapharyngeal abscess is suggested by the clinical findings and confirmed radiographically. Symptoms disproportionate to physical examination findings should prompt further evaluation.
- CT scan of the neck ++++
- MR angiography ++++ to assess for vascular involvement

COMMENTS AND TREATMENT CONSIDERATIONS
Infections involving the deep spaces of the neck quickly spread through facial planes. The airway must be secured, antibiotics administered, and otolaryngology consultation obtained promptly for surgical drainage. Appropriate antibiotic regimens are similar to those for retropharyngeal abscess: ampicillin/sulbactam, clindamycin, or a third-generation cephalosporin with metronidazole.

REFERENCES
Sethi DS, Stanley RE: Parapharyngeal abscesses, *J Laryngol Otol* 105:1025, 1991.

 OROPHARYNGEAL OR LARYNGEAL TUMOR

Sore throat or hoarseness that persists for more than 3 weeks, particularly without signs of infection, should be referred to an otolaryngologist for a complete examination to rule out malignancy or other serious cases.

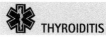
THYROIDITIS

Thyroiditis can cause anterior neck pain; see Chapter 29, Palpitations and Tachycardia.

CHAPTER 35

Syncope and Near-Syncope
Richelle J. Cooper and Eric A. Savitsky

Syncope is defined as an acute, transient loss of consciousness with loss of postural tone and accounts for approximately 1% to 3% of all ED visits and 6% of hospital admission. Near-syncope should be approached in a similar fashion to syncope, as both entities share similar etiologies. The differential diagnosis is broad, and although the etiology is benign for the majority of patients experiencing syncope, in a small percentage of patients the cause is life threatening. In addition, even benign causes for syncope can lead to falls and significant injury, particularly in the elderly. In the ED evaluation of the patient with syncope, the primary goal is to distinguish patients at low risk who can safely be discharged from those who are at increased risk and should be hospitalized. For evaluation, management, and prognosis, it is useful to divide syncope into one of two etiologic categories: cardiogenic and noncardiogenic. One-year mortality for cardiogenic syncope is 18% to 35% if untreated, as opposed to 6% for noncardiogenic syncope.

Approximately 50% of cases of syncope have an identifiable cause. The history and physical examination obtained in the ED are the most useful diagnostic tools. Nevertheless, specific diagnostic studies selected on the basis of the history and physical increase diagnostic yield. The cause is determined in only a small minority of patients in whom the ED workup is inconclusive. Recent investigations have attempted to create clinical prediction rules that could be used to identify a cohort of patients who are at such low risk that they can be discharged for outpatient evaluation. To date, however, there are no sufficiently validated prediction rules to use in practice. Until further research provides more definitive guidance, it is prudent to consider admission for any patient at risk for cardiac syncope who lacks a clearly identified, benign etiology for syncope.

Seizures are also characterized by transient loss of consciousness. In practice, distinguishing between an unwitnessed seizure and syncope may be difficult. Certain features of the history and physical examination, such as a preceding aura, postictal period, or neurologic abnormality, make a diagnosis of seizure more likely. When a clear differentiation between a syncopal event and a seizure is not possible, patients are often hospitalized and evaluated for both conditions.

See Chapter 32, Seizure, Adult and Chapter 33, Seizure, Pediatric.

CARDIOGENIC SYNCOPE

Important categories of cardiogenic syncope include arrhythmias, left ventricular outflow obstruction, right ventricular compromise, and pump failure (Fig. 36–1). Suspected or known cardiac disease is the strongest predictor of cardiogenic syncope, and thus patients with unexplained syncope in whom cardiac disease is a concern should be admitted to a telemetry unit for further evaluation.

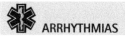 **ARRHYTHMIAS**

Arrhythmias are a frequent cause of cardiogenic syncope and may predispose patients to recurrent syncope or sudden death. Tachyarrhythmias capable of inducing syncope include sustained

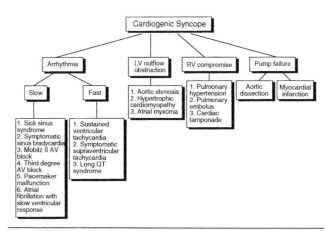

Fig. 36–1 Categories of cardiogenic syncope.

ventricular tachycardias and rapid supraventricular tachycardias. Bradyarrhythmias associated with syncope include sick sinus syndrome, sinus pause >3 seconds, sinus bradycardia <40 bpm, Mobitz II AV block, third-degree AV block, pacemaker malfunction, and atrial fibrillation with a slow ventricular response.

See Chapter 29, Palpitations and Tachycardia.

SYMPTOMS AND SIGNS
Vary depending on the rhythm. Syncope may occur while sitting or supine or may be associated with exertion. Patients may report weakness, fatigue, palpitations, chest discomfort, or dyspnea.

WORKUP
- Initial monitoring yields a diagnosis in 2% to 11% of patients.
- In preselected populations, 24-hour monitoring diagnoses an arrhythmia in 14% of patients. Cardiac event and external loop recorders are twice as likely to produce diagnostic rhythm strips as continuous 48-hour monitoring. In selected cases, monitoring with an implantable loop recorder has been shown to be valuable in diagnosis, cost effective, and safe.
- Electrophysiologic studies are warranted in only a small percentage of patients.

COMMENTS AND TREATMENT CONSIDERATIONS
Patients with a history of prolonged QT interval or Brugada syndrome should be considered at high risk for cardiogenic syncope and evaluated accordingly. In a study of patients with syncope and a history of pacemaker use, only 6.5% of the time was pacemaker malfunction the cause of syncope. Patients with pacemakers have underlying cardiac disease and should also be admitted for evaluation of cardiogenic syncope.

REFERENCES
Benditt DG, Ermis C, Pham S, et al: Implantable diagnostic monitoring devices for evaluation of syncope, and tachy- and brady-arrhythmias, *J Interv Card Electrophysiol* 9:137, 2003.

Farwell DJ, Freemantle N, Sulke AN: Use of implantable loop recorders in the diagnosis and management of syncope, *Eur Heart J* 25:1257, 2004.

Gibson TC, Heitzman MR: Diagnostic efficacy of 24-hour electrocardiographic monitoring for syncope, *Am J Cardiol* 53:1013, 1984.

Kinlay S, Leitch JW, Neil A, et al: Cardiac event recorders yield more diagnoses and are more cost-effective than 48-hour Holter monitoring in patients with palpitations: a controlled clinical trial, *Ann Intern Med* 124:16, 1996.

MYOCARDIAL INFARCTION

COMMENTS AND TREATMENT CONSIDERATIONS

Syncope is a presenting complaint in a small minority of all myocardial infarctions but becomes more common in the elderly. In patients older than 85, dyspnea is the most common complaint during myocardial infarction, followed by chest pain, syncope, stroke, or altered mental status. Patients with acute coronary syndromes who present with syncope or symptoms other than chest pain are more likely to be misdiagnosed and therefore experience increased morbidity.

See Chapter 7, Chest Pain.

REFERENCES

Bayer AJ, Chadha JS, Farag RR, et al: Changing presentation of myocardial infarction with increasing old age, *J Am Geriatr Soc* 34:263, 1986.

Bosker G: Assessment and triage of elderly patients with acute coronary ischemia, *Emerg Med Rep* 9:25, 1988.

Brady WJ: Missing the diagnosis of acute MI: challenging presentations, electrocardiographic pearls, and outcome-effective management strategies, *Emerg Med Rep* 18:91, 1997.

AORTIC DISSECTION

Syncope occurs in about 5% to 10% of cases of aortic dissection and may indicate aortic rupture or cardiac tamponade. Isolated syncope without other symptoms and signs suggestive of aortic dissection is rare.

See Chapter 7, Chest Pain.

REFERENCES

Rigolin VH, Harrison JK, Wilson JS, et al: Update on aortic dissection, *Emerg Med Rep* 17:35, 1993.

Slater EE, DeSanctis RW: The clinical recognition of dissecting aortic aneurysm, *Am J Med* 60:625, 1976.

Spittell PC, Spittell JA, Joyce JW, et al: Clinical features and differential diagnosis of aortic dissection: experience with 236 cases (1980 through 1990), *Mayo Clin Proc* 68:642, 1993.

CHAPTER 36

PULMONARY EMBOLUS

Syncope occurs in up to 10% of patients with pulmonary embolus. In these patients syncope is usually a sign of massive pulmonary embolus, with commonly more than 50% of the pulmonary circulation obstructed. Patients typically have marked acute right ventricular overload and have symptoms such as shortness of breath, chest pain, and signs of cardiovascular collapse. Two-dimensional echocardiography may be diagnostically useful in these patients.

See Chapter 7, Chest Pain.

 AORTIC STENOSIS

Syncope in the presence of aortic stenosis (AS) indicates advanced disease and unless the AS is corrected portends a poor prognosis. Mean survival after the onset of angina is 5 years, after the onset of syncope 3 years, and after congestive heart failure (CHF) symptoms 2 years. Symptoms typically develop when the valve area is less than 1 to 1.5 cm^2 and valve gradients exceed 50 mm Hg. The incidence of sudden death is high after the onset of symptoms.

SYMPTOMS
- Angina
- Dyspnea
- Orthopnea
- Peripheral edema
- Syncope
- Symptoms are often exertional.

SIGNS
- Cardiac auscultation: normal S1, soft A2 or single S2, loud S4, and a harsh crescendo-decrescendo systolic murmur at the right upper sternal border radiating to the carotids. Loudness of the murmur may diminish and length may increase as the stenosis becomes more severe.
- Classic delayed and diminished carotid upstrokes are often not present in the elderly because of the inelasticity of the vascular system in this population.
- Narrow pulse pressure may be noted.

WORKUP
- ECG commonly shows evidence of left ventricular hypertrophy and possibly left atrial enlargement.

- Echocardiography is a rapid diagnostic test that can demonstrate abnormal valve function and estimate gradients across the valve.
- Chest x-rays are nondiagnostic. A calcified aortic valve is often seen in the elderly but often indicates benign aortic sclerosis.
- Cardiac catheterization is the "gold standard" for determining the degree of stenosis and valve area.

COMMENTS AND TREATMENT CONSIDERATIONS
Any patient with a suspected AS–related syncope should be hospitalized pending a cardiology evaluation. Caution should be taken when treating angina or symptoms of CHF because overdiuresis or nitrate-induced preload reduction may lead to dramatic and potentially irreversible hypotension.

REFERENCES
Freeman RV, Crittenden G, Otto C: Acquired aortic stenosis, *Expert Rev Cardiovasc Ther* 2:107, 2004.

Wilson JS, Hearne SE, Harrison JK, et al: How to recognize—and manage—aortic stenosis in the elderly, *J Crit Illness* 9:42, 1994.

CHAPTER 36

 HYPERTROPHIC CARDIOMYOPATHY

Hypertrophic cardiomyopathy is a condition characterized by a hypertrophied, nondilated left ventricle. It is the most common cause of sudden death in young athletes.

SYMPTOMS
- Dyspnea +++
- Angina +++
- Syncope ++
- Symptoms are typically exertional.

SIGNS
- Cardiac auscultation: mimics aortic stenosis with normal S1, normal S2, and dynamic crescendo-decrescendo, harsh systolic murmur that is heard best between the apex and left sternal border. The murmur is classically accentuated with decreased preload (standing or Valsalva) and is softer with increased preload (squatting).
- Carotid upstrokes are brisk, unlike those in aortic stenosis.

WORKUP
- ECG may show evidence of left ventricular hypertrophy. Q waves in the precordial leads +++ represent depolarization of the hypertrophied myocardial septum.
- Chest x-rays demonstrate cardiomegaly +++.

- Two-dimensional echocardiography: definitive, demonstrating a thickened ventricular wall with hyperdynamic ejection and abnormal relaxation phase.
- Holter monitoring frequently detects arrhythmias, most often ventricular +++.
- Stress testing may be valuable because of the exertional nature of symptoms.

COMMENTS AND TREATMENT CONSIDERATIONS

The etiology of hypertrophic cardiomyopathy–related syncope is multifactorial, and it may be associated with outflow obstruction, arrhythmia, or ischemia. Inherited and sporadic forms of this disease exist. This diagnosis is often not considered in the elderly; however, one third of cases occur in patients older than 60 years.

REFERENCES

Baughman KL: Hypertrophic cardiomyopathy, *JAMA* 267:846, 1992.
Germann CA, Perron AD: Sudden cardiac death in athletes: a guide for emergency physicians, *Am J Emerg Med* 23:504, 2005.
Spirito P, Seidman CE, McKenna WJ, et al: The management of hypertrophic cardiomyopathy, *N Engl J Med* 336:775, 1997.

 PULMONARY HYPERTENSION

Primary pulmonary hypertension occurs in familial and sporadic forms and has been linked to the use of certain diet pills. Secondary pulmonary hypertension occurs as a result of many disorders including COPD, chronic hypoventilation, sleep apnea, left ventricle dysfunction, mitral stenosis, small multiple pulmonary emboli, and congenital cardiac shunts. The majority (65% to 80%) of cases of primary pulmonary hypertension occur in women. Symptoms are often present for 1 to 3 years before diagnosis.

SYMPTOMS

- Dyspnea +++ is the most common presenting symptom and occurs in all patients as the disease progresses.
- Syncope or near-syncope +++, particularly with exertion
- Fatigue ++
- Chest pain ++
- Raynaud's phenomenon +

SIGNS

- Cardiac auscultation: loud P2; may have a systolic ejection murmur, S3 or S4
- Signs of right ventricular failure (late)

WORKUP

- Electrocardiography often shows evidence of right ventricular hypertrophy.
- Chest x-rays may demonstrate right ventricular hypertrophy and often reveal enlarged central pulmonary arteries.
- Echocardiography helps to rule out valvular and congenital cardiac lesions as well as provide an estimate of pulmonary artery systolic pressure.
- Right heart catheterization is diagnostic for pulmonary hypertension.

COMMENTS AND TREATMENT CONSIDERATIONS

Patients with pulmonary hypertension and right ventricular dysfunction are at increased risk for pulmonary thromboembolic events, which may also cause syncope. Standard treatment includes anticoagulant therapy with warfarin (Coumadin) and furosemide for fluid retention caused by right-sided heart failure. Advances in vasodilator therapy, including the use of bosentan and sildenafil, have been shown to relieve symptoms and prolong life.

REFERENCES

Hughes JD, Rubin JL: Primary pulmonary hypertension: an analysis of 28 cases and a review of the literature, *Medicine (Baltimore)* 65:56, 1986.

Humbert M, Sitbon O, Simonneau G: Treatment of pulmonary arterial hypertension, *N Engl J Med* 351:1425, 2004.

Rubin JL: Primary pulmonary hypertension, *N Engl J Med* 336:111, 1997.

 CARDIAC TAMPONADE

See Chapter 7, Chest Pain.

NONCARDIOGENIC SYNCOPE

Noncardiogenic syncope can be subdivided into several categories (Fig. 36–2).

 NEUROCARDIOGENIC (VASOVAGAL) SYNCOPE

SYMPTOMS

- A history of previous similar episodes.
- An identifiable triggering event, including pain, emotional stress, or anxiety related to "fight-or-flight" situation.

CHAPTER **36**

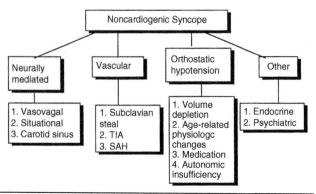

Fig. 36–2   Categories of noncardiogenic syncope.

- Presyncopal or prodromal phase lasting a few seconds to a few minutes is often reported.
- Symptoms during the prodrome include a sense of lightheadedness +++, diaphoresis ++, headache or visual changes ++, epigastric discomfort, nausea, and vomiting ++.

SIGNS
- Normal physical examination is most often noted.
- Decreased heart rate and low blood pressure are noted if the patient is still symptomatic.

WORKUP
- Complete history and physical examination to rule out life-threatening causes of syncope.
- Head-upright, tilt-table testing is advocated by some to confirm diagnosis; however, the accuracy of these tests is controversial.

COMMENTS AND TREATMENT CONSIDERATIONS
Episodes typically occur while the patient is standing and are uncommon in the supine or seated position. The diagnosis of vasovagal disorder in new-onset syncope should be made with hesitation in patients at risk for cardiac disease.

There is no clearly effective drug therapy, and trials of pacemakers have produced mixed results but pacemakers cannot be recommended. The mainstay of management is education. Patients should be warned that syncope might recur when they are exposed to similar inciting triggers. The syncopal event can be aborted if the patient lies down during the prodromal phase.

REFERENCES

Grubb BP, Kosinski D: Current trends in etiology, diagnosis, and management of neurocardiogenic syncope, *Curr Opin Cardiol* 11:32, 1996.

Kapoor W: Evaluation and management of the patient with syncope, *JAMA* 268:2553, 1992.

Kapoor WN: Is there an effective treatment for neurally mediated syncope? *JAMA* 289:2272, 2003.

 CAROTID SINUS SYNCOPE

Carotid sinus hypersensitivity can lead to episodes of acute decrease in blood pressure. Attacks of syncope are precipitated by shaving, sudden turning of the head, or a tight collar and typically occur in elderly patients. Not all patients with carotid sinus hypersensitivity are symptomatic.

WORKUP

- Carotid massage: The patient is placed in the supine position, with ECG and blood pressure monitoring, and the carotid artery is massaged for 5 to 40 seconds. A decline in systolic blood pressure of >50 mm Hg or asystole >3 seconds is considered diagnostic. This test is infrequently done in the ED setting. Both carotids should not be massaged simultaneously.

COMMENTS AND TREATMENT CONSIDERATIONS

Patients with carotid sinus syncope often have a scar or a tumor arising from the carotid body, parotid gland, thyroid gland, or lymph node. Evidence supports the use of permanent cardiac pacing to prevent recurrent syncope in patients with clearly identified carotid sinus syncope.

REFERENCES

Brignole M: Randomized clinical trials of neurally mediated syncope, *J Cardiovasc Electrophysiol* 14(9 Suppl):S64, 2003.

Healey J, Connolly SJ, Morillo CA: The management of patients with carotid sinus syndrome: is pacing the answer? *Clin Auton Res* 14(Suppl 1):80, 2004.

Kapoor WN: Current evaluation and management of syncope, *Circulation* 106:1606, 2002.

 TRANSIENT ISCHEMIC ATTACKS

Transient ischemic attacks (TIAs) refer to cerebrovascular insufficiency leading to transient neurologic dysfunction. Isolated syncope is an uncommon presentation of a stroke syndrome. Typically, symptoms associated with vertebrobasilar artery insufficiency accompany the syncopal event. Basilar artery insufficiency is one of several causes of "drop attacks," an event characterized by sudden, brief periods of paresis that cause the patient to fall down. Drop attacks are not true syncopal events because consciousness is not lost.

See Chapter 9, Dizziness (Vertigo), and Chapter 44, Weakness and Fatigue.

REFERENCES

Baloh R: Vertebrobasilar insufficiency and stroke, *Otolaryngol Head Neck Surg* 112:114, 1995.

Fields WS, Lemak NA: Joint study of extracranial arterial occlusion, VII subclavian steal—a review of 168 cases, *JAMA* 222:1139, 1972.

 SUBARACHNOID HEMORRHAGE

Up to 50% of patients have a transient loss of consciousness after rupture of an intracranial aneurysm. These patients commonly exhibit other signs and symptoms of subarachnoid hemorrhage, which can be elicited during a careful history and physical examination.

See Chapter 18, Headache.

REFERENCES

Edlow JA: Diagnosis of subarachnoid hemorrhage, *Neurocrit Care* 2:99, 2005.

Sedat J, Dib M, Rasendrarijao D, et al: Ruptured intracranial aneurysms in the elderly: epidemiology, diagnosis, and management, *Neurocrit Care* 2:119, 2005.

U-King-Im JM, Koo B, Trivedi RA, et al: Current diagnostic approaches to subarachnoid haemorrhage, *Eur Radiol* 15:1135, 2005.

 ORTHOSTATIC HYPOTENSION

Syncope caused by orthostatic hypotension occurs immediately after rising from a sitting or supine position and is often associated with weakness, diaphoresis, headache, visual changes, and epigastric discomfort. Often the result of hypovolemia, the associated signs and symptoms vary depending on the etiology of volume loss. Life-threatening causes of intravascular volume depletion (e.g., acute blood loss, severe dehydration) must be considered.

Other causes include antihypertensives and neurologic diseases including Parkinson's disease and diabetic neuropathy.

See Hypovolemia in Chapter 44, Weakness and Fatigue.

REFERENCES

Atkins D, Hanusa B, Sefcik T, et al: Syncope and orthostatic hypotension, *Am J Med* 91:179, 1991.

Hajjar I: Postural blood pressure changes and orthostatic hypotension in the elderly patient: impact of antihypertensive medications, *Drugs Aging* 22:55, 2005.

Kapoor W: Syncope in older persons, *J Am Geriatr Soc* 42:426, 1994.

Task Force on Syncope, European Society of Cardiology: Guidelines on management (diagnosis and treatment) of syncope—update 2004. Executive summary, *Eur Heart J* 25:2054, 2004.

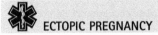 **ECTOPIC PREGNANCY**

See Chapter 41, Vaginal Bleeding.

CHAPTER 36

Toxic Exposure, Approach to
Michael J. Burns and Michael Levine

More than 5 million poison exposures occur annually in the United States and account for 5% to 10% of all emergency department (ED) visits and approximately 5% of intensive care unit admissions.

Not infrequently, the ED physician is faced with an uncooperative, unreliable, or unresponsive poisoned patient and must rapidly assess the severity of illness, make a diagnosis, and provide sound initial treatment, often without the results of an adequate history or extensive laboratory tests. A systematic and consistent approach to the evaluation and treatment of poisoning is therefore necessary. Evaluation involves poisoning recognition, identification of agents involved, assessment of severity, and prediction of toxicity. Treatment involves the provision of supportive care, prevention of poison absorption, and, when necessary, administration of antidotes and enhancement of poison elimination. The tempo, sequence, methods, and priorities of treatment are determined by the agent or agents involved and the presenting and predicted severity of poisoning. The American Association of Poison Control Centers' local poison center, which can be reached at (800) 222-1222, is an excellent resource to assist in the management of poisoned patients.

STEPWISE APPROACH TO ALL SIGNIFICANTLY POISONED PATIENTS

1. ABCs with ACLS measures as necessary
2. Maintain in-line cervical immobilization in those patients with suspected coexisting trauma.
3. IV, O_2, cardiac monitoring, ECG
4. Rapid initial screening physical examination: vital signs (including pulse oximetry and rectal temperature), mental status, skin (color, moisture), and pupillary assessment

5. For those with altered mental status
   a. Immediate bedside glucose determination. If unavailable, empirical glucose administration is indicated. Dose: adults: 50 ml D50 IV; children: 2 to 4 ml/kg D25 IV
   b. Thiamine 100 mg IV (alcoholics or those at risk for vitamin deficiency)
   c. Consider naloxone (adult: 0.4 to 2.0 mg IV; children: 0.1 mg/kg with a maximal single dose of 2 mg), particularly in the presence of bradypnea or miosis. For synthetic opioids (i.e., propoxyphene and methadone), which may have a longer half-life or greater affinity for the opioid receptor than naloxone; up to 10 mg may be necessary for reversal. Naloxone can induce opiate withdrawal in opioid-dependent patients, and the use of naloxone has been associated with hypertension, tachycardia, ventricular arrhythmias, pulmonary edema, and seizures.

6. Flumazenil is *not* recommended for routine use in patients with nonspecific coma. Flumazenil can be used cautiously in those with known isolated benzodiazepine ingestions and the presence of CNS or respiratory depression, provided that the QRS interval <100 msec on the ECG. Flumazenil is dosed at 0.01 mg/kg IV (maximum 0.2 mg initial dose) with subsequent doses given every 30 to 60 seconds to a maximum of 0.05 mg/kg or 1 mg IV. Flumazenil may precipitate seizures in those with mixed ingestions (i.e., cointoxication with cocaine, isoniazid [INH], and tricyclic antidepressants [TCAs]), underlying seizure disorder, and in those given a complete coma-reversing dose (i.e., precipitate acute benzodiazepine withdrawal).

7. Endotracheal intubation is recommended for those with altered mental status who are unable to protect their airway.

8. Detailed history and physical (see Signs and Symptoms)

9. Directed toxicologic laboratory evaluations (see Workup)

10. Initiate patient decontamination as clinically indicated (e.g., removal of contaminated clothing, topical irrigation, activated charcoal [AC], gastric lavage, whole bowel irrigation [WBI], and endoscopic or surgical removal). Gastric lavage may be considered but is rarely indicated for most toxic ingestions (see Comments and Treatment Considerations) (Table 37–1).

11. Antidote administration, as indicated (Table 37–2)

12. Enhanced elimination techniques as indicated (e.g., forced diuresis, urinary pH manipulation, multidose AC, hemodialysis, hemoperfusion, hemofiltration, exchange transfusion, hyperbaric oxygen [HBO]) (Table 37–3)

13. Supportive care

CHAPTER 37

TABLE 37-1
GASTROINTESTINAL DECONTAMINATION METHODS

METHOD	INDICATION	CONTRAINDICATION	DOSING/TECHNIQUE	COMPLICATION
Activated charcoal	Most poison ingestions unless clearly nontoxic*	Bowel obstruction/perforation Depressed mental status and unprotected airway (intubate first) Relative: corrosive and low-viscosity hydrocarbon ingestions	1 g/kg AC OR 10:1 (g:g) AC to toxicant	Nausea/vomiting Abdominal cramps Diarrhea (with sorbitol) Constipation (aqueous suspensions) Aspiration
Whole bowel irrigation (WBI)	Toxic foreign bodies (e.g., cocaine or heroin packets) SR or EC drug preparations Heavy metals (e.g., As, Fe, Li, Hg, Zn) Suspected drug concretions	Bowel obstruction or perforation, bleeding, or ileus Depressed mental status with unprotected airway (intubate first)	Polyethylene glycol EG-3350 (e.g., CoLyte) NGT administration recommended 1–6 yr: 500 ml/hr 6–12 yr: 1 L/hr >12 yr: 1–2 L/hr	Nausea and vomiting Abdominal cramps and bloating Aspiration
Gastric lavage	Obtunded, intubated patients with life-threatening ingestion; if it can be performed in <1 hr of ingestion Life-threatening ingestion of agent not bound by AC*	Corrosive ingestion Low-viscosity hydrocarbon ingestion Depressed mental status and unprotected airway (intubate first) Patient noncompliance Significant esophageal or gastric pathology	Left lateral decubitus or supine 24–28 Fr tube (pediatric) 36–40 Fr tube (adult) Gravity instillation and drainage of up to 5 L of tap water or NS	Aspiration Esophageal perforation Tracheal lavage GI bleeding Hypoxia and hypercapnia Laryngospasm Fluid and electrolyte disturbance

Syrup of ipecac†	Home or prehospital setting	0–6 mo: none	Protracted vomiting (delays
	Alert patient within	6–12 mo: 10 ml	administration of AC or antidotes)
	15–60 min of ingestion	12 mo–12 yr: 15 ml	Lethargy
		(may repeat)	Aspiration
		>12 yr: 30 ml	
		(may repeat)	
	CNS depression		
	Corrosive ingestion		
	Low-viscosity hydrocarbons		
	Agents that may rapidly		
	compromise airway		
	Debilitated patients		
	Third trimester pregnancy		
Cathartics	Adjunct to first dose of AC	Sorbitol (70%): 1 g/kg	Nausea/vomiting
		or 1–2 ml/kg for all	Abdominal cramps and bloating
		>2 yr	Dehydration
		Magnesium citrate:	Hypotension
		4 ml/kg	Hypernatremia
		MgSO₄: 250 mg/kg	Hypermagnesemia
	Bowel obstruction, perforation,		
	or ileus		
	Electrolyte imbalance		
	Hypotension		
	Mg cathartics to those with		
	renal failure		
Endoscopic surgery	Pharmacobezoars		Aspiration
	Heavy metals in stomach		Viscus perforation
	Surgery for those with		
	suspected ruptured		
	cocaine packets		
	Endoscopy should not be used		
	to remove drug packets (high		
	risk of iatrogenic rupture)		
Dilution	Corrosive agent	5 ml/kg water or milk	Vomiting and increased toxic exposure
	Vomiting patient	(up to 250 ml)	

*See text for agents that are not absorbed by charcoal.
†The use of syrup of ipecac is no longer recommended.

CHAPTER 37

TABLE 37-2
POISONS AND THEIR ANTIDOTES

POISON	ANTIDOTE	DOSE
Acetaminophen	N-Acetylcysteine (po) (Mucomyst 20%) N-Acetylcysteine (IV) (Acetadote)	Initial dose: 140 mg/kg followed by 70 mg/kg q4h × 17 doses Initial dose: 150 mg/kg in 200 ml D5W over 15 min; then 50 mg/kg in 500 ml D5W over 4 hr; then 100 mg/kg in 1000 ml D5W over 16 hr This terminal rate continued indefinitely for patients with hepatic failure
Anticholinergic agents*	Physostigmine (Antilirium)	Initial dose: 0.5-2.0 mg IV over 3-5 min; children 0.02 mg/kg
Benzodiazepines*	Flumazenil (Romazicon)	Initial dose: 0.1-0.2 mg IV over 30-60 sec. Repeat at 0.1-0.2 mg IV every minute prn up to 1 mg
Beta-blockers	Glucagon Calcium Insulin + dextrose	Initial dose: 5-10 mg IV bolus, then 2-10 mg/hr IV infusion; Children: 50-100 µg/kg IV bolus initially, then 0.07 mg/kg/hr IV Calcium chloride 10%: 1 g (10 ml) IV, repeat as necessary Insulin load: 0.5-1.0 U/kg IV bolus, then 0.5-1.0 U/kg/hr IV; dextrose 10% IV (with KCl), titrate to euglycemia
Calcium channel blockers	Calcium Glucagon Insulin + dextrose	Calcium chloride 10%: 1-4 g (10-40 ml) IV, repeat as necessary; children 20 mg/kg initially Initial dose: 5-10 mg IV bolus, then 2-10 mg/hr IV infusion Insulin load: 0.5-1.0 U/kg IV bolus, then 0.5-1.0 U/kg/hr; dextrose 10% IV (with KCl), titrate to euglycemia
Carbon monoxide	Oxygen ± hyperbaric oxygen	100% oxygen by ventilator or NRB high-flow oxygen by tight-fitting face mask

Crotalid snakebite[†]	Crotalidae ovine polyvalent immune Fab (CroFab)	Initial dose: 4-6 vials reconstituted in 250 ml NS. Infuse 50 ml/hr for first 10 min. If no allergic reaction, give remaining 200 ml over 50 min (for both adult and pediatric patients) Subsequent dosing: repeat initial dose of antivenin hourly until envenomation syndrome controlled
	Wyeth polyvalent Crotalidae equine antivenin	Mild: 3-5 vials; moderate 6-10 vials; severe 10-20 vials. Mix reconstituted antivenin in 1000 ml NS over 4-6 hr
Cyanide	amyl nitrate pearls Sodium nitrate (3% solution) Sodium thiosulfate (25%)	1 ampule by inhalation for 15-30 sec, q3-4min 10 ml (300 mg) IV over 3 min; children 0.33 ml/kg 50 ml (12.5 g) IV over 10 min, children: 1.65 ml/kg IV
Digoxin (cardiac glycosides)	Digoxin Immune Fab (Digibind)	Number of mg ingested × 0.8 / 0.6 = number of vials needed Digoxin concentration (in ng/ml) × 5.6 × kg (weight)/600 = number of vials Empirical dose: 10 vials (acute poisoning) or 1-3 vials (chronic poisoning) Reconstitute Digibind in NS and administer IV over 5-30 min
Ethylene glycol[†]	Fomepizole (4-methylpyrazole) (Antizol), hemodialysis Ethanol 10% in D5W, hemodialysis	Initial load: 15 mg/kg IV over 30 min, then 10 mg/kg IV q12h over 30 min × 4 doses, then 15 mg/kg until level <20 mg/dl. Rebolus during hemodialysis Initial load: 10 ml/kg IV of 10% ethanol over 30 min, then 1.5 ml/kg IV infusion (titrate to serum ethanol of 100 mg/dl). Double to triple infusion during hemodialysis
Heparin	Protamine sulfate	1 mg neutralizes 90-115 mg heparin. Initial dose: 1 mg/min to total dose of 20 mg in 2 hr

Continued

CHAPTER 37

501

TABLE 37-2
POISONS AND THEIR ANTIDOTES—CONT'D

POISON	ANTIDOTE	DOSE
Hydrofluoric acid	Calcium gluconate	Topical calcium gluconate gel 3% applied for 1-2 days or intradermal or SQ calcium gluconate injection 5% at burn site (0.5 ml per cm² burn area) Regional intravenous (Bier block): 10 ml 10% in 40 ml NS injected locally in venous system × 20-30 min Intra-arterial calcium gluconate 10%: 10-20 ml in 40 ml NS over 4 hr; repeat as necessary until pain relief
Iron	Deferoxamine (Desferal)	10-15 mg/kg/hr IV infusion until urine color clears or until patient clinically well. Do not exceed 6 g/24 hr
Isoniazid	Pyridoxine (vitamin B₆)	Initial dose: 1 g pyridoxine for every g INH ingested or empirical 5 g IV over 10 min if amount ingested unknown
Lead†	2,3-Dimercaptosuccinic acid (DMSA) (Succimer); 100 mg capsules	30 mg/kg po in three divided doses × 5 days, then 20 mg/kg in twice daily doses × 14 days; repeat therapy prn after 2 wk rebound
Mercury†, arsenic†, lead†, gold‡	British antilewisite, dimercaprol (BAL); in peanut oil	Initial dose: 4-6 mg/kg IM q4-6h × 2 days
Methemoglobinemia	Methylene blue (1% solution)	Initial dose: 1-2 mg/kg (0.1 ml/kg) IV over 5 min; repeat prn

Opiates	Naloxone (Narcan). Others: nalmefene, naltrexone	Initial dose: 0.1-2.0 mg IV push. Opioid-dependent patients should receive 0.1 mg IV every 30-60 sec until clinical response; synthetic opiates may need up to 10 mg for initial reversal dose. Children: 0.1 mg/kg IV
Organophosphates, carbamates, nerve agents	Atropine	Initial dose: 0.5-2.0 mg IV; repeat every 3-5 min until sweat and secretions clear. Children: 0.05 mg/kg IV
	Pralidoxime (2-PAM) (Protopam)	Initial dose: 1 g IV over 15 min, then IV infusion of 3-4 mg/kg/hr for 24-72 hr or until clinical toxicity resolves; children: 25-50 mg/kg IV initially Alternative dosing: 30 mg/kg IV initially, then 8 mg/kg/hr infusion
Sulfonylurea, meglitinides	Octreotide (Sandostatin) + dextrose	Initial dose: 50-100 µg SQ or IV, then 50 µg q12 hours until euglycemia maintained without supplemental dextrose; children: 1-2 µg/kg SQ initially
Tricyclic antidepressants	Sodium bicarbonate (NaHCO₃)	Initial dose: 1-2 ampules (50-100 mEq) IV push, then IV infusion to maintain blood pH 7.45-7.55 and Pco_2 approximately 30 mm Hg (usual drip: 3 ampules NaHCO₃ in 1 L D5W infused at 200-250 ml/hr); children: 1 mEq/kg IV bolus initially

*Risks may outweigh benefits; consultation with toxicologist recommended.
†Consultation with a toxicologist is recommended.

CHAPTER 37

TABLE 37-3
ENHANCED ELIMINATION TECHNIQUES

TECHNIQUE	DOSING TECHNIQUE REQUIREMENTS	COMPLICATIONS	AGENTS FOR WHICH EFFECTIVE
Multiple dose AC	0.5–1.0 g/kg AC q2-h Requires bowel sounds	Nausea, vomiting, diarrhea, constipation, bowel obstruction and infarction, aspiration	Carbamazepine, **phenobarbital, theophylline,** quinine, nadolol, dapsone, meprobamate, salicylates, valproate, SR and EC preparations
Forced diuresis	Isotonic fluid (e.g., NS or LR) at 500 ml/hr Requires normal kidney and cardiac functioning Requires urinary catheterization	Fluid overload, pulmonary edema	Barium, bromides, chromium, cisplatin, iodine, fluoride, calcium, lithium, potassium
Urinary alkalization	D5W or $\frac{1}{2}$ NS + 50–150 mEq NaHCO$_3$/L at 500 ml initially (adults). Goal: urine flow 3 ml/kg/hr and urinary pH >7.5	Fluid overload, pulmonary edema, cerebral edema, hypernatremia, hypokalemia, alkalemia, ionized hypocalcemia	Chlorpropamide, **salicylates,** barbiturates, methotrexate, fluoride, sulfonamides
Hemodialysis	Requires poison with molecular weight <500 d, low protein binding, high water solubility, low endogenous clearance, and a small volume of distribution	Hypotension, bleeding, hypothermia, air embolus, central venous access complications	Barbiturates, bromides, chloral hydrate, **alcohols, lithium,** procainamide, theophylline (hemoperfusion better), **salicylates,** atenolol, sotalol

Hemoperfusion	Requires drug to be bound by AC	Charcoal embolization, hypocalcemia, hypoglycemia, thrombocytopenia, leukopenia, hypotension, bleeding, hypothermia	Barbiturates, meprobamate, glutethimide, phenytoin, carbamazepine, valproate, **theophylline**, disopyramide, paraquat, procainamide, *Amanita* mushrooms, methotrexate
Hemofiltration	Can be run continuously	Clotting of filter, bleeding	Aminoglycosides, vancomycin, metal chelate complexes, procainamide
Exchange transfusion	Double or triple volume exchanges usually performed	Transfusion reactions, ionized hypocalcemia, hypothermia	Arsine, sodium chlorate, methemoglobinemia, sulfhemoglobinemia, neonatal drug toxicity

Note: Agents in **bold** more commonly require the specified enhanced elimination technique.

CHAPTER 37

SIGNS AND SYMPTOMS

Symptoms obtained by history and signs obtained on physical examination may be used to help establish and confirm a diagnosis of poisoning. A group of signs and symptoms that are often associated with a particular poison or type of poison is referred to as a toxidrome. Familiarity with common toxidromes is important to the practicing ED physician and allows clinical recognition of toxin patterns (Table 37–4).

HISTORY

- The history may be unreliable when obtained from the patient. It is important, therefore, to try to corroborate the history with family, friends, police, prehospital personnel, and the patient's physician and pharmacist.
- Be sure to inquire specifically about over-the-counter (OTC) drugs.
- Thoroughly search exposure environment for pill bottles, suicide note, or drug paraphernalia.
- Obtain source, nature, time, route, amount, and location of and reason for exposure.
- Inquire about treatment provided prior to hospital arrival.
- Correlate history with physical examination and ancillary test results.

PHYSICAL EXAMINATION

1. Vital signs, mental status, skin findings, and papillary signs are most useful and allow patient classification into a state of physiologic stimulation or depression.
2. Physiologic stimulation (increased HR, BP, T, RR, agitation, seizures, and mydriasis) commonly results from:
   a. Sympathomimetics
   b. Anticholinergics
   c. Central hallucinogens
   d. Drug withdrawal states
3. Physiologic depression (decreased HR, BP, T, RR, lethargy, coma, and miosis) commonly results from:
   a. Sympatholytics
   b. Cholinergics
   c. Opiates
   d. Sedative-hypnotics, alcohols, skeletal muscle relaxants, anticonvulsants
   e. Simple asphyxiants (e.g., inert gases)
4. Mixed physiologic effects can be observed with:
   a. Polysubstance overdoses
   b. Metabolic poisons (e.g., hypoglycemic agents, salicylates, toxic alcohols)

TABLE 37–4
TOXIDROMES

TOXIDROME	SYMPTOMS	SIGNS	EXAMPLES OF TOXIC AGENTS
Sympathomimetic	Agitation Hallucinations Headache Nausea/vomiting Palpitations Paranoia Tremor	CNS: **Agitation**, hyperalert, delirium, seizures, coma VS: **Hypertension**, widened pulse pressure, **tachycardia**, tachypnea, hyperpnea, hyperthermia Pupils: **Mydriasis** Other: **Diaphoresis**, hyperreflexia, tremors, flushed or pale skin	Cocaine Amphetamines Ephedrine Pseudoephedrine Phenylpropanolamine Theophylline Caffeine Albuterol Methylphenidate
Anticholinergics	Agitation Hallucinations Mumbling speech Unresponsive	CNS: **Agitation**, **delirium**, hypervigilance, mumbling speech, hallucinations, coma VS: Hyperthermia, **tachycardia**, hypertension, tachypnea Pupils: **Mydriasis** Other: **Dry flushed skin**, **dry mucous membranes**, decreased bowel sounds, urinary retention, myoclonus, choreoathetosis, picking behavior, seizures (rare) Mnemonic: "**Dry as a bone, red as a beet, blind as a bat, hot as a hare, mad as a hatter**"	Antihistamines Tricyclic antidepressants Cyclobenzaprine Orphenadrine Antiparkinson agents Antispasmodics Phenothiazines Atropine Scopolamine Belladonna alkaloids (e.g., Jimson weed)

Continued

CHAPTER **37**

507

TABLE 37-4
TOXIDROMES—CONT'D

TOXIDROME	SYMPTOMS	SIGNS	EXAMPLES OF TOXIC AGENTS
Hallucinogenic	Hallucinations Perceptual disorientations Depersonalization Synesthesia Agitation	CNS: **Hallucinations**, depersonalization, agitation VS: Hyperthermia, tachycardia, hypertension, tachypnea Pupils: Mydriasis (usually) Other: Nystagmus	Phencyclidine Ketamine Dextromethorphan *Salvia divinorum* LSD Mescaline Psilocybin Designer amphetamines (e.g., MDMA, MDEA, STP, DOM, 5-MeO-DIPT)
Opioid	Lethargy Confusion Unresponsive	CNS: **Lethargy**, coma, confusion VS: **Bradypnea**, hypothermia, bradycardia, hypotension, hypopnea Pupils: **Miosis** (usually) Other: Hyporeflexia, pulmonary edema, **needle marks**	Heroin Morphine Meperidine Methadone Oxycodone Hydrocodone Fentanyl Hydromorphone Diphenoxylate Loperamide Propoxyphene Pentazocine

Sedative hypnotics	Confusion Stupor Unresponsive Slurred speech	CNS: **Lethargy**, coma, confusion, dysarthria, ataxia VS: Hypothermia, bradycardia, hypotension, hypopnea, **bradypnea** Pupils: Miosis (usually) Other: Hyporeflexia, nystagmus	Benzodiazepines Barbiturates Carisoprodol Meprobamate Glutethimide Alcohols Zolpidem
Cholinergic	Confusion Unresponsive SOB Cramps Nausea/vomiting Diarrhea Weakness Seizures Drooling	CNS: **Agitation**, coma, confusion, seizures VS: **Bradycardia**, hypertension or hypotension, tachypnea or bradypnea Pupils: Miosis (not universal) Other: **Salivation, urination and fecal incontinence**, diarrhea, **emesis,** **diaphoresis, lacrimation,** GI cramps, bronchoconstriction, muscle fasciculations, weakness	Organophosphate and carbamate insecticides Nerve agents Nicotine Pilocarpine Physostigmine Edrophonium Bethanechol Urecholine Neostigmine Pyridostigmine
Serotonin syndrome	Lethargy Confusion Agitation Tremulous	CNS: Agitation, lethargy, coma, **confusion**, delirium VS: **Hyperthermia**, tachycardia, hypertension, tachypnea Pupils: Mydriasis Other: Tremor, myoclonus, hyperreflexia, clonus, diaphoresis, flushing, trismus, rigidity, diarrhea	MAOIs alone or with: SSRIs, meperidine, L-tryptophan, Trazodone, TCAs, nefazodone, dextromethorphan

CHAPTER 37

Continued

TABLE 37-4
TOXIDROMES—CONT'D

TOXIDROME	SYMPTOMS	SIGNS	EXAMPLES OF TOXIC AGENTS
Cyclic antidepressants	Confusion Agitation Unresponsive Slurred speech	CNS: Lethargy, coma, confusion, seizures VS: Hyperthermia, **tachycardia**, hypertension then hypotension, hypopnea Pupils: **Mydriasis** Other: **Dry skin, myoclonus**, choreoathetosis, cardiac arrhythmias and conduction disturbances	Amitriptyline Nortriptyline Imipramine Clomipramine Desipramine Doxepin Trimipramine
Sympatholytic	Lethargy Confusion Unresponsive	CNS: Lethargy, confusion, coma, seizures (uncommonly) VS: **Bradycardia**, hypotension, bradypnea, hypopnea Pupils: **Miosis** (often)	Alpha-adrenergic antagonists (e.g., prazosin) Beta-blockers (e.g., propranolol) Calcium channel blockers (e.g., verapamil, diltiazem) Alpha$_2$-adrenergic agonists (e.g., clonidine, tizanidine)

| Digitalis and other cardiac glycosides | Anorexia
Nausea/vomiting
Diarrhea
Lethargy
Weakness
Dizziness
Vertigo
Visual disturbances (xanthopsia, chromatopsia)
Syncope | CNS: Normal or lethargy and confusion
VS: Bradycardia, hypotension
Pupils: Normal
Other: **Cardiac arrhythmias and conduction disturbances** | Digoxin
Digitoxin
Digitalis purpurea (foxglove)
Digitalis lantana
Nerium oleander (oleander)
Thevetia peruviana (yellow oleander)
Convallaria majalis (lily of the valley)
Urginea maritime (red squill)
Bufonidae toads (e.g., Colorado River toad) |
| Extrapyramidal
Dystonia
Akathisia
Parkinsonism | Anxious
Inability to talk | CNS: Alert and oriented, anxious, dysarthria, mutism
VS: Normal
Pupils: Normal
Other: **Oculogyric crisis, facial grimacing, torticollis, buccolingual spasm,** tremor, rigidity, involuntary movements, opisthotonus, bradykinesia, masked facies, akathisia | Antipsychotics (e.g., haloperidol, phenothiazines, molindone)
Antiemetics (e.g., droperidol, prochlorperazine, metoclopramide |

Terms in **bold** are common findings.

CHAPTER 37

c. Heavy metals (e.g., arsenic, iron, lead, lithium, mercury)
d. Membrane-active agents (e.g., volatile inhalants, antiarrhythmics, local anesthetic agents)
e. Agents with multiple mechanisms of actions (e.g., cyclic antidepressants)
f. Cellular asphyxiants (e.g., CO, cyanide [CN], methemoglobinemia)

5. Normal vital sign and mental status may be evidence of a nontoxic exposure, or that insufficient time has passed from exposure to the patient's presentation and evaluation.

WORKUP

- Ancillary studies may be used to confirm, establish, or refute poisoning diagnosis. Tests ordered should be guided by history and physical examination.
- ECG is recommended for intentional poisonings, those with hemodynamic instability, or those exposed to cardiotoxic agents. The ECG provides clues for diagnosis (e.g., sinus tachycardia with widened QRS interval or tall R in aVR suggests cyclic antidepressant poisoning).
- Symptomatic patients or those with unreliable or unknown history should generally have measurements of serum electrolytes (calculate anion gap), BUN, creatinine, glucose, and urinalysis.
- Routine urine pregnancy testing is recommended in all women of childbearing age.
- ABG, cooximetry, serum osmolality, and lactate measurements are recommended in patients with potential acid-base, cardiovascular, neurologic, or respiratory disturbance.
- The presence of an anion gap metabolic acidosis should prompt measurements of serum calcium, creatinine, glucose, ketones, lactate, osmolality (suggesting toxic alcohols, ethylene glycol), salicylates, quantitative toxic alcohol levels where indicated, and examination of the urine for crystals.
- Liver function tests (LFTs) and PT (INR) should be performed following acetaminophen ingestion or exposure to other hepatotoxic agents; LFT elevations may be significantly delayed.
- Toxic screening should minimally include serum measurements of acetaminophen and salicylate in those with intentional poisoning or uncertain history because acetaminophen is completely asymptomatic in the early treatable phase and salicylate symptoms may be overlooked.
- Comprehensive toxic screening is rarely necessary or indicated, particularly when patients are asymptomatic or have clinical findings consistent with history. A toxicologic screen (i.e., immunoassay) for drugs of abuse is also generally unnecessary.

512

TABLE 37–5
DRUGS FOR WHICH QUANTIFICATION OF LEVEL MAY BE USEFUL

Acetaminophen
Antiepileptic agents
 Carbamazepine
 Phenobarbital
 Phenytoin
 Valproic acid
Carboxyhemoglobin
Digoxin
Ethanol
Ethylene glycol
Heavy metals
 Iron
 Lead
 Mercury
Lithium
Methanol
Methemoglobin
Paraquat
Salicylates
Theophylline

Serum alcohol levels may help reassure clinicians in the early phases of evaluation of altered patients as an explanation of symptoms, although alcoholics may also have concurrent head injury or other causes for altered mental status.

- At times, obtaining quantitative levels of toxins is necessary to determine or predict the severity of poisoning and guide treatment (Table 37–5).

COMMENTS AND TREATMENT CONSIDERATIONS

Management strategies are dictated by the poison involved, presenting and predicted severity of illness, and time of presentation in relation to time of exposure. Supportive care, in conjunction with decontamination procedures, is sufficient for the majority of patients. Some patients may require admission for observation given delayed absorption (if extended-release products are consumed or if taken in conjunction with another substance that may alter gastric emptying time).

POISON DECONTAMINATION (see Table 37–1)

- The sooner decontamination is performed, the more effective it is at preventing poison absorption, although its efficacy in many circumstances has been questioned.
- For dermal and ocular exposures, contaminated clothing and particulate matter should be immediately removed and exposed areas should be irrigated copiously with normal saline or tap water.

- For inhalation exposures, the patient should be immediately removed from the contaminated area and given supplemental oxygen.
- GI decontamination is recommended for poison ingestions, unless the exposure was clearly nontoxic. These recommendations are largely based on theoretical grounds, however, as there are few data to demonstrate clear benefit from GI decontamination more than 1 hour after ingestion.
- AC administration alone is the preferred means of GI decontamination for the majority of poison ingestions. Caution should be taken, however, if giving charcoal to lethargic individuals, as fatal cases of charcoal aspiration have been reported.
- AC does not effectively adsorb hydrocarbons, corrosives (i.e., acids and alkalis), alcohols, heavy metals, inorganic ions, boric acid, and essential oils.
- Gastric lavage (in addition to AC) may be useful and, thus, considered for life-threatening ingestions (e.g., intubated, obtunded patients with a lethal toxin not bound by AC), provided it can be performed within 60 minutes of ingestion.
- Whole bowel irrigation is useful for patients who have ingested heavy metals (e.g., arsenic, iron, and lithium), drug packets ("body stuffer" or "body packer"), or sustained-release or enteric-coated preparations or those who are suspected to have drug concretions (pharmacobezoars).
- Syrup of ipecac is not recommended for hospital use, and the American Academy of Pediatrics no longer recommends its use in children.

ANTIDOTES
Antidotes are not available for most toxic agents and are used in approximately 1% of all poison exposures. Common antidotes and their doses are listed in Table 37–2. It is appropriate to administer an antidote when the expected benefits of therapy outweigh the associated risks.

ENHANCED ELIMINATION (see Table 37–3)
In approximately 1% of poison exposures, it becomes necessary to accelerate the removal of absorbed toxins using enhanced elimination techniques. In a few selected cases, an aggressive approach to elimination can be lifesaving. Enhanced elimination techniques should be considered when a patient fails (or is considered unlikely to respond to) maximal supportive care and the predicted benefit of the intervention outweighs its risks of complications. Consultation with a toxicologist is recommended.

TOXIC TIME BOMBS (see Table 37–6)

Both actual and predicted toxic effects determine the patient's disposition. Certain poisons produce delayed toxic manifestations, usually secondary to toxic metabolites, and few, if any, early signs may be present following lethal doses of these agents. If history, physical examination, or initial laboratory testing is suggestive of delayed toxicity, a prolonged period of observation or treatment is required, even if the patient initially appears well.

TABLE 37–6

SUBSTANCES WITH DELAYED CLINICAL TOXICITY

Acetaminophen
Antimetabolites
    Alkylating agents
    Colchicine
    Methotrexate
Carbon tetrachloride
Cyanogenic glycosides
Drug packet ingestion (heroin, cocaine)
Elapid snake envenomations
Enteric-coated preparations
    Aspirin
Ergotamines
Fat-soluble organophosphate insecticides
Heavy metals
    Lead
    Mercury
    Thallium
Lomotil
MAOIs
Methylene chloride (metabolized to CO)
Mushrooms
    Amanita (amatoxin)
    Lepiota (amatoxin)
    Gyromitra (gyromitrin)
    Cortinarius (orellanine/orelline)
Oral hypoglycemic agents
Paraquat/diquat
Pennyroyal oil
Warfarin/superwarfarin
    Brodifacoum
Sustained-release preparations
    Beta-blockers
    Calcium channel blockers
    Lithium
    Theophylline
Toxic alcohols
    Ethylene glycol
Methanol

SUPPORTIVE CARE

Supportive care is frequently all that is necessary to effect a good outcome for the patient.

Hypertension

Hypertension is best treated initially with nonspecific sedation (e.g., benzodiazepines such as lorazepam dosed at 0.1 mg/kg IV). When it is associated with end-organ dysfunction, hypertension is best treated with calcium channel blockers (e.g., verapamil), phentolamine, or a combination of nitroprusside with a beta-blocker. Beta-blockers should *not* be used alone in sympathomimetic states (e.g., cocaine) because they may precipitate unopposed alpha-adrenergic vasoconstriction.

Hypotension

Numerous poisons can deplete the endogenous catecholamine stores, thus causing hypotension. Intravenous fluid is the first-line treatment, but occasionally vasopressors (e.g., norepinephrine) may be needed. Antidotes and other specific treatments should be administered as indicated.

Agitation

Agitation is generally best treated with benzodiazepines, supplemented as necessary with neuroleptics (e.g., haloperidol). Physostigmine (0.02 mg/kg IV, maximum 2 mg/ initial dose) may be appropriate for some patients with agitated delirium secondary to the anticholinergic syndrome. Caution should be used when administering physostigmine because of the potential for seizures and severe bradycardia or asystole; toxicology consultation is recommended. Physostigmine is contraindicated in patients with prolonged PR or QRS intervals (as seen in TCA ingestions).

Ventricular Arrhythmias

Standard doses of antiarrhythmics (e.g., lidocaine) are recommended for treatment of ventricular arrhythmias. Sodium bicarbonate (1 to 2 mEq/kg IV bolus) is indicated for wide complex tachycardias resulting from TCA overdose and other membrane-active agents. Other antidotes (i.e., digoxin-specific Fab fragments [Digibind]) may be indicated for certain drug-associated ventricular arrhythmias.

Bradyarrhythmias with Hypotension

Treatment of bradyarrhythmias with hypotension is drug specific. Standard doses of atropine are recommended. Management of calcium channel blocker, beta-blocker, and digoxin poisonings is discussed separately at the end of the chapter.

Seizures

A bedside blood glucose determination should be performed on all seizure patients and dextrose administered as necessary. Generally, seizures are best treated with benzodiazepines followed by phenobarbital. Pyridoxine (vitamin B_6) is indicated for INH or *Gyromitra* mushroom–induced seizures (see Table 37–2 for dosing). The routine use of phenytoin is not recommended for most toxin-induced seizures; its use could worsen arrhythmias and hypotension (e.g., TCAs and theophylline).

SPECIFIC AGENTS

 ACETAMINOPHEN (TYLENOL OR PARACETAMOL)

Acetaminophen (APAP) is the most common cause of pharmaceutical-associated poisoning and death each year in the United States. Patients may be asymptomatic or demonstrate non-specific clinical effects (i.e., nausea and vomiting) early after APAP overdose. Thus, measurement of a serum APAP concentration is recommended for all suspected ingestions. *N*-Acetylcysteine (NAC) should be administered empirically to patients (1) who may have ingested a toxic amount of APAP *and* (2) for whom the estimated time of ingestion is close to or greater than 8 hours and the delay while waiting for a level will result in treatment beginning more than 8 hours after ingestion.

SYMPTOMS

- Early (0 to 24 hours)—initial toxicity is often mild or overlooked, consisting of anorexia, nausea, vomiting, and malaise.
- Late: (>24 hours)—right upper quadrant pain, symptoms of liver failure (recurrent nausea, vomiting, malaise, lethargy, confusion)

SIGNS

- Stage I (0 to 24 hours): none
- Stage II (24 to 72 hours): right upper quadrant tenderness, elevation of hepatic transaminases and bilirubin, prolongation of pro-thrombin time and INR, deteriorating renal function
- Stage III (72 to 96 hours): sequelae of hepatic necrosis (jaundice, coagulation defects, renal failure, hepatic encephalopathy, asterixis metabolic acidosis, and tachypnea). Death can result. These effects occur in those not treated or treated too late with antidote.
- Stage IV (>96 hours to 2 weeks): complete resolution of toxic effects

WORKUP

- Plasma APAP concentrations measured from 4 to 24 hours after single, acute overdose can be plotted on the modified

517

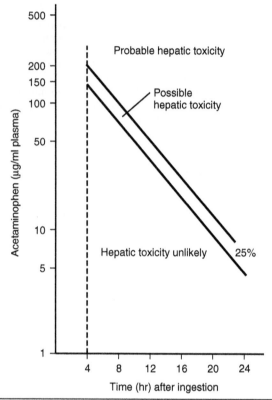

Fig. 37-1 Rumack-Matthew nomogram for acetaminophen poisoning. (From Rumack BH, Matthew H: Acetaminophen poisoning and toxicity, Pediatrics 55:871, 1975.)

Rumack-Matthew nomogram to predict the risk of subsequent hepatotoxicity and the need for NAC antidotal treatment (Fig. 37–1). If a sustained-release product (e.g., Tylenol ER) was ingested, repeated APAP levels need to be obtained and plotted on the nomogram every 4 hours until the levels are declining. Perform baseline and daily BUN, creatinine, LFTs, and PT/INR.

COMMENTS AND TREATMENT CONSIDERATIONS

Patients with a level greater than the line connecting 150 µg/ml at 4 hours and 5 mg/L at 24 hours ("possible hepatic toxicity" line) currently receive antidotal therapy with NAC in the United States (see Table 37–2 for dosing). Treatment is nearly 100% effective at preventing APAP toxicity if it is initiated within 8 hours of ingestion. Effectiveness progressively diminishes with further delay of treatment. A decision to initiate or forgo antidotal treatment in those (1) with multiple subtoxic ingestions, (2) who have ingested sustained-release preparations, or (3) who are more susceptible to hepatotoxicity (e.g., alcoholics, Gilbert's disease, chronic antiepileptic therapy) should be made in conjunction with a toxicologist. In addition, consider toxicologic consultation in admitted patients when abbreviated treatment (<72 hours) is being considered.

Previously in the United States, NAC was available only as a 20% oral solution. This solution has an unpleasant taste and smell, which are best masked in cola or juice. Nausea and vomiting are common side effects of both APAP toxicity and NAC therapy. Thus, antiemetic therapy with ondansetron or metoclopramide is recommended. In 2004, however, an intravenous form of NAC (Acetadote) was approved for use by the FDA. The intravenous form may be given to patients who are unable to tolerate oral or nasogastric dosing. Intravenous administration is preferred in patients with APAP-associated hepatic failure.

If a patient presents late to the hospital and hepatotoxicity has occurred, NAC should be continued until (1) the transaminases return to near-normal levels and/or the INR is decreasing and less than 2.0, (2) the patient receives a liver transplant, or (3) death ensues. Any patient with evidence of hepatic damage following an APAP ingestion should be considered for transfer to a center capable of performing liver transplantation. Consultation with a toxicologist is recommended.

CALCIUM CHANNEL BLOCKERS AND BETA-BLOCKERS

The toxic effects from and treatment for calcium channel blockers (CCBs) and beta-blockers (BBs) are largely similar and are discussed together.

CCBs are competitive antagonists of slow, voltage-dependent (L-type) calcium channels. These agents block phase II (plateau) and phase IV (spontaneous depolarization) of the action potential in membranes of cardiac and smooth muscle vasculature cells. Electrophysiologic effects include decreased cardiac contractility, vasomotor tone, heart rate, and atrioventricular nodal conduction. The CCBs fall into three major classes: (1) phenylalkylamines (e.g., verapamil), (2) dihydropyridines (e.g., nifedipine and amlodipine), and (3) benzothiazepines (e.g., diltiazem). At therapeutic doses, the phenylalkylamines have greater negative inotropic effect and the dihydropyridines have greater vasodilatory effect. In overdose, tissue selectivity is lost and all tissue effects are prominent. Insulin release

519

in the pancreas is a calcium channel–mediated process; toxicity with CCBs may be associated with hyperglycemia.

BBs are competitive antagonists of beta-adrenergic receptors. BBs produce decreased contractility, heart rate, and atrioventricular conduction. In contrast to that with CCB toxicity, vasomotor tone is increased with BB toxicity. BBs can be classified on the basis of their selectivity for the beta-1 receptor. The agents that are predominantly beta-1 receptor specific (e.g., atenolol, esmolol, and metoprolol) are considered cardioselective; those that work on both the beta-1 and beta-2 receptors (e.g., propranolol, sotalol) are nonselective and, thus, produce more peripheral effects at therapeutic doses. In overdose, cardioselectivity may be largely lost. Certain BBs have quinidine-like antiarrhythmic effects (e.g., acebutolol, propranolol). Agents that are highly lipophilic (e.g., propranolol) have a significant propensity for producing CNS toxicity (e.g., CNS depression, seizures). Unlike CCBs, BBs are associated with hypoglycemia related to beta$_2$-adrenergic antagonism.

SYMPTOMS
- Lethargy
- Slurred speech
- Confusion
- Nausea, vomiting
- Seizures

SIGNS
- Cool skin for BBs and warm skin for CCBs
- Hypotension, shock
- Arrhythmias (bradycardias, variable AV nodal blockade with nodal or ventricular escape rhythms, bundle branch blockade, asystole)
- Reflex tachycardia (early after dihydropyridines only)
- Respiratory arrest
- Mesenteric and myocardial ischemia
- Hyperglycemia (with CCBs)
- Hypoglycemia and hyperkalemia (with BBs)
- QRS prolongation (verapamil, propranolol, acebutolol)
- QT prolongation and torsades de pointes (with sotalol)
- Bronchospasm (with noncardioselective BBs)
- Pulmonary edema
- Elevated anion gap metabolic (lactic) acidosis
- Ileus
- Coma

WORKUP
- Electrolytes, BUN/creatinine, glucose, ECG, ABG, Ca^{2+}
- Blood levels of these agents are neither available nor helpful for management.

COMMENTS AND TREATMENT CONSIDERATIONS

It is important to recognize the combination of bradyarrhythmias and hypotension as the hallmarks of CCB and BB poisoning. AC administration is recommended following poisoning with these agents. When sustained-release preparations are ingested, adjunctive WBI may be beneficial and is also recommended. The differential diagnosis for toxicologic etiologies of hypotensive and bradycardic patients with altered mental status should also include overdose of opiates, cardiac glycosides, clonidine and imidazolines, lithium, organophosphates, cyanide, and chloroquine. Patients with hyperkalemia and hypermagnesemia may also present similarly.

There are numerous specific pharmacotherapies that are available and potentially beneficial for patients with symptomatic BB and CCB toxicity. Dose recommendations are similar for both agents and are detailed in Table 37–2. For bradycardias, recommended therapies include atropine, calcium salts, glucagon, catecholamines and other pressors, and electrical pacing. For hypotension with or without bradycardia, available therapies include IV crystalloid, calcium salts, glucagon, catecholamines and other pressors, hyperinsulinemia-euglycemia treatment, intra-aortic balloon pump, and cardiopulmonary bypass therapy. Treatments should be dictated and guided by physical findings (e.g., pulse, blood pressure, peripheral pulse, and skin examination), urine output, ECG findings, and more advanced hemodynamic monitoring techniques (e.g., echocardiogram, pulmonary artery catheter, central venous catheter). Patients with significant poisoning often require numerous simultaneous therapies to achieve an acceptable pulse and blood pressure.

Although atropine is commonly used for treatment of the bradycardia, it is frequently not beneficial; it inconsistently raises the heart rate and rarely increases the blood pressure.

When administered, catecholamine pressors are often needed in supraphysiologic doses.

Glucagon acts on a distinct glucagon receptor, which increases adenyl cyclase, resulting in increased intracellular cyclic adenosine monophosphate (cAMP) through a second-messenger system. The increase cAMP results in an influx of calcium ions through calcium channels. This mechanism occurs independently of beta cells and thus works for both CCB and BB overdoses

Administration of exogenous insulin along with dextrose (hyperinsulinemia-euglycemia) is a recently recognized, effective therapy for refractory shock associated with either BB or CCB toxicity. Concurrent administration of potassium may be necessary. Insulin increases cytosolic calcium in cardiac myocytes (positive inotropic effect) and increases substrate uptake into cardiac myocytes, which become carbohydrate dependent with BB and CCB toxicity.

CHAPTER 37

521

If seizures occur, hypoglycemia should be excluded as an etiology. Benzodiazepines are recommended as first-line treatment for seizures.

 CARBON MONOXIDE

Carbon monoxide (CO) is an odorless, tasteless, and colorless gas produced by the incomplete combustion of any carbon-containing material. Common scenarios where CO is encountered include automobile exhaust fumes (especially with inadequate ventilation), poorly ventilated charcoal grills, exposure to paint thinners containing methylene chloride, gas or kerosene heaters, and smoke inhalation from fires. The use of pulse oximetry is inaccurate and does not provide a valid measurement of cellular oxygenation status in CO poisoning.

CO exerts its toxicity largely by binding tightly to and inhibiting the function of many cytochromes, such as hemoglobin, myoglobin, cytochrome oxidase (a-a_3), and guanylate cyclase. CO binds to hemoglobin with 240 times greater affinity than oxygen. The binding of CO to hemoglobin produces a conformational change in the tetramer and results in a leftward shift of the oxyhemoglobin dissociation curve. Further oxygen is inhibited from binding to hemoglobin and its release into tissues is impaired. The CO binding to myoglobin impairs oxygen uptake into myocardial tissue and binding to cytochrome oxidase impairs cellular respiration. Cellular ischemia and hypoxia produced by CO result in a subsequent cascade of reperfusion events (e.g., lipid peroxidation and free radical production) that result in further tissue injury.

SYMPTOMS

Symptoms correlate variably with the carboxyhemoglobin (COHb) concentration. The COHb concentration in nonsmoking adults is 2% to 4% and in smoking adults is nearly 10%. After a brief, acute exposure, COHb concentrations may correlate with symptoms.

- 10%-20%: headache, dizziness, chest pain, dyspnea
- 20%-30%: visual disturbance, confusion
- 30%-40%: syncope
- 40%-50%: seizures, coma
- >55%: death

After prolonged, indolent exposure, patients may exhibit severe toxicity with only mildly elevated COHb levels.

SIGNS

- Physical findings include tachycardia, tachypnea, confusion, coma, and respiratory depression.

- Cardiac arrhythmias, pulmonary edema, and hypotension may occur.
- The findings of cutaneous and mucosal erythema, retinal hemorrhages, and bullae on the skin are rarely observed.

WORKUP
- COHb concentrations (can be venous or arterial) often confirm exposure.
- ABG analysis: may show metabolic acidosis. Readings of the oxygen saturation are falsely normal if calculated from the PaO_2. Thus, it must be measured directly by cooximetry to be accurate.
- ECG: may show nonspecific repolarization or ischemic changes and tachyarrhythmias.
- Chest x-ray: CO does not change the chest x-ray itself, but the chest x-ray may reflect changes resulting from smoke inhalation, such as nonspecific findings of interstitial or alveolar edema, atelectasis, perivascular/bronchial cuffing, and peripheral opacities.

COMMENTS AND TREATMENT CONSIDERATIONS
The initial treatment should be with 100% oxygen (if intubated) or high-flow oxygen by nonrebreather face mask (if not intubated). The elimination half-life of COHb is 4 to 6 hours when breathing room air at normobaric pressure and drops to 60 minutes when breathing 100% oxygen at normobaric pressure and 20 to 40 minutes when breathing 100% oxygen at 2.5 to 3.0 atmospheric pressure. Oxygen therapy should be continued until COHb levels are <10% (4 to 6 hours) and symptoms have resolved. The exact benefit of HBO is controversial because the two largest studies have demonstrated conflicting results, especially with regard to preventing late neurologic sequelae. Accepted indications for HBO include altered mental status, a history of loss of consciousness or syncope, coma, seizures, focal neurologic deficits, and pregnancy with evidence of fetal distress. Considerations for HBO include those with metabolic acidosis, cardiac end-organ effects, COHb level >25%, abnormal neuropsychometric testing, and pregnancy with COHb level >15%.

 CYANIDE

Cyanide intoxication is an uncommon but highly dangerous poisoning. Cyanide salts and hydrocyanic acid are commonly used in industrial processes, such as jewelry and metal cleaning, electroplating, and precious metal extraction. Sodium nitroprusside releases cyanide during its metabolism, and prolonged exposure to sodium nitroprusside can result in clinically significant cyanide intoxication. Cyanogenic glycosides are present in the seeds of certain fruits (e.g., cherry, plum, peach, apricot). Lastly, cyanide poisoning can result from smoke inhalation. Smoke exposure victims, especially in confined spaces, can develop both cyanide and carbon monoxide poisoning, and these poisonings have synergistic toxic effects. Numerous reports of aircraft accident–related fatalities have occurred where the cause of death was not the trauma but rather cyanide and carbon monoxide intoxication.

Cyanide binds to the ferric ion (Fe^{3+}) in cytochrome oxidase (in complex IV), thereby preventing electron transport and further oxidation of NADH. The cell's ability to utilize oxygen in oxidative phosphorylation is inhibited and the cell undergoes anaerobic metabolism. Lactic acid production is greatly increased, and an anion gap metabolic acidosis develops.

SYMPTOMS
- Headache
- Anxiety, irritability, agitation
- Nausea/vomiting
- Dyspnea

SIGNS
- Hyperpnea and tachypnea
- Tachycardia
- Diaphoresis
- Seizures
- Dilated pupils, which are either sluggishly reactive or nonreactive
- Rapid loss of consciousness and coma
- Hypertension or hypotension
- Lactic acidosis
- Respiratory failure
- Ventricular arrhythmias and bradyasystole
- Noncardiogenic pulmonary edema
- Bitter almond smell (rare)

WORKUP
- The diagnosis is made by history and physical examination.
- Continuous cardiac monitoring and pulse oximetry should be implemented.
- ECG
- Arterial and venous blood gases and serum lactate, electrolytes, and bicarbonate should be obtained. Significantly elevated lactate concentrations (i.e., >10 mmol/L) and anion gap metabolic acidosis can be used as surrogate markers for CN poisoning.
- A red blood cell cyanide level should be ordered, but results are usually not immediately available and, thus, do not assist in treatment.
- Chest x-ray should be obtained if pulmonary edema is suspected.

COMMENTS AND TREATMENT CONSIDERATIONS

Cyanide-exposed patients who manifest anxiety, hyperventilation, or headache but no metabolic abnormalities do not require any specific treatment other than 100% oxygen. Any exposed skin or eyes should be copiously irrigated with water or normal saline. Patients with metabolic abnormalities should be treated with the Taylor Cyanide Kit (formerly called the Lilly Cyanide Kit).

The Taylor kit consists of amyl nitrite, sodium nitrite, and sodium thiosulfate. Amyl nitrite pearls can be broken into a gauze pad and placed over the nose of patients who are spontaneously breathing. If the patient is not breathing, they can be placed into the lip of a face mask or inside the bag-valve mask of patients who are being artificially ventilated. Each pearl should be inhaled for 30 seconds, and a new pearl should be replaced every 3 to 4 minutes until intravenous access is established. When an IV is in place, amyl nitrite should be discontinued and sodium nitrite should be administered. Sodium nitrite is administered as a 300-mg bolus (3% of a 10 ml ampule) for adults or 0.33 ml/kg for pediatric patients. Sodium nitrite can cause hypotension; the incidence of hypotension can be reduced by slowing the rate of administration. Because the mechanism of sodium nitrite is to induce methemoglobinemia, dangerously high levels of methemoglobin are possible. Methemoglobin levels should be obtained frequently, and levels greater than 30% to 40% should be avoided. Sodium nitrite should be followed by sodium thiosulfate (adult dose is 12.5 g or one 50-ml ampule of 25% solution; pediatric dosage is 1.65 ml/kg). A repeated dose of sodium nitrite and sodium thiosulfate can be administered at one half the initial dose if clinical response is inadequate after 30 minutes.

For cases of severe smoke inhalation with carbon monoxide poisoning and suspected cyanide poisoning, sodium thiosulfate and 100% supplemental oxygen should be administered initially. In these cases, administration of amyl nitrite and sodium nitrite should be avoided because the combination of methemoglobinemia and carboxyhemoglobinemia can be deadly. It is recommended that amyl nitrite be avoided entirely and sodium nitrite not be administered until the patient is in an HBO chamber at desired pressure.

Patients who are asymptomatic after apparent minimal exposure should be observed for 6 hours and then can be safely discharged if they remain asymptomatic with normal laboratory studies. Patients who are exposed to nitrile compounds, however, need observation for at least 12 hours, even if asymptomatic. Patients with serious toxicity should be administered all antidotes and then observed in an intensive care until for at least 24 hours.

CHAPTER 37

CYCLIC ANTIDEPRESSANTS

Cyclic antidepressants (CAs) block presynaptic reuptake of monoamine neurotransmitters in the CNS (norepinephrine, serotonin, and dopamine). TCAs have additional effects, which include (1) antagonism of H1 histamine receptors, (2) antagonism of alpha$_1$-adrenergic receptors, (3) antagonism of M1 muscarinic acetylcholine receptors, (4) quinidine-like (type Ia) antiarrhythmic effects, and (5) variable blockade of gamma-aminobutyric acid receptors in the CNS.

SYMPTOMS
- Lethargy to coma
- Seizures
- Confusion

SIGNS
- Mydriasis (anticholinergic) or miosis (alpha-adrenergic blockade)
- Dry skin and mucous membranes
- Tachycardia
- Lethargy to coma
- Seizures
- Hypotension
- Agitated delirium
- Urinary retention, ileus
- Ventricular arrhythmias, tachycardia with aberrant intraventricular conduction, terminal bradycardia

WORKUP
- ECG: may show sinus tachycardia with atrioventricular and intraventricular conduction disturbances (e.g., prolonged QRS, R in a VR [rightward axis of terminal 40 msec of limb lead QRS]), ventricular tachycardia, and ventricular fibrillation. The lack of sinus tachycardia early after acute overdose is a good sign because anticholinergic manifestations typically appear early after overdose.
- Quantitative TCA levels are not recommended in the acute overdose setting.

COMMENTS AND TREATMENT CONSIDERATIONS
All but the most trivial poisonings require close cardiac monitoring because patients can rapidly deteriorate in the first few hours after ingestion. If patients remain or become asymptomatic after 4 to 6 hours of observation following an ingestion of an immediate release product, they are unlikely to have a complication related

to cyclic antidepressant ingestion. AC should be administered early by mouth or nasogastric tube.

Death is most commonly caused by refractory hypotension or ventricular arrhythmias. A QRS >100 msec or R in aVR >3 mm predicts serious toxicity (i.e., seizures and VT/VF) and warrants ICU admission, close monitoring, and sodium bicarbonate administration. Sodium bicarbonate, which overcomes the fast sodium channel blockade, is given in 1 to 2 mEq/kg intravenous boluses until the arterial pH is 7.45 to 7.55. This degree of alkalinization decreases the toxic cardiac effects (attenuates the conduction disturbances and provides positive inotropic support). Hyperventilation is also recommended in those requiring intubation as adjunctive therapy to sodium bicarbonate (target Pco_2 of 30 mm Hg). Type Ia, Ic, and III antiarrhythmic agents are contraindicated for ventricular arrhythmias associated with TCAs as they can potentiate cardiotoxicity.

 DIGOXIN

Digoxin is a cardiac glycoside that inhibits the sodium-potassium adenosine triphosphatase (Na^+, K^+-ATPase) exchanger in the heart and results in an intracellular increase of Na^+ and Ca^{2+} and decrease of potassium. Increased cytosolic Ca^{2+} enhances excitation-contraction coupling and improves myocardial contractility. In toxic doses, digoxin results in decreased automaticity of the SA node, decreased AV nodal conduction, and enhanced automaticity in atrial and ventricular myocytes. Clinical manifestations include bradyarrhythmias and triggered tachyarrhythmias. Poisoning with cardioactive steroids can also occur following consumption of certain plants (e.g., foxglove, lily of the valley, oleander).

SYMPTOMS
- Nausea/vomiting
- Anorexia
- Headache
- Fatigue
- Confusion
- Hallucinations
- Visual blurring, scotomata, xanthopsia, chromatopsia (altered color perception)

SIGNS
- Delirium
- CNS depression
- Hypotension
- Bradyarrhythmias (e.g., sinus arrest, AV blocks)

- Tachyarrhythmias (e.g., premature ventricular contractions, paroxysmal atrial tachycardia, accelerated junctional tachycardia, VT, VF)
- Sagging (scooped-out) ST depression with a short QT interval
- Combination of supraventricular tachycardia with AV block or bidirectional VT is highly suggestive of cardiac glycoside toxicity

WORKUP

- Serum studies should include electrolytes, BUN/creatinine, and digoxin level.
- An ECG should be obtained.
- In the *acute* overdose setting, the serum K^+ concentration is indicative of the magnitude of the Na^+,K^+-ATPase inhibition and correlates closely with mortality without antidotal treatment. For example, a serum K^+ >5.0 mEq/L is associated with a 50% mortality rate without antidotal treatment.

COMMENTS AND TREATMENT CONSIDERATIONS

AC is the preferred method of GI decontamination.

Calcium salt administration is relatively contraindicated in the setting of known or suspected cardiac glycoside toxicity. Exogenous calcium salt administration to treat associated or coexisting hyperkalemia may potentiate the cardiac toxicity from cardiac glycosides.

For hemodynamically stable patients with mildly elevated digoxin levels who are free of significant arrhythmias, treatment should consist of holding further doses of digoxin and observing the patient in a closely monitored setting.

The treatment of choice for life-threatening digoxin toxicity is the administration of digoxin-specific polyclonal antibody (Fab) fragments (Digibind). These fragments bind to and neutralize digoxin directly. Fab fragments reverse the tissue binding of digoxin and increase the speed of the digoxin excretion. The indications for Digibind administration include (1) any immediately life-threatening tachyarrhythmia, bradyarrhythmias, or conduction disturbance; (2) serum K^+ concentration >5.0 mEq/L in the setting of *acute* poisoning; (3) ingestion of >10 mg of digoxin in an adult or >4 mg in a child; and (4) serum digoxin level >10 ng/ml at any time. Monitored serum digoxin levels after the administration of Digibind are not accurate and erroneously high unless the assay is performed on an ultrafiltrate of serum. If given, the total dose should be infused over 15 to 30 minutes, with clinical improvement noted from 20 to 60 minutes later. See Table 37–2 to calculate needed dose. In general, 1 to 3 vials are often sufficient to treat chronic digoxin toxicity, whereas 10 to 20 vials may be necessary to treat acute poisoning.

Alternative or adjunctive treatments for ventricular arrhythmias include lidocaine, phenytoin, and magnesium. Alternative treatments for bradyarrhythmias include atropine and catecholamine pressors. The use of electrical pacing for bradyarrhythmias is not recommended over Fab fragment therapy for it may precipitate malignant ventricular arrhythmias. Electrical cardioversion for ventricular arrhythmias is not recommended over Fab fragment therapy. If necessary, electrical cardioversion should be performed at the lowest effective energy level.

 LITHIUM

Lithium is an alkali metal that interferes with endogenous cations during transmembrane ion transport, thus altering excitability of various tissues. Lithium also interferes with adenylate cyclase, Na^+,K^+-ATPase, and biogenic amine (norepinephrine and serotonin) release.

SYMPTOMS
- Mild or early: nausea, vomiting, and diarrhea
- Moderate or intermediate: agitation, confusion, lethargy, slurred speech
- Severe or late: marked confusion, coma, seizures

SIGNS
- Mild or early: dysarthria, ataxia, tremor, muscle weakness, hyperreflexia
- Moderate or intermediate: confusion, agitation, hypertonia, myoclonus, fasciculations, bradycardia or tachycardia
- Severe or late: coma, choreoathetosis, seizures, muscle rigidity, hyperthermia, hypotension, cardiovascular collapse

WORKUP
- Lithium level, electrolytes, BUN/creatinine, and ECG
- Abnormal laboratory parameters include leukocytosis, hyperglycemia, albuminuria, glucosuria, nephrogenic diabetes insipidus, elevated creatinine from acute renal failure, and elevated serum chloride (falsely low anion gap).
- ECG changes include sinus bradycardia, flattened or inverted T waves, AV block, and a prolonged QT interval.
- Lithium level, in conjunction with history (acute or chronic ingestion) and neurologic examination (e.g., mental status, neuromuscular examination), is used to determine severity of poisoning and appropriate treatment strategy.

COMMENTS AND TREATMENT CONSIDERATIONS
GI decontamination may necessitate WBI following ingestion of sustained-release preparations. AC does not adsorb lithium.

CHAPTER 37

The oral administration of the ion-exchange resin Kayexalate is unproven as treatment to prevent the GI absorption of lithium.

Treatment involves restoration of sodium and water balance (rehydration with intravenous normal saline in dehydrated patients) and hemodialysis for those with severe poisoning. Hemodialysis is recommended for patients with coma, seizures, persistent confusion, and acute renal failure.

 ## SALICYLATES

Salicylates are a common cause of poisoning in the United States. Salicylates are readily available in OTC products such as aspirin, Pepto-Bismol (bismuth subsalicylate), Ben-Gay, and oil of wintergreen (methyl salicylate). Salicylate poisoning is frequently misdiagnosed, particularly when chronic poisoning exists. Symptoms or signs, especially in chronic salicylate intoxication, are often nonspecific, and erroneous diagnoses such as sepsis, altered mental status, gastroenteritis, or CHF sometimes occur.

SYMPTOMS
- Mild or early poisoning (1 to 2 hours after acute ingestion): nausea, vomiting, abdominal pain, headache, tinnitus, dizziness, and fatigue
- Moderate or intermediate poisoning (12 to 24 hours after acute ingestion): fever, sweating, deafness, lethargy, confusion, hallucinations, breathlessness
- Severe or late poisoning (more than 24 hours after acute ingestion or unrecognized, untreated chronic ingestion): coma, seizures, fever

SIGNS
- Mild or early: lethargy, ataxia, mild agitation, hyperpnea, mild abdominal tenderness
- Moderate or intermediate: fever, asterixis, diaphoresis, deafness, pallor, confusion, slurred speech, disorientation, agitation, hallucinations, tachycardia, tachypnea, orthostatic hypotension
- Severe or late: dehydration, coma, seizures, hypothermia, hyperthermia, tachycardia, hypotension, respiratory depression, pulmonary edema, arrhythmias, papilledema

WORKUP
- Obtain electrolytes, glucose, BUN/creatinine, urinalysis (particularly urine pH), ABG, salicylate level, LFT, CBC, PT/INR, and calcium for severe poisoning.
- Acid-base disturbances: respiratory alkalosis (mild or early poisoning), respiratory alkalosis with metabolic acidosis (moderate or intermediate poisoning), and metabolic acidosis with or without

respiratory acidosis (severe or late poisoning). Children younger than 4 years tend to have a more prominent metabolic component; older children and adults tend to have a predominant respiratory component.

- Serum salicylate concentration, in conjunction with history (acute or chronic ingestion) and severity and phase of poisoning, determines appropriate treatment strategy.

COMMENTS AND TREATMENT CONSIDERATIONS

Treatment consists of GI decontamination (multidose AC); correction of acid-base, fluid, and electrolyte disturbances; and enhanced elimination with serum alkalinization (see Table 37–3). Alkalinization of the urine is indicated for symptomatic patients or those with serum salicylate concentrations >30 mg/dl (see Table 37–3). Hemodialysis is indicated for those with severe toxicity (salicylate concentration >100mg/dl in acute intoxication and >60 mg/dl in chronic intoxication, altered mental status, refractory acid-base disturbances, and deterioration despite maximal supportive care).

Noncardiogenic pulmonary edema is more common in chronic salicylate intoxication than acute intoxication. Severe chronic salicylate intoxication occurs at lower plasma salicylate levels than acute intoxication, and clinical features correlate poorly with serum concentrations. Supportive therapy and urinary alkalinization are the same as for acute toxicity, but the extracorporeal techniques to enhance elimination should be instituted at lower serum concentrations than in acute intoxication.

TOXIC ALCOHOLS (ETHYLENE GLYCOL, METHANOL, AND ISOPROPANOL)

Poisonings by ethylene glycol and methanol cause significant morbidity and mortality. Patients require early diagnosis and treatment to prevent accumulation of their toxic acid metabolites and subsequent development of profound metabolic acidosis and end-organ complications. Ethylene glycol is commonly found in antifreeze, coolants, and glass cleaners. Common sources of methanol include antifreeze, windshield washer fluid, Sterno and related fuels, and contaminated moonshine. Isopropyl alcohol is found in rubbing alcohol and glass cleaners and is generally less toxic. Toxicity results predominantly from ingestion. Isopropyl alcohol intoxication has occurred in pediatric patients given isopropanol sponge baths; it is unclear whether poisoning resulted from transdermal absorption or inhalation in these cases.

SYMPTOMS

- Early (1 to 12 hours): anorexia, nausea, vomiting, abdominal pain, headache, vertigo, weakness, lethargy, and coma

531

- Late (6 to 36 hours): progressive visual disturbances (e.g., blurred vision, diplopia, scotoma, "snowfields," tunnel vision, blindness), shortness of breath, confusion, lethargy, seizures, coma, hematemesis, flank pain

SIGNS
- Early: CNS inebriation (e.g., slurred speech, nystagmus, lethargy, coma, ataxia)
- Late: progressive visual field and acuity deficits, optic disc hyperemia, papilledema, mydriasis nonreactive to light, confusion, agitation, delirium, coma, myoclonus, tetany, seizures, tachypnea, hyperpnea, ketotic breath, sinus tachycardia, hypertension or hypotension

WORKUP
- Serum electrolytes (to determine anion gap), BUN/creatinine, glucose, amylase, calcium, ketones, osmolality, lactate, ABG, urinalysis
- Serum concentration of solvents (e.g., ethanol, ethylene glycol, isopropanol, and methanol)
- Calculate the osmolar gap.
  Osmolar gap = [measured serum osmolality] – [calculated serum osmolality]
  Calculated serum osmolality = $2(Na^+)$ + (glucose/18) + (BUN/2.8) + (EtOH/4.6) + (MeOH/3.2) + (EtGly/6.2) + (Iso/6), where sodium is measured in mEq/L and all other variables are measured in mg/dl:
  Early: Elevated osmolal gap without anion gap (common)
  Late: Elevated anion gap with or without elevated osmolal gap (common)
  Normal osmolal gap (early or late) does not exclude toxic alcohol poisoning
- Ketosis (serum and urinary acetone) without acidosis is commonly seen in isopropanol poisoning.
- Elevated serum creatinine with normal BUN is a clue to isopropyl alcohol poisoning. This artifactual elevation of serum creatinine is due to interference of acetone with colorimetric creatinine autoanalyzers.
- Serum hypocalcemia, urinary calcium oxalate crystals, acute tubular necrosis (microscopic hematuria, proteinuria, oliguria), elevated BUN/creatinine, bronchopneumonia on chest x-ray, and cerebral edema demonstrated by head CT may be seen in ethylene glycol poisoning.

COMMENTS AND TREATMENT CONSIDERATIONS
Conventional treatment of ethylene glycol and methanol poisoning includes sodium bicarbonate administration for metabolic acidosis, ethanol or fomepizole (4-MP) infusion to inhibit metabolism to

toxic acid metabolites (see Table 37–2 for dosing), vitamin administration to enhance metabolite elimination, and hemodialysis to remove rapidly toxic alcohol and its metabolites. For methanol, the vitamins administered are folinic acid followed by folate to assist the conversion of formic acid to carbon dioxide and water. For ethylene glycol, the vitamins administered are thiamine with magnesium and pyridoxine administration to assist in the conversion of glyoxylic acid into alpha-keto-beta-hydroxyadipate and glycine, respectively.

Fomepizole or ethanol therapy is indicated for those with suspected ingestion by history or laboratory data (e.g., ethylene glycol or methanol levels >20 mg/dl or osmolal gap >10 mOsm/L). Hemodialysis is typically recommended for those with (1) ethylene glycol or methanol concentrations >50 mg/dl, (2) pH <7.20, or (3) significant end-organ toxicity (e.g., renal insufficiency, visual impairment, or seizures). Fomepizole, although more expensive per dose than ethanol, may be more cost effective. Fomepizole is easier to administer and does not require frequent serum ethanol and glucose concentrations as are needed with ethanol therapy. Unlike ethanol therapy, fomepizole therapy does not cause CNS depression, pancreatitis, gastritis, or habituation.

The treatment for isopropyl alcohol intoxication is supportive. Hemodialysis has been recommended for patients with hypotension or serum concentrations >400 mg/dl.

REFERENCES

American Academy of Clinical Toxicology, European Association of Poison Centers and Clinical Toxicologists: Position statements, *J Toxicol Clin Toxicol* 35:695, 1997.

American Academy of Clinical Toxicology: Position paper: whole bowel irrigation, *J Toxicol Clin Toxicol* 42:843, 2004.

American Academy of Clinical Toxicology. Position paper: ipecac syrup, *J Toxicol Clin Toxicol* 42:133, 2004.

American Academy of Pediatrics: Policy statement, poison treatment in the home, *Pediatrics* 112:1182, 2003.

Barceloux DG, Bond GR, Krenzelok EP, et al: American Academy of Clinical Toxicology practice guidelines on the treatment of methanol poisoning, *J Toxicol Clin Toxicol* 40:415, 2002.

Barceloux DG, Krenzelok EP, Olson K, et al: American Academy of Clinical Toxicology practice guidelines on the treatment of ethylene glycol poisoning. Ad hoc committee, *J Toxicol Clin Toxicol* 37:537, 1999.

Boyer WE, Shannon M: Treatment of calcium-channel-blocker intoxication with insulin infusion, *N Engl J Med* 344:1721, 2001.

Brent J, McMartin K, Phillips S, et al: Fomepizole for the treatment of ethylene glycol poisoning, *N Engl J Med* 340:832, 1999.

Burns MJ, Linden CH: Insulin for beta-blocker toxicity, *Ann Emerg Med* 30:11, 1997.

Cox RD, Phillips WJ: Ethylene glycol toxicity, *Mil Med* 169:660, 2004.

Goodman LS. Digitalis. In: Haddad LM, Shannon MW, Winchester JF (eds): *Clinical management of poisoning and drug overdose*, ed 3. Philadelphia, 1998, WB Saunders, pp 1001-1020.

Hoffman RS, Goldfrank LR: The poisoned patient with altered consciousness: controversies in the use of a "coma cocktail," *JAMA* 274:562, 1995.

Kerns W 2nd, Schroeder D, Williams C, et al: Insulin improves survival in a canine model of acute beta-blocker toxicity, *Ann Emerg Med* 29:748, 1997.

Krenzelok EP, Kerr F, Proudfoot AT: Salicylate toxicity. In: Haddad LM, Shannon MW, Winchester JF (eds): *Clinical management of poisoning and drug overdose*, ed 3. Philadelphia, 1998, WB Saunders, pp 675-687.

Marques I, Gomes E, de Oliveria J: Treatment of calcium channel blocker intoxication with insulin infusion: case report and literature review, *Resuscitation* 57:211, 2003.

Mycyk MB, Leikin JB: Antidote review: fomepizole for methanol poisoning, *Am J Ther* 10:68, 2003.

Pearigen PD: Calcium channel blocker poisoning. In: Haddad LM, Shannon MW, Winchester JF (eds): *Clinical management of poisoning and drug overdose*, ed 3. Philadelphia, 1998, WB Saunders, pp 1020-1031.

Perry H, Shannon MW. Acetaminophen. In: Haddad LM, Shannon MW, Winchester JF (eds): *Clinical management of poisoning and drug overdose*, ed 3. Philadelphia, 1998, WB Saunders, pp 664-674.

Rumack BH, Matthew H: Acetaminophen poisoning and toxicity, *Pediatrics* 55:871, 1975.

Salhanick SD, Shannon MW: Management of calcium channel antagonist overdose, *Drug Saf* 26:65, 2003.

Scheinkestel CD, Bailey M, Myles PS, et al: Hyperbaric or normobaric oxygen for acute carbon monoxide poisoning: a randomized controlled clinical trial, *Med J Aust* 170:203, 1999.

Watson WA, Litovitz TL, Klein-Schwartz W, et al: 2003 annual report of the American Association for Poison Control Centers Toxic Exposure Surveillance System, *Am J Emerg Med* 22:335, 2004.

Weaver LK, Hopkins RO, Chan KJ, et al: Hyperbaric oxygen for acute carbon monoxide poisoning, *N Engl J Med* 347:1057, 2002.

Wolf LR. Beta adrenergic blocker toxicity. In: Haddad LM, Shannon MW, Winchester JF (eds): *Clinical management of poisoning and drug overdose*, ed 3. Philadelphia, 1998, WB Saunders, pp 1031-1040.

Yuan TH, Kerns WP, Tomaszewski CA, et al: Insulin-glucose as adjunctive therapy for severe calcium channel antagonist poisoning, *Clin Toxicol* 37:463, 1999.

CHAPTER 38

Transplant Patient, Approach to
Zachary A. Gray

The rising incidence of organ transplantation ensures that emergency physicians will increasingly be required to evaluate and treat post-transplant patients. The spectrum of disease specific to these patients includes technical surgical complications, infection, rejection, graft failure, and medication toxicity. In addition, chronically immune-suppressed patients pose a challenge because those with serious underlying pathology often present with subtle signs and symptoms. One study of 290 emergency department (ED) visits by liver transplant patients found that of those later diagnosed with serious infections, 51% were afebrile at presentation and 71% had normal or low white blood cell counts. The potential for serious illness with often minimal and nonspecific manifestations necessitates a low threshold for comprehensive diagnostic testing, early consultation with the patient's transplant physician, and frequently empirical therapy. It is also important to recognize that transplant patients often have multiple, coexistent, and interdependent pathologic processes contributing to their clinical condition.

REFERENCES
Savitsky EA, Votey SR, McCain S, et al: A descriptive analysis of 290 liver transplant patient visits to an emergency department, Acad Emerg Med 7:898, 2000.

INFECTION IN THE TRANSPLANT PATIENT
The infections transplant patients experience vary with the time since transplantation. There are three distinct periods: the first post-transplantation month, months 2 to 6, and after 6 months (Table 38–1). It is important to recognize that this framework applies when graft rejection does not preclude the normal tapering of immunosuppressives.

TABLE 38-1
TIMING OF INFECTIONS IN ORGAN TRANSPLANT PATIENTS

	VIRAL	FUNGAL	BACTERIAL	MYCOBACTERIAL	PARASITIC
0–1 month	HSV, HBV, HCV	*Aspergillus*, routine postoperative fungal infections	Routine postoperative bacterial infections, drug-resistant nosocomial bacteria		
1–6 months	CMV, EBV, HSV, VZV, RSV, influenza	*Aspergillus*, *Pneumocystis*, *Cryptococcus*	*Listeria*, *Nocardia*	*M. tuberculosis, M. avium*	*Toxoplasma*, *Strongyloides*
6+ months	CMV (retinitis, colitis), HPV	Geographically restricted endemic fungi			

CHAPTER **38**

Infection in the First Month

Although opportunistic infections related to the intense immunosuppression of the early post-transplantation period do occur, routine postoperative infections are more common. Organisms are typically bacterial or candidal and involve the surgical site, the graft itself, the lungs, the urinary tract, and indwelling vascular catheters. They are managed in the usual fashion, with the caveat that these highly immune-suppressed patients may initially present with minimal symptoms despite having overwhelming and rapidly progressive infections. In addition to severe septic shock and associated graft failure, such early disseminated infections in transplant patients can result in mycotic aneurysms at sites of vascular anastomosis that can precipitously rupture. Fortunately, such early, aggressive infections are rarely encountered in the ED. A thorough inquiry into the postoperative course, especially when evidence of acute graft failure is present, may enable the emergency physician to identify those at risk. Of particular importance in this period is invasive aspergillosis, which carries a mortality rate approaching 90% and peaks in incidence toward the end of the first post-transplantation month. Risk factors for *Aspergillus* disease include poor graft function and hemodialysis use.

Infection in Months 2 to 6

Opportunistic infections are the principal concern during this period, with cytomegalovirus (CMV) being particularly important. Disease may result from primary infection of the recipient by an infected allograft or from reactivation of prior infection because of immune suppression. CMV infection may present as *CMV disease* (characterized by fever, myalgias, elevated transaminase levels, and pancytopenia) or it may manifest as *tissue-invasive CMV disease* affecting the pulmonary, gastrointestinal, or central nervous system. Epstein-Barr virus (EBV) is another important viral pathogen. Both CMV and EBV disease are thought to cause immune dysregulation, which further predisposes the patient to opportunistic infection and rejection. Other important opportunistic pathogens may be bacterial (*Nocardia* and *Listeria*), fungal (*Aspergillus*, *Pneumocystis carinii*, *Cryptococcus*, and *Candida*), mycobacterial (*M. tuberculosis* and *M. avium complex*), or parasitic (*Toxoplasma* and *Strongyloides*). The respiratory tract is the most common site of infection, but any organ system—especially that involving the allograft—may be affected.

Infections after the First 6 Months

The risk of serious opportunistic infection returns to near-normal levels as immune-suppressive regimens are gradually tapered. Patients who experience problems with rejection requiring prolongation of higher dose immunosuppressives remain at increased risk. In addition, transplant patients remain at a significantly higher risk for nosocomial infections such as *Pseudomonas*, methicillin-resistant *Staphylococcus aureus*, and vancomycin-resistant enterococci.

SYMPTOMS

- Up to half of transplant patients with serious infections are afebrile at presentation.
- Many patients have only nonspecific symptoms such as lethargy, nausea, or anorexia.

WORKUP

- Transplant patients evaluated during the first 6 post-transplantation months require a thorough search for an underlying infectious process unless a definitive alternative diagnosis is present.
- Workup for infection should include symptom-based studies such as urinalysis, chest radiography, and computed tomography of the chest, abdomen, or pelvis as indicated.
- In addition to bacterial and fungal cultures of blood and urine, cultures of cerebrospinal fluid, T-tube drainage, indwelling vascular catheters, and the surgical site should be obtained when clinically warranted.
- Other considerations include viral cultures and serum titers for CMV, EBV, and HSV.

COMMENTS AND TREATMENT CONSIDERATIONS

After cultures of blood, urine, and other sites as indicated, empirical treatment should include broad-spectrum antibiotics with coverage of gram-positive organisms, gram-negative organisms (including *Pseudomonas*), and anaerobic organisms. In clinically stable patients, monotherapy with carbapenems, extended-spectrum penicillins (piperacillin/tazobactam), or selected third-generation cephalosporins (ceftazidime, cefepime) is appropriate. Acutely ill patients require combination therapy with double coverage for gram-negative organisms including *Pseudomonas*. Those with indwelling vascular catheters require enhanced gram-positive coverage such as vancomycin or oxacillin. Patients in the first 6 post-transplantation months or those with signs of active CMV disease should be considered for empirical treatment with ganciclovir. Given its potential for toxicity, empirical antifungal therapy is not routinely indicated in the ED. Empirical antibiotic choices should be modified in accordance with known institutional patterns of microbial resistance. Immunosuppressed transplant patients with possible infection require admission for further observation and treatment.

CHAPTER 38

REFERENCES

Fishman JA, Rubin RH: Infections in organ-transplant recipients, *N Engl J Med* 338:1741, 1998.

Pizzo PA: Fever in immunocompromised patients, *N Engl J Med* 341:893, 1999.

MEDICATION TOXICITY

Corticosteroids

Transplant patients experience risks similar to those of others using corticosteroids in moderate to high doses for extended periods of time. Complications include adrenal insufficiency, immunosuppression, diabetes, osteopenia, avascular necrosis of the femoral head, and steroid psychosis. Of note are the distinct patterns of skeletal disease. Up to 38% of liver transplant patients experience a vertebral compression fracture. In renal transplant patients, the bones of the feet are at increased risk of fracture. Bone scan or MRI may be required to diagnose insufficiency fractures in renal transplant patients with unexplained foot pain. Early consideration of the need for stress-dose steroids (hydrocortisone 100 mg IV) in the critically ill transplant patient can be lifesaving.

Nephrotoxicity Caused by Immunosuppressants

Cyclosporine (Sandimmune), tacrolimus (FK-506, Prograf), and sirolimus (Rapamune) may cause dose-dependent nephrotoxicity. Nephrotoxicity typically occurs in the setting of elevated drug levels but can occur at therapeutic levels. Meaningful levels are trough levels measured prior to a scheduled dose. Many routinely used medications have the potential to elevate serum levels of immunosuppressives (Table 38–2). Avoidance of medications known to affect immunosuppressive levels and nephrotoxic agents (e.g., aminoglycosides, amphotericin) is prudent. Prompt consultation with the transplant physician is indicated when drug-induced nephrotoxicity is suspected. Withdrawal of the offending agent may result in recovery of baseline renal function. Any change in dosage of these medications must be made in consultation with the transplant physician.

Other Toxic Effects of Immunosuppressants

Cyclosporine and azathioprine (Imuran) can cause reversible hepatotoxicity. Azathioprine is also a potent inhibitor of lymphocyte proliferation and may cause dose-related bone marrow suppression with resultant leukopenia and thrombocytopenia. OKT3 (muromonab-CD3) is a monoclonal antibody that suppresses T cells and may cause bronchospasm, pulmonary edema, and an aseptic meningitis syndrome. Virtually all of the immunosuppressives, with the exception of azathioprine, are also known to cause

TABLE 38–2
CLINICALLY SIGNIFICANT IMMUNOSUPPRESSIVE DRUG INTERACTIONS

IMMUNOSUPPRESSIVE	INTERACTING DRUG	ADVERSE EFFECT
Cyclosporine, tacrolimus, or sirolimus	Diltiazem, verapamil, amiodarone, azole antifungals, and macrolide antibiotics	Nephrotoxicity caused by increased immunosuppressive blood levels
Cyclosporine or tacrolimus	Aminoglycosides, amphotericin B, and iodinated contrast material	Increased risk of nephrotoxicity without change in blood level
Cyclosporine, tacrolimus, or sirolimus	Phenobarbital, phenytoin, carbamazepine, rifampin, and isoniazid	Increased rejection risk caused by lowered immunosuppressive blood levels

a variety of neurologic and gastrointestinal side effects including seizures, altered mentation, headache, paresthesias, nausea, vomiting, and diarrhea. These effects may be significant enough to limit compliance.

REFERENCES

Haagsma EB, Thijn CJP, Post JG, et al: Bone disease after orthotopic liver transplantation, *J Hepatol* 6:94, 1988.

Savitsky EA, Üner AB, Votey SR: Evaluation of orthotopic liver transplant recipients presenting to the emergency department, *Ann Emerg Med* 31:507, 1998.

Venkat KK, Venkat A: Care of the renal transplant recipient in the emergency department, *Ann Emerg Med* 44:330, 2004.

THE LIVER TRANSPLANT PATIENT

The Organ Procurement and Transplantation Network (OPTN) reported that 68,000 orthotopic liver transplantations (OLTs) have been performed in the United States since 1988, with more than 5000 each year since 2000. Infection, graft failure, vascular complications, biliary complications, rejection, and medication toxicity are all common causes of ED visits by OLT patients. A high index of suspicion for serious illness is necessary because OLT patients often present early in the course of their illness with relatively nonspecific symptoms. In a study of 321 consecutive OLT patients' deaths, infection (64%), liver failure (12%), pulmonary failure (10%), multiorgan system failure (8%), and cardiovascular disease (6%) were determined to be responsible at autopsy.

GRAFT FAILURE

Failure of allograft function may be usefully divided into failure that occurs in the first post-transplantation year and that which occurs later. Early graft failure is responsible for 75% of allograft failure; late graft failure is responsible for the remaining 25%. Causes of early graft failure include primary graft failure (39%), ischemic graft failure with or without overt vascular injury (47%), and acute rejection (14%). Primary graft failure is an idiopathic condition affecting transplant patients in the first post-transplantation week that is thought to be related to graft ischemia time and reperfusion injury. Early graft failure is characterized by profound hypoglycemia, coagulopathy, metabolic acidosis, and progressive encephalopathy. These patients can deteriorate rapidly. Late graft failure is typically the result of chronic rejection (48%), recurrence of primary liver disease (30%), or other miscellaneous causes (22%).

SYMPTOMS
- Fatigue
- Jaundice, pruritus, dark urine, clay-colored stools
- Nausea, vomiting, abdominal pain
- Decreased T-tube output
- Confusion

SIGNS
- Jaundice
- Petechiae, ecchymosis
- Abdominal tenderness
- Peripheral edema, anasarca
- GI bleeding, hypotension
- Altered mental status, commonly from hypoglycemia or hepatic encephalopathy

WORKUP
- Bedside glucose testing is mandatory in the setting of AMS to exclude hypoglycemia.
- CBC with WBC differential may be helpful but is not sensitive for infection.
- Serum chemistry, with particular attention to creatinine, bicarbonate, and glucose
- PT/INR to assess hepatic synthetic function and need for fresh frozen plasma (FFP)
- AST, ALT, total and conjugated (direct) bilirubin are useful as markers of severity of acute liver injury.
- Type and screen (include crossmatch in the patient with hypotension or obvious bleeding)

- If infection is suspected, chest x-ray and urinalysis should be obtained, along with cultures of blood, urine, wound drainage, and T-tube output where appropriate.
- In the setting of early graft failure, prompt imaging of the graft is required to discover reversible vascular complications. Institutional practices vary, but both duplex ultrasound and helical CT have reported sensitivities above 90%. Angiography may be required in equivocal cases.

COMMENTS AND TREATMENT CONSIDERATIONS

Diagnosis and treatment should focus on supportive care and prompt discovery of reversible conditions. Hypoglycemia, shock secondary to hemorrhage, severe coagulopathy, and sepsis are conditions with specific treatments that complicate acute graft failure. Acute graft failure necessitates early consultation with the transplant service and admission, generally to a monitored bed. The majority of patients with evidence of new or worsening chronic rejection also require admission.

- Prompt intravenous dextrose for hypoglycemia. A continuous infusion of dextrose is typically required.
- Early insertion of two large-bore IV catheters in the potentially unstable patient
- Fresh Frozen Plasma (FFP) is often required for severe coagulopathy and/or active bleeding. Appropriate dosing is 15 to 30 ml/kg (size of "unit" varies between 200 and 400 ml; consult your blood bank).
- Prompt replacement of blood loss by transfusion is required to minimize ischemic damage to the vulnerable graft and prevent multiorgan system failure.

 VASCULAR EMERGENCIES

Structural vascular complications are an important cause of early graft failure, accounting for 10% of graft failure in adults and 30% in children and infants. These include hepatic artery thrombosis (HAT), portal vein thrombosis (PVT), and hepatic artery rupture. HAT and PVT tend to occur early in the post-transplantation period, usually within the first month. They may also occur later as a result of rejection. Both present with evidence of graft failure. It is important to recognize that these descriptions of the common vascular complications in OLT patients represent a simplification of a complex spectrum of disease. Emergency physicians should maintain a high index of suspicion for vascular complications in the early post-transplantation period.

SYMPTOMS

- HAT is characterized by abrupt onset of symptoms and rapid development of life-threatening illness.

CHAPTER 38

543

- PVT follows a more indolent course.
- Patients with hepatic artery rupture usually present in hypovolemic shock, often preceded by a varying interval of abdominal symptoms. Abrupt onset of shock, abdominal pain, peritonitis, and increased abdominal girth suggest hepatic artery rupture.

WORKUP
- Early diagnostic imaging with either duplex ultrasound or helical CT with intravenous contrast
- Typically the workup outlined for graft failure is undertaken simultaneously.

COMMENTS AND TREATMENT CONSIDERATIONS
Treatment of acute vascular complications in the OLT patient is often surgical, and early consultation with the liver transplant service is appropriate. When HAT is suspected, early coordination with interventional radiology is advised because emergent angiography and vascular intervention may be required to restore hepatic artery flow. When hepatic artery rupture is suspected, early communication with blood bank personnel is essential as transfusion requirements can be large.

 BILIARY COMPLICATIONS

Biliary complications, typically bile leak or obstruction to flow, occur in roughly one quarter of OLT patients. Bile leaks are often complicated by peritonitis, which may be chemical or infectious. Infections are often polymicrobial and usually involve typical biliary tract pathogens (*Enterobacter*, *Enterococcus*, *Bacteroides*, and *Clostridium* species). Abscess formation is common. Biliary obstruction may be caused by stent malfunction, stent dislocation, sludging with stone formation, or biliary stricture. Biliary obstruction typically presents with jaundice, bilirubinemia, and varying degrees of abdominal pain.

WORKUP
- Ultrasound or CT scan, especially when abscess is suspected
- Definitive diagnosis usually requires cholangiography.
- Routine laboratory tests should include CBC, LFTs, PT, and serum electrolytes, BUN, and creatinine.
- Febrile patients should undergo infection workup.

COMMENTS AND TREATMENT CONSIDERATIONS
Early bile leaks often result in more severe illness and often require surgical intervention. Empirical therapy for peritonitis should be

broad spectrum including coverage for gram-positive, gram-negative (including *Pseudomonas*), and anaerobic organisms. Biliary complications can often be managed by endoscopic retrograde cholangiopancreatography (ERCP) with stenting or balloon dilatation. Consultation with the transplant surgery service and admission is necessary.

REJECTION IN THE LIVER TRANSPLANT PATIENT

Immune-mediated injury to a transplanted organ may be classified as hyperacute, acute, and chronic. In OLT patients, only acute rejection and chronic rejection occur with any frequency. Acute and chronic rejections have similar clinical features, with chronic rejection being distinguished by a more gradual and prolonged deterioration. OLT patients with chronic rejection typically have persistently elevated LFTs and progressively declining liver function. Although the timing and histology of these two processes differ, it is important to recognize that they probably represent opposite ends of a more continuous spectrum of graft dysfunction. Between 60% and 80% of patients experience at least one episode of acute rejection and chronic rejection develops in approximately 5% to 9%.

CHAPTER 38

SYMPTOMS
- Malaise
- General weakness
- Progressive jaundice, pruritus, clay-colored stools, dark urine
- Abdominal pain
- Fever

SIGNS
- Jaundice
- Right upper quadrant tenderness
- Fever

WORKUP
- Alkaline phosphatase, AST, ALT. Initial elevation of the alkaline phosphatase and bilirubin followed by a rise in AST and ALT is characteristic of but not specific for rejection.
- PT and serum albumin serve as important markers of synthetic function.
- Definitive diagnosis is made by liver biopsy.
- Patients with fever require simultaneous evaluation for infection.

COMMENTS AND TREATMENT CONSIDERATIONS

Treatment of rejection is with high-dose intravenous methylprednisolone. Given the need for biopsy to confirm the diagnosis, this therapy is rarely instituted in the ED. Acute rejection has a favorable prognosis, with up to 85% of patients recovering with functional grafts. Chronic rejection is less responsive to immunosuppressive therapy and often necessitates retransplantation. It is important to continue to consider infection and other complications in cases of suspected rejection because multiple complications may coexist.

REFERENCES

Eckhoff DE, D'Alessandro AM, Knechtle SJ, et al: 100 consecutive liver transplants in infants and children: an 8 year experience, *J Pediatr Surg* 213:48, 1991.

Legmann P, Costes V, Tudoret L, et al: Hepatic artery thrombosis after liver transplantation: diagnosis with spiral CT, *AJR Am J Roentgenol* 164:97, 1995.

Lopez RR, Benner KG, Ivancev K, et al: Management of biliary complications after liver transplantation, *Am J Surg* 163:519, 1991.

Lowes JR, Hubscher SG, Neuberger JM, et al: Chronic rejection of the live allograft, *Gastroenterol Clin North Am* 22:401, 1993.

O'Shaughnessy DF, Atterbury C, Williamson LM, et al: Guidelines for the use of fresh-frozen plasma, cryoprecipitate and cryosupernatant, *Br J Haematol* 126:11, 2004.

Pinson CW, Lopez RR, Brenner KG, et al: Initial two year results of the Oregon liver transplant program, *Am J Surg* 161:606, 1991.

Quiroga J, Colina I, Demetris AJ, et al: Cause and timing of first allograft failure in orthotopic liver transplantation: a study of 177 consecutive patients, *Hepatology* 14:1054, 1991.

Savitsky EA, Üner AB, Votey SR: Evaluation of orthotopic liver transplant recipients presenting to the emergency department, *Ann Emerg Med* 31:507, 1998.

Shaw BW, Gordon RD, Iwatsuki S, et al: Hepatic retransplantation, *Transplant Proc* 17:264, 1985.

The Organ Procurement and Transplantation Network Website: www.optn.org.

Torbenson M, Wang J, Nalesnik MA, et al: Causes of death in autopsied liver transplantation patients, *Mod Pathol* 11:37, 1998.

THE RENAL TRANSPLANT PATIENT

The prevalence of end-stage renal failure and the relative success of cadaveric renal transplantation have made renal transplantation the most common transplant procedure in the United States. OPTN documented almost 200,000 renal transplants performed in the United States since 1988, with 14,633 in 2004 alone. In general, the transplanted kidney is placed in the right or left lower quadrant of the abdomen. Arterial supply is obtained from the internal or external iliac artery with venous drainage to the internal or external iliac vein. The donor ureter is typically attached directly to the host bladder.

 VASCULAR COMPLICATIONS

Anastomotic thrombosis and hemorrhage are the most frequent vascular complications in the renal transplant patient. Thrombosis may result from an underlying hypercoagulable state or an anatomic cause such as vascular compression by an external structure or renal artery dissection. External compression by abscess, hematoma, or urinary leak may also cause compromise of the vascular supply and subsequent allograft failure. In addition to acute vascular occlusion, chronic rejection can produce progressive renal artery stenosis leading to secondary hypertension and renal failure.

Acute Vascular Occlusion

Thrombosis or failure of the anastomosis causing acute occlusion of the transplant renal artery or vein is rare (incidence <1%) and most often occurs in the first post-transplantation week. It should be suspected in the recent transplant patient who presents with oliguria or anuria and acute renal failure. Doppler ultrasonography is the study of choice to demonstrate lack of vascular flow. ED management consists of urinary catheterization to assess renal function, measurement of BUN/creatinine, prompt imaging, and early contact with the transplant surgeon. Although prompt surgical exploration may result in salvage in a minority of cases, the overall prognosis for the graft is poor. Case reports and small series suggest a possible role for intra-arterial fibrinolytic administration in some patients.

CHAPTER 38

Peritransplantation Hemorrhage

Serious perioperative bleeding in the renal transplant patient has an incidence of approximately 2% to 3% and is typically the result of failure of one of the vascular anastomoses. The clinical presentation is one of severe pain over the allograft, anemia, and worsening renal failure. Hypovolemic shock may develop rapidly in the setting of active arterial bleeding. ED management consists of fluid resuscitation and transfusion as indicated, catheterization to monitor urinary output, CT imaging to identify the source of bleeding, and early consultation with the transplant surgeon. Immediate surgery is indicated as soon as the diagnosis is made. Although some allografts can be salvaged with timely surgical repair, nephrectomy is usually required.

OTHER SURGICAL COMPLICATIONS

Urinary leak, lymphocele, and obstructive uropathy are the most common noninfectious urinary complications encountered in the renal transplant patient. Lymphocele is one of the more common postsurgical complications in the renal transplant patient.

Urinary Leak

Failure of the ureteral anastomosis leads to collection of urine outside the urinary tract. This collection can compress the ureter, causing urinary obstruction, or the renal vasculature, compromising perfusion. Patients with urinary leak typically present early in the postoperative period with pain over the graft, oliguria, and renal failure. Ultrasonographic or CT imaging can demonstrate a fluid collection, but percutaneous aspiration of fluid with analysis of BUN and creatinine levels is often required to make the diagnosis. ED management includes Foley catheter drainage, appropriate imaging, and consultation with the transplant surgeon to arrange for surgical repair.

Lymphocele

Approximately 5% to 15% of renal transplant patients experience symptoms resulting from postoperative lymphatic leaks and lymphocele formation. Manifestations include lower extremity edema, urinary frequency related to bladder compression, and obstructive uropathy from compression of the ureter. Larger lymphoceles can compromise vascular flow and threaten graft viability. In addition, they can predispose the patient to deep venous thrombosis and subsequent pulmonary embolism through compression of the large pelvic veins. As with urinary leak, ultrasonography or CT imaging can identify a fluid collection, but aspiration may be required to determine whether the fluid collection is urine or lymph. ED management consists of imaging to establish diagnosis, placement of a Foley catheter if urinary obstruction is suspected, and consultation with the transplant surgeon to facilitate surgical or percutaneous drainage. Lymphoceles causing obstructive uropathy or vascular compression represent true emergencies requiring prompt intervention to preserve allograft function and avert thromboembolic complications.

Obstructive Uropathy

Approximately 3% to 6% of renal transplant patients experience urinary outflow obstruction resulting in renal failure. In the early post-transplantation period, urinary obstruction can be caused by technical problems with the ureteral anastomosis or external compression of the ureter by hematoma, urine collection, or lymphocele. Ultrasonography is the modality of choice for evaluating the graft for hydronephrosis and the ureters for evidence of external compression. Hematoma, urinary leak, or lymphocele resulting in obstructive uropathy requires emergent surgical intervention to relieve the compression. ED management consists of Foley catheterization, ultrasonography, and early consultation with the transplant surgeon. Although definitive treatment often requires laparotomy, temporizing measures include cystoscopy with retrograde stenting of the ureter and percutaneous nephrostomy.

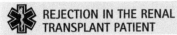

REJECTION IN THE RENAL TRANSPLANT PATIENT

Current immunosuppressive regimens have reduced the incidence of rejection in the first post-transplantation year to between 15% and 25%. Clinical features of acute rejection include fever, tenderness over the allograft, and acute renal failure. The same clinical features may also be present in graft infection. In contrast, chronic rejection results in minimal symptoms and is characterized by a slow progressive decline in renal function. Chronic rejection accounts for 40% to 50% of graft failure after the first post-transplantation year. ED management centers on treatment of the life-threatening complications of renal failure and exclusion of other reversible causes.

SYMPTOMS OF ACUTE REJECTION
- Oliguria, anuria
- Fever
- Abdominal pain, often localized to the graft site

SIGNS OF ACUTE REJECTION
- Fever
- Elevated blood pressure
- Tenderness and swelling over the allograft

WORKUP
- Serum chemistries: elevated BUN and creatinine and, possibly, hyperkalemia
- Urinalysis may reveal pyuria and proteinuria.
- CBC may show mild leukocytosis but is neither sensitive nor specific.
- Chest x-ray may demonstrate signs of volume overload (cephalization, pulmonary venous congestion, and pulmonary edema).
- ECG may show signs of acute hyperkalemia (peaked T waves).
- Doppler ultrasound to assess vascular flow and exclude hydronephrosis suggestive of urinary outflow obstruction

CHAPTER 38

549

COMMENTS AND TREATMENT CONSIDERATIONS

Foley catheterization is important to eliminate any element of lower urinary tract obstruction and to monitor urine output. The renal transplant patient who presents with fever, pyuria, and worsening renal function should be presumed to have an infection and empirical treatment with non-nephrotoxic broad-spectrum antibiotics begun. Renal biopsy is required to make the definitive diagnosis of allograft rejection. High-dose methylprednisolone is the treatment of choice for proven rejection, but its initiation is typically left to the nephrologist. Acute or chronic rejection that results in severe renal failure may require emergent dialysis for severe hyperkalemia or fluid overload.

 CARDIOVASCULAR COMPLICATIONS

Renal transplant patients are three to five times more likely to experience atherosclerotic vascular disease than the general public, and cardiovascular disease accounts for up to half of all deaths of renal transplant patients after the first post-transplantation year. It is imperative that symptoms that may indicate ischemic cardiac disease be taken seriously even if atypical. Renal transplant patients are also at increased risk for hypertension and its sequelae. The calcium channel blockers diltiazem and verapamil inhibit the hepatic metabolism of cyclosporine, tacrolimus, and sirolimus and should be avoided in the treatment of hypertension in renal transplant patients.

REFERENCES

Briganti EM, Russ GR, Mcneil JJ, et al: Risk of renal allograft loss from recurrent glomerulonephritis, *N Engl J Med* 347:103, 2002.

Fahlenkamp D, Raatz D, Schonberger B, et al: Laparoscopic lymphocele drainage after renal transplantation, *J Urol* 150:316, 1993.

Kasiske BL: Cardiovascular disease after renal transplantation, *Semin Nephrol* 20:176, 2000.

Mignat C: Clinically significant drug interactions with new immunosuppressive agents, *Drug Saf* 16:267, 1997.

Rouviere O, Berger P, Lyonnet D, et al: Acute thrombosis of renal transplant artery: graft salvage by means of intra-arterial fibrinolysis, *Transplantation* 73:403, 2002.

The Organ Procurement and Transplantation Network Website: www.optn.org.

Venkat KK, Venkat A: Care of the renal transplant recipient in the emergency department, *Ann Emerg Med* 44:330, 2004.

THE HEART TRANSPLANT PATIENT

According to the OPTN, there were 1866 heart transplantations in the United States in 2004, which brings the cumulative total to 36,345 since 1988. In addition to problems with infection, rejection, and graft failure common to all transplant patients, heart transplant recipients have clinically important differences in their cardiac physiology.

PHYSIOLOGIC DIFFERENCES IN THE TRANSPLANTED HEART

The transplanted heart lacks any vagal input, resulting in a resting heart rate of approximately 100 beats per minute. The response to endogenous catecholamines is preserved, however, allowing the heart rate to increase to approximately 70% of maximum predicted for age in response to stress or exercise. The lack of vagal input to the transplanted heart renders atropine ineffective in the treatment of bradycardia or AV block. In addition, denervation-induced AV nodal hypersensitivity may result in prolonged AV nodal block and subsequent cardiovascular collapse in response to standard adenosine doses (6 to 12 mg/kg IV in adults or 0.05 to 0.1 mg/kg in children). Although some authors recommend reducing dosage by a factor of 10, the safest course is synchronous DC cardioversion in the heart transplant patient with paroxysmal supraventricular tachycardia (PSVT). The ECG of the heart transplant recipient reveals two P waves, one from the donor SA node, which is conducted through the AV node to the ventricles, and a redundant impulse from the native SA node.

CHAPTER 38

REJECTION IN THE HEART TRANSPLANT PATIENT

Acute rejection most frequently occurs within the first post-transplantation month but continues to occur throughout the first year and subsequently. By the end of the first post-transplantation year, virtually every heart transplant patient has experienced an episode of acute rejection. Patients with acute rejection may present with vague constitutional symptoms such as lethargy and fatigue or obvious physiologic derangements such as overt heart failure or a dysrhythmia. ED management of suspected rejection includes treatment of its acute complications and a diligent search for treatable conditions such as infection, pericardial tamponade, or myocardial infarction. Definitive diagnosis is made by biopsy. Treatment is with high-dose steroids, and it is typically instituted at the direction of the transplant cardiologist.

GRAFT CORONARY ARTERY DISEASE

Atherosclerotic disease is a major problem in heart transplant patients, with a prevalence of up to 50% by the fifth post-transplantation year. Despite agreement that this accelerated atherosclerosis has an immunologic origin, advances in immuno-suppressive therapy have had limited impact. For the emergency physician, identifying myocardial ischemia in the heart transplant patient presents a particular problem because the denervation of the allograft precludes the development of angina as a symptom. Instead, heart transplant patients typically present late in the course of their infarction with shortness of breath and severe cardiac dysfunction. A high index of suspicion for disease is warranted, and consultation with the treating cardiologist is advised.

REFERENCES

Kubo SH, Naftel DC, Mills RJ, et al (Cardiac Transplant Research Database Group): Risk factors for late recurrent rejection after heart transplantation: a multiinstitutional, multivariable analysis, *J Heart Lung Transplant* 14:409, 1995.

Miniati DN, Robbins RC, Reitz BA: Heart and lung transplantation. In Braunwald E, Zipes DP, Libby P, et al: *Heart disease: a textbook of cardiovascular medicine, ed 6*. Philadelphia, 2001, WB Saunders, pp 615-630.

Poston RS, Griffith BP: Heart transplantation, *J Intensive Care Med* 19:3, 2004.

The Organ Procurement and Transplantation Network Website: www.optn.org.

Toft J, Mortensen J, Hesse B: Risk of atrioventricular block during adenosine pharmacologic stress testing in heart transplant recipients, *Am J Cardiol* 82:696, 1998.

Trauma, Approach to

Charles N. Pozner, Hilarie Hartel Cranmer,
and Michael Levine

Trauma is the leading cause of mortality for persons younger than 45 and accounts for nearly 60 million injuries and 9 million disabilities per year. Nearly half of all traumatic deaths occur instantly or within the first few minutes after injury, and 30% of deaths occur within the first few hours. This second group often dies from intracranial injuries or irreversible shock. The remaining 20% of traumatic deaths occur days or weeks after the initial injury and are the result of multiorgan system failure or sepsis. If a patient survives the first few minutes following the trauma, the survival of surgically remediable injuries is greatly enhanced if the patient is taken to the operating room within the first hour of the injury. Because the events occurring within this "golden hour" may make the difference between a person living or dying, the initial management of trauma is one of the most important functions for which the emergency physician (EP) must become both proficient and efficient. One of the EP's most important responsibilities is to recognize when the patient requires another venue, be it the operating room, the interventional radiology suite, or transfer to another facility, in order to receive the most appropriate management.

PREHOSPITAL CARE

The initial phase of trauma management begins at the scene of the injury.

- Triage: in multiple casualty incidents, triage is undertaken to determine which patients require immediate versus delayed care, whereas in a single-patient incident, triage refers to the determination of the most appropriate receiving facility and most efficient means of transporting the patient. Although circumstances dictate wide variability, an acceptable on-scene time for trauma patients is generally 10 minutes or less.

- Stabilization and prevention of additional injuries: airway management and ventilation, spine immobilization, and hemorrhage control
- Initiation of treatment: timely placement of IV lines, needle thoracostomy for suspected tension pneumothorax, and so forth
- Data collection: information about the scene, mechanism of injury, and estimated blood loss
- Advanced notification allows the assembly of the trauma team, anticipation of a patient's needs, preparation for procedures, timely consultations, operating room preparedness, blood bank, and critical care unit readiness.

OVERVIEW OF EVALUATION OF MULTIPLY INJURED PATIENTS

Although the care of the injured patient is described in a sequential fashion, many of the following steps should be performed simultaneously. Once detected, immediate life-threatening processes must be attended to before progressing to a detailed evaluation. Before the patient arrives in the trauma bay, the trauma team should be in place, with an identified leader. The trauma team leader must ensure that other members clearly understand their roles and responsibilities. Throughout the evaluation of the patient, it is important that the examining physician clearly articulate the findings of the examination to the rest of the trauma team. Upon arrival of the trauma patient, the following considerations must be addressed:

- EMS report: mechanism, age, injuries, prehospital treatment, status changes
- Primary survey. This includes *a*irway (A), *b*reathing (B), *c*irculation (C), a brief neurologic examination focused on *d*isability (D), and full *e*xposure of the patient to allow inspection for injuries (E). Interventions are made immediately if the primary survey identifies life-threatening abnormalities.
- Airway management assumptions: full stomach, cervical injury (if altered mental status, head injury, suggestive mechanism, or clinical suspicion). Definitive airway management should occur for airway protection, obstruction, respiratory failure, closed head injury, persistent hypotension, or refractory agitation (to facilitate evaluation).
- Breathing: adequacy of ventilation with bilateral breath sounds
- Circulation: establish presence or absence and quality (e.g., strong, weak/thready) of pulses. Identify hemorrhage requiring control with direct pressure, elevation (if possible), or compression of pressure points. MAST trousers may be considered for unstable pelvic fractures while awaiting definitive management.
- Disability: Glasgow coma score, papillary examination, movement of extremities, and presence or absence of posturing

- Exposure: completely undress the patient, but then protect against hypothermia.
- Simultaneously with the primary survey (if not already completed in the prehospital setting), the patient should be placed on cardiac and O_2 saturation monitors, two large-bore proximal IV lines placed, 100% oxygen administered by mask.

RESUSCITATION

Emergent surgical intervention is the primary treatment of exsanguinating hemorrhage. Volume resuscitation should be considered only a bridge to this definitive therapy.

- The initial fluid administered should be crystalloid (normal saline or lactated Ringer's). The initial infusion rate and volume should be 2 L wide open, unless the patient is unstable, whereupon 2 L should be administered by a rapid infuser if available.
- Type O negative blood (or O positive in male patients or postmenopausal females) should be given to the unstable patient immediately following the initial 2 L of crystalloids if the patient remains unstable or there is major ongoing blood loss.

SECONDARY SURVEY

The secondary survey, a thorough head-to-toe examination, is performed after initial stabilization. Priority is placed on identifying life threats. During the primary survey, some injuries may be missed, especially in unconscious patients and in those with dramatic injuries that distract attention from other, potentially more significant injuries. Throughout the secondary survey, the team leader should be aware of any changes in vital signs and regularly reassess the ABCs.

- HEENT: scalp, cranium, and midface (tenderness, stability, deformity, ecchymosis, or laceration), pupils, orbits, nose (blood/CSF, septal hematoma), oropharynx (teeth, bleeding), ears (otorrhea, hemotympanum, Battle's sign)
- Neck: airway injuries, subcutaneous emphysema, penetration, vascular injuries, vertebral step-offs, jugular venous distention
- Chest: penetration (possible cardiac injury if between right midclavicular line and left anterior axillary line and upper abdomen), abrasions and bruises, open wounds, flail chest, subcutaneous emphysema, and symmetry of chest expansion
- Abdomen: abrasions and ecchymosis, abdominal breathing, distention, bruits (possible vascular injury), tenderness, or guarding. A normal examination does not rule out significant intra-abdominal injury
- Pelvis: instability and fracture (may indicate source of occult bleeding), genitourinary bleeding

CHAPTER 39

- Rectal and urethral examination: examine the rectum for gross blood (not occult blood) and tone. Examine the urethral meatus for blood. The presence of a "high-riding" prostate, prostate tenderness/bogginess, or blood at the urethral meatus mandates a retrograde urethrogram prior to insertion of a Foley catheter.
- Extremities: hemorrhage, deformity, pulses, capillary refill
- Neurologic: LOC, agitation, tone, gross motor or sensory focality, priapism
- Back: log roll each patient to evaluate for vertebral step-offs, penetration, abrasions, and bruises (possible retroperitoneal injury).

SCREENING RADIOGRAPHS

Radiographs may be obtained concurrently with the head-to-toe examination (secondary survey) or between the primary and secondary surveys. Team members should wear lead protection to facilitate the process. Chest, pelvis, and cervical spine radiographs should be obtained. However, the patient's care should not be delayed pending radiographs. Intubation, if necessary, should occur with in-line immobilization prior to obtaining a radiograph of the cervical spine. Cervical spine precautions must be followed until the cervical spine is evaluated both radiographically and clinically.

- Supine anteroposterior chest x-ray should be obtained to evaluate for subcutaneous or pleural air; pneumothorax; evidence of hemothorax; naso/orogastric tube placement, evidence of hollow viscus above the diaphragm, or an abnormal hemidiaphragm (especially on the right) consistent with a diaphragmatic injury; a widened or abnormal mediastinum consistent with potential aortic injury; or air-space consolidations consistent with pulmonary contusion. A suspected tension pneumothorax should be treated empirically, without radiographic confirmation.
- Pelvic x-rays should be obtained to evaluate for pelvic fractures because pelvic fractures can be occult sites of major blood loss. Pelvic x-rays may be unnecessary in the asymptomatic, awake, alert, stable patient who can reliably be examined.
- Lateral cervical spine x-ray. This one view detects approximately 85% of cervical spine injuries. A minimum of three views is needed to better evaluate the cervical spine. Computed tomography, especially in elderly or obtunded patients, may be superior to plain films.

LABORATORY STUDIES AND TREATMENT

- Hemoglobin and hematocrit (H/H): may be normal in the setting of acute exsanguinations; initial H/H is useful to follow trends.
- Type and crossmatch blood, electrolytes, PT/INR, PTT.
- Urinalysis

- Pregnancy test (women of childbearing age)
- Other "trauma labs" may include toxicology screen, amylase/lipase, liver function test, blood gas (for base deficit), and lactate; use of these tests is controversial.
- Tetanus prophylaxis
- Prophylactic antibiotics if indicated (e.g., for open fracture)
- A Foley catheter should be inserted to evaluate for genitourinary hemorrhage and to follow urine output.
- Nasogastric or orogastric tube may be inserted to evaluate for gastrointestinal hemorrhage and minimize aspiration risk.

MANAGEMENT OF THE TRAUMA AIRWAY
Securing the airway and maintaining adequate ventilation are the first and highest priorities. Rapid sequence intubation (RSI) is the safest and most effective method of controlling the trauma airway. Care should be taken to maintain in-line cervical spine immobilization in all patients with potential cervical spine injuries.

Preparation (SOAP)
- **S**uction at the bedside
- Pre-**O**xygenate using nonrebreather mask.
- **A**irway equipment (tested): BVM, endotracheal tube (ETT) (two sizes), stylet, syringe, laryngoscope (two sizes of blade), endotracheal CO_2 detector, esophageal detection device (EDD) (optional)
- **P**harmaceuticals: intracranial pressure protectors (fentanyl, lidocaine), sedatives, induction agents (e.g., etomidate), and paralytics (e.g., succinylcholine)
- Cricothyrotomy equipment (or other backup airway equipment) should be immediately available.

Advanced Airway Techniques
1. Predictors of difficult airway include neck or lower facial injury, obese habitus (consider awake intubation with airway anesthesia and sedation).
2. Orotracheal intubation (method of choice)
   a. Suspected cervical spine injuries: use in-line immobilization
   b. Contraindications: not feasible because of patient's anatomy or tracheal disruption
3. Rapid sequence intubation
   a. Consider alternatives to paralysis if difficulty with the BVM is anticipated (e.g., large open facial wounds, difficult anatomy).
   b. Pretreatment: consider lidocaine (1.5 mg/kg) and/or fentanyl (1 µg/kg) in head-injured patients
   c. Consider defasciculating dose of nondepolarizing agent (e.g., vecuronium 0.01 mg/kg).

CHAPTER 39

   d. Induction: etomidate (0.3 mg/kg) is the drug of choice because of its favorable hemodynamic effects; fentanyl (3 µg/kg) and midazolam (0.1 to 0.3 mg/kg) are alternatives.

   e. Paralysis: succinylcholine (1 to 2 mg/kg) is preferred because of its rapid onset and short duration. Contraindicated in patients with significant crush or burns >24 hours after injury, hyperkalemia, history of malignant hyperthermia, or chronic neuromuscular disease. If succinylcholine is contraindicated, the newer nondepolarizing agents (e.g., rocuronium 0.6 mg/kg) or higher dose of standard nondepolarizing agents (e.g., vecuronium, 0.15 mg/kg) can be used.

   f. Confirm ETT placement by CO_2 detection, auscultation, chest x-ray; reliance on other indicators of endotracheal placement (e.g., condensation in the tube) is contraindicated.

4. Nasotracheal intubation

   a. Higher complication and failure rate than orotracheal intubation

   b. Contraindications include respiratory arrest, intracranial hypertension (relative), cribriform plate injury (relative).

5. Surgical airway. Indications include unfeasible or failed intubation.

6. Other options: fiberoptic intubation, retrograde intubation, light wand–guided intubation, Bullard laryngoscope, laryngeal mask airway (classic or intubating), or Combitube

HEAD AND NECK INJURIES

Head and neck injuries may be isolated or associated with multisystem trauma. Most patients with suspected head injuries should undergo head CT as soon as hemodynamic stability has been assured. If other life-threatening injuries take priority and CT scanning of the head must be deferred, neurosurgical consultation should be pursued. Placement of a ventriculostomy for intracranial pressure monitoring may be considered.

   Identification of cervical spine injuries, particularly spinal cord injuries, is also a priority in patients with multiple injuries. Nevertheless, other life-threatening injuries may take precedence, and radiographs may be deferred. In these cases protection of the cervical spine throughout the stabilization process (including trauma-related surgery) is mandatory. The physical examination is not adequately sensitive to exclude spinal injuries in patients with multiple injuries.

 SEVERE TRAUMATIC BRAIN INJURY

It is critical to determine whether an intracranial injury is present and the extent of that injury and to prevent the progression of

secondary injury. Significant intracranial injuries may occur without external signs of injury. Traumatic brain injury patients have traditionally been classified into three groups: severe (GCS <8), moderate (GCS 9-13), and mild (GCS 13-15). Patients with a GCS of 13, however, have a significantly higher incidence of abnormal CT scans than those with a GCS of 14 to 15. Thus, the definition of minor head trauma is now usually accepted as that producing a GCS of 14 to 15. If hypotension is detected at any time during the evaluation of a patient with head trauma, another source should be sought. With the exception of profound blood loss from scalp laceration or bleeding into an epidural or subgaleal hematoma (only in young children, with unfused suture lines), hypotension is almost always caused by another source.

SIGNS

- GCS <15 or altered mental status even with a GCS of 15
- Asymmetric or abnormal pupils
- Otorrhea and/or rhinorrhea
- Loss of skull integrity
- Battle's sign
- Periorbital ecchymosis ("raccoon eyes")
- Posturing

 HERNIATION SYNDROMES

When the intracranial pressure (ICP) exceeds the CNS's natural compensatory abilities, the intracranial contents may shift and herniate through various foramina.

- Uncal herniation is the most common herniation following traumatic injury. The uncus is forced through the tentorial hiatus. The first findings are anisocoria, ptosis, and abnormal extraocular movements related to third cranial nerve compression. Contralateral hemiparesis and decerebrate posturing may also occur.
- Central transtentorial herniation occurs as a result of an expanding hematoma at the vertex or frontal or occipital poles. Manifestations may be subtle, including bilateral pinpoint pupils and minor mental status changes. Increased muscle tone and positive Babinski signs may present. As the syndrome progresses, the pupils may become midpoint and lose responsiveness. Cheyne-Stokes breathing (hyperpnea and tachypnea) and posturing may develop subsequently.
- Upward transtentorial herniation occurs in the setting of an expanding posterior fossa lesion. The patient may present with rapidly declining LOC with pinpoint pupils gazing downward.

39

CHAPTER

559

- Cerebellotonsillar herniation occurs as a result of a cerebellar or large central vertex lesion causing the cerebellar tonsils to herniate through the foramen magnum. Flaccid quadriplegia and sudden cardiorespiratory collapse may occur because of medullary impingement.

 FOCAL LESIONS

- Traumatic subarachnoid hemorrhage (TSAH) is the most common post-traumatic intracranial hemorrhage. Headache and photophobia are common. The CSF may be bloody. The amount of blood seen on CT correlates directly with outcome and inversely with the presenting GCS. Isolated TSAH does not carry a poor prognosis, but post-traumatic cerebral vasospasm may occur 48 hours after the initial injury.
- Subdural hematoma (SDH) develops between the dura mater and the brain and is usually caused by movement of the brain relative to the skull (e.g., acceleration-deceleration injuries) resulting in laceration of superficial bridging veins. The clinical presentation depends on the amount of blood and the rate of expansion. Acute SDH produce symptoms within 24 hours; subacute SDH produce symptoms between 24 hours and 2 weeks. Chronic SDH produces symptoms after 2 weeks.
- Epidural hematoma (EDH) is usually a result of a laceration of the middle meningeal artery and hematoma formation between the skull and the dura mater. Classically, the patient has a decreased level of consciousness soon after the trauma, followed by a lucent interval that occurs before a second episode of decreased consciousness.

MANAGEMENT
- Maintaining perfusion and oxygenation of the injured brain is essential if a good neurologic outcome is to be achieved; the ABCs must be addressed immediately and effectively.
- Neurosurgical consultation
- Although evidence is limited, many authorities continue to recommend elevating the head of the bed to 30 degrees (if possible).
- Hyperventilation of patients with traumatic brain injury is controversial; hyperventilation to a $Paco_2$ of 35 torr may be appropriate if elevated ICP is suspected. Hyperventilation to a $Paco_2$ of <30 torr should be avoided.
- Mannitol (0.5 to 1 g/kg) may be considered.
- Anticipate coagulopathy.
- Seizure prophylaxis with phenytoin 18 mg/kg over 20 minutes

• Open fractures require antibiotic prophylaxis (e.g., cefazolin 1 g). Routine use of antibiotics for patients with otorrhea or rhinorrhea caused by a basilar skull fracture is not recommended.

FACIAL TRAUMA

Once airway patency is assured, deforming injuries of the face should never distract from attending to other, more serious life-threatening conditions.

SIGNS
• Hemorrhage
• Enophthalmos, exophthalmos
• Ecchymosis
• Disconjugate gaze
• Deformity
• Asymmetry
• Instability
• Malocclusion
• Palpable bone step-offs
• Crepitus
• Septal hematoma

MANAGEMENT
• CT scan, panoramic radiograph view of mandible
• Repair may be delayed if there are other injuries requiring attention.
• Antibiotics should be considered.

SPECIAL CONSIDERATIONS
Le Fort fractures:
I—maxilla at nasal fossa
II—maxilla at nasal bones, medial aspects of orbits
III—maxilla, zygoma, nasal bones, ethmoids, vomer, lesser bones of cranial base

Neck Injuries

Life-threatening injuries to the neck may be subtle, leading to dangerous delays in diagnosis. The most immediate threats to life are airway compromise, hemorrhage, and cervical spine injury. Vascular and airway injuries may initially be occult, especially in blunt trauma.

BLUNT NECK INJURY

SIGNS
- Hematoma
- Ecchymosis
- Dyspnea
- Stridor
- Bruit
- Dysphagia
- Focal neurologic deficits
- Subcutaneous emphysema
- Horner's syndrome (miosis, ptosis, and anhidrosis)

MANAGEMENT
- Early intubation if there is any risk of airway compromise
- Timely ENT consultation
- Cervical spine and chest x-rays, fiberoptic bronchoscopy, esophagram and/or upper endoscopy, angiography, or Doppler ultrasound of major neck vessels may be indicated.
- Hospital admission for observation

SPECIAL CONSIDERATIONS
Vascular injury (intimal tear, thrombosis, pseudoaneurysm) may present as hemiparesis or may be initially asymptomatic. Vascular injuries are frequently the result of minor blunt trauma and must always be considered. Complications include airway compromise, air embolus, intravascular thrombus, or dissection.

 PENETRATING NECK INJURIES

Penetrating injuries to the anterior neck may damage major blood vessels, trachea, or esophagus. Penetrating injuries to the posterior neck may produce damage to the spinal cord or vertebral artery.

SIGNS
- Hematoma
- Ecchymosis
- Dyspnea
- Stridor
- Bruit
- Dysphagia
- Focal neurologic deficits
- Subcutaneous emphysema
- Horner's syndrome
- Hemoptysis
- Absent pulse

MANAGEMENT

1. Airway: early intubation if indicated
2. Hemorrhage: pressure, oropharyngeal packing
3. Timely ENT consultation. Unstable patients necessitate operative repair.

SPECIAL CONSIDERATIONS

Penetrating injuries to the neck are classified into one of three zones:

Zone I—below the cricoid cartilage

Zone II—cricoid cartilage to the angle of mandible

Zone III—above the angle of mandible

The management of penetrating neck injuries that pierce the platysma remains controversial. In general, however, zone II injuries require surgical exploration, and zone I and III injuries can be evaluated nonsurgically. The nonsurgical evaluation of zone I and III injuries includes lateral neck film, chest x-ray, bronchoscopy, esophagoscopy, esophagography, and angiography. Intravenous antibiotics are indicated for all neck injuries penetrating the platysma, as is 24 hours of observation.

SPINE TRAUMA

Spinal injuries may be blunt or penetrating and can involve either the bone elements of the spinal column, the spinal cord itself, or both. Motor vehicle collisions account for the majority of spinal injuries. Complete cord lesions result in total loss of motor and sensory function below the level of the lesion; incomplete lesions result in some preservation of motor or sensory function and portend a better prognosis.

SIGNS

- Decreased or absent sensation
- Decreased or absent movement
- Decreased or absent rectal tone

MANAGEMENT

A radiographic evaluation of the cervical spine is mandatory for patients with suspected spine or cord injuries.

- At minimum, three views of the cervical spine should be obtained with plain radiography. Radiographic evaluation of the cervical spine should never delay other more pressing aspects of the evaluation or treatment of the multiply injured patient. Cervical immobilization is required regardless of the results of the radiographs.
- Indications for using computed tomography of the cervical scan include (1) inadequate plain films, (2) suspicious findings on

CHAPTER 39

563

plain films, (3) fractures/displacement demonstrated by standard radiography, and (4) high clinical suspicion of injury despite normal plain film.

- If acute cord hemorrhage, cord edema, or cord contusion is suspected, an MRI should be obtained.
- If any abnormalities are detected on CT or plain film, early neurosurgical consultation should be obtained.
- The patient with persistent neck pain, a normal neurologic examination, and negative imaging should remain in a hard cervical collar and have follow-up MRI or flexion-extension films.
- Patients with incomplete cord lesions (see later) may be treated with methylprednisolone (30 mg/kg IV bolus, followed by 5.4 mg/kg/hr for 23 hours if therapy is instituted within 3 hours of symptom onset; if therapy is instituted 3 to 8 hours after symptom onset, the continuous infusion should be continued for a total of 48 hours). Use of this therapy is controversial.

SPECIAL SITUATIONS
INCOMPLETE CORD LESIONS

- Anterior cord syndrome is caused by a cervical flexion injury resulting in injury to the anterior spinal artery or direct injury to the anterior spinal cord. Characterized by a loss of motor function and decreased pain and temperature sensation, with preservation of the vibratory, light touch, and position sense distal to the site of the lesion.
- Brown-Séquard syndrome occurs following hemisection of the cord, usually because of penetrating injuries or fractures of the lateral masses. Presents as ipsilateral loss of proprioception and vibration senses, contralateral loss of pain and temperature sensation, and ipsilateral paralysis distal to the lesion.
- Central cord syndrome is a hyperextension injury, particularly in patients with degenerative arthritis of the cervical spine. In this syndrome, the ligamentum flavum bends into the cord, resulting in a contusion of the central part of the cord. The upper extremities are affected more than the lower extremities. The damage occurs to the spinothalamic and pyramidal tracts.
- Cervical spine fractures can be classified as stable or unstable (see Table 39-1).

THORACIC TRAUMA

All life-threatening thoracic conditions must be quickly identified and treated. Patients must be constantly monitored for deterioration during subsequent examination and management. Both blunt and penetrating injuries can cause significant morbidity and mortality.

TABLE 39-1
STABILITY OF CERVICAL SPINE DISLOCATIONS AND FRACTURES

Atlantoaxial dislocation	Unstable
Atlantooccipital dislocation	Unstable
Bilateral facet dislocation	Unstable
Burst fracture of vertebral body	Stable
Clay shoveler's fracture	Stable
Extension teardrop fracture	Stable in flexion, unstable in extension
Flexion teardrop fracture	Extremely unstable
Jefferson fracture	Extremely unstable
Hangman fracture	Unstable
Odontoid fracture	Unstable
Subluxation	Potentially unstable
Transverse process fracture	Stable
Unilateral facet dislocation	Stable
Wedge fracture	Stable

CHAPTER 39

Rapid deceleration may also bring about subtle although potentially life-threatening processes (see tension pneumothorax, cardiac tamponade, traumatic aortic rupture in Chapter 7, Chest Pain).

POTENTIAL INJURIES
- Flail chest
- Open (sucking) chest wound
- Pneumothorax and tension pneumothorax
- Hemothorax
- Tracheobronchial tree disruption
- Esophageal injury
- Pulmonary contusion
- Myocardial or pericardial injury (tamponade, myocardial contusion)

- Great vessel injury
- Diaphragmatic injury

SIGNS
- Dyspnea
- Hypoxemia
- Shock
- Hemoptysis
- Decreased breath sounds
- Tracheal deviation
- Distended neck veins
- Asymmetric chest excursion
- Abrasions
- Contusions
- Dullness or hyperresonance to percussion
- Subcutaneous emphysema
- Irregular pulse
- Bowel sounds in chest

MANAGEMENT
1. Assess thoracic integrity, breath sounds, trachea, jugular venous distention.
2. Pulselessness
   a. Rapid IV fluid boluses
   b. Consider needle thoracostomies,
   c. Blunt injury: thoracotomy rarely indicated
   d. Penetrating injury: thoracotomy is indicated if vital signs were lost while the patient was in care of EMS or in the emergency department. If the patient was found without vital signs, thoracotomy is not indicated.
3. Cardiac tamponade necessitates pericardiocentesis and operative intervention. Beck's triad of jugular venous distention, hypotension, and tachycardia should be sought; however, jugular venous distention may be absent in the setting of profound hypovolemia.
4. Tension pneumothorax, if suspected, should be treated immediately, without waiting for radiographic confirmation. Initial treatment involves insertion of a 14-gauge 2-inch needle into the second intercostal space at the midclavicular line. Definitive treatment involves placing a 28 to 36 Fr chest tube into the fifth intercostal space, along the anterior axillary line.
5. Hemothorax: decreased breath sounds, hypoxemia, effusion on chest x-ray
   a. Chest tube: 32 to 38 Fr chest tube into the fifth intercostals space, along the anterior axillary line, directed posteriorly. If available, an autotransfuser may be used.

b. If more than 1000 to 1500 ml of blood is evacuated initially, or more than 200 ml per hour of blood is evacuated in the first 3 hours, or the patient remains hypotensive despite adequate volume resuscitation, operative intervention is indicated.

6. Open pneumothorax: apply a loose dressing (taped only on three sides to prevent conversion of the open pneumothorax into a tension pneumothorax), as a bridge to thoracostomy.

7. Supine anteroposterior chest x-ray
   a. Normal, but hypotensive: consider tamponade or extrathoracic source of shock.
   b. Abnormal:
      i. Tension pneumothorax, pneumothorax, hemothorax → thoracostomy
      ii. Mediastinal abnormality: possible aortic injury
      iii. Infiltrate: possible pulmonary contusion
      iv. Pneumomediastinum: possible tracheobronchial injury
      v. Abnormal hemidiaphragm (most often left): possible diaphragmatic disruption
      vi. Lower rib fractures: consider abdominal injury.

8. ECG: myocardial contusion may result in ischemic changes or dysrhythmia.

CHAPTER 39

ABDOMINAL TRAUMA

Eliciting the mechanism of injury is critical in the assessment of abdominal trauma. Blunt trauma can occur without external physical signs, resulting in life-threatening intra-abdominal injuries being overlooked during the initial assessment and treatment. In penetrating trauma, it is important to determine whether the peritoneum was violated as well as to consider the likely path of the penetrating object. Consider the anatomic site, number of wounds, type and size of weapon, and angle of approach of the weapon. Projectiles often have unpredictable paths and most often necessitate surgical exploration to assess the extent of injury. Because of the diaphragm's changing position with inspiration, penetrating thoracic injuries below the nipple line anteriorly and the tip of the scapula posteriorly may directly injure intra-abdominal organs. Wounds that appear to enter the abdomen may traverse the diaphragm and enter the thorax. Blunt trauma can cause pelvic fractures, which may lead to significant hemorrhage. Bladder or urethral injuries may occur in both blunt and penetrating trauma.

POTENTIAL INJURIES
- Solid organ
- Hollow viscus

- Vascular (including mesentery)
- Fracture (pelvis)
- Upper: diaphragm, stomach, liver, spleen, gallbladder, bowel
- Lower: bowel, colon
- Retroperitoneal: pancreas, kidneys, ureters, aorta, inferior vena cava (IVC), spinal cord, duodenum
- Pelvis: fracture, rectum, bladder, blood vessels, genitalia

SIGNS
- Hemodynamic instability
- Abrasions
- Contusion
- Penetrating wounds (must log roll)
- Guarding
- Distention
- Hematemesis
- Hematochezia
- Hematuria

MANAGEMENT
1. Pulseless
   a. Blunt injury: thoracotomy rarely indicated
   b. Penetrating injury: thoracotomy with cross-clamping of aorta and then operative intervention is indicated if vital signs were lost while the patient was in care of EMS or in the emergency department. If the patient was found without vital signs, thoracotomy is not indicated.
2. Hemodynamically unstable, persistent shock
   a. Blunt: FAST (focused abdominal sonography for trauma) scan to confirm free intraperitoneal fluid, then emergent laparotomy
   b. Penetrating trauma: emergent laparotomy
3. Stable
   a. Emergency laparotomy: impaled object, evisceration, peritoneal signs, diaphragm injury, pneumoperitoneum, rectal or nasogastric tube blood
   b. Penetrating injury:
      i. Gunshot wounds: emergent laparotomy generally performed if peritoneum violated (through-and-through wounds or if missile observed on plain film), flank injury. Selective management utilized at some centers; algorithms vary, including local exploration, diagnostic peritoneal lavage (DPL) (emergency laparotomy if >5000 RBC), CT, or laparoscopy. Observation if negative workup.

      ii. Other penetrating wounds: local wound exploration (must extend wound as necessary): if intact peritoneum, observe; if peritoneum violated, surgery is usually indicated.

  c. Blunt injury

      i. The FAST scan has largely replaced DPL as a means to evaluate the abdomen in trauma patients. FAST specifically looks only for free intraperitoneal fluid using four areas for ultrasound analysis.

      ii. CT: intraperitoneal and retroperitoneal injuries can be detected; also useful to detect pelvic and spine fractures; less reliable for hollow viscus injury. Depending on the injury, a positive CT results in surgery; however, stable patients with liver or spleen injuries are often observed. If negative, observe. CT should include rectal contrast if there is concern for colon injury.

      iii. DPL: laparotomy indicated for gross blood, >100,000 RBC in blunt trauma (5000 if lower chest wound with possible diaphragmatic injury), stool/urine, elevated amylase/alkaline phosphatase, or food material observed. If negative, CT scan or observe.

      iv. Laparoscopy

SPECIAL CONSIDERATIONS

Pelvic fractures can be a source of major bleeding. External pelvic fixation and radiographic embolization are used to control bleeding from pelvic fractures causing hemodynamic instability.

EXTREMITY TRAUMA

Vessel, nerve, and orthopedic injury can occur as a result of either blunt or penetrating mechanisms. Open fractures require prompt orthopedic consultation and operative irrigation and fixation. Patients with diminished distal pulses also require emergent relocation and splinting (and typically angiography to assess integrity of the vasculature). Patients with evidence of impaired distal circulation require immediate reduction of the fracture or dislocation, often before radiographic documentation of the injury.

POTENTIAL INJURIES
- Fracture
- Dislocation
- Laceration
- Puncture wound

CHAPTER **39**

- Crush injury
- Compartment syndrome
- Neurovascular injury
- Soft tissue injury

SIGNS
- Deformity
- Hematoma
- Lacerations
- Abrasions
- Pulselessness
- Pain
- Paralysis
- Paresthesia
- Bruit or thrill (a "buzzing" or "tingling" sensation felt over the vessel)

MANAGEMENT
1. Reduce and splint major deformities in anatomic position.
2. Vascular
   a. Risk stratification
      i. High risk: pulsatile bleed, absent pulse, shotgun wound, neurologic deficit, hematoma, bruit, major tissue defect, delayed capillary refill, ankle-brachial indices (ABIs) <1.00 (see Chapter 13, Extremity Pain and Numbness)
      ii. Low risk: normal examination, ABI >1.00
   b. Workup
      i. High risk: arteriography; operating room if gross arterial bleeding
      ii. Low risk: observation

SPECIAL CONSIDERATIONS
- Serial assessment with arteriography or duplex scanning of minor vessel injury may be an alternative to surgical repair in some cases.
- Antibiotics (e.g., cefazolin, gentamicin) for open fractures
- Maintain a low threshold for compartment pressure measurement and emergent fasciotomy, if indicated.

TRAUMA IN PREGNANCY
Trauma remains the leading cause of nonobstetric morbidity and mortality in pregnant patients. The EP must be aware of several of the physiologic changes that occur throughout pregnancy, as these

changes can significantly alter the presentation of the pregnant patient. These changes include the following:

1. Maternal blood volume increases from week 10 through week 28, resulting in hypervolemia and relative physiologic anemia. Thus, the pregnant woman can lose 30% to 35% of the circulating blood volume before manifesting hypotension or clinical signs of shock.
2. Heart rate is increased by 10 to 20 beats in the second trimester.
3. Decrease in systolic and diastolic blood pressures of 10 to 15 torr in the second trimester
4. The uterus becomes an intra-abdominal organ after the 12th week of pregnancy and the bladder moves more anterior in the third trimester, increasing their risk of injury.
5. Increased uterine blood flow (>600 ml/min in late pregnancy), making severe hemorrhage from uterine injury possible
6. The gravid uterus can compress the IVC (by 18 to 20 weeks of gestation), causing hypotension when the mother is supine.

The most common cause of fetal death is maternal death, and the second most common cause of fetal death is placental abruption. Placental abruption usually complicates 1% to 5% of minor trauma and 40% to 50% of major trauma. Findings consistent with placental abruption include abdominal pain, vaginal bleeding, and tetanic uterine contractions. It is classically described as painful vaginal bleeding in the third trimester. Complications include fetal loss, DIC, and amniotic fluid embolism.

Direct fetal injury is relatively rare in blunt abdominal trauma during the first trimester, but when it occurs, it is usually the result of a displaced maternal pelvic fracture penetrating the fetal head.

Uterine rupture is also relatively rare but can occur during the late second and third trimesters. It should be suspected by loss of the uterine contour on abdominal examination or palpation of fetal parts in the abdomen.

TREATMENT

Because fetal survival is unlikely if the mother dies, all initial efforts should be directed toward adequate resuscitation of the mother. Although the initial management is the same as for the non-pregnant patient, there are several exceptions:

- Changes in fetal heart rate occur before changes in pulse or blood pressure in the mother and are a more sensitive indicator of early maternal shock.
- All pregnant women should receive 100% oxygen during the trauma resuscitation, regardless of the pulse oximetry.
- Aggressive fluid resuscitation should occur, and an additional 50% crystalloid volume may be required to account for the additional plasma volume during pregnancy.

CHAPTER 39

571

- In patients who need to be in spinal immobilization, a wedge should be paced under the right hip to move the gravid uterus off the IVC.
- Fetomaternal hemorrhage should be suspected if there is uterine tenderness, contractions, vaginal bleeding, or direct (or indirect) abdominal trauma. For Rh-negative mothers, Rh_0 immune globulin (RhoGAM) should be administered empirically if fetomaternal hemorrhage is suspected. If the mother is at <12 weeks of gestation, 50 μg of RhoGAM should be administered; 300 μg should be administered for all other gestational ages. Additional doses of RhoGAM may be indicated on the basis of the Kleihauer-Betke (KB) test.
- Tetanus prophylaxis should be administered as one would provide to a nonpregnant patient.
- Radiographs should be taken, as necessary. Doses <10 rads are not associated with adverse fetal effects.
- A sterile pelvic examination is indicated. Fluid with pH <7 is suggestive of amniotic fluid, whereas a pH of 5 is consistent with vaginal secretions. The presence of pooling or ferning is also suggestive of amniotic fluid.
- Assessment of the fetal heart rate by Doppler stethoscope should occur during the secondary survey, as the initial fetal heart rate has prognostic implications. The normal fetal heart rate is 120 to 160 beats per minute.
- The indications for DPL or laparotomy do not differ from those for the nonpregnant patient. However, if DPL is to be performed, it should be performed by an open, supraumbilical technique.
- Early fetal tocodynamometry for a minimum of 4 hours is recommended to observe for evidence of placental abruption. If more than three contractions are observed per hour or if there is an abnormal fetal heart tracing, a minimum of 24 hours of continuous monitoring is required.

REFERENCES

American College of Surgeons: *Advance trauma life support instructors manual*. Chicago, 1997, American College of Surgeons.

Fan JY: Effect of backrest position on intracranial pressure and cerebral perfusion pressure in individuals with brain injury: a systematic review, *J Neurosci Nurs* 36:278, 2004.

Gin-Shah SL, Jorden RC: Multiple trauma. In Marx JA, Hockberger RS, Walls RM (eds): *Rosen's emergency medicine: concepts and clinical practice*, ed 5. St. Louis, 2002, Mosby, p 242.

Hockberger RS, Kirshenbaum KJ: Spine. In Marx JA, Hockberger RS, Walls RM (eds): *Rosen's emergency medicine: concepts and clinical practice*, ed 5. St. Louis, 2002, Mosby, p 329.

Shaffer MA, Doris PE: Limitation of the cross table lateral view in detecting cervical spine injuries: a retrospective analysis, *Ann Emerg Med* 10:508, 1981.

Stocchetti N, Maas AI, Chieregato A, van der Plas AA: Hyperventilation in head injury: a review, *Chest* 127:1812, 2005.

Tang N, White D: Trauma in pregnancy. In Tintinalli JE, Klein GD, Stapczynski JS (eds): *Emergency medicine: a comprehensive study guide*, ed 6. New York, 2004, McGraw-Hill, p 1553.

39

CHAPTER

Trauma, Burns
Charles N. Pozner, Resa Lewiss, and Michael Levine

Despite tremendous improvements in care over the past quarter-century, burns continue to be a major source of morbidity and mortality. The incidence of burns follows a bimodal distribution, with peaks occurring in children younger than 5 years and again during the third decade of life. Nearly two thirds of burns occur in males. In children younger than 4, most burns are scald injuries, caused by hot liquids falling on the patient. In older children, burns are frequently caused by mischievous activities. Most burns in adults are due to flame injuries, and up to one third are work related.

Burns often occur in the context of additional trauma. Although burns require specific treatment and can cause significant morbidity and mortality, it is essential that initial care be directed to all potentially life-threatening injuries. Patients with serious burns are often most effectively managed at a burn center.

 INHALATIONAL INJURIES

Inhalational burns can be immediately and overtly life threatening but may be occult. If significant airway injury is suspected (based on singed nasal hairs, soot around the airway, or exposure to intense heat), the patient should be given 100% humidified oxygen until the airway can be directly visualized or secured by early endotracheal intubation. Carbon monoxide and cyanide exposure should be considered.

SYMPTOMS
- Initially may be minimal or absent
- Hoarse voice
- Brassy cough

SIGNS

- Initially may be minimal or absent
- Stridor
- Dysphonia
- Singed nasal or facial hairs
- Carbonaceous sputum
- Mouth or nose burns
- Airway edema or erythema

 THERMAL BURNS

A rapid and accurate assessment of a patient's burn injury is a crucial determinant of management and disposition. Severity of thermal burns is judged by depth, location, and body surface area (BSA) affected. Burns can be divided into epidermal burns; superficial partial-thickness, deep partial-thickness, and full-thickness burns; and those extending beyond the skin. There are several important historical questions that need to be answered in caring for the burn patient (Table 40–1).

TABLE 40–1
IMPORTANT HISTORICAL INFORMATION IN BURN ASSESSMENT

Mechanism
Scenario (e.g., blast injuries can create additional injuries)
Type of burn (e.g., flame, scald, electrical)
Accidental or intentional
Did burn occur in enclosed space (increases risks of inhalational injury)?
Substance burning (e.g., cyanide poisoning can occur from nitrogen-containing polymers, such as vinyl, wool, silk)

Exact Injury
If scald burn: What was the liquid? Was a solute in the liquid (solutes raise the boiling temperature and therefore create potential for more severe burn)?
If electrocution: What was the voltage? Was power source AC or DC? Was there a flash or arc?
If chemical: What was the chemical? Was it powder or liquid? Is the pH known?

Timing
How long was the patient exposed to the agent?
What time did the burn occur?

Treatment
Was anything applied to the burn surface?
What IV fluids and how much were given prior to arrival?
When was last tetanus vaccination?

BURN DEPTH

FIRST-DEGREE BURNS

Also called epidermal burns, first degree burns are the most superficial burns. Most sunburns are first degree burns.

- Redness
- Tenderness and pain
- Absence of blisters
- Intact neurovascular examination

SECOND-DEGREE BURNS

Superficial partial-thickness burns; involve epidermis and papillary dermis

- Red, moist skin
- Capillary refill intact
- Tenderness and pain
- Thin-walled, fluid-filled blisters

Deep partial-thickness burns; involve epidermis, papillary dermis, and reticular dermis

- Red and blanched white skin (capillary refill decreased)
- Thick walled, fluid-filled blisters (frequently ruptured)
- Diminished two-point discrimination
- Pressure sensation intact

THIRD-DEGREE BURNS

Third degree burns, also called full-thickness burns, involve the epidermis and entire dermis.

- White or leathery appearance
- Decreased pressure sensation (often no pain at all)

FOURTH-DEGREE BURNS

Involve destruction of skin, subcutaneous tissue, and often fascia, muscle or bone.

BODY SURFACE AREA DETERMINATION

The "rule of nines" is frequently employed (Fig. 40–1) to estimate the magnitude of the surface area burned. The area of the patient's palm represents approximately 0.8% of the BSA. The rule of nines for infants differs from that for adults owing to the disproportionately large size of the infant's head compared with an adult's head. If used correctly, the Lund and Browder chart is the most accurate method for calculating BSA, as this method takes into account variation in body shape with age.

BURN SEVERITY

MAJOR BURNS

1. Partial thickness burn >25% BSA in patients aged 10 to 50 (or >20% BSA in all other age groups)

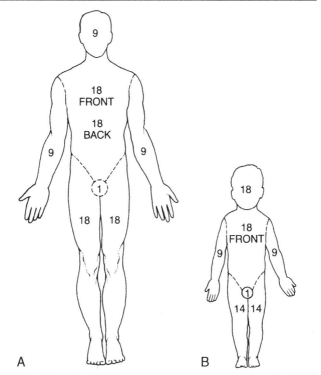

Fig. 40-1 Rule of nines. **A**, Adult. **B**, Infant. (From Rosen P, Barkin RM, Hockberger RS, et al [eds]: *Emergency medicine: concepts and clinical practice*, vol 2, ed 4. St. Louis, 1998, Mosby; from Roberts JR, Hedges J [eds]: *Clinical procedures in emergency medicine*, ed 4. Philadelphia, Saunders, 2004.)

2. Full thickness involving >10%
3. Burns to the hands/feet, face, ears, perineum
4. Burns caused by caustic chemicals
5. High-voltage electrical injury
6. Burns associated with inhalation injuries or major trauma
7. Burns in patients with underlying debilitating illnesses

MODERATE BURNS
1. Partial-thickness burns of 15% to 25% BSA in patients aged 10 to 50 (or 10% to 20% BSA in all other ages)
2. Full-thickness burns that do not create functional or cosmetic impairments of the face, hands/feet, or perineum, with BSA of 2% to 10%

577

MINOR BURNS

1. Partial-thickness burns <15% BSA in patients aged 10 to 50 (or <10% BSA in all other age groups)
2. Full-thickness burns <2% BSA that do not present a serious functional or cosmetic threat to the face, hands/feet, or perineum

 ELECTRICAL BURNS

Electrical injuries may produce significant internal injuries despite the presence of relatively few signs of external injury. The extent of damage depends on numerous factors, including the type of current, duration of exposure, and the voltage. Because alternating current (AC) causes sustained muscle contraction resulting in longer contact with the electrical current, AC injuries are generally more severe. Direct current (DC) results in a single muscle contraction with rapid release and subsequently shorter contact with the electrical current. High voltage (>1000 V) is associated with more harm than lower voltage. It is said that people with electrical injuries "die three times." The first significant cause of death following electrical exposure results from instantaneous lethal arrhythmias, such as ventricular fibrillation. In addition, the exposure may result in muscle tetany, including the diaphragm. Thus, the "second death" results from apnea. Lastly, significant electrical injuries can result in severe neurologic injury or muscle injury, the latter of which may produce compartment syndromes and rhabdomyolysis with subsequent renal failure.

 CHEMICAL BURNS

Chemical agents continue to burn until the agent is removed; therefore, immediate removal of the caustic agent is essential. If the caustic agent is a solid, it should be wiped away before placing water near the agent. If the agent is a liquid, decontamination with copious amounts of water should be employed unless contraindicated by the specific nature of the chemical. The decontamination team should don protective attire, appropriate for the specific chemical agent. The patient's clothes should be removed and placed in a plastic bag.

If exposure involves the eye, prompt irrigation (often through a Morgan lens) is required. The pH should be checked and the eye irrigated until the pH returns to normal. Alkaline burns tend to be more severe than acidic burns because alkaline burns undergo liquefactive necrosis whereas acidic burns undergo coagulative necrosis. Following irrigation, a thorough ophthalmologic examination is required, including slit lamp and fluorescein stain. Any fluorescein uptake necessitates reevaluation within 24 hours.

TREATMENT

The initial management of a burn patient is similar to that of any other trauma patient.

A. Airway. Assess whether the airway is compromised or at risk. If signs of inhalational injury are present (e.g., full-thickness burns to the face, neck, or upper torso, carbonaceous sputum, singed nasal hair, dysphonia, stridor), the patient should be intubated. Airway burns may become edematous after several hours, particularly after fluid resuscitation is begun. Thus, it is always better to secure an airway early if there is any suspicion of an airway injury.

B. Breathing. All burn patients should receive 100% oxygen through a humidified nonrebreather mask. Deep burns to the chest wall may limit chest wall expansion. Blast injuries may produce blunt or penetrating injuries, resulting in pneumothoraces or pulmonary contusions. Smoke inhalation may cause bronchospasm as well as impair the normal ciliary action. Carbon monoxide poisoning may result from smoke inhalation; therefore, determination of carboxyhemoglobin (COHb) levels is essential, especially if the burn occurred in an enclosed space. Hyperbaric oxygen should be considered for patients with (1) COHb >25%, (2) any elevation of the COHb in pregnancy, or (3) altered mental status including seizures. The diagnosis of cyanide poisoning should be entertained if the patient is persistently dyspneic, hypoxic, and not improving with oxygen (see Chapter 37, Toxic Exposure, Approach to).

C. Circulation. Two large-bore IVs should be established at an uninvolved site. Any circumferential burn may impair distal circulation when swelling occurs. Fluid resuscitation should begin employing the Parkland formula (4 ml/kg/BSA) or the Brook Army formula (2 ml/kg/hr). Both the Parkland and Brook Army formulas estimate the fluid requirement during the first 24 hours. Half of the fluid should be replaced in the first 8 hours from the burn, and the second half should be replaced in the remaining 16 hours.

D. Disability. Mental status should be assessed and graded according to the Glasgow Coma Scale.

E. Exposure. It is crucial to expose the entire patient to evaluate burns and assess for concomitant injuries. Burn patients should be promptly re-covered because they are at high risk for the development of hypothermia.

F. A Foley catheter should be inserted into all patients to monitor urine output.

Circumferential burns that restrict ventilation or blood flow may require emergent escharotomy.

Major burns require admission and early surgical referral and are best managed at a designated burn center. If the patient is to

CHAPTER 40

be transferred to a burn center, wounds should be simply wrapped in a clean, dry sheet. In all other cases, however, the wounds should be cleaned with a sterile saline or commercial cleaning product containing poloxamer 188 (e.g., Shur-Clens). Topical antibacterial creams can be applied to the burns. These creams include silver sulfadiazine (Silvadene), mafenide acetate (Sulfamylon), and bacitracin. Mafenide is preferred for burns to cartilaginous areas. Prophylactic administration of systemic antibiotics has not been shown to be beneficial in preventing systemic infections. Moderate burns require admission and early surgical referral but not necessarily transfer to a designated burn center. Minor burns can often be managed on an outpatient basis. All patients experiencing pain should receive appropriate analgesia. The administration of intravenous opiates is often necessary. Tetanus prophylaxis should be provided, if indicated.

REFERENCES:

Edlich RF, Bailey TL, Bill TJ: Thermal burns. In Marx JA, Hockberger RS, Walls RM (eds): *Rosen's emergency medicine: concepts and clinical practice*, ed 5. St. Louis, 2002, Mosby, pp 801-813.

Hettiaratchy S, Dziewulski P: ABC of burns. Introduction, *BMJ* 328:1366, 2003.

Hettiaratchy S, Dziewulski P: ABC of burns. Pathophysiology and types of burns, *BMJ* 328:1427, 2003.

Hettiaratchy S, Papini R: ABC of burns. Initial management of a major burn: I—overview, *BMJ* 328:1555, 2003.

Hettiaratchy S, Papini R: ABC of burns. Initial management of a major burn: II—assessment and resuscitation, *BMJ* 329:101, 2004.

Rapini R: ABC of burns. Management of burn injuries of various depths, *BMJ* 329:158, 2004.

Schwartz LR, Balakrishnan C: Thermal burns. In Tintinalli JE, Klein GD, Stapczynski JS (eds): *Emergency medicine. A comprehensive study guide*, ed 6. New York, 2003, McGraw-Hill, pp 1220-1226.

Sheridan RL: Burn care. Results of technical and organizational progress, *JAMA* 290:719, 2003.

Vaginal Bleeding
Vena Ricketts

The most important factor in assessing vaginal bleeding in any woman in the reproductive years of life is pregnancy status. History alone is not sufficient to determine pregnancy status; patients may be unaware or not admit that they are pregnant. A urine or blood pregnancy test is mandatory in all cases (urine qualitative pregnancy tests are generally very accurate as a pregnancy screen). Vaginal bleeding is an important symptom in both intrauterine and ectopic pregnancy and should prompt a thorough evaluation.

Excluding normal menstruation, causes of vaginal bleeding in nonpregnant women fall in two main categories: anatomic lesion and hormonal (estrogen and/or progesterone) imbalance. Gynecologic cancers are a potential cause of vaginal bleeding, particularly in postmenopausal women. Although bleeding in nonpregnant women can occasionally be severe and cause hemodynamic compromise, most of these women are stable and can be referred for gynecologic follow-up after ED evaluation.

COMPLICATIONS OF EARLY PREGNANCY

 ECTOPIC PREGNANCY

The most important diagnosis to exclude in the pregnant patient with vaginal bleeding is ectopic pregnancy (EP). Despite a 90% decrease in the mortality related to improved methods of detection and management, EP remains the leading cause of pregnancy-related deaths in the first trimester. In the United States, EP rates are still rising. EP must be considered in any woman of reproductive age presenting with pelvic pain, vaginal bleeding, or syncope and a positive pregnancy test. Although risk factors for EP have been identified (these include previous EP, previous abdominal surgery, tubal ligation, tubal pathology, in vitro fertilization, and a history of pelvic inflammatory disease), half of all patients with EP have no identified risk factor. Heterotopic pregnancy (coexisting intrauterine and EP) occurs in approximately 1 in 4000 patients.

SYMPTOMS
- Pelvic or abdominal pain ++++
- Vaginal bleeding ++++ is usually present but is minimal in most cases.
- Amenorrhea +++
- Dizziness +++, syncope ++
- Nausea and vomiting ++
- Asymptomatic ++
- Vaginal passage of tissue +
- Shoulder pain may indicate ruptured EP with blood in the peritoneal cavity.

SIGNS
- Abdominal or pelvic tenderness ++++
- Adnexal tenderness ++++
- Adnexal mass +++. Occasionally an EP can be found on the opposite side of a palpable adnexal mass (20%). This finding is due to a corpus luteum cyst.
- Uterine enlargement ++
- Orthostatic changes in pulse or blood pressure ++
- Fever +
- Hemodynamic compromise if rupture has occurred

WORKUP
- Urine pregnancy test +++++ (most assays are highly sensitive even in very early pregnancy)
- Quantitative serum βHCG; if a woman of reproductive age presents with pelvic pain, vaginal bleeding, or other symptoms potentially consistent with EP and a screening urine pregnancy test is positive, a quantitative serum βHCG and pelvic ultrasound should be performed.
- Pelvic ultrasound; transvaginal ultrasound is preferred in the first trimester because of its superior visualization of the features of early pregnancy compared with transabdominal ultrasound.
- Hematocrit, hemoglobin, or CBC
- Rh assay; all pregnant women having vaginal bleeding must have their Rh status determined, and those who are Rh negative must be treated with $Rh_0(D)$ immune globulin intramuscularly (MICRhoGAM 50 μg when <13 weeks pregnancy and RhoGAM 300 μg if >13 weeks).
- Type and crossmatch for transfusion if clinically indicated.

- Serum progesterone level does not provide additional clinically important information.

COMMENTS AND TREATMENT CONSIDERATIONS

Unstable patients with EP require emergent operative management. Hypotension, tachycardia, a low or falling hematocrit, an acute abdomen, and ultrasonographic evidence of intraperitoneal fluid are indications for surgery. ED care of these patients should be brief, concentrating on stabilization of the patient (ABCs, monitoring, two large-bore intravenous lines, fluid resuscitation) and obtaining the necessary laboratory studies.

For stable patients, the results of transvaginal ultrasound and serum βHCG are considered. Ultrasound usually provides information on location of pregnancy, gestational age, and viability as indicated by the presence or absence of fetal cardiac activity. An empty uterus in a woman with a positive pregnancy test suggests an EP but is also consistent with a very early pregnancy (<3 weeks gestational age) or a completed abortion. With technologic improvements in ultrasonographic identification of an intrauterine gestational sac, the diagnosis of an intrauterine pregnancy (IUP) can be made at a βHCG level as low as 1200 to 1500 mIU/ml. This level is referred to as the discriminatory zone. For stable patients with a βHCG level below this and without evidence of an IUP or EP by ultrasound, close obstetric outpatient follow-up with a recheck of βHCG level in 2 days should be considered. The diagnosis of EP is generally made in patients with a βHCG level below the discriminatory zone with ultrasound evidence of EP or in those with a βHCG level above the discriminatory zone and without signs of IUP on ultrasound. Note that rarely early twin gestations may lead to βHCG above the discriminatory zone and not yet show definitive signs of IUP on ultrasound. Treatment of EP may be surgical (laparotomy laparoscopy), medical (methotrexate), or expectant. Choice of therapeutic modality is often institution specific. Obstetrics/gynecology consultation is required.

Pregnant women having vaginal bleeding and who are Rh negative should receive Rh_0(D) immune globulin intramuscularly (MICRhoGAM 50 μg when <13 weeks pregnancy and RhoGAM 300 μg if >13 weeks).

REFERENCES

Barnhart KT, Simhan H, Kamelle SA: Diagnostic accuracy of ultrasound above and below the βhCG discriminatory zone, *Obstet Gynecol* 94:583, 1998.

Buster JE, Pisarsk MD: Medical management of ectopic pregnancy, *Clin Obstet Gynecol* 42:23, 1999.

Cacciatore B, Stenman UH, Ylostalo P: Diagnosis of ectopic pregnancy: vaginal ultrasonography in combination with a discriminatory serum βhCG levels and ultrasonograph findings, *Br J Obstet Gynaecol* 97:904, 1994.

Carson SA, Buster JE: Ectopic pregnancy, *N Engl J Med* 329:1174, 1993.

Cohen MA, Sauer MV: Expectant management of ectopic pregnancy, *Clin Obstet Gynecol* 42:48, 1999.

Hajenius PJ, Engelsbel S, Mol BW, et al: Randomized trial of systemic methotrexate vs. laparoscopic salpingostomy in tubal pregnancy, *Lancet* 350:774, 1997.

Kaplan BC, Dart RG, Moskos M, et al: Ectopic pregnancy: prospective study with improved diagnostic accuracy, *Am Emerg Med* 28:10, 1996.

Lau S, Tulandi T: Conservative medical and surgical management of interstitial ectopic pregnancy, *Fertil Steril* 72:207, 1999.

SPONTANEOUS ABORTION (THREATENED, INCOMPLETE/INEVITABLE, COMPLETE, MISSED, AND SEPTIC)

Vaginal bleeding occurs in the first trimester in 25% to 40% of pregnancies and spontaneous abortion or miscarriage occurs in 5% to 15% of diagnosed pregnancies. Most pregnancies that survive the first trimester continue to term. Spontaneous abortion is a process that is described in three or four stages (threatened, incomplete/inevitable, complete). Missed and septic abortions are complications of this process. History should include the last menstrual period (LMP), the estimated gestational age (EGA), presence and course of symptoms (bleeding, abdominal or pelvic pain, fever), and results of prior pelvic ultrasound, if any. EP is usually in the differential diagnosis unless a prior ultrasound has documented an intrauterine pregnancy, and even then a heterotopic pregnancy remains a possibility.

Threatened Abortion

Any degree of vaginal bleeding without passage of tissue and a closed internal cervical os in early (<20 weeks) intrauterine pregnancy is defined as a threatened abortion.

SYMPTOMS
- Vaginal bleeding +++++, may be minimal (spotting) to occasionally severe. Clots may be present, but no tissue.
- Abdominal or pelvic pain, may radiate to back or perineum.

SIGNS
- Cervical os is closed.
- Uterine or cervical motion tenderness may be present but raises concern for EP or septic abortion.
- Fetal heart tones may be present.

WORKUP

- Urine pregnancy test +++++; if positive, a quantitative serum βHCG should be sent.
- Urinalysis is frequently performed because of the belief that UTI is a common cause of spontaneous abortion.
- Hemoglobin, hematocrit, or CBC if blood loss is a concern
- RH assay
- If pelvic examination produces material suspected of being products of conception, send tissue to the laboratory for identification (consent is required in some states). What appear on visual examination to be products of conception can actually be a molar pregnancy or a decidual cast associated with an EP.
- Pelvic ultrasound, preferably transvaginal. Indications: potential for EP (the most common and important indication), moderate to severe pain or bleeding, open cervical os, cervical motion tenderness, discrepancy between expected (based on LMP) and actual uterine size, pelvic mass, and discrepancy between expected and measured βHCG levels.
- Type and crossmatch for transfusion if clinically indicated.

COMMENTS AND TREATMENT CONSIDERATIONS

In most cases after evaluation for a potential EP has been completed, women with the diagnosis of threatened abortion can be referred to obstetrics/gynecology for follow-up as outpatients. For patients in whom EP cannot be completely ruled out because of a βHCG below the discriminatory zone, follow-up should be arranged at 2 days to assess resolution of symptoms and ensure appropriate rise in the βHCG.

Incomplete/Inevitable Abortion

An incomplete/inevitable abortion is defined as pregnancy at <20 weeks with dilation of the cervix without expulsion of products of conception. In the past, incomplete abortion and inevitable abortion were classified as distinct entities. Currently, however, they are considered the same stage of spontaneous abortion. Patients typically present with more severe vaginal bleeding than in threatened abortion and may have seen passage of tissue. Transvaginal ultrasound shows retained fetal products.

SYMPTOMS

- Vaginal bleeding +++++; clots and tissue may be present.
- Abdominal or pelvic pain, may radiate to back or perineum

SIGNS

- Cervical os is open

CHAPTER **41**

WORKUP
See Threatened Abortion.

COMMENTS AND TREATMENT CONSIDERATIONS
Most women found to have an incomplete abortion expel all fetal tissue and complete their abortion without complication. Although in years past all patients diagnosed with an incomplete abortion had dilation and curettage (D&C), most patients may be discharged for expectant management by obstetrics/gynecology. Patients should be advised to return for significant bleeding or other signs/symptoms of blood loss and have close follow-up. The occasional patient with more severe bleeding requires immediate fluid resuscitation and emergent obstetrical consultation. An emergent D&C and blood transfusion are sometimes necessary for these patients.

Completed Abortion
The diagnosis of completed abortion is made when all products of conception have passed from the uterus and abdominal pain and vaginal bleeding have subsided.

SYMPTOMS
- Vaginal bleeding +++++; clots and tissue may be present.
- Abdominal or pelvic pain, may radiate to back or perineum

SIGNS
- Vaginal bleeding is minimal to moderate and decreases with time.
- Cervical os is closed.
- No fetal heart tones

WORKUP
See Threatened Abortion.

COMMENTS AND TREATMENT CONSIDERATIONS
Definitively diagnosing complete abortion in the ED can be difficult unless an intact gestational sac was expelled or a patient known to have an IUP documented on ultrasound is found to have an empty uterus following an episode of vaginal bleeding. Nevertheless, if the uterus is empty on ultrasound, there is no concern for EP, and the patient is stable, no further treatment is necessary in the ED and the patient can be referred for follow-up with obstetrics/gynecology. Pregnancy tests should be repeated on an outpatient basis to be sure that the diagnosis is correct (i.e., that the test becomes negative) and an abnormal pregnancy is not present.

Missed Abortion
Missed abortion is defined as in utero death of the embryo or fetus before the 20th week of gestation with retained products

of conception. Missed abortion is usually an ultrasonographic diagnosis, intrauterine fetal demise (IUFD).

SYMPTOMS
- May be asymptomatic
- Vaginal bleeding or spotting
- Abdominal or pelvic pain

SIGNS
- Cervical os is closed.
- Uterus may be enlarged.
- No fetal heart tones

WORKUP
See Threatened Abortion.

COMMENTS AND TREATMENT CONSIDERATIONS
Although in the past D&C was performed in most cases of missed abortion, management is currently generally expectant. Patients require strict precautions regarding bleeding and infection as well as close follow-up with obstetrics/gynecology.

Septic Abortion
Septic abortion is defined as spontaneous or therapeutic abortion complicated by a pelvic infection. The incidence of septic abortion has decreased dramatically with the availability of therapeutic abortions performed by medical professionals under sterile conditions.

SYMPTOMS
- Abdominal or pelvic pain
- Fever
- Vaginal bleeding and/or discharge

SIGNS
- Cervical os may be open or closed.
- Uterine and/or cervical motion tenderness

WORKUP
See Threatened Abortion.
- Patients suspected of having a septic abortion should have a cervical culture and blood cultures.

COMMENTS AND TREATMENT CONSIDERATIONS
Septic abortion is a gynecologic emergency, requiring parenteral antibiotics, hospitalization, and urgent obstetrics/gynecology consultation.

CHAPTER 41

REFERENCES

Coppola PT, Coppola M: Vaginal bleeding in the first 20 weeks of pregnancy, *Emerg Med Clin North Am* 21:667, 2003.

Everett C: Incidence and outcome of bleeding before the 20th week of pregnancy: prospective study from general practice, *BMJ* 315:32, 1997.

Scott JR: Early pregnancy loss. In *Danforth's obstetrics and gynecology*, ed 8. Philadelphia, 1999, Lippincott Williams & Wilkins, pp 143-153.

Turner LM: Vaginal bleeding during pregnancy, *Emerg Med Clin North Am* 12:45, 1994.

MOLAR PREGNANCY

Molar pregnancy results from abnormal proliferation of trophoblastic tissue and encompasses several disorders, all of which can arise from a normal pregnancy, EP, or spontaneous abortion. In the United States and Europe, *hydatidiform mole* occurs in approximately 1 of 1000 pregnancies, more commonly in women < 20 years of age or > 40 years of age. It can be partial (fetal tissue with trophoblastic tissue) or complete (no fetal tissue). Hydatidiform mole has a high rate of spontaneous remission (80% to 85%) and fatalities are rare. Complications include development of a trophoblastic malignancy, hemorrhage, and sepsis. *Invasive mole* (chorioadenoma destruens) occurs in 1 of 12,000 pregnancies and is a progressive form of hydatidiform mole that has invaded the myometrium or other structures. Although metastases are uncommon, mortality is higher than with hydatidiform mole. *Choriocarcinoma* is a trophoblastic tissue malignancy that occurs in 1 of 40,000 pregnancies. Spontaneous remission is rare, metastases (lung, brain, liver, kidney, bowel) are common, and fatalities occur. Approximately half of choriocarcinomas are preceded by a hydatidiform mole and a quarter each by spontaneous abortion and term pregnancy. Timely diagnosis of molar pregnancy is important because early treatment is highly effective.

SYMPTOMS

- Molar pregnancy often has no specific clinical characteristics to distinguish it from a normal pregnancy in the early stages of gestation.
- Vaginal bleeding +++++
- Hyperemesis +++, can be severe
- Abdominal pain ++

SIGNS

- Absent fetal heart tone +++++
- Vaginal bleeding +++, may see "grape clusters" of hydatid vesicles

- Uterine enlargement may be disproportionately large for the gestational age +++.
- Preeclampsia in pregnancy less than 24 weeks' gestation ++
- Enlarged ovaries because of theca lutein cysts ++
- Hyperemesis gravidarum, which is frequently severe and protracted compared with normal pregnancy ++
- Anemia secondary to vaginal bleeding
- Signs of hyperthyroidism + and pulmonary trophoblastic emboli +

WORKUP
- Quantitative serum βHCG: abnormally high levels for dates with a continuous rise
- Ultrasonography is the technique of choice to confirm the diagnosis of molar pregnancy.
- Evaluate for metastases (chest x-ray; consider head and abdominal CT scanning).
- CBC with platelets
- PT/INR and PTT

COMMENTS AND TREATMENT CONSIDERATIONS
Initial treatment focuses on stabilization of the patient, including transfusion and correction of coagulopathy as needed. Obtain emergent obstetrical consultation. Subsequent management must take into consideration the stage of the disease, the age of the patient, and the desire for fertility. The choice is between D&C and hysterectomy. Subsequently chemotherapy may be necessary. Extended monitoring of serum βHCG levels is imperative.

REFERENCES
Freeman RS, Tortolero-Luna G, Pandey DK, et al: Gestational trophoblastic disease, *Obstet Gynecol Clin North Am* 23:548, 1996.
McKennett M, Fullerton JT: Vaginal bleeding in pregnancy, *Am Fam Physician* 53:639, 1995.
Viera AJ, Clenny TL, Shenenberg DW: Vaginal bleeding at 16 weeks, *Am Fam Physician* 59:649, 1999.

THIRD TRIMESTER BLEEDING
Bleeding in the third trimester of pregnancy can be a major cause of maternal and fetal morbidity and mortality. Placental abruption and placenta previa are the diagnoses of concern. Care providers must recognize the potential danger of third trimester bleeding and realize that the patient may be more ill than she first appears.

 PLACENTAL ABRUPTION

Placental abruption is the premature separation of the whole or part of a normally implanted placenta from the uterus. Abruption results in hemorrhage, which may occasionally be external with painless bleeding from the separated edges of the placenta draining through the placenta and into the vagina via the cervix. Alternatively, there may be concealed hemorrhage in which retroplacental bleeding results in blood pooling in the uterus without any avenue of escape.

SYMPTOMS
- Abdominal and pelvic pain/cramping ++++
- Vaginal bleeding in third trimester ++++

SIGNS
- Uterus hypertonic (fails to relax after contraction) and tender ++++
- Vaginal bleeding ++++; the amount of external bleeding may not correlate with the severity of abruption.
- Painful uterine contraction +++
- Back pain +++
- Fetal distress (tachycardia, bradycardia)
- Preterm labor ++
- Maternal shock with variable degrees of hypotension and tachycardia
- Fetal demise
- Hematuria, bruising

WORKUP
- Diagnosis is clinical.
- PT/PTT and DIC panel
- Hematocrit (frequently normal) +++
- Type and crossmatch blood.
- Rh assay
- Ultrasound, often nondiagnostic even in critical cases +++

COMMENTS AND TREATMENT CONSIDERATIONS
Insert two large-bore intravenous lines, and initiate fluid resuscitation as needed. Place the patient on cardiac and fetal monitoring. Obtain emergent obstetric consultation. Observe for cessation of contractions, fetal distress, and a rapidly enlarging uterus or maternal shock. All Rh-negative women must be treated with $Rh_0(D)$ immune globulin intramuscularly (RhoGAM 300 μg). Disseminated intravascular coagulation (DIC) is a common complication (see Chapter 6, Bleeding).

 PLACENTA PREVIA

Placenta previa results from implantation of the placenta over the cervical os. In most cases, low-lying placentas seen in early pregnancy "migrate" away from the cervical os as the pregnancy progresses.

Occasionally, the placenta remains partially or completely over the cervical os. Placenta previa should be considered in all women presenting with vaginal bleeding in the third trimester, and ultrasound should be performed before a pelvic examination is performed because of the theoretical risk of inducing bleeding.

SYMPTOMS
- May be asymptomatic
- Vaginal bleeding in late second/third trimester ++++, often sudden, painless, and profuse
- Contractions may occur simultaneously with the bleeding.

SIGNS
- Vaginal bleeding
- Hypotension and tachycardia
- Uterus may be soft and nontender.
- Normal fetal heart tones are often present.

WORKUP
- Ultrasound is diagnostic +++++.
- Hematocrit
- Type and crossmatch blood.
- Rh assay

COMMENTS AND TREATMENT CONSIDERATIONS
If active bleeding is occurring, preparations for aggressive fluid and blood resuscitation should be made as obstetrical consultation is obtained. Apply oxygen, start two large-bore intravenous lines, and place the patient on cardiac and fetal monitoring. It is important that the ED physician not perform a pelvic examination in the ED in a patient with third trimester bleeding. The pelvic examination should be performed by an obstetrician in the operating room, with the physician fully prepared to perform an immediate cesarean delivery. $Rh_0(D)$ immune globulin (RhoGAM) should be given to pregnant Rh-negative women with vaginal bleeding.

REFERENCES
Frederiksen MC, Glassenberg R, Stika CS: Placenta previa: a 22-year analysis, *Am J Obstet Gynecol* 180:1432, 1999.

Nyberg DA, Mack LA, Benedetti TJ, et al: Placental abruption and placental hemorrhage: correlation of sonographic findings with fetal outcome, *Radiology* 358:357, 1987.

Scott JR: Placenta previa and abruption. In *Danforth's obstetrics and gynecology*, ed 8. Philadelphia, 1999, Lippincott Williams & Wilkins, pp 407-418.

CHAPTER 41

NONPREGNANT PATIENTS

Nonpregnant patients with vaginal bleeding rarely present with life-threatening conditions and are generally managed as outpatients. Pelvic tumors (benign and malignant) can cause vaginal bleeding, and stable patients should receive return precautions and close follow-up.

 DYSFUNCTIONAL UTERINE BLEEDING

Anovulation is the most frequent cause of dysfunctional uterine bleeding, which by definition is unrelated to organic or anatomic lesions of the uterus.

SYMPTOMS
• Vaginal bleeding +++++

SIGNS
• Vaginal bleeding +++++
• Normal pelvic examination

WORKUP
• Pregnancy test; pregnancy must be excluded prior to making this diagnosis.
• Hematocrit, type and crossmatch if unstable
• Endometrial biopsy to rule out endometrial cancer if patient is older than 35 to 40 years or is otherwise at high risk. Patients can generally be referred to gynecology for this procedure.

COMMENTS AND TREATMENT CONSIDERATIONS
Dysfunctional uterine bleeding is a diagnosis of exclusion. For severe bleeding, patients may require intravenous hormonal treatment, curettage, or, rarely, hysterectomy. Stable patients are generally treated as outpatients, with hormonal therapy such as medroxyprogesterone (Provera) 10 mg po for 7 to 10 days. Patients should be counseled that they will have withdrawal bleeding after completing the course of treatment. Gynecologic follow-up is advised.

REFERENCES
Bayer SR, DeCherney AH: Clinical manifestation and treatment of dysfunctional uterine bleeding, *JAMA* 269:1823, 1993.

Choung CJ, Brenner PF: Management of abnormal uterine bleeding, *Am J Obstet Gynecol* 175:787, 1996.

Wathen PI, Henderson MC, Witz CA: Abnormal uterine bleeding, *Med Clin North Am* 79:329, 1995.

Vision, Change in
Joseph S. Englanoff

The etiologies of nontraumatic loss of vision are diverse and include anatomic, vascular, infectious, toxicologic, autoimmune, and psychogenic causes. With many ophthalmologic emergencies, particularly central retinal artery occlusion, retinal detachment, and temporal arteritis, time is of the essence. Immediate action needs to be taken to correct the current loss of vision and to prevent further loss of vision.

It is important to obtain a history that focuses on the extent and time interval of the loss as well as any associated symptoms. The physical examination should include visual acuity, evaluation for foreign body, pupillary, funduscopic, and slit-lamp evaluations, as well as intraocular pressure measurement.

The characteristics of visual field loss help to localize the causative lesion. Lesions in front of the optic chiasm (optic nerve and retina) cause monocular symptoms. Lesions behind the chiasm produce homonymous hemianopias (loss of right or left visual field in both eyes). Chiasm lesions affect both eyes in different ways, such as bitemporal hemianopia (loss of temporal visual fields in both eyes).

An afferent pupillary defect (APD) is present when direct pupillary constriction to light in the affected eye is less than the consensual response when light is shined in the unaffected eye. Moving the light from the unaffected to the affected eye therefore leads to pupillary dilation. An APD suggests pathology of an afferent structure of vision (e.g., retina or optic nerve) in the affected eye.

Emergency department ophthalmologic consultation is required for all patients with acute loss of vision related to disorders of the eye itself. Other emergent consultations may be required depending on the etiology of the visual loss. In addition to a routine examination, indirect funduscopic examination (usually done by an ophthalmologist) is required in most cases.

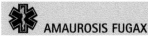

AMAUROSIS FUGAX

Amaurosis fugax is unilateral loss of vision usually caused by an atheromatous plaque at the carotid bifurcation that either embolizes or causes a temporary reduction in retinal circulation.

SYMPTOMS
- Completely painless process (unless associated with a migraine)
- Monocular complete or partial loss of vision that may last seconds to (occasionally) 1 to 2 hours
- Visual loss may be described as a "curtain lowering" in eye.

SIGNS
- Normal eye and funduscopic examination (except if coexisting disease)
- Occasionally, signs of central retinal artery occlusion are seen on funduscopic examination.
- Concomitant contralateral arm or leg weakness or numbness may be present if this is an embolic phenomenon to a larger more proximal vessel.

WORKUP
- Complete history, detailing the event and determining whether the visual loss is truly monocular or possibly binocular. Previous episodes, transient ischemic attacks (TIA), cerebrovascular accidents, heart or valvular disease, and intravenous drug abuse should be investigated.
- Complete ophthalmologic evaluation including visual field tests and dilated funduscopic examination
- Depending on the history and clinical findings, other tests may be appropriate.
- A CBC with platelet count may be helpful to rule out polycythemia or thrombocytosis.
- Carotid duplex may be helpful to determine origination of embolus.
- Cardiac echocardiogram may be helpful to determine origination of embolus.
- CT or MRI may be helpful if a postchiasmic lesion is suspected or if other neurologic signs or symptoms accompany monocular visual loss.

COMMENTS AND TREATMENT CONSIDERATIONS
Because amaurosis fugax is a form of TIA, it should be investigated and treated as such, with emphasis on rapid detection of extracranial arterial disease, cardiac abnormalities, and hematologic disorders. In one study, 16% of patients with amaurosis fugax eventually

suffered a stroke or permanent loss of vision in the affected eye, or both.

See Chapter 44, Weakness and Fatigue.

REFERENCES

Benavente O, Eliasziw M, Streifler JY, et al: Prognosis after transient monocular blindness associated with carotid-artery stenosis, *N Engl J Med* 345:1084, 2001.

Burde RM: Amaurosis fugax: an overview, *J Clin Neuroophthalmol* 9:185, 1989.

Lord RS: Transient monocular blindness, *Aust N Z J Ophthalmol* 18:299, 1990.

Wakakura M, Ishikawa S: Neuro-ophthalmic aspects of vascular disease, *Curr Opin Ophthalmol* 5:18, 1994.

 RETINAL DETACHMENT

Retinal detachment is separation of the inner neuronal layer of the retina from the outer pigment epithelial layer. It is more common in patients with diabetes, the elderly (average age of onset is in the fifth decade), trauma patients, and individuals with previous retinal detachment.

SYMPTOMS
- Painless event
- Monocular complaints of flashes of light, floaters (specks of pigment or blood), or a "curtain" moving over the field of vision
- Loss of vision or a visual field defect varies and may be gradual or sudden in onset.
- Visual acuity remains normal until the macula is involved.

SIGNS
- Normal anterior chamber
- Afferent pupillary defect may be present.
- Blood in the vitreous may occur because bleeding is common with retinal detachment.
- Retina may appear to have an elevation, flap, hole, or an undulatory appearance; direct ophthalmoscopy demonstrates that portions of the retina are in focus while other portions are not.

WORKUP
- Indirect ophthalmoscopy by an ophthalmologist is mandatory.
- Ultrasound is frequently used to evaluate the retina because a concomitant vitreous hemorrhage may prevent visualization of the retina.

CHAPTER 42

COMMENTS AND TREATMENT CONSIDERATIONS

Retinal detachment is a true emergency requiring immediate ophthalmologic intervention, which aims to reattach the detached portion, thereby restoring retinal blood supply, and to prevent further undermining and detachment. If left untreated, it may progress to complete loss of vision, especially if the macula becomes separated. Treatment consists of air or silicon oil injections, cryotherapy, photocoagulation, diathermy, and scleral buckling.

REFERENCES

Cavallerano AA: Retinal detachment, *Optom Clin* 2:25, 1992.
Classe JG: Clinicolegal aspects of vitreous and retinal detachment, *Optom Clin* 2:113, 1992.
Reichel E: Vitreoretinal emergencies, *Am Fam Physician* 52:1415, 1995.

 CENTRAL RETINAL ARTERY OCCLUSION

Central retinal artery occlusion is frequently caused by an embolism from carotid artery disease and primarily affects the elderly, with an increased incidence in men.

SYMPTOMS

- Monocular
- Painless
- Sudden and complete or partial loss of vision

SIGNS

- Pale fundus (compared with the other eye) with a cherry red spot in the center of the macula (Fig. 42–1)
- Afferent pupillary defect to some degree is almost always present.
- Retinal arterioles may have a "boxcar" appearance, that is, segmentation of the blood column in the arterioles.

WORKUP

- Full dilated funduscopic examination (including indirect by an ophthalmologist), which should exclude other causes of painless, monocular loss of vision such as retinal detachment and vitreous hemorrhage
- Orbit or brain CT, ESR, and WBC counts are of no benefit.

COMMENTS AND TREATMENT CONSIDERATIONS

Early intervention and treatment may relieve the occlusion; vision is permanently lost if the process persists for more than 2 hours. Immediate ophthalmologic consultation is critical.

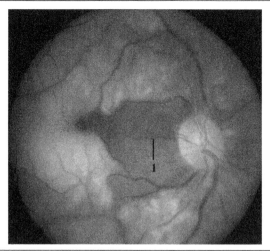

Fig. 42–1 Central retinal artery obstruction with a patent cilioretinal artery (1) sparing the fovea. Diffuse retinal whitening from retinal ischemia appears several hours after the arterial occlusion. The normal-appearing retina between the optic nerve and fovea is perfused by the centrally located cilioretinal arteriole. (From Palay DA, Krachmer JH: *Ophthalmology for the primary care physician.* St Louis, 1997, Mosby.)

While awaiting the ophthalmologist's arrival, the emergency physician should attempt to dislodge the embolus by applying digital pressure to the globe repeatedly for 5 seconds and releasing for 5 seconds. Furthermore, using a technique called enhanced external counterpulsation, which entails inflating in sequences pressure cuffs around the legs, has shown some limited promise.

Increasing Pco_2 by having the patient breathe into a brown paper bag for 10 minutes each hour may relieve vasospasm. Acetazolamide (Diamox) 500 mg po may be given in addition to timolol 0.5% eye drops. Sublingual nitroglycerin may cause vascular dilation. The ophthalmologist may attempt an anterior chamber paracentesis to decompress the globe and dislodge the embolus. The use of intra-arterial fibrinolysis is quite controversial, with the majority of studies showing no added benefit.

Retinal vein occlusion can also occur and cause visual impairment or loss (Fig. 42–2).

REFERENCES

Atebara NH, Brown GC, Cater J: Efficacy of anterior chamber paracentesis and Carbogen in treating acute nonarteritic central retinal artery occlusion, Ophthalmology 102:2029, 1995.

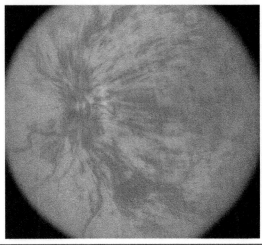

Fig. 42–2 Central retinal vein occlusion in a patient with 20/400 visual acuity. Note the dramatic retinal hemorrhages in all four quadrants. Significant venous dilation and tortuosity are present. Mild to moderate ischemia is seen with diffuse cotton-wool spots. The optic disc is blurred with peripapillary hemorrhage. (From Palay DA, Krachmer JH: *Ophthalmology for the primary care physician.* St Louis, 1997, Mosby.)

Butz B, Strotzer M, Manke C, et al: Selective intraarterial fibrinolysis of acute central artery occlusion, *Acta Radiol* 44:680, 2003.

Framme C, Spiegel D, Roider J, et al: Central retinal artery occlusion. Importance of selective intra-arterial fibrinolysis, *Ophthalmologe* 98:725, 2001.

Schmidt DP, Schulte-Monting J, Schumacher M: Prognosis of central retinal artery occlusion: local intraarterial fibrinolysis versus conservative treatment, *Am J Neuroradiol* 23:1301, 2002.

Werner D, Michalk F, Harazny J, et al: Accelerated reperfusion of poorly perfused retinal areas in central retinal artery occlusion and branch retinal artery occlusion after a short treatment with enhanced external counterpulsation, *Retina* 24:541, 2004.

 TEMPORAL (GIANT CELL) ARTERITIS

The loss of vision itself is a painless process; that is, the eye is not painful, but the surrounding structures may be painful. It is usually a sudden, nearly complete, monocular loss of vision that may become bilateral.

See Chapter 18, Headache.

VITREOUS HEMORRHAGE

Vitreous hemorrhage should be considered in patients with diabetes mellitus, hypertension, and trauma.

SYMPTOMS
- Painless event
- Gradual or sudden loss of vision that may vary from normal vision to only light perception
- Black spots with flashing lights that move with eye movement are a common complaint. Some patients report seeing a red haze.
- Usually a unilateral process, but bilateral involvement has been reported.

SIGNS
- Anterior chamber, usually normal
- Mild afferent pupillary defect may be present (possibly associated with retinal detachment).
- Red light reflex may be decreased or absent.
- Inability to visualize the fundus is common with large vitreous hemorrhages.

WORKUP
- Clinical diagnosis can be confirmed by performing a full dilated posterior pole examination.
- Indirect ophthalmoscopy or ultrasound is used to rule out retinal detachment.

COMMENTS AND TREATMENT CONSIDERATIONS
Vitreous hemorrhage may be easily discovered, yet the cause of the hemorrhage must be ascertained. Treatment depends on the cause. Retinal detachment must be definitively ruled out, and ED ophthalmologic consultation is essential.

If no cause can be found and the area of hemorrhage is large, the patient may be admitted to the hospital. Aspirin, NSAIDs, and other anticlotting agents are avoided. Bed rest with the head of the bed elevated for 2 to 3 days is recommended. Some patients require cryotherapy, laser photocoagulation, or vitrectomy.

REFERENCES
Benson WE, Spalter HF: Vitreous hemorrhage, *Surv Ophthalmol* 15:297, 1971.

Dana MR, Werner MS, Viana MA, et al: Spontaneous and traumatic vitreous hemorrhage, *Ophthalmology* 100:1377, 1993.

Spraul CW, Grossniklaus HE: Vitreous hemorrhage, *Surv Ophthalmol* 42:3, 1997.

CHAPTER 42

OPTIC NEURITIS

Optic neuritis causes loss of vision that is usually unilateral (more common in adults) but is sometimes bilateral (more common in children). It is caused by demyelination of the optic nerve and has a gradual onset (hours to days). Optic neuritis is a common finding in multiple sclerosis (MS). In some patients it is related to a previous (4 to 6 weeks), nonspecific viral illness. Other possible causes should be investigated, including sarcoidosis, SLE, toxoplasmosis, Lyme disease, HIV, cytomegalovirus (CMV), and syphilis.

SYMPTOMS
- Loss of vision can range from minimal loss to no light perception.
- Loss of vision is usually associated with decreased color vision and light intensity perception.
- Pain with eye movement is very common.

SIGNS
- Afferent pupillary defect (varying degrees)
- Central scotoma or arcuate visual field defects are possible.
- Optic nerve head may appear swollen with edema and possible retinal hemorrhages.
- Optic nerve head may appear normal if retrobulbar optic neuritis is present (more common in adults).

WORKUP
- Diagnosis is clinically based and often is one of exclusion. A history confirming the course of vision loss and occurrence of any previous episodes is useful. A list of past and current medication use may be helpful (ethambutol and tamoxifen use should be solicited).
- Complete ophthalmologic evaluation including a dilated funduscopic examination and visual field test
- Complete and thorough neurologic examination is essential.
- MRI may assist in diagnosing MS and in ruling out an intracranial or orbital tumor that is compressing the optic nerve.

COMMENTS AND TREATMENT CONSIDERATIONS
The treatment of optic neuritis is controversial. Many suggest observation only; others recommend systemic steroids. The association between monocular optic neuritis and the development of MS in many patients is well established, with MS developing in the majority within 4 years. Information concerning steroid use is conflicting, but steroids may diminish the chance for subsequent development of MS. IV immunoglobulin, once thought to have possible therapeutic benefit, has since been shown to be of no benefit.

However, trials with the use of interferon have shown substantial benefit. Consultation with a neurologist or ophthalmologist who will observe the patient is an essential part of management. Recovery ensues within 4 to 6 weeks for approximately 90% of patients.

REFERENCES

Beck RW, Cleary PA, Anderson MM, et al: A randomized, controlled trial of corticosteroids in the treatment of acute optic neuritis. The Optic Neuritis Study Group, *N Engl J Med* 326:581, 1992.

Beck RW, Cleary PA, Trobe JD, et al: The effect of corticosteroids for acute optic neuritis on the subsequent development of multiple sclerosis, *N Engl J Med* 329:1764, 1993.

CHAMPS Study Group: Interferon beta-1a for optic neuritis patients at high risk for multiple sclerosis, *Am J Ophthalmol* 132:463, 2001.

McDonald WI: Optic neuritis and its significance, *Clin Exp Neurol* 26:1, 1989.

Roed HG, Langkilde A, Sellebjerg F, et al: A double-blind, randomized trial of IV immunoglobulin treatment in acute optic neuritis, *Neurology* 64:804, 2005.

Wray SH: Optic neuritis: guidelines, *Curr Opin Neurol* 8:72, 1995.

CHAPTER 42

Vomiting, Pediatric
Alisa McQueen, Frances McCabe, and Neal Peeples

There are numerous causes of vomiting in infants and children. In most cases the cause is benign, the vomiting attributable to viral gastroenteritis or a food poisoning, and the principal concern maintenance of normal hydration. Less commonly, vomiting is a sign of a more serious disease. It is crucial to distinguish the child who is vomiting because of a serious illness from the many children whose illness is self-limited. This chapter reviews a number of serious conditions in which vomiting is caused by a primary abnormality of the gastrointestinal tract. In addition to the entities discussed in this chapter, there are numerous other conditions in which vomiting can be a presenting symptom, particularly in the pediatric patient. Vomiting can be a manifestation of poisoning, medication effect, testicular torsion, neurologic disease (e.g., head injury or any cause of elevated intracranial pressure), metabolic or endocrine disease (e.g., inborn errors of metabolism or new-onset diabetes mellitus), or infection (e.g., pyelonephritis or meningitis). Hematemesis is discussed in Chapter 6, Bleeding.

 POISONINGS
See Chapter 37, Toxic Exposure, Approach to.

 TESTICULAR TORSION
See Chapter 31, Scrotal Pain.

 HEAD INJURY
See Chapter 18, Headache and Chapter 39, Trauma, Approach to.

MENINGITIS

See Chapter18, Headache.

 PYELONEPHRITIS

See Chapter 4, Back Pain, Lower, and Urinary Tract Infection in Chapter 22, The Irritable Child.

MALROTATION AND VOLVULUS

Malrotation occurs when the embryonic midgut fails to rotate either partially or completely and is frequently associated with additional GI tract abnormalities, including Hirschsprung's disease and intestinal atresias. Midgut volvulus (MGV) associated with malrotation most commonly presents in the first month of life but is occasionally seen in infants 1 to 6 months of age. Rarely, MGV develops later in childhood and even in adulthood, and patients may give a history of nonspecific gastrointestinal symptoms for years. MGV can result in obstruction and bowel ischemia if unrecognized. Based on several series, mortality is about 5% but has generally decreased in recent years as a result of early surgical intervention.

CHAPTER 43

SYMPTOMS
- Bilious (green) vomiting ++++; most common in patients younger than 1 month. Nonbilious vomiting and irritability and pain are less common.
- Intermittent vomiting
- Poor feeding
- Abdominal bloating

SIGNS
- Abdominal distention may or may not be present because obstruction may be proximal.
- The presence or absence of bowel sounds is neither sensitive nor specific for malrotation and volvulus.
- Blood in the stool (gross or occult) ++ is an ominous sign that may signal bowel ischemia.
- Lethargy, with or without vomiting, may be present and may be the only clue to shock and significant acidosis from compromised intestinal blood flow.

WORKUP
- Bilious vomiting in a neonate must be considered a surgical emergency. Infants who are highly suspected of having MGV or

an acute abdominal condition require rapid operative intervention to prevent bowel necrosis and death. Obtaining extensive diagnostic workups on these patients leads to undue and potentially dangerous delays.

- Abdominal x-rays +++; may show evidence of obstruction, loops of small bowel overriding the liver, double-bubble sign of duodenal obstruction, gastric dilatation, and possibly limited gas distal to the obstruction.
- Upper gastrointestinal tract series is the study of choice.

COMMENTS AND TREATMENT CONSIDERATIONS

MGV is associated with high morbidity if the diagnosis is missed or delayed. Patients suspected of MGV should have a nasogastric tube placed for gut decompression and receive fluid resuscitation to make up for fluid and electrolyte losses caused by vomiting and bowel edema. The importance of early surgical consultation and repair cannot be overstated.

REFERENCES

Andrassy RJ, Mahour GH: Malrotation in the midgut in infants and children: a 25-year review, *Arch Surg* 116:158, 1981.

Kamal IM: Defusing the intra-abdominal ticking bomb: intestinal malrotation in children, *CMAJ* 162:1315, 2000.

Kimura K, Loening-Baucke V: Bilious vomiting in the newborn: rapid diagnosis of intestinal obstruction, *Am Fam Physician* 61:2791, 2000.

Millar AJ, Rode H, Cywes S: Malrotation and volvulus in infancy and childhood, *Semin Pediatr Surg* 12:229, 2003.

Pumberger W, Dinhobl I, Dremsek P: Altered consciousness and lethargy from compromised intestinal blood flow in children, *Am J Emerg Med* 22:307, 2004.

 NECROTIZING ENTEROCOLITIS

Necrotizing enterocolitis (NEC) is the most common and lethal surgical abdominal emergency in the newborn. The cause of NEC is unclear. Prematurity is the greatest risk factor (++++); however, term infants with risk factors for ischemic bowel (cardiac disease, infection, perinatal hypoxic ischemic insults, aggressive enteral feedings) are also at risk. Although this disease is seen almost exclusively in the neonatal intensive care unit, as more infants are sent home earlier in life, NEC presentations to the ED may increase. Extremely premature infants (<28 weeks) remain at high risk until they reach the postconceptual age of 35 to 36 weeks.

SYMPTOMS
- Vomiting and poor feeding ++
- Lethargy
- Irritability
- Episodes of apnea

SIGNS
- Abdominal distention ++++, may evolve over time
- Blood in the stools, gross or occult ++++
- Fever is uncommon.
- Red or dark streaks on the abdomen are occasionally seen in advanced cases.

WORKUP
- Abdominal x-rays are the primary diagnostic tool for establishing NEC. X-rays may be normal or show mild ileus pattern early in the course. Pneumatosis intestinalis makes the definitive diagnosis of NEC. Free air indicates intestinal perforation.
- Electrolytes for metabolic acidosis and other derangements from vomiting and bowel edema
- CBC may demonstrate anemia and thrombocytopenia. Leukocytosis may or may not be present, and leukopenia indicates severe disease.

COMMENTS AND TREATMENT CONSIDERATIONS
Treatment of NEC is based on severity, but all infants in whom this diagnosis is suspected should be hospitalized in an institution with neonatology and pediatric surgical subspecialty consultation available. Generally, enteral feedings are discontinued. Intravenous antibiotics, nasogastric decompression, and vigorous hydration constitute initial management, with surgical intervention for patients who develop signs of intestinal perforation.

REFERENCES
Caplan MS, Jilling T: New concepts in necrotizing enterocolitis, *Curr Opin Pediatr* 13:111, 2001.

Ng SC: Necrotizing enterocolitis in the full-term neonate, *J Paediatr Child Health* 37:1, 2001.

Ostlie DJ, Spilde TL, St Peter SD, et al: Necrotizing enterocolitis in full-term infants, *J Pediatr Surg* 38:1039, 2003.

 INCARCERATED INGUINAL HERNIA

Inguinal hernias occur in 1% to 4% of children; approximately 10% of these become incarcerated. The male/female ratio is 4:1, but the incarceration rate is higher in girls.

SYMPTOMS
- Irritability
- Vomiting
- History of a scrotal mass that comes and goes

SIGNS
- Tender scrotal mass
- Abdominal distention
- Fever
- Irritability

WORKUP
- Thorough physical examination is sufficient to make the diagnosis in most cases.
- Ultrasound may occasionally be useful in differentiating hernia from other scrotal pathology.
- Abdominal x-rays can be used to rule out obstruction.

COMMENTS AND TREATMENT CONSIDERATIONS
Reduction of an incarcerated hernia is necessary, followed by definitive surgical repair. Emergent surgical intervention is required for a nonreducible hernia or if infarcted bowel is present. An easily reducible hernia without incarceration can be electively repaired in consultation with a surgeon.

REFERENCES
Abantanga FA: Groin and scrotal swellings in children aged 5 years and below: a review of 535 cases, *Pediatr Surg Int* 19:446, 2003.

Sheldon CA: The pediatric genitourinary examination: inguinal, urethral, and genital diseases, *Pediatr Clin North Am* 48:1339, 2001.

 PYLORIC STENOSIS

Pyloric stenosis is the idiopathic hypertrophy of smooth muscle of the pylorus that leads to gastric outlet obstruction in infants. It is an acquired disease, usually presenting between 2 and 4 months of age (median age 6 weeks). The etiology us unknown but probably involves some combination of genetic predisposition and environmental exposure. The male/female ratio is 4:1. First-born infant boys are most commonly affected, and a positive family history is common. An association between erythromycin in early infancy and the development of pyloric stenosis has been described, and this finding has been corroborated in multiple series.

SYMPTOMS
- Vomiting described as projectile and nonbilious +++++. Median duration of vomiting before diagnosis is 7 days.
- An infant may appear hungry and feed vigorously between episodes unless, or until, he or she becomes severely dehydrated.

SIGNS
- Epigastric or right upper quadrant mass +++, classically known as the "olive," is more easily palpable with the child in prone position or by elevating the child's legs and palpating during a feed just after the stomach has been emptied. Although classically described, it is only occasionally palpable, and its absence does not exclude the diagnosis of pyloric stenosis.
- Volume depletion +++

WORKUP
- Electrolyte measurement may demonstrate hypokalemic and hypochloremic metabolic acidosis.
- Ultrasound +++++ has nearly replaced upper GI series in the evaluation of pyloric stenosis.
- Upper GI series is generally more time consuming and less sensitive and specific than ultrasound for pyloric stenosis.
- Endoscopy is more invasive than ultrasound, and limited data exist on its use in this setting.
- Plain abdominal x-rays are of little value when the diagnosis is suspected.

COMMENTS AND TREATMENT CONSIDERATIONS
Intravenous hydration and electrolyte and dextrose replacement should be administered as guided by clinical volume status and serum electrolytes. Approximately 60% of infants with pyloric stenosis also have a hypochloremic metabolic alkalosis. Although studies suggest that atropine administered intravenously may obviate the need for surgical repair, pyloromyotomy is commonly performed in most institutions. Emergent repair is not necessary, but infants should be hospitalized for parenteral hydration and correction of metabolic abnormalities.

REFERENCES
Cooper WO, Griffin MR, Arbogast P, et al: Very early exposure to erythromycin and infantile hypertrophic pyloric stenosis, *Arch Pediatr Adolesc Med* 156:647, 2002.

Honein MA, Paulozzi LJ, Himelright IM, et al: Infantile hypertrophic pyloric stenosis after pertussis prophylaxis with erythromycin: a case review and cohort study, *Lancet* 354:2101, 1999.

CHAPTER **43**

Kawahara H, Imura K, Nishikawa M, et al: Intravenous atropine treatment in infantile hypertrophic pyloric stenosis, *Arch Dis Child* 87:71, 2002.

Nagita A, Yamaguchi J, Amemoto K, et al: Management and ultrasonographic appearance of infantile hypertrophic pyloric stenosis with intravenous atropine sulfate, *J Pediatr Gastroenterol Nutr* 23:172, 1996.

 GASTROESOPHAGEAL REFLUX

Gastroesophageal reflux is more common early in infancy and slowly declines in incidence over the first year of life. Nearly all infants have some degree of reflux, but the symptoms vary greatly in severity. Reflux becomes medically important when it causes respiratory symptoms and failure to thrive. The association of reflux with respiratory symptoms (reactive airway disease, stridor, pneumonia, and apnea) is less well substantiated than the GI symptoms. However, occasional resolution of respiratory symptoms with reflux treatment has been demonstrated.

SYMPTOMS
- Irritability
- Regurgitation and nonprojectile vomiting
- Recurrent cough, wheeze, or stridor
- In infants, reflux may be the underlying etiology of an apparent life-threatening event (ALTE).

SIGNS
- There are few clinical signs of reflux.
- Sandifer's syndrome describes abnormal movements of the head, neck, and trunk related to reflux in the infant.
- Abdominal examination is normal.
- Failure to thrive is seen in severe cases.
- Lethargy and dehydration are rare and should prompt an investigation of other, more serious diagnoses.

WORKUP
- Observation of feeds can be helpful in the evaluation of reflux. Upper GI series may be helpful if more serious diseases are a diagnostic consideration.

COMMENTS AND TREATMENT CONSIDERATIONS
Patients should generally be referred for outpatient evaluation after conditions requiring emergent treatment have been ruled out.

REFERENCES

Rudolph CD, Mazur LJ, Liptak GS, et al.: Guidelines for evaluation
and treatment of gastroesophageal reflux in infants and children:
recommendations of the North American Society for Pediatric
Gastroenterology and Nutrition, *J Pediatr Gastroenterol Nutr*
32:S1, 2001.

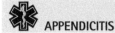 **APPENDICITIS**

See Chapter 1, Abdominal Pain.

Weakness and Fatigue
Richard T. Griffey and Jonathan S. Ilgen

There are innumerable causes of weakness, and patients can mean very different things when they complain of feeling "weak." In considering potential causes, the clinician should consider the patterns of symptoms and signs that suggest potential causes referable to the neurologic system (brain, spinal cord, peripheral nerves, and neuromuscular junction), muscles (myositis, rhabdomyolysis, etc.), or systemic disorders (endocrinologic, metabolic, medication effects, infectious, etc.).

The first step in identifying the cause of a patient's complaint of weakness is distinguishing a generalized sense of weakness involving the entire body from focal weakness involving only a portion of the body, such as a hemiparesis involving one side of the body but sparing the other. Although the pattern of weakness described by the patient (localized, in a particular distribution, or diffuse) is not a perfect indicator of the underlying cause, it provides a crucial clue to direct further evaluation. Focal weakness may indicate a stroke but has a broader differential including spinal cord and peripheral nerve injury.

Next, one should attempt to distinguish a subjective sense of fatigue or energy loss, which can result from a multitude of systemic processes, such as infections, metabolic disorders, or myocardial infarction, from actual decreased motor strength, typically caused by abnormalities of muscle, nerve, or neuromuscular junction. Patients are often unable to make this distinction, which can remain uncertain even after a good history and physical examination. The patient's mental status may help make the distinction. The lethargic and globally weak patient is more likely to have systemic illness such as sepsis. The fully alert and cognitively intact patient who is having difficulty swallowing and standing is unlikely to have a systemic illness and more likely to have a neurologic or neuromuscular disorder. The presence or absence of other symptoms and onset and duration of signs and symptoms (acute, gradual, or chronic) are also helpful in ordering the differential diagnosis and prioritizing the patient's evaluation.

NEUROLOGIC DISEASE

Weakness caused by neurologic disease generally follows patterns corresponding to the level of injury. When weakness is due to a *cortical lesion*, symptoms and signs are typically contralateral to the lesion and thus localized to one side of the body; they are also frequently associated with other concordant neurologic deficits. Alterations in the quality or coordination of muscle movements can result from *cerebellar dysfunction* of the ipsilateral side and also typically occur along with other cerebellar and posterior fossa findings. Lesions in the *spinal cord* typically produce a motor or sensory "level" below which neurologic deficits are pronounced, with normal function above the lesion. Some spinal cord diseases are characterized by changing levels over a variable period of time. *Nerve root* lesions produce findings limited to the distribution served by the involved roots, but because of significant overlap in the innervation of individual muscles, motor findings are typically subtle if only a single root is involved. Multiple nerve distributions may be affected with processes that involve an anatomic area containing multiple roots, such as the brachial plexus or the cauda equina. *Peripheral nerve* damage eventually leads to lower motor neuron signs (atrophy, flaccid paralysis, fasciculations, and depressed reflexes) as well as weakness isolated to the muscles served by the involved nerve. Disorders of the *neuromuscular junction* (NMJ) often result in weakness in the muscles innervated by the cranial nerves (extraocular, facial, and bulbar) as well as skeletal muscles.

In addition to the entities discussed in detail here, the differential diagnosis for neurologic etiologies of weakness should also consider transverse myelitis and multiple sclerosis.

 ACUTE UNILATERAL WEAKNESS (STROKE)

Although not the only cause of acute unilateral weakness, stroke is the most common cause of this presentation. In the past there was no effective treatment for stroke, but recent data suggest that prompt evaluation and therapy may improve outcome. A doctor faced with this clinical picture in the ED should focus on a rapid evaluation and be aware of the treatment options.

Stroke can be ischemic or hemorrhagic. Ischemic stroke occurs when interruption of blood flow to the brain leads to critical hypoperfusion resulting in loss of function and eventually brain infarction. Ischemic stroke is generally caused by thrombosis or embolism and may become secondarily hemorrhagic. Spontaneous intracerebral hemorrhage (ICH) makes up approximately 15% of strokes. There is no reliable way to differentiate an ischemic stroke from an ICH by clinical examination.

Ischemic stroke and transient ischemic attack (TIA) are essentially the same pathophysiologic process and are impossible to separate on initial evaluation. Stroke causes a sustained or permanent neurologic dysfunction. TIA is distinguished from stroke by the resolution of symptoms within minutes to hours. The rate of stroke recurrence is not different in patients who are diagnosed with a TIA instead of a stroke.

In the evaluation of a patient with acute unilateral weakness, it is important to consider other entities that may mimic stroke. These entities account for a significant minority of patients with unilateral weakness and must be differentiated from stroke. This differentiation can be very difficult or even impossible on a clinical basis. Neuroimaging is often necessary, and occasionally even this is not definitive.

- Hypoglycemia may result in focal neurologic symptoms or signs, with or without mental status changes. A finger stick blood glucose is an essential part of the evaluation of the patient with sudden-onset unilateral weakness or other acute focal neurologic deficits.
- Postictal paralysis, also known as Todd's paralysis, is transient, often unilateral, paralysis that follows a generalized tonic-clonic seizure and resolves over minutes to hours.
- Epidural and subdural hemorrhage can cause focal neurologic deficits, including unilateral weakness.
- Although a common cause of neurologic deficits in the form of visual disturbances, migraines are also a rare cause of unilateral weakness. Weakness may precede or accompany headache. Patients presenting with their first episode cannot be dependably distinguished from stroke by history and examination.
- Brain tumors can cause gradual or occasionally acute onset of focal neurologic deficits mimicking stroke.
- Acute peripheral facial nerve (cranial nerve VII) dysfunction, known as Bell's palsy causes unilateral weakness of the facial muscles of both the forehead and lower face. In contrast, a stroke almost always involves the lower face only. A brain stem stroke involving the facial nerve to the upper and lower face results in abnormal eye movements and other neurologic findings.
- Rarely, psychiatric illness (e.g., conversion reaction) can manifest with symptoms suggestive of a stroke. A psychiatric basis for neurologic symptoms should be considered only after neurologic causes have been excluded.

SYMPTOMS

- Acute unilateral weakness (++++) in any combination of face, arm, and leg (except face and leg without arm)
- Aphasia or impaired language
- Dysarthria or slurred speech
- Anosognosia or unawareness of neurologic deficits to the point of denial of illness, commonly associated with left-sided weakness from right hemisphere stroke
- Visual symptoms: visual field deficits in hemispheric stroke, diplopia in brain stem stroke
- Headache, more commonly with ICH
- Nausea and vomiting, particularly in ICH and posterior fossa stroke

History should be obtained from family, prehospital care personnel, or other observers in addition to the patient. Patients with anosognosia or severe aphasia may not be able to communicate accurate historical information. Patients with severe dysarthria may only be able to communicate by writing.

In addition to eliciting the patient's symptoms, it is important to ascertain the time of onset. This is defined as the last time the patient was known to be symptom free. Stroke risk factors (prior stroke or TIA, hypertension, diabetes, coronary artery disease, atrial fibrillation, hyperlipidemia, peripheral vascular disease, and smoking) are also routinely elicited.

SIGNS

- Focal neurologic signs (weakness is dominant) ++++; specific signs vary according to vascular territory involved.
- Weakness may be minimal to the point of being difficult to detect on examination, moderate, or so profound as to result in total paralysis of the affected part. Distribution of weakness caused by ischemic stroke reflects the areas of the brain perfused by specific arteries (Fig. 44–1). For example, patients with infarction in the territory of the anterior cerebral artery present with weakness involving the leg more than the arm or face. In contrast, patients with infarction in the territory of the middle cerebral artery present with weakness of the face and arm greater than the leg. Branch artery occlusion can cause more delimited weakness, involving only part of a limb or the face alone. Occlusion of small penetrating arteries deep in the brain result in a variety of stroke syndromes called lacunar strokes. Lacunar strokes may present with varying degrees and patterns of weakness, including a *pure motor stroke*, with face, arm, and leg weakness and *clumsy hand-dysarthria syndrome* presenting with slurred speech and unilateral hand weakness and ataxia.

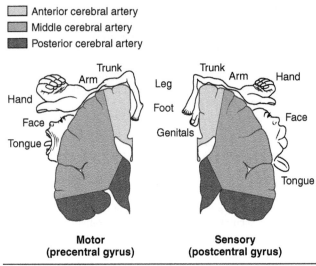

Anterior cerebral artery
Middle cerebral artery
Posterior cerebral artery

Trunk   Trunk
    Arm   Arm   Hand
Hand   Leg
          Foot
Face   Face
          Genitals
Tongue   Tongue

Motor   **Sensory**
(precentral gyrus) **(postcentral gyrus)**

Fig. 44–1   Arterial perfusion in relation to the homunculus.

- Aphasia (impaired language) is associated with dominant hemisphere strokes (typically left brain and right-sided weakness).
- Dysarthria (slurred speech) can be associated with facial weakness.
- Diplopia, vertigo, and vomiting often accompany brain stem strokes.
- Cranial nerve and cerebellar findings in posterior circulation stroke
- Blood pressure is typically elevated on presentation, but tends to decline spontaneously towards normal with sequential measurement.
- Cardiac irregularity associated with atrial fibrillation
- Diminished carotid pulses or carotid bruits

The National Institutes of Health Stroke Scale (NIHSS) is an examination tool that can be used to delineate neurologic deficits and repeated to quantify improvement or worsening (Table 44–1).

WORKUP

- All patients suspected of having a stroke should undergo timely neuroimaging. *Noncontrast CT* scan has high sensitivity and specificity for identifying hemorrhage, but a CT scan done in the first few hours after a nonhemorrhagic (ischemic) stroke is

TABLE 44–1

NATIONAL INSTITUTES OF HEALTH STROKE SCALE (NIHSS)

SECTION	MEASURE	SCORE
1a. Level of consciousness (LOC)	0 = Alert, 1 = Easily arousable, 2 = Difficult to arouse, 3 = Unresponsive	
1b. LOC questions	0 = Both correct, 1 = One correct, 2 = Both incorrect	
1c. LOC commands	0 = Both correct, 1 = One correct, 2 = Both incorrect	
2. Best gaze	0 = Normal, 1 = Partial gaze deviation, 2 = Forced gaze deviation	
3. Visual fields	0 = No visual loss, 1 = Partial hemianopia, 2 = Complete hemianopia, 3 = Blind	
4. Facial palsy	0 = Normal, 1 = Minor paralysis, 2 = Partial paralysis, 3 = Complete paralysis	
5. Motor arm 5a. Left arm 5b. Right arm	0 = No drift, 1 = Drift, 2 = Some effort against gravity, 3 = No effort against gravity, 4 = No movement	a. b.
6. Motor leg 6a. Left leg 6b. Right leg	0 = No drift, 1 = Drift, 2 = Some effort against gravity, 3 = No effort against gravity, 4 = No movement	a. b.
7. Limb ataxia	0 = Absent, 1 = Present in one limb, 2 = Present in two limbs	
8. Sensory	0 = Normal, 1 = Mild to moderate sensory loss, 2 = Severe sensory loss	
9. Best language	0 = No aphasia, 1 = Mild to moderate aphasia, 2 = Severe aphasia, 3 = Mute	
10. Dysarthria	0 = Normal, 1 = Mild to moderate dysarthria, 2 = Severe dysarthria	
11. Extinction and inattention	0 = Normal, 1 = Visual, tactile, auditory, or personal inattention, 2 = Profound hemi-inattention	

Adapted from the National Institute of Neurological Disorders and Stroke, National Institutes of Health: NIH Stroke Scale, revised 2003.

CHAPTER 44

typically normal, and abnormalities may not be identifiable on CT scan for 12 to 24 hours. A CT angiogram can identify occlusion of the large arteries, and a CT perfusion study can identify regions of the brain at risk of infarction. *MRI* is comparable to CT scanning for identifying acute hemorrhage if appropriate sequences are used and has greater sensitivity for detecting ischemic stroke, particularly in the first hours after symptom onset and strokes occurring in the in the posterior fossa.

- Bedside finger stick blood glucose
- ECG: to evaluate for arrhythmia and acute coronary syndrome. Atrial fibrillation is strongly associated with thromboembolic stroke. Stroke may be complicated by an associated myocardial infarction, and myocardial infarction may be complicated by stroke.

The American Heart Association guidelines for the evaluation of patients with acute ischemic stroke also recommend blood samples for baseline studies: chemistry panel; complete blood count including platelet count; and coagulation studies. A pregnancy test for all women having childbearing potential and a chest x-ray are also commonly recommended. Although most clinicians routinely act in accordance with these recommendations, their utility in the management of stroke patients has not been systematically validated.

COMMENTS AND TREATMENT CONSIDERATIONS

Immediate neurosurgical consultation is indicated for patients with a spontaneous ICH and operative intervention may be necessary.

Supportive care has long been the mainstay of management of patients with ischemic stroke and higher quality supportive care has been shown to improve outcomes. Airway, breathing, and circulation must be vigilantly monitored and maintained. It is important to avoid aspiration. Hypoxia would be expected to worsen the ischemic injury. Supplemental oxygen is therefore mandatory in the setting of hypoxia, but is not necessary for stroke patients who have normal oxygen saturation.

Moderate hypertension is common on presentation and should not be treated. Hypotension induced by antihypertensives is a greater risk to the patient. Areas of brain injury have impaired autoregulation of blood flow and are dependent on systemic pressure for perfusion. Thus, hypotension would be expected to diminish flow and thereby exacerbate ischemic injury. Hypotension is uncommon and if present should raise concern for a non-neurologic cause including aortic dissection and myocardial infarction.

Maintenance of euvolemia with isotonic solutions such as normal saline helps to ensure adequate cerebral perfusion. Intravenous solutions containing dextrose should be avoided because elevated serum glucose levels are associated with worse outcome from stroke, independent of whether there is a history of diabetes.

Aspirin and heparin have long been used in the management of stroke and TIA, although until recently there was a paucity of outcome data. Two recent large trials of aspirin treatment within 48 hours of symptom onset of ischemic stroke demonstrated a small but consistent reduction of deaths and recurrent strokes. Conversely, data does not currently support the use of heparin in stroke patients. Clinical trials of emergent anticoagulation with heparin have not shown benefit, including among patients with cardioembolic stroke, intracardiac or intra-arterial thrombus, vertebrobasilar artery occlusion or arterial dissection, In addition heparin anticoagulation has been associated with an increased risk of hemorrhagic transformation of stroke and major hemorrhage.

Therapeutic interventions with the goal of reducing disability in acute ischemic (non-hemorrhagic) stroke have been an area of intense research for over a decade. In particular, intravenous thrombolytic therapy has been the subject of extensive study and controversy. Intravenous administration of recombinant tissue plasminogen activator (TPA) in patients with ischemic stroke

---

CHARACTERISTICS OF PATIENTS WITH ISCHEMIC STROKE WHO COULD BE TREATED WITH TPA

Inclusion Criteria
- Clinical Diagnosis of ischemic stroke causing measurable neurological deficit
- Onset of symptoms know to be <3 hours before beginning treatment
- The patient or family understand the potential risks and benefits from treatment

Exclusion Criteria
History:
- Symptoms suggestive of a subarachnoid hemorrhage
- Seizure at time of onset (suggestive of postictal residual neurological impairments)
- Head trauma or prior stroke in previous 3 months
- Myocardial infarction in the previous 3 months
- Gastrointestinal or urinary tract hemorrhage in previous 21 days
- Major surgery or serious trauma in the previous 14 days
- Arterial puncture at a noncompressible site in the previous 7 days
- History of intracranial hemorrhage

Continued

CHARACTERISTICS OF PATIENTS WITH ISCHEMIC STROKE WHO COULD BE TREATED WITH TPA—CONT'D

- History of AVM, intracerebral aneurysm, or brain tumor
- Use of heparin in previous 48 hours, and prolonged PTT
- Use of an oral anticoagulant, and INR ≥ 1.7

Examination:
- Neurological signs resolving spontaneously
- Neurologic signs minor and isolated (e.g., minimal weakness, ataxia alone, dysarthria alone, sensory deficit alone)
- Caution should be exercised in treating a patient with major deficits
- Evidence of active bleeding or acute trauma (e.g., fracture) on examination
- Blood pressure elevated (systolic >185 mm Hg and diastolic >110 mm Hg)

Laboratory:
- Blood glucose concentration <50 mg/dL (2.7 mmol/L)
- Platelet count <100 000 mm^3
- Female patient with a positive pregnancy test or other definitive evidence of pregnancy.

Cerebral Imaging:
- Hemorrhage or possible hemorrhage of any degree or type
- Findings suggestive of multilobar infarction (hypodensity >⅓ cerebral hemisphere)

Modified from: Adams H, Adams R, Del Zoppo G, Goldstein LB: Guidelines for the early management of patients with ischemic stroke: 2005 guidelines update a scientific statement from the Stroke Council of the American Heart Association/American Stroke Association, *Stroke* 36:916, 2005.
AVM=arteriovenous malformation, INR=International Normalized Ratio, PTT=partial thromboplastin time

within 3 hours of symptom onset is employed in many medical centers in the United States, based in large part on the results of the National Institute of Neurological Disorders and Stroke (NINDS) TPA trial. The interpretation of the results of this study and the benefit of intravenous TPA in general have, however, been questioned by some authorities in the United States and around the world who believe the literature to date suggests that the risk of cerebral hemorrhage from thrombolysis outweighs potential treatment benefits. Notably, outcomes have differed in different settings. Clinicians should become informed of the accepted stroke management strategies in their institution and make treatment decisions collaboratively with appropriate consultants.

The risks of TPA include fatal ICH and other major bleeding. TPA should not be administered to any patient with a hemorrhagic stroke and therefore treating centers must have available expertise in neuro imaging interpretation. If TPA is to be used, adherence to the treatment guidelines, particularly inclusion and exclusion criteria, is critical because deviation is associated with an increased risk of ICH.

More recently human clinical trials have begun on a number of endovascular interventions, including the use of lasers, ultrasonography, angioplasty, microsnares, and a variety of clot retrieval devices. To date, the role of these therapies has not been established.

REFERENCES

Adams H, Adams R, Del Zoppo G, Goldstein LB: Guidelines for the early management of patients with ischemic stroke: 2005 guidelines update a scientific statement from the Stroke Council of the American Heart Association/American Stroke Association, *Stroke* 36:916, 2005.

Albers GW, Amarenco P, Easton JD, et al: Antithrombotic and thrombolytic therapy for ischemic stroke: the Seventh ACCP Conference on Antithrombotic and Thrombolytic Therapy, *Chest* 126(3 Suppl):483S, 2004.

Albers GW, Caplan LR, Easton JD, et al: Transient ischemic attack—proposal for a new definition, *N Engl J Med* 347:1713, 2002.

Brott T, Bogousslavsky J: Treatment of acute ischemic stroke, *N Engl J Med* 343:710, 2000.

Bruno A, Levine SR, Frankel MR, et al: Admission glucose level and clinical outcomes in the NINDS rt-PA Stroke Trial, *Neurology* 59:669, 2002.

CAST (Chinese Acute Stroke Trial) Collaborative Group: CAST: randomised placebo-controlled trial of early aspirin use in 20,000 patients with acute ischaemic stroke, *Lancet* 349:1641, 1997.

Goldstein LB, Samsa GP: Reliability of the National Institutes of Health Stroke Scale: extension to non-neurologists in the context of a clinical trial, *Stroke* 28:307, 1997.

Goldstein LB, Simel DL: Is this patient having a stroke? *JAMA* 293:2391, 2005.

Hacke W, Kaste M, Fieschi C, et al: Intravenous thrombolysis with recombinant tissue plasminogen activator for acute hemispheric stroke: the European Cooperative Acute Stroke Study (ECASS), *JAMA* 274:1017, 1995.

International Stroke Trial Collaborative Group: The International Stroke Trial (IST): a randomized trial of aspirin, subcutaneous heparin, both, or neither among 19435 patients with acute ischaemic stroke, *Lancet* 349:1569, 1997.

Katzan IL, Hammer MD, Furlan AJ, et al: Quality improvement and tissue-type plasminogen activator for acute ischemic stroke: a Cleveland update, *Stroke* 34:799, 2003.

CHAPTER 44

Kidwell CS, Alger JR, Di Salle F, et al: Diffusion MRI in patients with transient ischemic attacks, *Stroke* 30:1174, 1999.

Kidwell CS, Chalela JA, Saver JL, et al: Comparison of MRI and CT for detection of acute intracerebral hemorrhage, *JAMA* 292:1823, 2004.

Kidwell CS, Starkman S, Eckstein M, et al: Identifying stroke in the field: prospective validation of the Los Angeles Prehospital Stroke Screen (LAPSS), *Stroke* 31:71, 2000.

Leys D, et al: Misdiagnoses in 1250 consecutive patients admitted to an acute stroke unit, *Cerebrovasc Dis* 7(Suppl 5): 284, 1997.

Libman RB, Wirkowski E, Alvir J, Rao TH: Conditions that mimic stroke in the emergency department: implications for acute stroke trials, *Arch Neurol* 52:1119, 1995.

Madhavan R, Jacobs BS, Levine SR: Stroke trials: what have we learned? *Neurol Res* 24(Suppl 1):S27, 2002.

The National Institute of Neurological Disorders and Stroke rt-PA Stroke Study Group: Tissue plasminogen activator for acute ischemic stroke, *N Engl J Med* 333:1581, 1995.

Ronning OM, Guldvog B: Should stroke victims routinely receive supplemental oxygen? A quasi-randomized controlled trial, *Stroke* 30:2033, 1999.

Scott PA, Silbergleit R: Misdiagnosis of stroke in tissue plasminogen activator-treated patients: characteristics and outcomes, *Ann Emerg Med* 42:611, 2003.

Singh V: Critical care assessment and management of acute ischemic stroke, *J Vasc Interv Radiol* 15:S21, 2004.

Stone J, Zeman A, Sharpe M: Functional weakness and sensory disturbance, *J Neurol Neurosurg Psychiatry* 73:241, 2002.

Wardlaw JM, Warlow CP, Counsell C: Systematic review of evidence on thrombolytic therapy for acute ischaemic stroke, *Lancet* 350:607, 1997.

 GUILLAIN-BARRÉ SYNDROME

Guillain-Barré syndrome (GBS) is an acute autoimmune demyelinating peripheral polyneuropathy. The signs and symptoms of GBS depend on the extent of axonal and myelin sheath involvement. Accordingly, patients can present with both motor and sensory complaints in either a generalized or more local distribution, although motor weakness is generally the principal complaint. Although the antecedent causes of GBS are diverse, the disease typically follows a bacterial or viral infection. Two thirds of patients report an upper respiratory or gastrointestinal illness prior to the onset of their neurologic symptoms. *Campylobacter jejuni*, a major cause of enteritis worldwide, remains the most frequent preceding pathogen and is associated with a more severe form of the disease.

SYMPTOMS
- Weakness commonly beginning in the distal legs is the most common presentation, but proximal muscles may appear more affected.
- Possible progression of weakness to trunk and arms
- Facial involvement, possibly asymmetric
- Bulbar muscle weakness less common ++
- Sensory complaints are less prominent but common and include paresthesias and numbness.
- Pain in the back, buttocks, thighs, or shoulders

SIGNS
- Distal muscle weakness (most common)
- Diminished or absent reflexes in the affected muscles
- Sensorium intact
- Cranial nerve abnormalities +++, involving in decreasing order of frequency facial, bulbar palsies, muscles of mastication, ocular. Unlike extremity weakness, facial weakness may be asymmetric.
- Autonomic dysfunction manifesting as labile blood pressure and heart rate and occasionally bowel or bladder disturbances ++
- There are several less common variants of GBS including the Miller-Fischer variant, which starts with ophthalmoplegia, areflexia, and ataxia followed by a descending paralysis.
- Loss of position and vibratory sense may occur.
- Respiratory muscle weakness is the most serious manifestation ++.

WORKUP
- The ED diagnosis of GBS is largely clinical.
- Respiratory status should be evaluated both clinically and by pulmonary function tests. Forced vital capacity and pulse oximetry are most often followed. A forced vital capacity <12 to 15 ml/kg or <1 L in an adult may be considered an indication for intubation, although most ED airway decisions are made on a clinical basis.
- A lumbar puncture may show albuminocytologic dissociation. Protein content of >400 mg/L and a cell count of <10 cells/ml (all mononuclear) would be confirmatory. LP is often normal early in the disease but eventually shows this profile.

COMMENTS AND TREATMENT CONSIDERATIONS
All patients should be admitted. Those with severe weakness, rapid progression, or respiratory compromise should be admitted to an ICU. Thirty percent may require mechanical ventilation. Depolarizing agents for intubation (e.g., succinylcholine)

should be avoided. GBS patients are also exquisitely sensitive to vasoactive substances. Only short-acting medicines should be used to treat high or low blood pressure and should be avoided if possible.

Plasma exchange and IV immunoglobulin may be considered. Steroids have been shown to be of no benefit and may be detrimental.

REFERENCES
Fulgham JR, Wijdicks EF: Guillain-Barré syndrome, *Crit Care Clin* 13:1, 1997.

Hahn AF: Guillain-Barré syndrome, *Lancet* 352:635, 1998.

Jacobs BC, Rothbard PH, van der Meche FG, et al: The spectrum of antecedent infections in Guillain-Barré syndrome: a case-control study, *Neurology* 51:1110, 1998.

Pascuzzi RM, Fleck JD: Acute peripheral neuropathy in adults: Guillain-Barré syndrome and related disorders, *Neurol Clin* 15:529, 1997.

Rees JH, Soudain SE, Gregson NA, Hughes RA: *Campylobacter jejuni* infection and Guillain-Barré syndrome, *N Engl J Med* 333:1374, 1995.

DISORDERS OF NEUROMUSCULAR TRANSMISSION

 MYASTHENIA GRAVIS

Myasthenia gravis (MG) is an autoimmune disease in which antibodies against nicotinic acetylcholine receptors (ACh-R) both decrease the number of receptors and change the morphology of the NMJ. The trigger for the autoimmune response is unknown, but a drug-induced form is reversible. Incidence follows a bimodal distribution occurring in women in their second and third decades and in men in their sixth and seventh decades. Adults with MG often have lymphoid hyperplasia in the thymus. Approximately 15% develop thymomas, which are generally benign and encapsulated but can be invasive.

SYMPTOMS
- Blurry vision and eyelid weakness ++++
- Generalized weakness ++++
- Other bulbar muscles become affected resulting in dysarthria, dysphagia, weakness in the muscles of mastication, and a charac-teristic nasal-sounding voice. The muscles of the neck, diaphragm, and proximal extremity then become involved in a descending fashion.

SIGNS

- Weakness of bulbar muscles, particularly eyelid weakness
- Reflexes are usually normal.
- Sensation and mental status are intact.
- Affected muscles are easily fatigable: prolonged upward gaze is one useful test.

WORKUP

- The Tensilon (edrophonium) test is the primary diagnostic test. Atropine should be available in case of severe bradycardia or other severe cholinergic effect induced by edrophonium. A predetermined muscle should be tested using both a placebo and edrophonium. Onset of improved strength begins within 30 seconds and lasts 5 minutes. A test is considered positive if there is unequivocal increase in strength.
- Immunodiagnosis can be made in many patients by testing for ACh-R antibody.
- Electromyography (EMG) studies have been used to help confirm the diagnosis.
- A CT scan of the chest can help exclude a concurrent thymoma but is not necessary in the ED.

COMMENTS AND TREATMENT CONSIDERATIONS

As with all disorders of neuromuscular transmission, assessment and management of the patient's airway and ventilation are the top priorities. A myasthenic crisis is defined as a life-threatening impairment of ventilation. A vital capacity of less than 1 L is indicative of impending respiratory failure and is more sensitive than the development of hypercapnia.

Cholinesterase inhibitors, most commonly pyridostigmine (Mestinon), are the first-line agents for MG. Immunosuppressive therapy (steroids, azathioprine, and cyclosporine), thymectomy, plasmapheresis, and intravenous IgG are other treatment modalities employed in severe cases.

Patients with known MG can present with weakness caused by insufficient medication (myasthenic crisis) or excessive treatment with pyridostigmine (cholinergic crisis). The muscle paralysis produced by the two states is indistinguishable, but patients with cholinergic crisis should also have symptoms of cholinergic (muscarinic) excess such as hypersecretion, diarrhea, and bradycardia. Further treatment with cholinesterase inhibitor in cholinergic crisis is contraindicated. Ventilatory support is the key intervention in myasthenic crises.

REFERENCES

Engstrom JW: Myasthenia gravis: diagnostic mimics, *Semin Neurol* 24:141, 2004.

CHAPTER 44

Keesey JC: Clinical evaluation and management of myasthenia gravis, *Muscle Nerve* 29:484, 2004.

Meriggioli MN, Sanders DB: Myasthenia gravis: diagnosis, *Semin Neurol* 24:31, 2004.

Saperstein DS, Barohn RJ: Management of myasthenia gravis, *Semin Neurol* 24:41, 2004.

 LAMBERT-EATON MYASTHENIC SYNDROME

Lambert-Eaton myasthenic syndrome (LEMS) is a rare autoimmune disease in which antibodies develop to the presynaptic acetylcholine-releasing terminal of the NMJ and parasympathetic effector junction, resulting in decreased acetylcholine release. Although a primary form exists, LEMS is often a paraneoplastic disorder. Age of onset is typically 40 to 80 years. All races are affected.

SYMPTOMS
- Presents insidiously as proximal muscle weakness, especially of the thighs and hips.
- Autonomic dysfunction +++ includes dry mouth, impotence, and postural hypotension.
- Bulbar muscles are generally spared, but ptosis has been reported in up to 25% of patients.
- Respiratory weakness may be seen but is generally neither common nor severe. Prolonged paralysis may develop in some patients postoperatively with the use of neuromuscular blocking agents.

SIGNS
- Proximal muscle weakness ++++.
- Initial weak grip strength may improve over a few seconds only to deteriorate again as grip is continued.
- Hyporeflexia, which follows the weakness
- Waddling gait because of hip weakness++
- Sensation and sensorium are normal.
- Dry mouth, postural hypotension, and ptosis may be found +++.

WORKUP
- A Tensilon test should be performed in equivocal cases, along with ACh-R and LEMS antibody titers, because LEMS is often difficult to distinguish from MG.
- Because LEMS is associated with cancer in 40% to 60% of cases (usually small cell lung cancer), a search for malignancy should be performed if it is not known to be present; chest x-ray, CBC, and a chemistry panel are warranted.

COMMENTS AND TREATMENT CONSIDERATIONS

Patients without respiratory compromise or obvious cancer should be referred to a neurologist for EMG studies and to a primary care physician for a more extensive search for malignancy. CT scanning, bronchoscopy, and other diagnostic tests should be considered. Patients should be followed closely for at least 4 years after diagnosis.

Treatment options include immunosuppression with glucocorticoids, azathioprine or cyclosporine, 3,4-diaminopyridine (DAP), plasmapheresis, and intravenous immunoglobulin.

REFERENCES

Mareska M, Gutmann L: Lambert-Eaton myasthenic syndrome, *Semin Neurol* 24:149, 2004.

Sanders D: Lambert-Eaton myasthenic syndrome: diagnosis and treatment, *Ann NY Acad Sci* 998:500, 2003.

 BOTULISM

Botulism is a neurotoxin-mediated paralysis. *Clostridium botulinum*, a gram-positive, rod-shaped, spore-forming anaerobic bacterium that is ubiquitous in soil and water, produces the botulinum toxin. The toxin binds irreversibly to the presynaptic membrane and blocks release of acetylcholine at the NMJ and autonomic ganglion. *C. botulinum* spores germinate in an anaerobic media such as home-canned goods and are found in both soil and marine environments.

There are three naturally occurring forms of botulism: foodborne, wound, and infant/intestinal botulism. Symptoms and signs differ somewhat depending on the type of botulism. The diagnosis should be considered in patients with autonomic and cranial nerve (e.g., diplopia, dysarthria, and dysphagia) dysfunction and a symmetric descending flaccid paralysis. Rapid progression to ventilatory failure may occur. Patients are typically afebrile and have a clear sensorium.

Recently, attention has focused on the potential use of the botulinum toxin as a bioterrorism agent, dispersed in food or water to be ingested or aerosolized for inhalation. See Chapter 26, Mass Casualty Exposure.

FOODBORNE BOTULISM

Clinical manifestations of foodborne botulism result from ingestion of the preformed neurotoxin. The spectrum of disease is wide, ranging from mild gastrointestinal complaints to a severe form resulting in death within 24 hours. Onset is typically within 12 to 36 hours after ingestion and is heralded by cranial nerve involvement followed by symmetric descending paralysis. Progression is often rapid, and paralysis of ventilatory muscles can lead to ventilatory failure and death. Patients with shortness of breath and an impaired gag reflex have an increased risk of death.

SYMPTOMS
- Nonspecific early: nausea, vomiting, weakness, malaise, constipation
- Dysphagia +++++
- Other cranial nerve symptoms: diplopia, dysarthria, and dysphonia
- Fatigue +++
- Dry mouth
- Progressive weakness, initially in neck and upper extremities, extending to thorax, then legs
- Ventilatory failure

SIGNS
- Cranial nerve dysfunction: ptosis ++++, extraocular muscle weakness +++, miosis +++, fixed or dilated pupils
- Descending muscle weakness or paralysis
- Reflexes, normal +++ or decreased +++
- Sensation and sensorium are usually intact.

WOUND BOTULISM
Wound botulism occurs after the germination of *C. botulinum* spores in the anaerobic environment of a contaminated wound, including traumatic injuries (e.g., crush injuries) and surgical wounds (e.g., after cesarean delivery). Outbreaks have been described among intravenous drug users. The resultant organisms subsequently produce the neurotoxin, causing a constellation of symptoms very similar to those seen with foodborne botulism. Because of the prolonged incubation time, the onset of symptoms is typically approximately 10 days after exposure.

SYMPTOMS
- Similar to those in foodborne botulism except GI complaints are less prominent and onset is over days instead of hours.

SIGNS
- Abscess or other wound. The wound may appear completely benign.

INFANT/INTESTINAL BOTULISM
Infant botulism, also known as intestinal botulism, occurs after ingestion of spores, with subsequent germination and release of neurotoxin in the intestinal tract. Although most cases occur in infants (median age of onset is 2 to 4 months), botulism attributed

to the same mechanism has been described in older children and adults. The most commonly identified source of botulism spores are honey or corn syrup, but these account for a minority of cases. Infant botulism also occurs in breastfed babies. Approximately half of all cases in the United States occur in California, Pennsylvania, and Utah, presumably because of the high spore counts in the soil of these states. The presentation of infant botulism is similar to that of sepsis, meningitis, and dehydration. Botulism should be considered but only after a complete septic workup has been performed and antibiotics administered. If botulism is strongly suspected, aminoglycoside antibiotics are contraindicated because they potentiate the neuromuscular blockade of the toxin.

SYMPTOMS
- Poor feeding/sucking +++++
- Constipation over 3 days duration ++++
- Lethargy +++

SIGNS
- Poor head control +++++
- Hypotonia ++++
- Weak cry ++++
- Expressionless face +++
- Depressed reflexes
- Decreased gag
- Ventilatory failure may occur.

Foodborne, Wound, and Infant Botulism
WORKUP
- The diagnosis of botulism is clinical. Confirmatory tests should be done, but treatment must be started before the results become available.
- Rule out other causes of neurologic dysfunction, such as MG and GBS.
- Serum, stool, wound, or food samples should be sent to the CDC for toxin testing.

COMMENTS AND TREATMENT CONSIDERATIONS
Patients with botulism should be admitted to the ICU because most ultimately require mechanical ventilation, and ventilatory failure may occur quickly. Decontamination of the GI tract (gastric lavage, cathartic agents, or enemas) should be considered for foodborne botulism and wound débridement for wound botulism. The U.S. CDC recommends intravenous infusion of one vial of trivalent equine antitoxin as soon as the diagnosis of foodborne or

wound botulism is suspected. Antitoxin is not routinely given in infant botulism. In the United States, antitoxin is available from the CDC. The CDC botulism weekday phone number is (404) 639-2206 or 639-3311; nights and weekends (404) 639-2888.

REFERENCES

Arnon SS, Schechter R, Inglesby TV, et al: Botulism toxin as a biological weapon: medical and public health management, *JAMA* 285:1059, 2001.

Hatheway CL: Botulism: the present status of the disease, *Curr Top Microbiol Immunol* 195:55, 1995.

Shapiro RL, Hatheway C, Swerdlow DL: Botulism in the United States: a clinical and epidemiologic review, *Ann Intern Med* 129:221, 1998.

Sobel J, Tucker N, Sulka A, et al: Foodborne botulism in the United States, 1990-2000, *Emerg Infect Dis* 10:1606, 2004.

Varma JK, Katsitadze G, Moiscrafishvili M, et al: Signs and symptoms predictive of death in patients with foodborne botulism— Republic of Georgia, 1980-2002, *Clin Infect Dis* 39:357, 2004.

Wigginton JM, Thill P: Infant botulism: a review of the literature, *Clin Pediatr* 32:669, 1993.

 TICK PARALYSIS

Tick paralysis occurs most often in Australia, South Africa, and North America. Although primarily a veterinary problem, it also affects humans. In North America, the common dog tick *Dermacentor variabilis* and the female wood tick *Dermacentor andersoni* are responsible for most cases. Bites occur in the spring and summer months. The toxin resides in the salivary gland of the tick, and after entering the bloodstream via the bite it reaches the NMJ, where it blocks the peripheral motor neuron release of acetylcholine. The diagnosis should be considered in patients with symptoms and signs consistent with the disease who have recently traveled to a tick-infested area.

SYMPTOMS

- Onset 5 to 7 days after tick attachment +++
- Ataxia, irritability, and lethargy are the initial symptoms.
- Paresthesias ++
- Progressive ascending weakness

SIGNS

- Ataxia (truncal ataxia, appendicular ataxia, nystagmus, and wide-based staggering gait) is a frequent presenting sign, particularly in children +++.

- Ascending flaccid paralysis ensues shortly after initial symptoms, progressing over hours to days; progression is more rapid than the progression seen in GBS.
- Affected muscles are areflexic.
- Paralysis eventually reaches the cranial nerves and respiratory muscles if the tick is not removed.
- Sensation and sensorium remain intact.
- Pupils are reactive.
- An attached tick is found.

WORKUP
- Search for the tick. They are most often found in the scalp but also may reside in the axilla, pubic/perianal area, popliteal fossa, or ear canal.
- No other studies are necessary if a tick is found. If a tick is not found, other diagnoses must be considered. For ataxia consider the Miller-Fisher variant of Guillain-Barré and acute cerebellitis. For paralysis consider GBS and botulism (although the latter is generally a *descending* paralysis).

COMMENTS AND TREATMENT CONSIDERATIONS
Tick removal is curative for North American cases. The tick is grasped with forceps as close to the site of attachment as possible and is removed carefully to avoid leaving the head in the skin. Symptoms generally improve within several hours but may not completely resolve for several days. Death may occur, more commonly in children, if the tick is not located and removed.

REFERENCES
Li Z, Turner RP: Pediatric tick paralysis: discussion of two cases and literature review, *Pediatr Neurol* 31:304, 2004.

Tick paralysis—Washington, 1995, *MMWR Morb Mortal Wkly Rep* 45:325, 1996.

Vendanarayanan V, Sorey WH, Subramony SH: Tick paralysis, *Semin Neurol* 24:181, 2004.

MYOPATHY
Myopathy is defined as a muscle disease not attributable to nerve or NMJ dysfunction. There are many myopathies. Myopathies, whether primary or due to some other underlying cause (e.g., hypothyroidism or hyperthyroidism, toxic myopathy, hypokalemia, infectious), generally result in symmetric weakness that is most pronounced in large, proximal muscles. Extraocular, facial, and bulbar muscles are usually spared. Patients complain of difficulty getting out of a chair or raising their arms to brush their hair or put on a shirt. Many myopathies have a gradual onset.

CHAPTER 44

GENERALIZED WEAKNESS AND FATIGUE CAUSED BY SYSTEMIC ILLNESS

Systemic illnesses may cause acute fatigue interpreted by the patient as weakness (e.g., acute myocardial infarction) or may cause actual muscle weakness (e.g., thyrotoxic periodic paralysis).

 SEPSIS

Sepsis is an infection-induced syndrome of systemic inflammation. Presenting complaints are often nonspecific, and the source of the infection may be inapparent. Patients who are elderly, diabetic, asplenic, HIV positive, or otherwise immunocompromised are particularly susceptible to infectious insults and may show early compromise. Common sources for infection should be considered, including genitourinary, abdominal, CNS, and pulmonary, as well as any indwelling catheters or foreign bodies that could serve as a nidus for infection. Delay in identifying and treating sepsis can lead precipitously to the vasodilatory and redistributive phenomena characteristic of septic shock.

See Chapter 30, Rash for a discussion of toxic shock syndrome, a form of sepsis.

SYMPTOMS
- Symptoms specific to a focus of infection
- Generalized sense of weakness and fatigue
- Fever
- Chills and rigors
- Myalgias
- Headache
- Altered mental status
- Loss of appetite, nausea, and vomiting

SIGNS
- Signs specific to site of infection
- Fever >38.5° C (may be hypothermic in some septic patients)
- Rash (diffuse macular erythroderma in toxic shock syndrome; petechial rash may occur in meningococcemia)
- Shock: hypotension, tachycardia, tachypnea, respiratory distress

WORKUP
- Tests are directed at finding the source of infection and evidence of multiorgan involvement.
- Urinalysis
- Chest x-ray
- Blood and urine cultures

- Lumbar puncture when indicated
- Electrolytes, BUN, creatinine
- CT scanning or occasionally exploratory laparotomy may be indicated when the abdomen is considered a likely source.

COMMENTS AND TREATMENT CONSIDERATIONS

The mainstays of treatment in sepsis are oxygen, fluid resuscitation, and intravenous antibiotics. Early use of so-called goal-directed therapy, with aggressive fluid resuscitation, inotropic support, and blood transfusion guided by specific hemodynamic and other parameters, has been shown to benefit patients in severe sepsis or septic shock. The use of near-physiologic doses of corticosteroids in severe sepsis remains a controversial issue but may benefit some patients. Larger doses of steroids have been demonstrated to be detrimental. Intensive insulin therapy for hyperglycemia may also reduce mortality.

REFERENCES

Annane D, Sebille V, Charpentier C, et al: Effect of treatment with low doses of hydrocortisone and fludrocortisone on mortality in patients with septic shock, *JAMA* 288:862, 2002.

Minneci PC, Deans KJ, Banks SM, et al: Meta-analysis: the effect of steroids on survival and shock during sepsis depends on the dose, *Ann Intern Med* 141:47, 2004

Nguyen HB, Rivers EP, Havstad S, et al: Critical care in the emergency department: a physiologic assessment and outcome evaluation, *Acad Emerg Med* 7:1354, 2000.

Rivers E, Nguyen B, Havstad S, et al: Early goal-directed therapy in the treatment of severe sepsis and septic shock, *N Engl J Med* 345:1368, 2001.

 ACUTE MYOCARDIAL INFARCTION

Gender and age strongly influence the presenting signs and symptoms of acute myocardial infarction (AMI). Many women and elderly patients who have an AMI do not have chest pain. Between 20% and 30% of patients older than 70 who have an AMI have no chest pain and present with weakness alone. Similarly, the most frequent symptoms preceding an AMI in women are unusual fatigue (71%) and sleep disturbance (48%).

See Chapter 7, Chest Pain.

REFERENCES

Bayer AJ, Chadha JS, Farag RR, Pathy MS: Changing presentation of myocardial infarction with increasing old age, *J Am Geriatr Soc* 34:263, 1986.

CHAPTER 44

Calle P, Jordaens L, De Buyzere M, et al: Age-related differences in presentation, treatment, and outcome of acute myocardial infarction, *Cardiology* 85:111, 1994.

McSweeney JC, Cody M, O'Sullivan P, et al: Women's early warning symptoms of acute myocardial infarction, *Circulation* 108:2619, 2003.

HYPOVOLEMIA

Hypovolemia is a condition of intravascular fluid depletion, manifest by a sympathetic autonomic response and the signs and symptoms of decreased tissue perfusion. Depending on the rate of development and the underlying cause, hypovolemia is often associated with extracellular and intracellular fluid depletion. Causes of hypovolemia include acute blood loss; losses from the gastrointestinal or urinary system, skin, or lungs; inadequate fluid intake; and fluid loss into internal potential spaces ("third spacing"). The symptoms and signs vary according to its cause.

SYMPTOMS
- Symptoms of disorders that lead to hypovolemia (e.g., bleeding, vomiting, diarrhea, fever, burns, crush injury)
- Generalized weakness
- Dizziness (more correctly a sensation of lightheadedness or near syncope), typically on standing
- Altered mental status
- Rapid palpitations

SIGNS
- Dry mucous membranes
- Poor skin turgor (more accurate in younger patients; elasticity of the skin decreases with age)
- Tachycardia (may be blunted by beta-blockers)
- Orthostatic vital signs/tilt test; the sensitivity and specificity of orthostatic vital signs are poor. Patients who report feeling dizzy upon standing should be considered to have orthostatic hypotension even if their vital signs do not meet the classic criteria. Specificity is higher if pulse change >30; unnecessary to test in the presence of symptoms or tachycardia.
- End-organ hypoperfusion (e.g., low urinary output, abnormal mental status, chest pain)
- Decreased jugular venous pressure

WORKUP
- Hypovolemia is primarily a clinical diagnosis.
- Hematocrit: In acute blood loss the hematocrit remains normal until there is time for fluid equilibration; therefore, repeat the

hematocrit after fluid resuscitation to assess magnitude of blood loss more accurately.

- Thorough search for potential sites of blood loss (chest, abdomen, pelvis, retroperitoneum, and gastrointestinal tract)
- Serum electrolytes, BUN and creatinine, and urinalysis are sometimes helpful in patients with vomiting, diarrhea, or poor oral intake.

COMMENTS AND TREATMENT CONSIDERATIONS
Large-bore intravenous access and administration of isotonic fluids should generally be initiated as the source of hypovolemia is investigated. Placement of a Foley catheter can be helpful to monitor urinary output

See Chapter 39, Trauma, Approach to, and Chapter 6, Bleeding.

REFERENCES
Fuchs SM, Jaffe DM: Evaluation of the tilt test in children, *Ann Emerg Med* 16:386, 1987.
Knopp R, Claypool R, Leonardi D: Use of the tilt test in measuring acute blood loss, *Ann Emerg Med* 9:72, 1980.
McGee S, Abernethy WB 3rd, Simel DL: The rational clinical examination. Is this patient hypovolemic? *JAMA* 281:1022, 1999.

CHAPTER 44

 RENAL FAILURE AND UREMIA

Uremia is caused by renal failure. Generalized weakness with evidence of fluid overload on physical examination is common, but uremia may occur in nonoliguric renal failure and normal volume status. Renal failure patients are at risk for sepsis, AMI, and other causes of generalized weakness, and these diagnoses must be considered and excluded before attributing weakness to uremia.

SYMPTOMS
- Neurologic symptoms: confusion, somnolence, tremor, and generalized weakness
- Symptoms of advanced renal failure: oliguria, anuria, anorexia, nausea, vomiting, fatigue, edema, and shortness of breath
- Pruritus

SIGNS
- Neurologic: tremor, weakness, myoclonic twitching, muscle cramps, tetany, asterixis, hiccups, and altered mental status
- Signs of fluid overload: hypertension, edema, hepatosplenomegaly, rales, increased jugular venous distention, and an S3
- AV grafts and dialysis catheters in unconscious patients

WORKUP

- Patients with renal failure often exhibit multiple laboratory abnormalities (normochromic normocytic anemia, hyperkalemia, hypocalcemia, hyperphosphatemia, metabolic acidosis, elevated BUN and creatinine, hyperuricemia).
- ECG (examine for evidence of hyperkalemia)
- Chest x-ray to evaluate for fluid overload, manifested as pleural effusions, pulmonary vascular congestion, or pulmonary edema ("uremic lung") with perihilar infiltrates

COMMENTS AND TREATMENT CONSIDERATIONS

Dialysis is required for the treatment of uremia and should be done immediately in cases of life-threatening hyperkalemia after temporizing measures are initiated (e.g., calcium chloride 5 ml of 10% solution IV or calcium gluconate 10 ml of 10% solution IV given over 2 to 10 minutes depending on acuity; insulin 10 units regular IV with 1 ampule of D50; sodium bicarbonate 1 to 2 ampules). Sodium polystyrene sulfonate (Kayexalate) may also be used to lower potassium levels pending dialysis.

 ADRENAL INSUFFICIENCY

Adrenal insufficiency occurs most commonly in patients who have abruptly discontinued chronic treatment with glucocorticosteroids. These patients have a type of secondary adrenal insufficiency (failure of the hypothalamic-pituitary axis leading to decreased ACTH) due to suppression caused by the prolonged use of exogenous steroids. Primary adrenal insufficiency (Addison's disease) and other causes of secondary adrenal insufficiency are infrequently diagnosed in the ED. Stressors such as infection, trauma, burns, or surgery can precipitate acute adrenal insufficiency in patients who, in the absence of stress, have adequate adrenal function. Patients who are receiving chronic steroid treatment and who are acutely ill or injured should be treated with "stress-dose steroids" in addition to therapies directed at the primary medical or surgical condition.

SYMPTOMS

- Symptoms of primary illness when secondary to physiologic stressor
- Weakness +++++
- Fatigue +++++
- Anorexia +++++
- Weight loss +++++ (when chronic)
- Nausea and vomiting +++
- Abdominal pain +++
- Diarrhea or constipation ++

SIGNS
- Lethargy
- Hypotension ++++
- Hyperpigmentation +++++ (in chronic primary adrenal insufficiency)

WORKUP
- ED diagnosis is clinical.
- Electrolytes: hypoglycemia, hyponatremia, and hyperkalemia are frequently seen, particularly in chronic adrenal insufficiency. Hypercalcemia may also occur.
- Evaluation for a primary process (urinalysis, chest x-ray, ECG, CBC, and other tests as clinically indicated)
- ACTH stimulation test can confirm the diagnosis. Serum cortisol levels are drawn at predetermined intervals before and after ACTH is administered. Treatment may be delayed until after the test is completed, or the patient can be treated with dexamethasone phosphate 4 mg IV q6-8h, which does not interfere with the test. In critically ill patients a single plasma free cortisol may substitute for an ACTH stimulation test.

COMMENTS AND TREATMENT CONSIDERATIONS
Adrenal insufficiency is most frequently a consideration in ill ED patients with a history of chronic glucocorticosteroid use. These patients should be treated with hydrocortisone hemisuccinate 100 mg IV q6h. Intravenous fluids and glucose should be administered as needed. Diagnosis and treatment of any precipitating illness are necessary.

REFERENCES
Arlt W, Allolio B: Adrenal insufficiency, *Lancet* 361:1881, 2004.
Cooper MS, Stewart PM: Corticosteroid insufficiency in acutely ill patients, *N Engl J Med* 348:727, 2003.
Lamberts SWJ, Bruining HA, de Jong FH: Corticosteroid therapy in severe illness, *N Engl J Med* 337:1285, 1997.
Nieman LK: Dynamic evaluation of adrenal hypofunction, *J Endocrinol Invest* 26(7 Suppl):74, 2003.
Ten S, New M, Maclaren N: Clinical review 130: Addison's disease 2001, *J Clin Endocrinol Metab* 86:2909, 2001.

PERIODIC PARALYSES
Periodic paralyses (PPs) are a group of rare muscle diseases characterized by episodic flaccid muscle weakness. Primary PPs usually involve alterations in serum potassium related to defective ion channels, resulting in myotonia. The most common of these is

hypokalemic PP. Secondary PPs, the most common of which is thyrotoxic PP, although thought to have a genetic component, occur sporadically and present later in life. Signs and symptoms are similar to those of primary PPs.

Most of the patients with PP have similar clinical features, which include:

- Acute onset of ascending symmetric paralysis
- Eyelid myotonia
- Normal level of consciousness and normal sensation
- Proximal weakness may be chronic, especially with hypokalemic PP.
- Diminished deep tendon reflexes during attacks

HYPOKALEMIC PERIODIC PARALYSIS

Hypokalemic periodic paralysis (HPP) is an autosomal dominant inherited disorder with imperfect penetration. Attacks are characterized by weakness or paralysis of the limbs and trunk and usually occur after a large carbohydrate meal, with rest after strenuous exercise, in cold weather, or after sleep. A family history is common, but sporadic cases occur. First attacks generally occur before 16 years of age, but patients may rarely be as old as 30 years. Attacks last hours to days but generally not longer than 72 hours. Symptoms are severe and may recur frequently.

SYMPTOMS
- Limb and trunk weakness

SIGNS
- Episodic periods of weakness or paralysis affecting the limbs and trunk but sparing the bulbar and diaphragm muscles
- Slow to normal heart rate
- Diminished reflexes
- Sensation and sensorium are intact, but patients have been known to become agitated during attacks.
- Absence of signs of hyperthyroidism +++
- Occasional myotonic lid lag +

WORKUP
- Electrolytes to demonstrate hypokalemia and exclude other electrolyte disorders
- ECG may show evidence of hypokalemia: flat or inverted T waves, U waves, prolonged PR interval, or sagging ST segments.

COMMENTS AND TREATMENT CONSIDERATIONS
Patients are treated with oral potassium replacement (bulbar muscles and the ability to swallow remain intact). Because there is

not a body deficit of potassium, and hypokalemia results from intracellular shifts, it is easy to overcorrect the potassium and cause hyperkalemia. Treatment is started with 60 to 120 mEq of oral potassium. Acetazolamide is used to prevent attacks but is poorly tolerated. Daily potassium does not prevent attacks.

THYROTOXIC PERIODIC PARALYSIS

Thyrotoxic periodic paralysis (TPP) is the most common secondary hypokalemic PP. Patients are usually male (95%), Asian (90%), and between 20 and 39 years old (80%). The estimated prevalence in patients with thyrotoxicosis ranges from 0.1% to 0.2% in whites to 13% to 14% in Chinese. Triggers include hyperinsulinemia, a carbohydrate load, exercise, stress, alcohol, cold exposure, menses, trauma, and infection. Ninety-five percent of TPP cases are sporadic, although a genetic predisposition is suspected. There is seasonal variability, with increased number of attacks in the summer.

SYMPTOMS
- Similar to those of HPP
- Weakness usually precedes other manifestations of thyrotoxicosis.
- Episodic weakness progressing over hours, typically after awakening from sleep
- Diurnal pattern is common with attacks late at night or in the early morning.
- Paralysis lasts 3 to 6 hours and resolution is in opposite order of onset.

SIGNS
- Similar to those of HPP
- Weakness is proximal and progressive from lower to upper extremities.
- Bulbar muscles and diaphragm are usually spared, but, if severe, may involve bulbar or ventilatory muscles.
- Reflexes are absent or diminished.
- Sensation and sensorium are intact.
- The patient may also show signs of thyroid hormone excess: tremulousness, tachycardia, goiter, exophthalmos, lid lag, warm, moist skin, fever, elevated pulse pressure.
- Serious effects are rare but include dysrhythmias, ventilatory failure, and death.

WORKUP
- See HPP.
- Hypokalemia is present during attacks.
- Thyroid function studies (TSH, free T_4)

CHAPTER 44

COMMENTS AND TREATMENT CONSIDERATIONS

Treatment is oral potassium replacement. As with HPP, potassium should be given slowly to avoid hyperkalemia.

Once the hyperthyroidism is controlled, these patients do not have any further problems with weakness. Recent studies suggest that propranolol may be not only a useful prophylactic agent but also an effective therapy for acute attacks, resolving TPP more quickly, without the risk of a rebound hyperkalemia. Propranolol is not an effective therapy for HPP.

See Thyrotoxicosis in Chapter 29, Palpitation and Tachycardia.

REFERENCES

Bergeron L, Sternback GL: Thyrotoxic periodic paralysis, *Ann Emerg Med* 17:843, 1988.

Links TP, Smit AJ, Molenaar WM, et al: Familial hypokalemic periodic paralysis: clinical, diagnostic, and therapeutic aspects, *J Neurol Sci* 122:33, 1994.

Tassone H, Moulin A, Henderson SO: The pitfalls of potassium replacement in thyrotoxic periodic paralysis: a case report and review of the literature, *J Emerg Med* 26:157, 2004.

Clinical Formulas

- Alveolar-arterial oxygen gradient (sea level) = $P(A\text{-}a)O_2$ = $(FiO_2 \times 713) - (PaCO_2/0.8) - PO_2$
- Anion gap = serum Na − (serum Cl + serum HCO_3)
- Creatinine clearance (ml/min estimate) = $(140 - \text{age})$ (wt in kg)/$(72 \times \text{serum Cr})$
- Fractional excretion of sodium = (urine Na × serum Cr)/(serum Na × urine Cr) × 100
- Serum osmolality = $[(2 \times Na) + (\text{glucose}/18) + (BUN/2.8) + (\text{mannitol}/18) + (EtOH\ (mg/dl)/4.6)]$
- Osmolar gap = serum osmolality measured − $[(2 \times Na) + (\text{glucose}/18) + (BUN/2.8) + (\text{mannitol}/18) + (EtOH\ (mg/dl)/4.6)]$
- QTc = QT/square root (RR)
- Temperature conversion
  C = 5(F − 32)/9
  F = (C × 9)/5 + 32

Emergency Drug Reference

DRUG	DOSE
Adenosine	6 mg rapid IV push; may repeat with 12 mg rapid IV; 12 mg may be repeated once
Pediatric	0.1–0.25 mg/kg rapid IV; maximum single dose 12 mg
Amiodarone Arrest Wide complex tachycardia	300 mg IV push; consider additional 150 mg push in 3-5 min 150 mg IV over 10 min; may repeat 150 mg IV over 10 min
Atropine* Arrest Bradycardia *Pediatric*	1 mg IV push; may repeat q3-5min; maximum 0.04 mg/kg 0.5 mg IV; may repeat q3-5min to total 0.04 mg/kg 0.02 mg/kg IV; minimum 0.1 mg; maximum single dose 0.5 mg for child, 1 mg for adolescent; may be repeated once
Diltiazem	0.25 mg/kg IV (consider 10-20 mg initial adult dose); may repeat in 10-15 min as 0.35 mg/kg dose; maintenance drip 5-15 mg/hr
Dobutamine	2-20 µg/kg/min IV; titrate to effect
Dopamine	2-20 µg/kg/min IV; titrate to effect
Epinephrine* Arrest Bradyarrhythmia Anaphylaxis *Pediatric arrest* *Pediatric anaphylaxis*	1 mg IV (10 ml 1:10,000) q3-5min 2-10 µg/min IV drip *Subcutaneous*: 0.3 mg (0.3 mg of 1:1000); may repeat *IV*: 0.1 mg (1 ml of 1:10,000 or 10 ml 1:100,000) over 5 min (20 µg/min), then reduce to 10 µg/min. 0.01 mg/kg IV of 1:10,000 q3-5min; 0.1 mg/kg per ETT *Subcutaneous*: 0.01 mg/kg (1:1000); maximum single dose 0.3 mg; may repeat *IV*: 0.01 mg/kg (1:10,000 or 1:100,000) over 5 min; maximum single dose 0.1 mg; may repeat

DRUG	DOSE
Furosemide	0.5-1.0 mg/kg IV
Isoproterenol	2-10 µg/min; titrate to heart rate; use with caution
Lidocaine* Arrest *Pediatric*	 1.0-1.5 mg/kg q3-5min; maximum 3 mg/kg; maintenance drip 1-4 mg/min 1 mg/kg IV; infusion 20-50 µg/kg/min
Magnesium SO$_4$	1-2 g IV push over 2 min
Morphine SO$_4$ response	2-4 mg IV over 1-5 min; may repeat q5-15min to desired
Naloxone*	0.4-4.0 mg IV push
Nitroglycerin	1-2 sprays for 0.5-1 sec or 0.3-0.4 mg tablet SL; may repeat q3-5min; IV drip: begin 10-20 µg/min; titrate to effect; caution hypotension
Nitroprusside	0.1-5.0 µg/kg/min; titrate to desired blood pressure q3-5min
Norepinephrine	0.5-30 µg/min IV; titrate to blood pressure
Procainamide	20 mg/min IV; in arrest up to 50 mg/min; maximum 17 mg/kg
Sodium bicarbonate	0.5-1.0 mEq/kg IV
Verapamil	2.5-5.0 mg IV over 1-2 min; may repeat in 15-30 min with 5-10 mg IV; max dose 20 mg; consider pretreatment with calcium gluconate, 5 ml IV 10% solution

*Medications that may be given by endotracheal tube. Dose should be 2 to 2.5 × IV dose.

APPENDIX B

Pediatric Emergency References

Fluid bolus: 20 ml/kg normal saline rapid IV/IO
Glucose 0.5-1.0 mg/kg (2-4 ml/kg D25) IV/IO

	AGE					
	Premature	Newborn/ Small Infant	Infant	1-2 yr	5 yr	8-10 yr
Weight	2.5 kg	3-3.5 kg	6-9 kg	10-14 kg	16-18 kg	24-30 kg
Laryngoscope	0 straight	1 straight	1 straight	1 straight	2 straight or curved	2 or 3 straight or curved
Endotracheal tube (mm)	2.5-3.0	3.0-3.5	3.5-4.0	4.0-4.5	5.0-5.5	5.5-6.5
Chest tube (F)	10-12	12-16	14-18	16-24	20-28	28-32
Nasogastric tube (F)	5	5-8	8	10	10-12	14-18
Foley catheter (F)	5	5-8	8	10	10-12	12

Defibrillation and Cardioversion

Defibrillation
Pulseless ventricular tachycardia (VT)/
  ventricular fibrillation (VF), or
  polymorphic VT
	Adult: 200 J, 200-300 J, 360 J
	Pediatric: 2 J/kg, 2-4 J/kg, 4 J/kg

Synchronized Cardioversion
Monomorphic VT or atrial fibrillation
 	
Paroxysmal supraventricular tachycardia
  or atrial flutter
	Adult: 100 J, 200 J, 300 J, 360 J
	Pediatric: Begin at 0.5-1.0 J/kg,
	  may increase to 2 J/kg
	Adult: 50 J, 100 J, 200 J, 300 J, 360 J
	Pediatric: Begin at 0.5-1.0 J/kg,
	  may increase to 2 J/kg

Doses are for monomorphic waveforms; the clinically equivalent biphasic waveform energy dose may be substituted.

Defibrillation and Cardioversion

Index

651

Printed and bound by CPI Group (UK) Ltd, Croydon, CR0 4YY

07/10/2024

01041951-0001